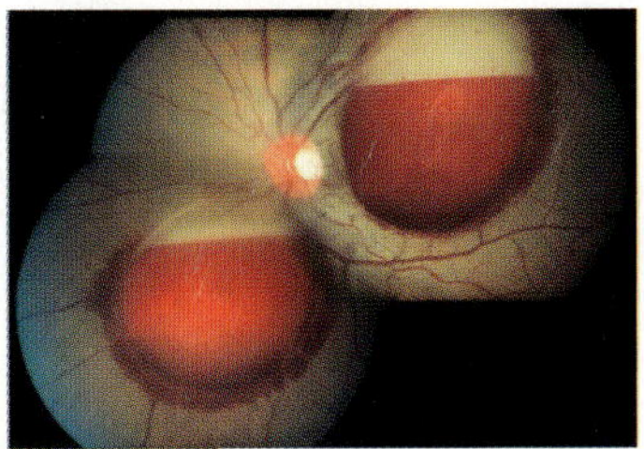

The Sankara Nethralaya

Atlas of Fundus Fluorescein Angiography

System requirement:

- Operating System – Windows XP or above
- Web Browser – Internet Explorer 8 or above, Google Chrome, Mozilla Firefox and Safari
- Essential plugins – Java & Flash player
  - Facing problems in viewing content – it may be your system does not have java enabled.
  - If Videos don't show up – it may be the system requires Flash player or need to manage flash setting
  - You can test java and flash by using the links from the troubleshoot section of the CD/DVD.
  - Learn more about flash setting from the link in the troubleshoot section.

Accompanying Photo CD/DVD-ROM is playable only in Computer and not in DVD player.

CD/DVD has Autorun function – it may take few seconds to load on your computer. If it does not work for you, then follow the steps below to access the contents manually:

- Click on my computer
- Select the **CD/DVD drive** and click open/explore – this will show list of files in the CD/DVD
- Find and double click file – "launch.html"

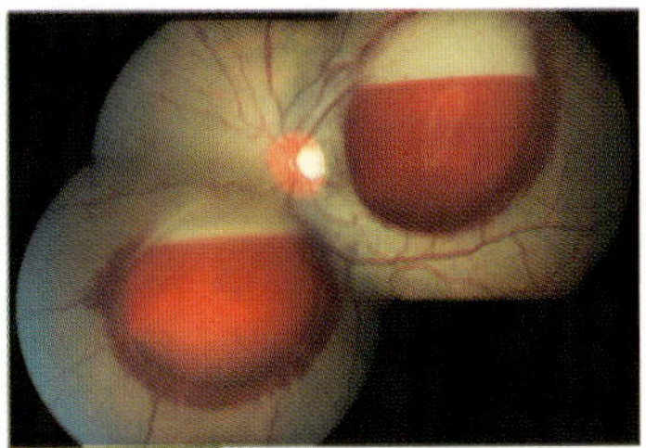

The Sankara Nethralaya

Atlas of Fundus Fluorescein Angiography

Second Edition

Pukhraj Rishi MS DO
Ekta Rishi MS
Tarun Sharma MD FRCSEd MBA
Muna Bhende MS
Parveen Sen MS
Dhanashree Ratra MS DNB FRCSEd
Pradeep Susvar DO DNB MBA FRCS (Glas)
Suchitra Pradeep DO
Chetan Rao MS
Vikas Khetan DO DNB
Vinata Rajendran MS
Rajesh P DNB
Suganeswari G MS
Rupak Ray MS
Rajeev Raman MS DNB
Kasinathan N DO DNB FRCS (Glas)
Lingam Gopal MS DNB FRCSEd

All Authors are Consultants of Sri Bhagwan Mahavir Vitreoretinal Service, Sankara Nethralaya, Chennai, Tamil Nadu, India or have served as faculty in the past

Foreword

Lawrence A Yannuzzi

SANKARA NETHRALAYA

JAYPEE - HIGHLIGHTS
MEDICAL PUBLISHERS, INC.

Jaypee Brothers Medical Publishers (P) Ltd

Headquarters
Jaypee Brothers Medical Publishers (P) Ltd
4838/24, Ansari Road, Daryaganj
New Delhi 110 002, India
Phone: +91-11-43574357
Fax: +91-11-43574314
Email: jaypee@jaypeebrothers.com

Overseas Offices

J.P. Medical Ltd.
83, Victoria Street, London
SW1H 0HW (UK)
Phone: +44-2031708910
Fax: +02-03-0086180
Email: info@jpmedpub.com

Jaypee-Highlights Medical Publishers Inc.
City of Knowledge, Bld. 237, Clayton
Panama City, Panama
Phone: +507-301-0496
Fax: +507-301-0499
Email: cservice@jphmedical.com

Jaypee Brothers Medical Publishers (P) Ltd.
17/1-B Babar Road, Block-B, Shaymali
Mohammadpur, Dhaka-1207
Bangladesh
Mobile: +08801912003485
Email: jaypeedhaka@gmail.com

Jaypee Brothers Medical Publishers (P) Ltd.
Shorakhute, Kathmandu
Nepal
Phone: +00977-9841528578
Email: jaypee.nepal@gmail.com

Website: www.jaypeebrothers.com
Website: www.jaypeedigital.com

Inquiries for bulk sales may be solicited at: jaypee@jaypeebrothers.com

The Sankara Nethralaya Atlas of Fundus Fluorescein Angiography

First Edition: 2004
Reprint: 2006
Second Edition: **2013**

ISBN 978-93-5025-577-3

Printed at: Ajanta Offset & Packagings Ltd., New Delhi

Dedicated to

Our dear patients who indeed are the source for our knowledge and experience.

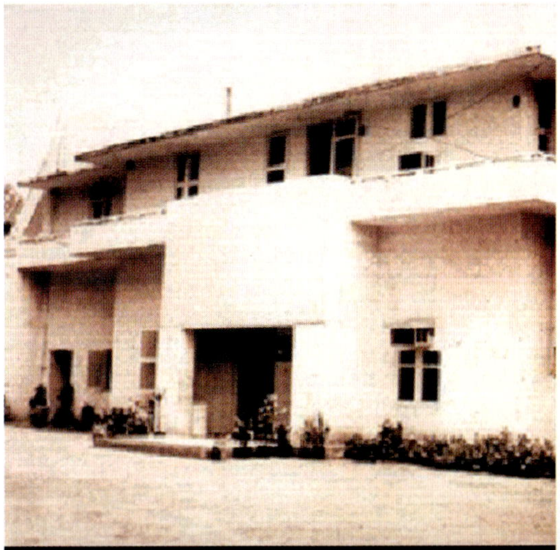

1978

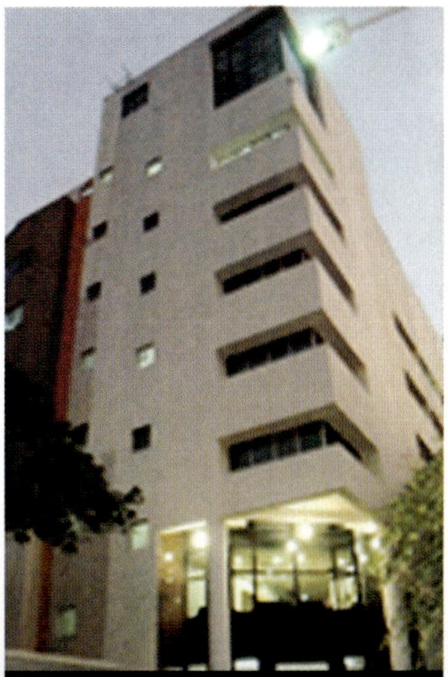

2012

The Sankara Nethralaya Philosophy

"Let the word *Sankara* of Sankara Nethralaya ever remind me and my associates
His Holiness' command that there be missionary spirit in the project.
Let the word *Nethralaya* constantly remind me and my colleagues that the place
of our work is an *alaya* (temple).
Work will be our worship which we shall do with sincerity,
dedication and utmost love."

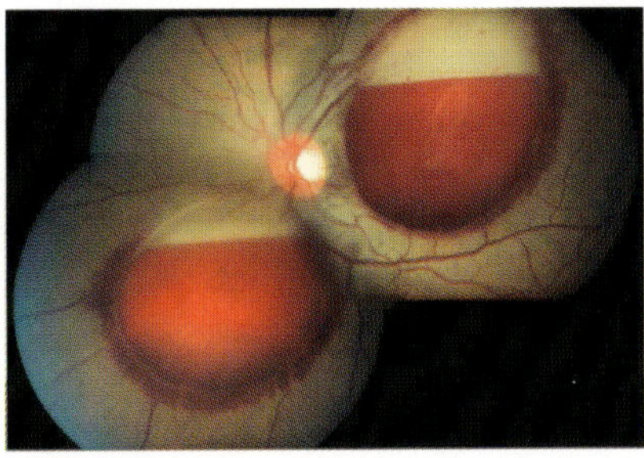

Foreword

For more than three decades, retinal specialists and ophthalmologists have enhanced their diagnostic and therapeutic skills through the diagnostic adjunct, fluorescein angiography. Numerous texts and atlases have been written on the interpretation of this procedure in English, French, Italian, German, and Japanese. The authors of this text have taken full advantage of their regional experience and encyclopedic knowledge of chorioretinal diseases by focusing on seven distinct divisions of retinal and macular disease in categorizing a myriad of abnormalities.

Thanks to them, there is for the first time an atlas on the subject of fluorescein angiography with a preferential emphasis on disorders prevalent in India. Arrays of excellent photographs have been used to fulfill this purpose, preceded by a section on technique and methodology to provide physicians-in-training and ophthalmic technicians, with the fundamentals needed to incorporate this discipline in their overall ophthalmic evaluations. The text is not meant for to describe new disease or new clinical manifestations and pathogenetic mechanisms in old disease. Nor does it provide an extensive bibliography to expand the potential for research of a given subject. The principal purposes are to introduce images for pattern recognition by clinicians to use in their practice, to enable a more accurate diagnosis, and in turn, to offer patients a more appropriate and effective treatment. Yet, the authors have in their preparation introduced new insight into pathophysiological mechanism of disease in the ocular fundus and offered unusual and challenging images which enhances our appreciation of these peculiar diseases.

In short, this volume represents a high level of industry, initiative, intuition, and intelligence by a group of skilled ophthalmologists and clinical scientists. Their efforts will be reciprocally rewarded by the gratitude of the ophthalmologists and retinal specialists who read this text and by the incalculable pleasure their photographs will bring, even to the casual and discerning reader.

Lawrence A Yannuzzi MD
Vice-Chairman
Department of Ophthalmology
and Director of Retinal Services
Manhattan Eye, Ear and Throat Hospital
Professor of Clinical Ophthalmology
College of Physicians and Surgeons
Columbia University, USA

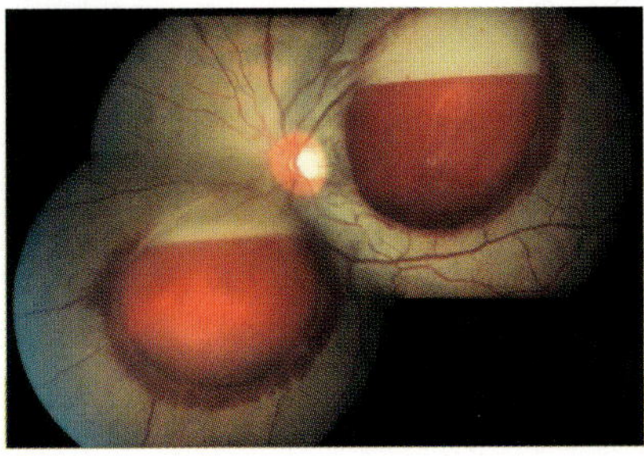

Preface to the Second Edition

A lot has changed in the field of vitreous-retina since the first edition of *The Sankara Nethralaya Atlas of Fundus Fluorescein Angiography* came out in 2004. Not only has our ability to investigate and diagnose clinical conditions improved but also the rapidly evolving treatment options have had a major impact on disease modulation. This has been possible due to the significant advances in multimodal retinal imaging, the advent of anti-VEGF era and path-breaking changes in drug delivery systems. A good knowledge of the changes occurring in the fluorescein angiogram is not only important for correct diagnosis and management of eye disorders, but also in determining treatment end-points. Even though OCT is fast emerging as a non-invasive retinal imaging tool, the role of FFA in diagnosis and treatment follow-up remains integral to the management of retinal conditions.

The aim of bringing out this Atlas is to have a comprehensive reference guide on the fluorescein angiographic findings in different disorders, so as to help the reader in understanding and managing these types of cases. The book is not intended to be a textbook on fluorescein angiography; the script has been kept to the minimum. This book intends to be a ready-reckoner for the practicing vitreoretinal surgeon/medical retina specialist as much as a reference guide for the vitreoretinal fellow. The same holds true for the Uvea specialists and fellows, respectively. Comprehensive ophthalmologists will find this atlas extremely useful in arriving at the correct diagnosis and appropriate management of their patients.

In this edition, we have added twenty-one new chapters and revised most of the previous ones. In doing so, we have preserved the original format of the chapters and the layout of the sections. A 'Self-test' chapter has been included in the end. Each section has been color coded which improves its user-friendliness while adding to the esthetic appeal of the book. Approximately, 400 new images have been added. References have been revised and updated. Also, in this edition we have included a Photo CD-ROM so that the tech-savvy user can browse the book 'on the go'.

Authors

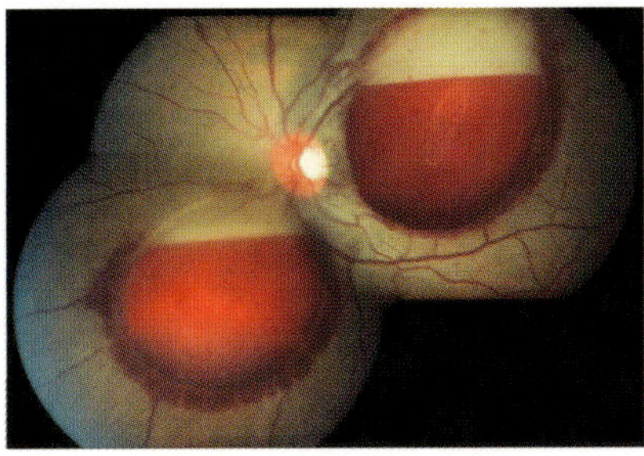

Preface to the First Edition

Fundus fluorescein angiography has played a crucial role in our understanding of different disease processes affecting the eye. A good knowledge of the changes occurring in the fluorescein angiogram is important for correct diagnosis and management of eye disorders. With this in mind, we decided to compile the cases seen at Sankara Nethralaya and publish it in the form of an Atlas. The aim of bringing out this Atlas is to have a comprehensive book on the fluorescein angiographic findings in different disorders, so as to help the reader in understanding the disorder and in managing these types of cases.

The vitreoretinal service at Sankara Nethralaya examines about 300 patients and undertakes 25 to 30 fluorescein angiography procedures everyday. These images are stored in the digital archival system, an excellent source for selecting cases for this Atlas. The meticulous manner in which records are maintained has greatly helped in making of this Atlas. All the cases, without exception, have been seen at Sankara Nethralaya, Chennai.

The book is not intended to be a textbook on fluorescein angiography; the script has been kept to the minimum. On the other hand, a color fundus photograph, a red free photograph and pictures of different phases of the angiogram are included for almost all cases. A detailed legend is given for all photographs.

The book has been divided into seven major sections with separate color coding for each. This was done to make the book as user-friendly as possible. Every attempt has been made to include as many representative cases as possible in each section.

Authors

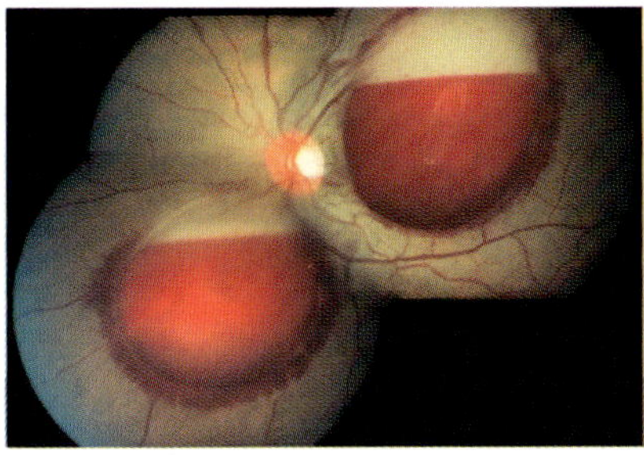

Acknowledgments

As in the first edition of this Atlas, Dr SS Badrinath has been the driving force in bringing out the second edition of this Atlas, too. His constant emphasis on maintaining good clinical records in the electronic medical record (EMR) era proved extremely useful in bringing out this edition. This Atlas is a testimony of the excellent teamwork involving all the Consultants and the Vitreoretinal fellows at Sankara Nethralaya. Cases published in this Atlas were contributed by the Consultants. Special thanks to Dr Jyotirmay Biswas and Dr Suchitra Pradeep from the Uvea department for their contributions. The vitreoretinal fellows helped in collecting and compiling the cases. Our sincere thanks and gratitude to all the following:

Consultants

Dr Jyotirmay Biswas
Dr Pramod Bhende
Dr Pratik Ranjan Sen
Dr Rajeev Raman
Dr Kasinathan N
Dr Pradeep S
Dr Suchitra Pradeep
Dr Chetan Rao
Dr Vikas Khetan
Dr Vinata R
Dr Rajesh P
Dr Suganeswari
Dr Rupak Ray
Dr Kumar Saurabh
Dr Sudipta Das

Vitreoretinal Fellows

Dr Sabyasachi Sen Gupta
Dr Harshali Kamat
Dr Sukant Pandey
Dr Bindu Appukuttan
Dr V Jaya Prakash
Dr Aditi Gupta
Dr Sayalee Lahane
Dr Sandhya Hegde
Dr J Sumanth Reddy
Dr Yogesh Patil

Special thanks go to our photography department headed by chief photographer, Mr MS Krishna and ably supported by Mr K Chidambaram, Mr CS Hariharan, Mr T Ravishankar, Mr M Thilak, Mr Shankar K (photographers), and Mrs Vanitha S and Shanthi P (Nursing staff). The entire credit for the quality of photographs goes to the photography team.

Mr Sampath Kumar, Mr Manavalan and their team from the IT department facilitated retrieval of images and provided easy solutions for data management.

Our sincere thanks to the publishers M/s Jaypee Brothers Medical Publishers (P) Ltd, New Delhi for their technical assistance and for printing and publishing the Atlas on time.

Last but by no means the least, we offer our humble gratitude to all our patients for trusting us and letting us participate in the management of their eye problems.

We thank Dr Nitin Shetty, Dr Mahesh Shanmugam, Dr Lekha Gopal, and Dr Preetam Samant for their efforts in bringing out the first edition to this Atlas.

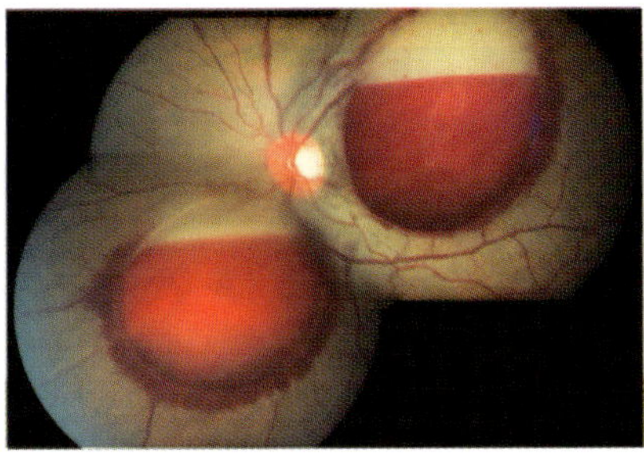

Contents

Section 1: Getting Started

Section 2: Macular Disorders

Section 3: Vascular Disorders

Section 6: Optic Nerve Disorders

Section 7: Tumors

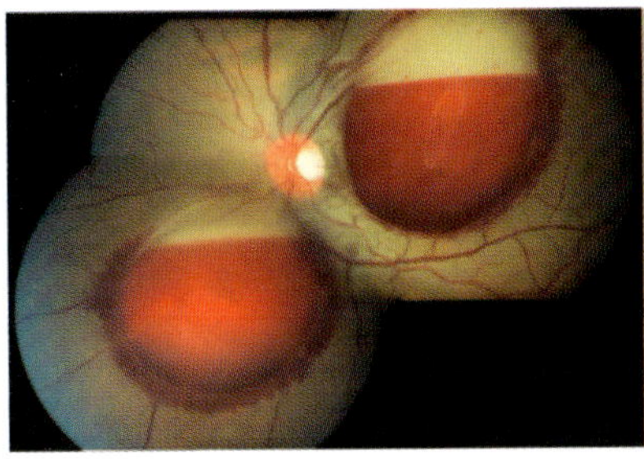

Section 1

Getting Started

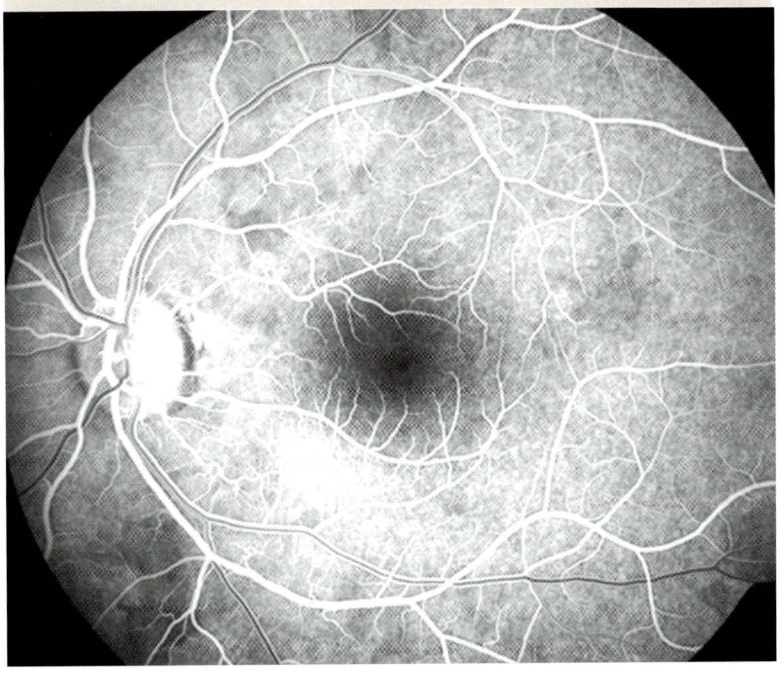

1 Chapter

Introduction

Luminescence

Emission of light from any source other than high temperature.

Fluorescence

Luminescence that is maintained only by continuous excitation.

Phosphorescence

Luminescence where the emission continues long after the excitation has stopped.

BASIC PRINCIPLES OF FLUORESCEIN ANGIOGRAPHY

- Sodium fluorescein is a fluorescent dye used for performing fundus fluorescein angiography. It absorbs light energy between 465 and 490 nm (blue) wavelength and emits light of 520 to 530 nm (green) wavelength. Hence, blue light is used to excite sodium fluorescein. It absorbs blue light and emits green light.
- A blue filter is placed in front of the flash of the fundus camera. This allows only the blue light to enter the eye.
- Sodium fluorescein dye is injected intravenously. Eighty percent of the dye is bound to plasma protein and is not available for fluorescence; the remaining 20 percent of unbound fluorescein is responsible for the fluorescence seen during the angiography procedure.
- The blue light from the fundus camera strikes the fluorescein molecules circulating in the retinal and choroidal blood vessels. It is absorbed and re-emitted as green light.
- In addition to the green light, a part of the blue light which is reflected from the fundus structures leaves the patient's eyes and travels back to the fundus camera.
- The reflected blue light is prevented from striking the film by placing a barrier filter in front of the film. This barrier filter allows only green light to pass through. Thus, the light that strikes the film is only true emitted fluorescent light.

BASIC PRINCIPLES OF INDOCYANINE GREEN ANGIOGRAPHY

- Indocyanine green is a fluorescent dye used for performing indocyanine green angiography. It absorbs light between 790 and 805 nm and emits light between 770 and 880 (peak 835) which fall in near infrared spectrum.
- Indocyanine green angiography provides better visualization of the choroidal circulation, as near infrared light penetrates retinal pigment epithelium better than fluorescein dye.
- Indocyanine green dye is injected intravenously. Ninety-three percent of the dye is bound to plasma protein and the leakage of the dye from choriocapillaris is minimal, which leads to better delineation of choriocapillaris.
- Two different types of fundus cameras are used and both give illumination in near infrared region:
  - With digital charge coupled device (CCD) for image recording.
  - Based on optics of scanning laser ophthalmoscope (SLO).
- Charge coupled device (CCD) cameras have high spatial resolution but temporal resolution is only few images in a second.
- Scanning laser ophthalmoscope (SLO) devices can record 20 to 30 images per second with lower spatial resolution.

2 Chapter

Checklist for Fluorescein Angiography

Fundus fluorescein angiography is one of the most commonly performed procedures for the diagnosis of posterior segment disorders.

It is a relatively safe procedure. However, ophthalmologists must be aware of the adverse effects associated with this procedure.

1. Inform patient about fluorescein angiography
2. Obtain written informed consent
3. Dilate patient's pupil
4. Arm board: To stabilize the patient's arm
5. Tape: To secure the needle at injection site
6. Alcohol swabs: To cleanse the injection site
7. Tourniquet
8. Gloves
9. Syringe and filter: To withdraw fluorescein dye from the vial
10. Butterfly infusion set of 21G/23G needle
11. Adhesive bandage/sterile cotton swab: To cover the site of venipuncture
12. Bin with plastic bag: Should the patient become nauseated
13. Prepare fluorescein solution
14. Prepare fundus camera
15. Record patient data.

Physician should be available on the premises while the procedure is going on.

SIDE EFFECTS OF FLUORESCEIN ANGIOGRAPHY

1. Unavoidable side effects of dilatation drops.
2. Adverse effects of the procedure itself can be categorized as:

Most Common

- Red after-image of photograph flash
- Temporary tan or yellow color of the dye
- Extravasation of dye
- Fluorescent discoloration of urine
- Interference with chemical tests performed by fluorescent method
- Transient nausea
- Occasional vomiting
- Excessive sneezing.

Less Common

- Hives
- Asthmatic symptoms
- Syncope.

Least Common

- Laryngeal edema
- Anaphylaxis to fluorescein
- Myocardial ischemia
- Pulmonary edema
- Seizure
- Cardiorespiratory arrest.

EMERGENCY DRUGS TO BE KEPT READY

S. No.	Description	Qty
	Intubation Items	
1.	Adhesive Tape	1
2.	Adult Suction Tubes (For Oral and ET Tube)—Each	1
3.	Airways (Adult)—all sizes	1
4.	Ambu Bag with O_2 Connector/Adult Mask	1
5.	Endotracheal Tubes (Cuffed) (Sizes 2.5, 3, 3.5, 4, 4.5, 5 ,5.5.,6,.6.5,7,7.5,8,8.5)—Each	1
6.	Gauze Pieces	10
7.	Gloves (7.5 Size)—Pair	1
8.	Laryngoscope with Blades (Adult)—Set	1
9.	Lignocaine Jelly	1
10.	Magills Forceps	1
11.	Stillete	1
12.	Syringe (10 CC)	1
	O_2 Administration Items	
1.	Adult O_2 Mask	1
2.	Adult O_2 Nasal Prongs	1
3.	Plain O_2 Catheter	1
	Cannulation Items	
1.	IV Cannulas (18 G, 20 G, 22 G, 24 G)—Each	2
2.	Scalp Vein Sets (21 G, 22 G, 23 G)—Each	1
3.	Syringes (2 ml, 5 ml, 10 ml, 20 ml)—Each	2
4.	Syringe (1 ml)	5
5.	Blood Set	2
6.	IV Set	6
7.	LP Needle (20G)	2

Contd...

Contd...

1.	Adrenaline—Ampoule	2
2.	Aminophylline—Ampoule	2
3.	Atropine—Ampoule	2
4.	Avil—Ampoule	2
5.	Betnesol—Ampoule	2
6.	Calcium Gluconate—Ampoule	2
7.	DNS—Pouch	2
8.	Decadron—Vial	2
9.	Deriphyllin—Ampoule	2
10.	Dextrose 25%—Ampoule	2
11.	Dextrose 5%—Pouch	2
12.	Dextrose 50%—Ampoule	2
13.	Dopamine—Ampoule	2
14.	Efcorlin/Cort-S	2
15.	Ephedrine—Ampoule	2
16.	Glycopyrrolate—Ampoule	2
17.	Isolyte—E	1
18.	Isolyte—P	1
19.	Lasix—Ampoule	2
20.	Mannitol—Pint (350 CC)	2
21.	Mephentine—Vial	1
22.	Nitroglycerine—Ampoule	2
23.	Potassium Chloride—Ampoule	2
24.	Ringer Lactate—Pint	2
25.	Sodium Bicarbonate—AMPOULE	2
26.	Sodium Chloride (10 ml)	2
27.	Sodium Chloride (500 ml)	2
28.	Verapamil/Dilzem	2
29.	Xylocard 2% — Vial	1
30.	Heparin—Vial	1
31.	Tab. Clopilet	10

SPECIAL SITUATIONS

1. **Pregnancy:** Some controversy exists concerning administration of fluorescein dye to a pregnant or lactating woman. Fluorescein does not cross the placenta. Fluorescein angiography has been performed in pregnant patients with no significant adverse effects. Nevertheless, it is best avoided, especially during the first trimester.[1]
2. Fluorescein angiography is best avoided in juvenile asthmatics.
3. **Renal failure:** End stage renal disease involves a patient to be permanently dependent on renal replacement therapy (dialysis or transplantation) in order to avoid uremia. It does not appear that dose adjustments are required to patients with renal impairment undergoing retinal angiography with usual doses of fluorescein sodium.[2]
4. **Previous allergy to fluorescein:** Most of the patients who develop an adverse reaction to fluorescein sodium fall in the mild reaction group. Severe reactions are rare. However, an established plan for managing serious reactions to fluorescein must be in place. Patients with known history of adverse reaction must have a decreased volume of fluorescein dye injection by using a higher concentration of the dye. Premedication appears beneficial in patients with previous history of allergic reactions.[3] Inj. Perinorm 5 mg–IM-1 hour before the procedure can be given.
5. Patients requiring special caution during intravenous injection include those with skin changes, coagulopathies, impaired blood or lymphatic circulation (post-mastectomy) and patients who are dehydrated or underweight.

SANKARA NETHRALAYA **Medical Research Foundation** **SN Main**, 41/18 College Road. Chennai – 600 006 **JKCN**, 21, Pycrofts Garden Road. Chennai – 600 006. **NSN**, 73 Venkatakrishna Road. R.A. Puram. Chennai – 600 028 **C. U. Shah SN**, 8. G. S. T. Road, Si. Thomas Mount. Chennai – 600 016.	Name: Mr/Ms... .... MRD No. .... Age .... Sex : M/F Date: ....

CONSENT FOR FLUORESCEIN ANGIOGRAPHY/FLUORESCEIN OPHTHALMOSCOPY

This investigative procedure comprises of injecting a dye—sodium fluorescein into one of the veins in your arm and either taking rapid serial photographs of its passage within the inner structures of the eye—the retina and choroid or examining the inside of your eye with an instrument called the indirect ophthalmoscope with appropriate filters. The information obtained from a study of this procedure aids your doctor in making a diagnosis, planning your treatment or assessing the results of treatment particularly photocoagulation. There is no discomfort from this test apart from the needle prick and the flash of the camera which is harmless. You may have nausea (sensation of vomiting) a minute or so after injection. This usually passes off in about 30 seconds. Remaining calm and breathing deeply helps in overcoming this difficulty. You are advised to be on empty stomach 3 hours prior to this test. Your usual diet can be taken soon after the procedure. Fluorescein is a highly nontoxic drug. Rarely does it produce a mild allergic reaction which responds rapidly to appropriate medication. Serious life-threatening reactions are exceptionally rare but can however occur. This is not different from what can occur with any other medication. The skin and urine stain yellow for about 36 hours and is of no consequence. You must be accompanied by an adult attendant during this test.

Informed Consent

Having understood the nature of the test and the benefits as well as risks associated with the same, I give my consent to the performance on this test on me by the staff of Sankara Nethralaya.

	Signature	Name	Date	Time
Patient				
Witness				
Doctor				
Interpreter				

CONSENT OF PATIENT REPRESENTATIVE/SURROGATE

The patient is unable to consent because: ____ and I, (name/relationship to the patient), therefore, consent for the patient. I acknowledge that I have had an opportunity to discuss this procedure, as stated above, with the doctor or doctor's designee, and hereby consent to this procedure.

	Signature	Name	Date	Time
Patient Representative with relationship				
Witness				
Doctor				
Interpreter				

REFERENCES

1. Fluorescein and Indocyanine Green Angiography Technician and Interpretation. 2nd edn. Ophthalmology Monographs, San Francisco, AAO 1997.
2. UK Medicine Information Pharmacists for NHS Health Care Professionals, Dukes, 12th May 2010.
3. Kris A Kwiterovich, et al. Ophthalmology 1993; 1139-42.

Chapter 3

Photographic and Angiographic Artifacts

High quality fundus photographs can be obtained through mutual interaction and proper alignment of the patient, the camera and the photographer. If an error in any one of them alters the ideal image, then it is called an artifact.

Typical artifacts include yellow or orange crescents, white or blue haze at the edge of the photograph, blinks, dust on the front element and blurry, poor focus.

Characteristics of the artifacts are based on:

1. Color
2. Shape
3. Exposure
4. Sharpness and
5. Others.

Color

The artifacts may be of any color. White, yellow, orange and blue colored artifacts are common.

Blue Central Spectral Reflectance

This occurs when the camera is too close to the eye or in eyes with poor pupillary dilatation. The former is corrected by maintaining an optimum camera-to-cornea distance.

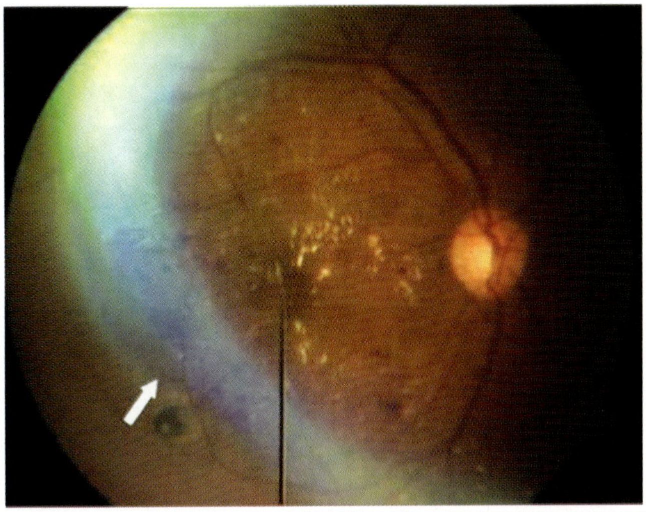

Right eye fundus showing centrally located spectral reflectance (arrow)

White or Orange Peripheral Crescent Artifact

This artifact occurs due to vertical and/or horizontal misalignment between the optical head of the camera, i.e. the illumination ring and patient's pupillary aperture. This is rectified by moving the camera in the opposite direction.

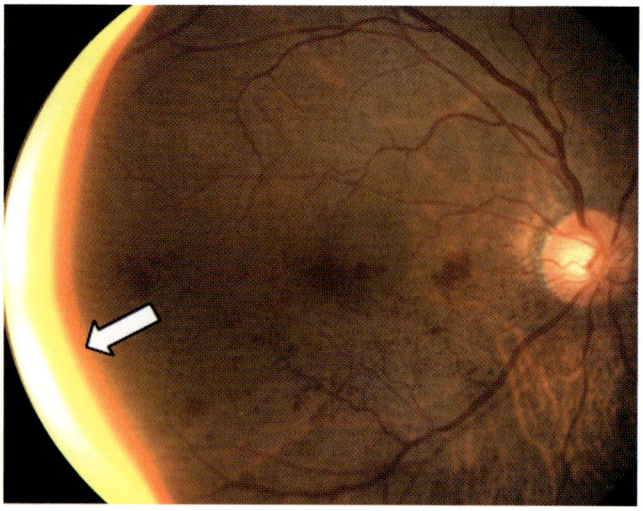

Right eye fundus showing white/orange crescent in the periphery (arrow)

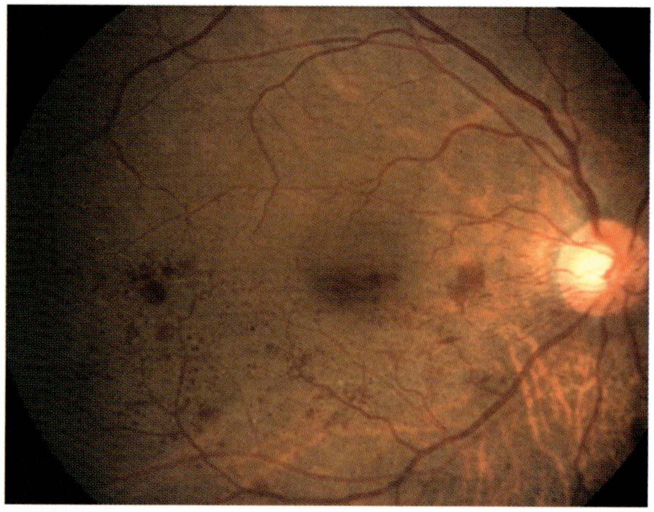

The same fundus image (as left) with the white/orange crescent artifact rectified

Shape

Circular, crescent or rectangular artifacts with sharp or blurry borders are possible.

Spotted Artifacts

This occurs due to particulate matter on the camera's objective lens. It is corrected by cleaning the lens prior to use.

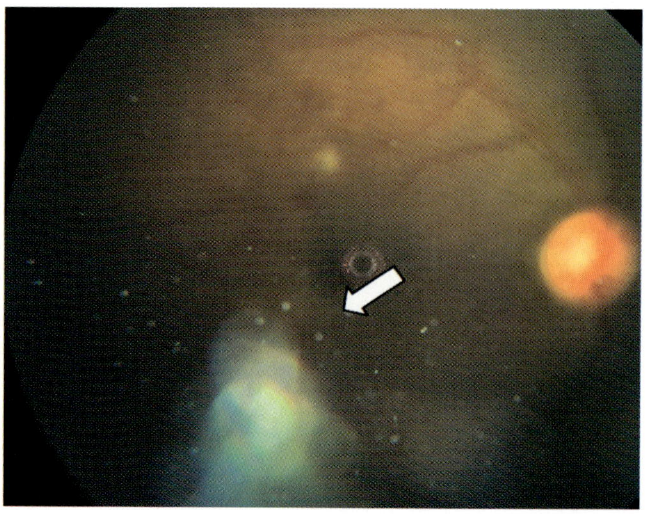

Right eye fundus showing spotted artifact (arrow)

Dark Spot Artifact

In a highly myopic fundus, when the photographer tries to focus, the central coating of the objective lens can result in a dark spot and sometimes may obscure the foveal region. This can be avoided by directing the patient to look temporally or superiorly so as to bring the central part of the macula into focus.

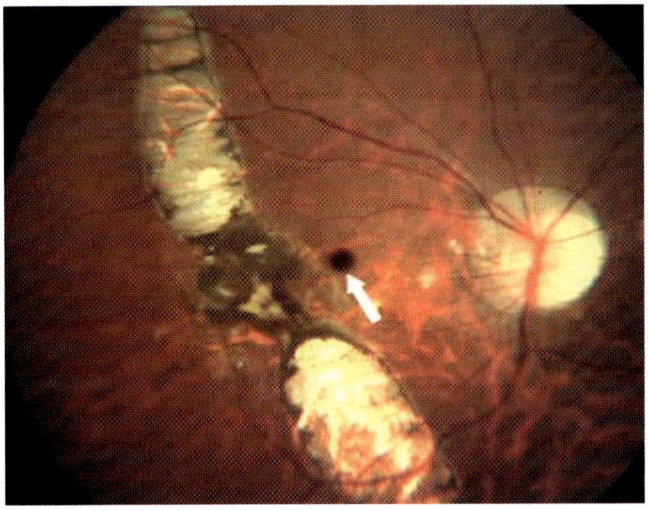

Right eye myopic fundus showing a dark spot artifact (arrow) near the foveal region

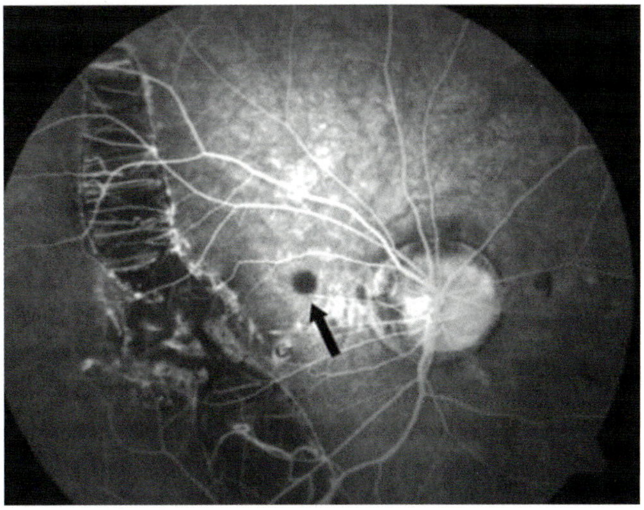

The same myopic eye (as left) in venous phase of FA showing a dark spot artifact (arrow) in the papillomacular bundle region

Exposure

The overall photograph may be too light or dark, or it may have a double exposure.

Double Exposure Artifact

This artifact occurs due to the combination of the present image over the pre-existing one. It is due to the improper functioning of the memory device in the fundus camera and also due to a poorly adjusted motor drive.

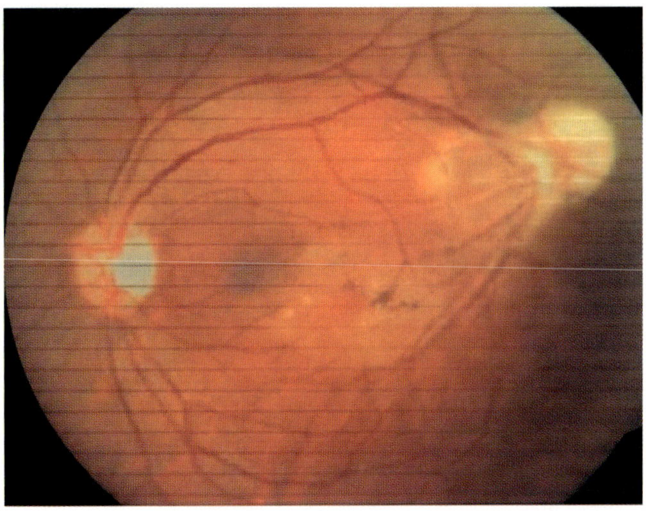

Fundus photo showing double exposure artifact

Blooming Effect Artifact

A localized area of marked hyperfluorescence is caused due to increased intensity of camera flash. This results in what is called the blooming effect which obscures the details of the region under scrutiny and gives a false impression of leakage and activity. This becomes better with reduced flash exposure.

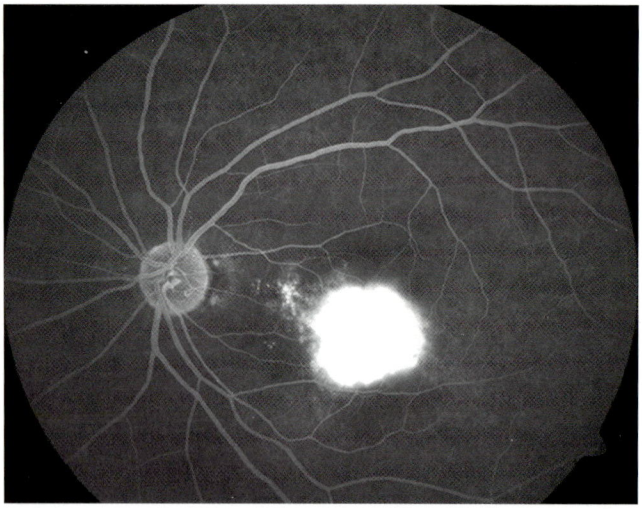

Left eye venous phase FA showing blooming effect artifact

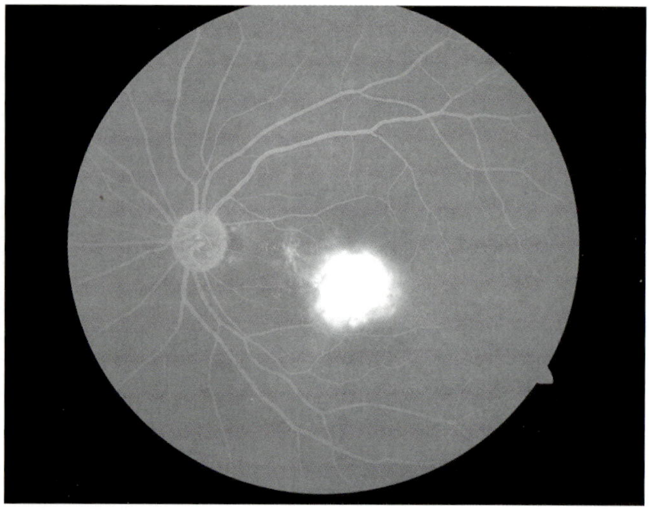

Blooming effect artifact reduced with reduced flash exposure

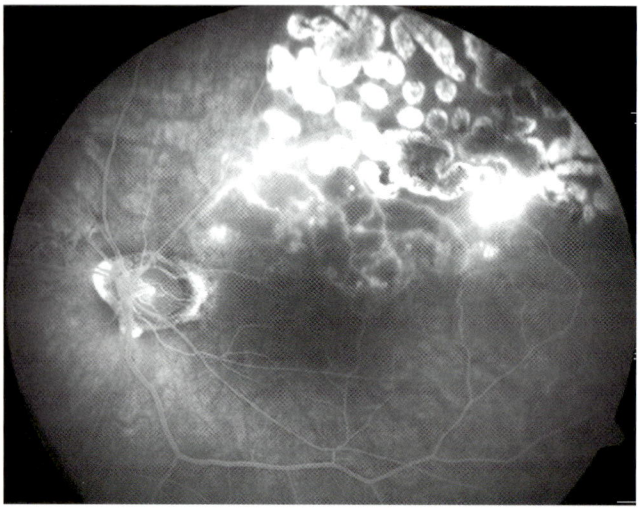

Left eye venous phase FA showing blooming effect artifact

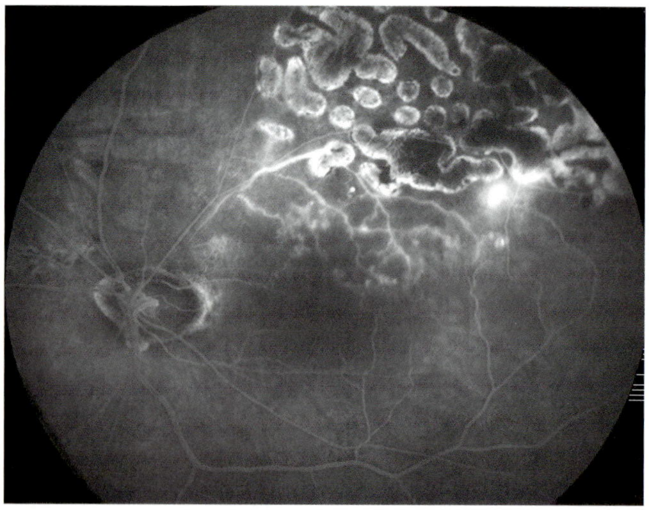

Blooming effect artifact reduced with reduced flash exposure

Sharpness

The entire photographed image may be sharp or blurred or some portions of it may be blurred.

Blurred Images

Blurred images can be caused by:

- Hazy media
- Eyelashes due to frequent blinking
- Incorrect eyepiece settings
- Failure to use diopteric compensation lens
- Failure to use astigmatic compensation device while filming retinal periphery.

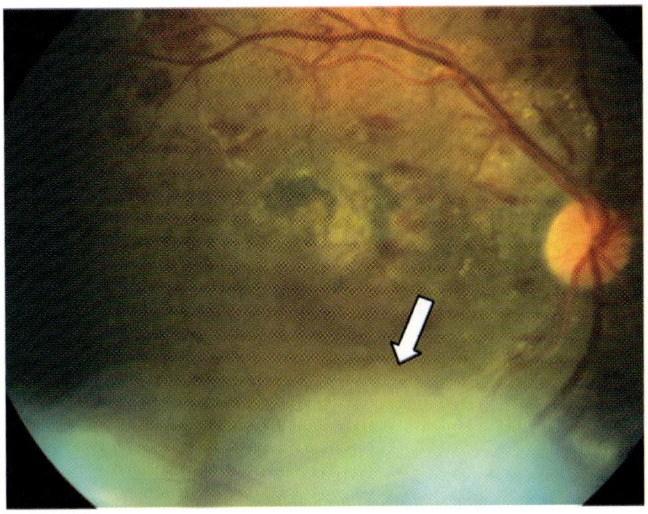

Right eye fundus showing blurred image inferiorly due to eyelashes (arrow)

Others

Double Image Artifact

This artifact is seen in partially gas filled eyes.

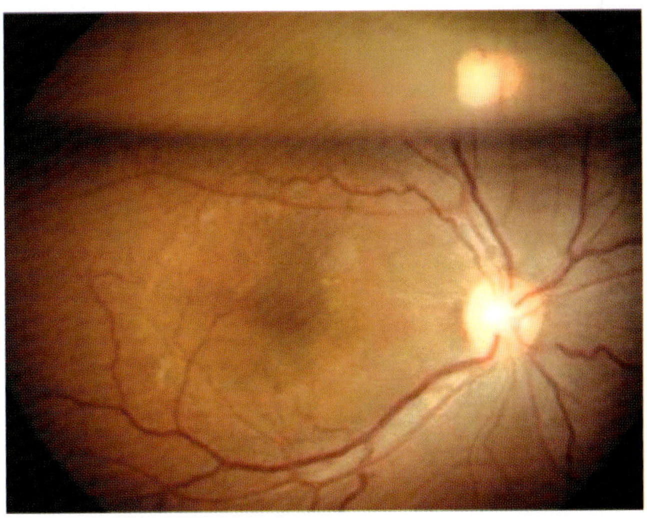

Right eye fundus showing double image artifact

Multiple Shiny Reflexes

Multiple shiny reflexes are seen in silicone oil filled eyes.

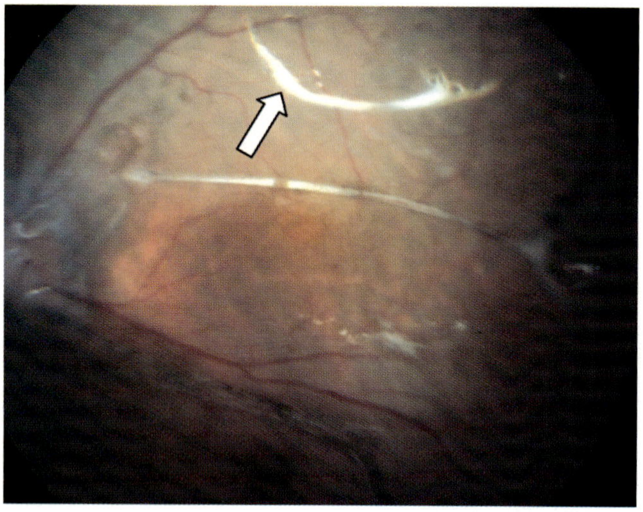

Silicone oil filled left eye fundus showing shiny reflexes (arrow)

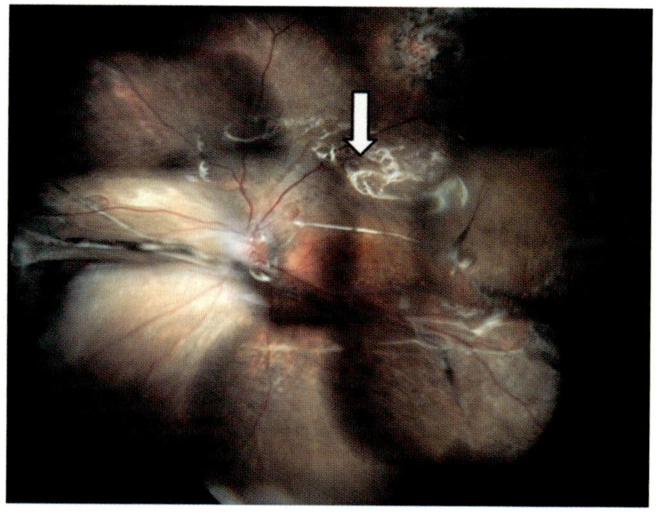

Montage photo of silicone oil filled left eye fundus showing multiple shiny reflexes (arrow)

BIBLIOGRAPHY

1. Busse B, Mittelman D. Use of Astigmatism Correction Device on the Zeiss Fundus Camera for Peripheral Retinal Photography. In. Justice Jr (Ed): Ophthalmic Photography. Boston: Little, Brown 1982:69-76.
2. Kelly MP. A superior method of achieving high myopic retinal focus. J Ophthal photog 1995;17:66.
3. Saine PJ, Tyler ME. Ophthalmic Photography. A Textbook of Retinal Photography, Angiography and Electronic Imaging. Butterworth-Heinemann 2002;13-98.
4. Schatz H, BurtonT,Yannuzi L, Rabb M. Interpretation of Fundus Fluorescein Angiography. St Louis: Mosby, 1978.
5. Tyler M. A way to sharper ophthalmic photography through astigmatic correction for the photographer. J Ophthal Photog 1981;4:20.

Chapter 4 Fundus Autofluorescence

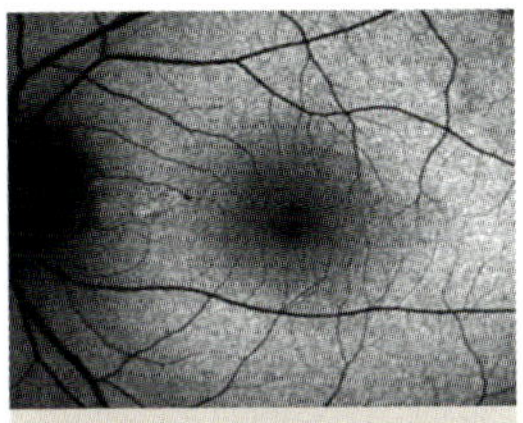

The property of intrinsically emitting fluorescence by a structure is called autofluorescence and in the eye, this property is exhibited by several structures including the lens, corneal epithelium and endothelium, optic nerve drusen and most importantly, the pigment in the RPE and macula.

Retinal pigment epithelium ingests the outer segment discs and the degeneration of these results in the collection of lipofuscin granules. Lipofuscin is a complex substance and contains many compounds, the most important of which is A2E (since, it is made from 2 molecules of vitamin A aldehyde and one of ethanolamine). A2E is the dominant fluorophore and possesses toxic properties. Lipofuscin is autofluorescent and is amenable for non-invasive detection.

Methods

Scanning laser ophthalmoscopy (SLO): This modality gives the best pictures of autofluorescence since it is easy to reduce the autofluorescence from other structures, due to the confocal nature of the system. Considering the low signals, there is tremendous stress on reducing the background noise. The SLO uses a blue laser excitation (488 nm) and a 500 nm barrier filter.

Using the fundus camera: By adjusting the wavelength of the exciting light and the barrier filter, the routine fundus camera could be adapted for autofluorescence, although the amount of light needed is lot more compared to the SLO. Excitation bandwidth of 535 to 580 nm and emission bandwidth of 615 to 715 nm is currently used to get the best results.[1] However, the contribution from the lens to the autofluorescence is not entirely eliminated. Hence, the quality of images degrades in eyes with age related yellowing and nuclear sclerosis of the lens. Hence, the autofluorescence image captured on SLO and fundus camera could differ significantly. For example, the optic disc is seen to be dark in SLO image while with fundus camera, it is brighter compared to rest of the retina.[2] Accumulation of excess amounts of lipofuscin will give rise to increased signals on FAF, while RPE cell loss results in reduced or absent FAF. Studies have shown that in geographic atrophy secondary to AMD, the central atrophic area has reduced FAF due to loss of RPE while the surrounding retina has increased FAF and this area is likely to become atrophic in the future.[3] Five FAF patterns have been described in geographic atrophy (dry AMD)- none, focal, banded, diffuse and patchy. The banded variety and diffuse variety were associated with greater risk of progression of AMD.[4] Studies in Stargardt's disease have shown that areas of increased FAF are actually associated with less risk of conversion to geographic atrophy. These authors also noted that there is focal remodeling of the fundus autofluorescence and no consistent conversion from increased fluorescence areas to decreased fluorescence areas. These features seem to indicate that the mechanism of damage may not be only lipofuscin toxicity as has been suggested so far.[5]

CASE 1

A 64-year-old lady presented with complaints of defective vision in both eyes since the last six months. Her BCVA was 6/9; N6 in the right eye and 6/7.5; N6 in the left eye. Clinical examination with FFA/OCT showed multiple RPE leaks with CSR in both eyes.

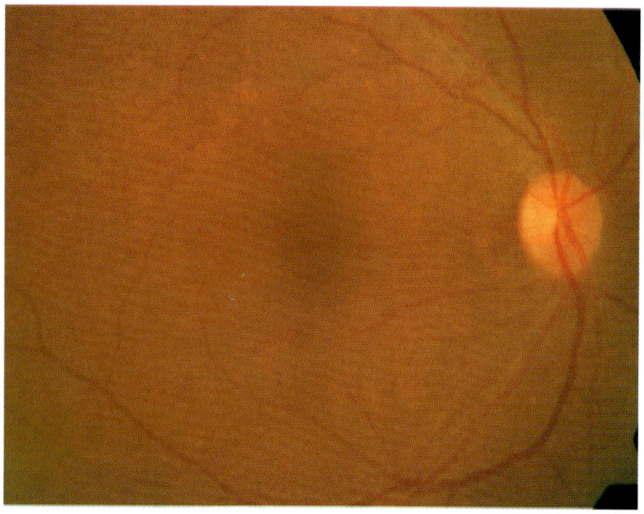

Color fundus photograph of the right eye reveals neurosensory detachment at the macula

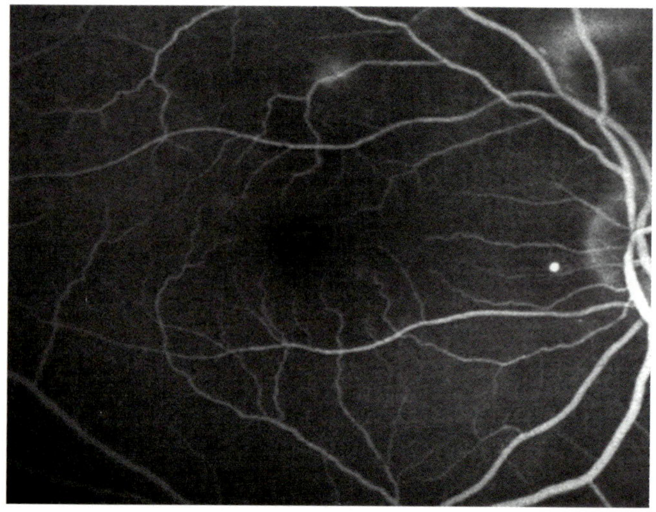

A-V phase angiogram reveals multiple leakages suggestive of multifocal CSR

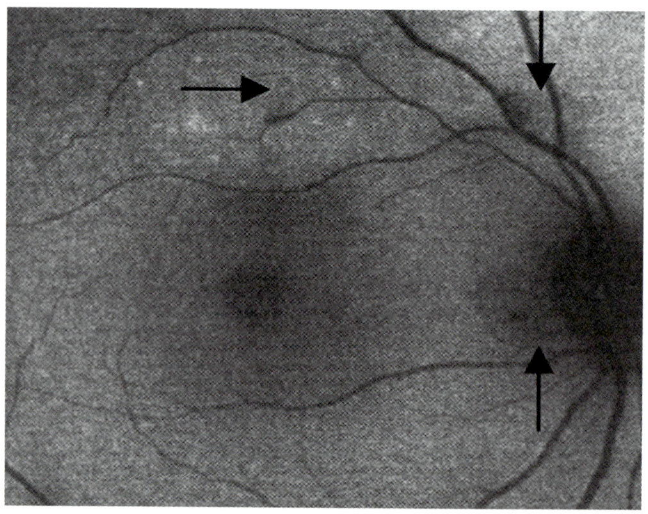

Areas of hypofluorescence (arrows) corresponding to the focal leaks on FFA are made out on fundus autofluorescence

CASE 2

A 45-year-old healthy male presented with poor central vision in the right eye since two years and in the left eye since the last two months. At presentation, his BCVA was 6/7.5; N6 in the right eye and 6/6; N6 in the left eye. Clinical and FFA/OCT findings revealed CSR in both eyes.

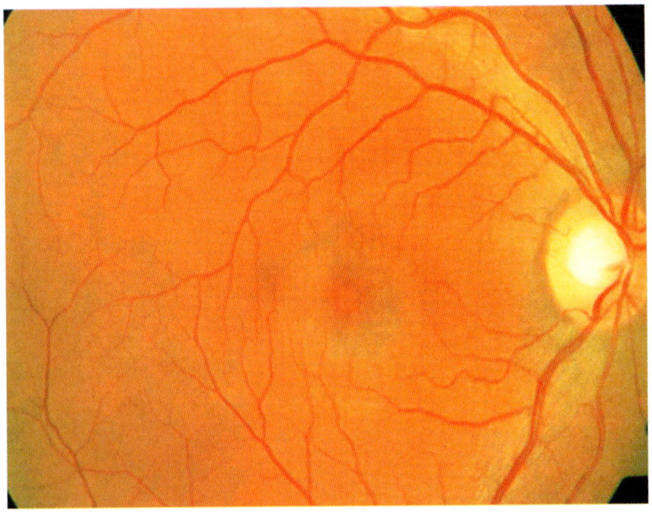

Color fundus photograph of the right eye reveals neurosensory detachment at the fovea with an oval area of RPE atrophy suggestive of chronic CSR

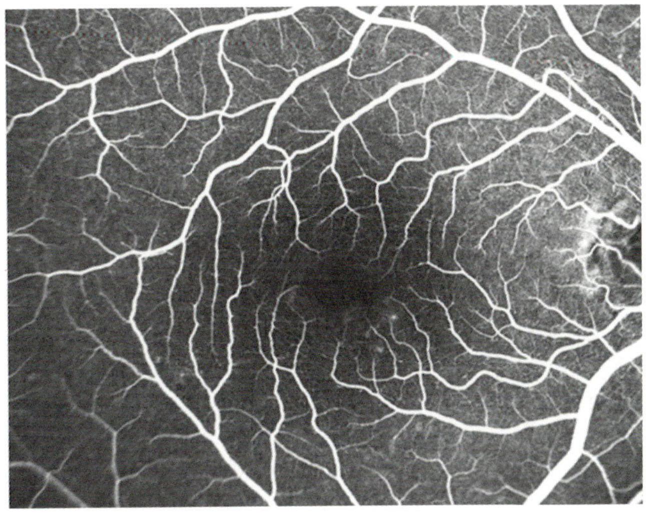

Early A-V phase angiogram reveals a point leakage inferonasal to the fovea

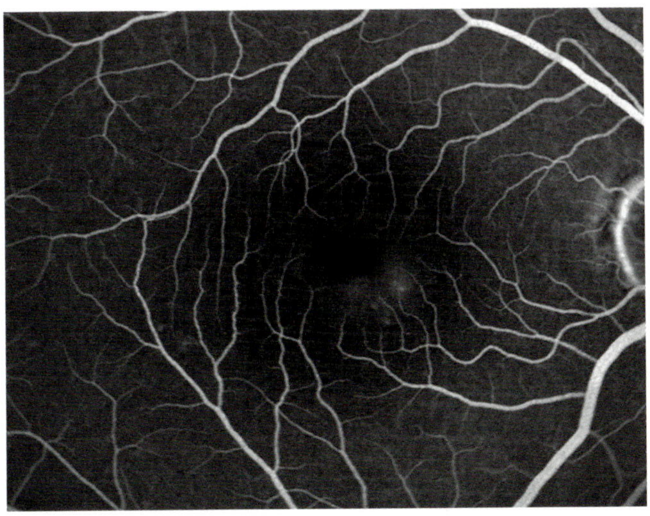

Late A-V phase angiogram reveals increased hyperfluorescence suggestive of spreading leakage inferonasal to the fovea

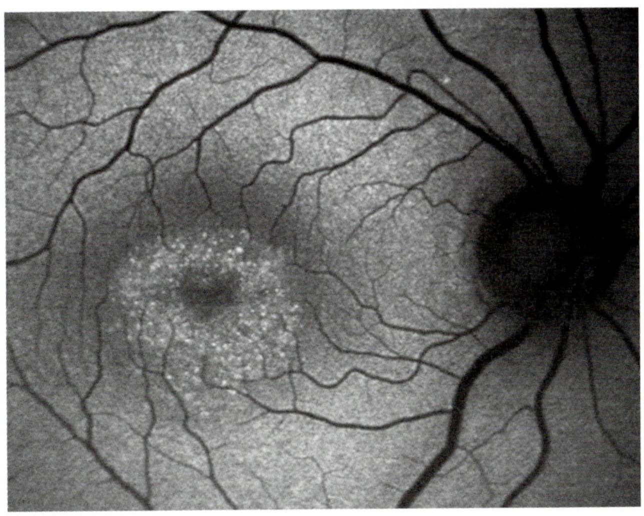

Autofluorescence image reveals speckled fluorescence corresponding to the oval area of RPE atrophy

CASE 3

A 43-year-old man presented with sudden blurring of central vision in the left eye since one week. His BCVA was 6/6; N6 in the right eye and 6/60; N36 in the left. Clinical evaluation showed CSR in both eyes with cystic macular changes in the left eye. FFA revealed single CSR leak in the right eye and multifocal CSR leaks in the left eye. Patient was on oral steroids and was asked to stop the medication. The patient was periodically reviewed. Four months later, right eye condition resolved while visual acuity in the left eye reduced to 3/36 <N36.

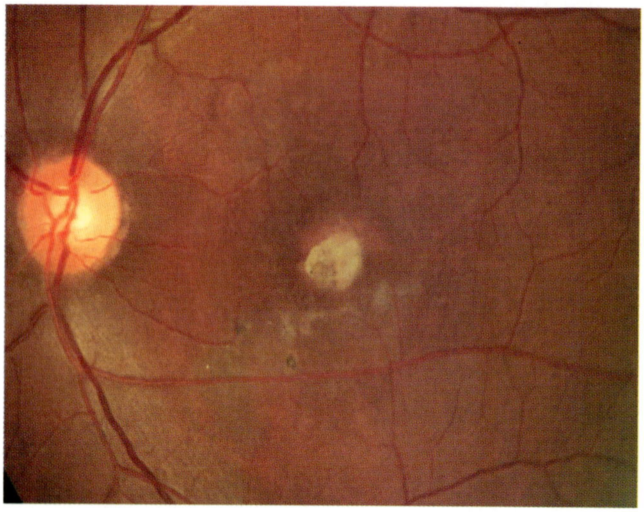

Color fundus photograph of the left eye reveals subretinal fluid with fibrin accumulated under the fovea with multiple atrophic patches suggestive of healing CSR

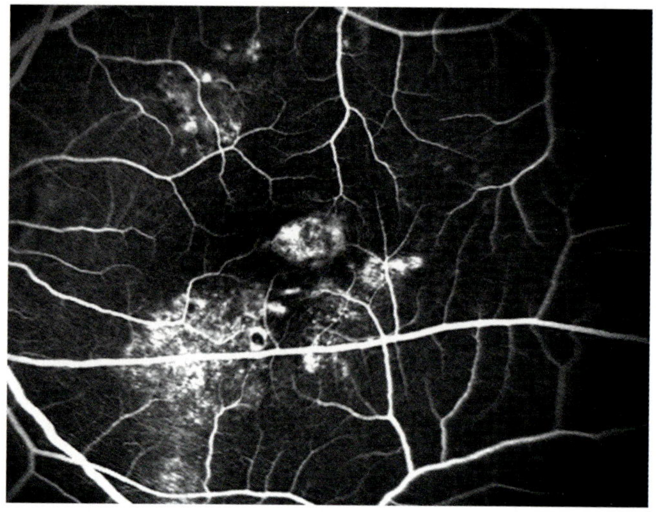

A-V phase angiogram reveals areas of pinpoint leakage superonasal to the fovea. RPE atrophic patches are seen inferior to the fovea. RPE atrophic tract is made out crossing the inferotemporal vascular arcades

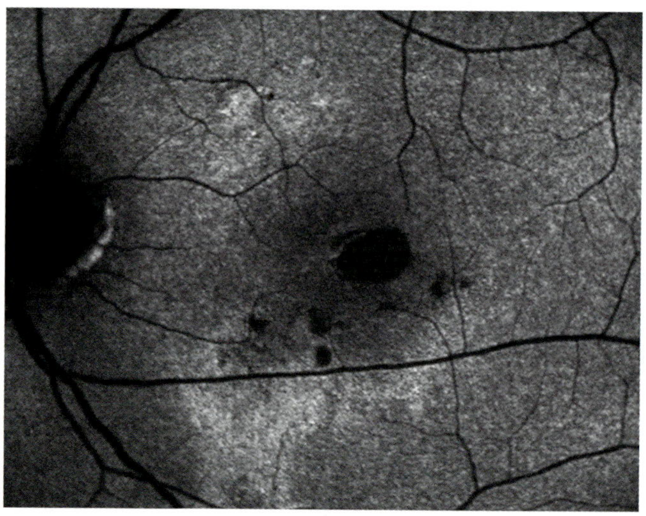

Autofluorescence image reveals hyperfluorescence corresponding to the areas of pinpoint leakage superonasal to the fovea and the RPE atrophic tract. Hypofluorescent spots corresponding to RPE atrophic patches are seen inferior to the fovea

POTENTIAL APPLICATIONS OF FUNDUS AUTOFLUORESCENCE

Macular and Retinal Dystrophies

1. *Best's disease:* Fundus autofluorescence (FAF) abnormalities are virtually pathognomonic and may aid in the diagnosis in questionable cases. The yellowish material ("egg-yolk") that accumulates in the macula is intensely hyperfluorescent and remains so during the vitelliruptive stages. In advanced Best's disease, when atrophy ensues, well-demarcated areas of decreased FAF may be observed.
2. *Stargardt's disease:* The pisiform subretinal lesions in these patients are hyperfluorescent. There are areas of decreased FAF centrally due to RPE atrophy.
3. *Cone and cone-rod dystrophies:* Have areas of central hypofluorescence surrounded by a penumbra of hyperfluorescence. The areas of decreased FAF represent areas of dead or absent RPE, whereas the ring of increased FAF is thought to represent the active edge of dysfunctional or injured photoreceptors. An inversed pattern is observed in patients with rod-cone degenerations with peripheral decreased AF and with increased AF at the center.

   In patients with retinitis pigmentosa and cone dystrophies, parafoveal rings of increased FAF have been identified in the absence of fundoscopically visible correlates, which tend to shrink or enlarge with disease progression, respectively. Interestingly, functional testing using microperimetry and electrophysiology indicates that these rings demarcate areas of preserved photoreceptor function.
4. *Pattern dystrophies.*

CSR

Patients with acute leaks imaged within the first month have minimal abnormalities other than a slight increase in autofluorescence of the serous detachment. Over time, the area of detachment increasingly exhibits levels of irregular increased autofluorescence. In some patients, discrete granules with increased intensity within the detachment are observed, which correspond with the pinpoint subretinal precipitates seen on fundoscopy. Patients with chronic disease have irregular levels of autofluorescence with markedly decreased intensity over areas of atrophy. A typical finding also is the visualization of fluid tracks in the inferior retina.

ARMD

1. *Dry ARMD:* Fundus autofluorescence (FAF) provides high contrast, identifying areas of RPE loss which are not evident clinically. In early dry ARMD, alterations at the level of the RPE may become visible in areas that appear normal on fundoscopy. Reticular pseudodrusen as a particular phenotype are readily visible on FAF images.

   FAF imaging is also useful in advanced ARMD. It has been demonstrated that areas with increased FAF signal, that might reflect excessive RPE lipofuscin build-up, precede the development of new areas or the enlargement of pre-existing atrophic patches in geographic atrophy secondary to AMD. Furthermore, the extension of abnormal FAF as well as the previously introduced FAF pattern classification have an impact on atrophy enlargement rates over time and may therefore serve as predictive determinants.
2. *Neovascular ARMD:* In patients with choroidal neovascularization, FAF abnormalities typically extend beyond the angiographically visible alterations indicating a more widespread disease. One recent study indicates that FAF changes better correlated with visual acuity than symptoms, length or lesion size. While early CNV typically manifested with patches of "continuous" or "normal" autofluorescence (corresponding with areas of hyperfluorescence on the comparative fluorescein angiograms), long-standing CNV exhibited more areas with decreased intensity. The latter observation was explained by photoreceptor loss and scar formation with increased melanin deposition. However, a decreased FAF signal does not necessarily mean irreversible retinal damage, as it might also be caused by subretinal fluid or hemorrhages. A possible predictive value of FAF imaging with regards to determination of therapeutic success by anti-VEGF treatment has been demonstrated. In particular, the development of visual acuity is less favorable in eyes with initially increased central FAF.

Chorioretinal Inflammatory Disorders

Fundus autofluorescence (FAF) findings have been studied in detail for serpiginous choroiditis. At a very early stage, the new lesions are slightly hypofluorescent, probably due to a masking effect by the deep retinal edema on the normal RPE autofluorescence. After two to five days, the active lesions develop a well-delineated hyperautofluorescence, indicating an accumulation of undegraded fluorescent material in a functionally altered RPE. This autofluorescence increases in the following days. A hypoautofluorescent border surrounds the hyperautofluorescent lesion soon afterwards (within a few days) and corresponds to depigmentation at the fundus examination. In the course of a few weeks, the central hyperautofluorescence changes from a granular to a speckled pattern. As the lesion heals, it becomes predominantly hypoautofluorescent. FAF findings can help the ophthalmologist to recognize activity or healing in serpiginous choroiditis and other chorioretinal disorders and consequently, to make better therapeutic decisions.

Macular Telangiectasia

Idiopathic parafoveal telangiectasia (IPT) type 2 is another condition with very characteristic FAF findings. Previously, IPT 2 was deemed to be a primary retinal vascular disease with subsequent secondary retinal neuronal damage. Recent observations, including FAF findings, however, suggest that retinal neuronal changes may be a component of the primary pathogenic process. Patients with IPT have depletion of macular luteal pigment, which manifests as loss of the normal foveal hypofluorescence on FAF imaging.

CLINICAL NUGGETS

1. Fundus autofluorescence (FAF) can demonstrate mottled areas of increased AF for detection of early evidence of hydroxychloroquine toxicity which without intervention can progress to a typical Bull's-eye configuration.
2. Measurements of atrophy by FAF have been shown to be reproducible and progression of atrophy has been suggested as a suitable endpoint for new dry AMD therapeutics.

REFERENCES

1. Holz FG, Bellman C, Staudt S, et al. Fundus autofluorescence and development of geographic atrophy in age related macular degeneration. Invest Ophthalmol Vis Sci. 2001;42:1051-6.
2. Holz FG, Bindewald-Wittich A, Fickenstein M, et al. Progression of geographic atrophy and impact of fundus autofluorescence patterns in age related macular degeneration. Am J Ophthalmol 2007;143:463-72.
3. Spaide RF. Autofluorescence imaging with the fundus camera in Holz FG, Scmitz-Valckenberg S, Spaide RF, Bird AC. (Eds): Atlas of autofluorescence imaging. Berlin Heidelberg, Springer 2007;pp.49-53.
4. Smith RT, Gomes NL, Narile G, Busuioc M, Lee N, Laine A. Lipofuscin and autofluorescence metrics in progressive Stargardt's disease. Invest Ophthalmol Vis Sci 2009;50;3907-14.
5. Valckenberg SS, Fleckenstein M, Scholl HPN, Holz HG. Fundus autofluorescence and progression of age related macular degeneration. Surv Ophthalmol 2009;54:96-117.

5 Chapter

Normal Fluorescein Angiogram

CHOROIDAL PHASE

- Begins 10 to 12 seconds after dye injection in young patients and 12 to 15 seconds after injection in older patients.
- Early choroidal fluorescence is faint, patchy and irregular: called *the choroidal flush*.
- Areas of choroidal filling and nonfilling become more distinct: called *patchy choroidal filling*.
- Cilioretinal artery fills during this phase.

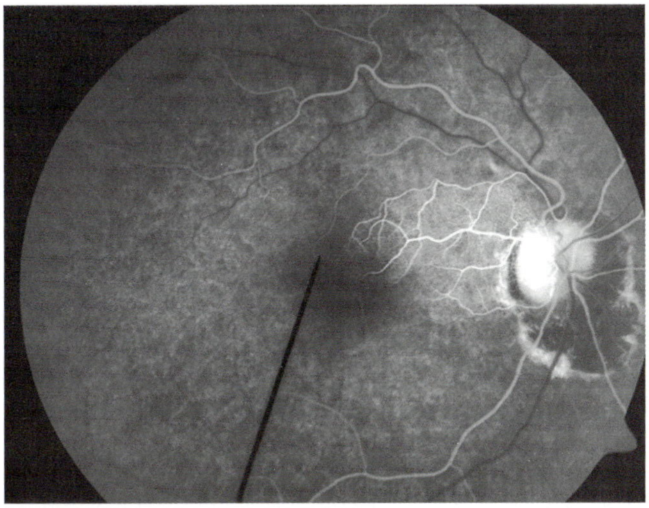

Cilioretinal artery (when present) fills in the choroidal phase before the filling of the retinal arteries. The dye is more brighter in the cilioretinal artery than the retinal arterioles that just begin to fill

ARTERIAL PHASE

- Starts 1 to 3 seconds after choroidal fluorescence with filling of the central retinal artery.
- After the central retinal artery begins to fill, the dye flows into the retinal arterioles, precapillary arterioles, the capillaries, the postcapillary venules, and finally the retinal veins.

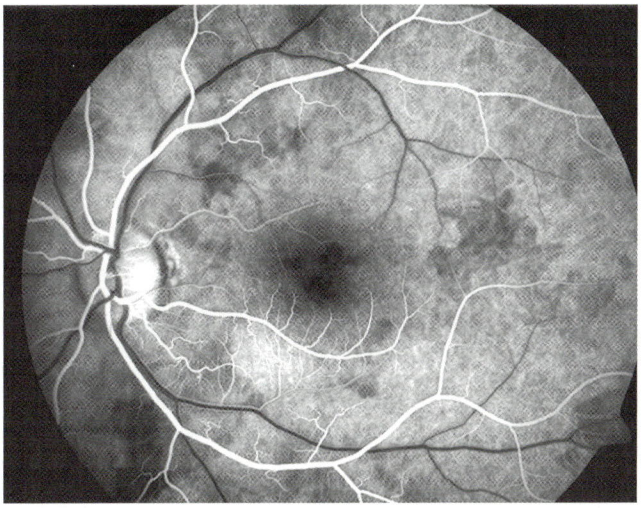

Arterial phase of the angiogram showing the filling of the arterioles; note the patchy background choroidal fluorescence

EARLY ARTERIOVENOUS PHASE

- The fluorescein dye from the smaller venules enters the veins along their walls resulting in a *laminar flow* of the dye in the vein.
- As the vascular flow is faster in the center of the vessel than on its side, the fluorescein dye sticks to the walls of the vein: another contributing factor for *laminar flow*.
- With time the laminae along the walls of the veins become thicker.
- At the junction of two veins, laminae of each vein merge creating a trilaminar flow.

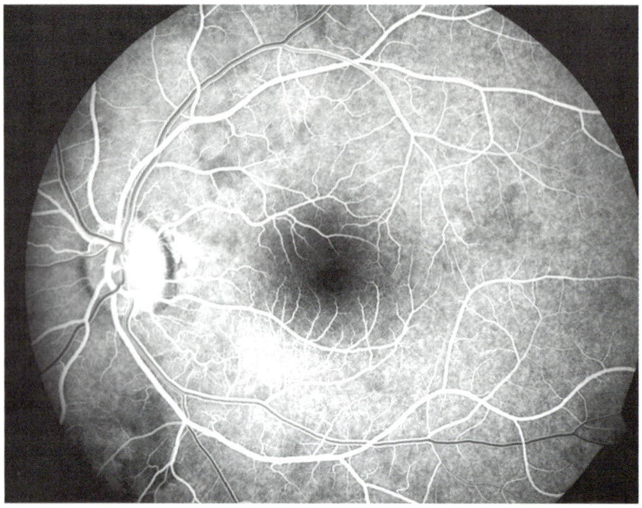

Early arteriovenous phase of angiogram showing laminar flow in the veins

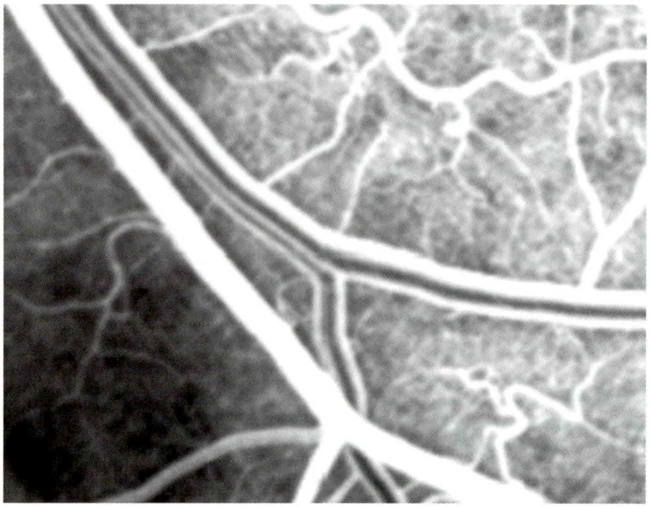

Magnified view showing the laminae along the walls of the tributaries joining to form a third central lamina—trilaminar flow-in the proximal vein

LATE ARTERIOVENOUS PHASE

- The dye completely fills the lumen of the vein.
- A perifoveal capillary network is best visualized at 20 to 25 seconds after the injection of the dye when the concentration of the dye is maximum.
- The fovea appears hypofluorescent because of the absence of blood vessels in the foveal avascular zone and due to blockage of the background choroidal fluorescence by the increased pigment in the tall RPE cells at the fovea.

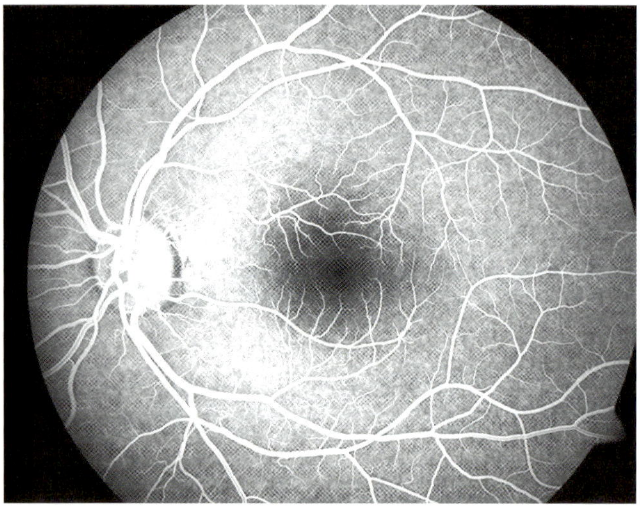

Arteriovenous phase of the angiogram showing complete filling of the veins

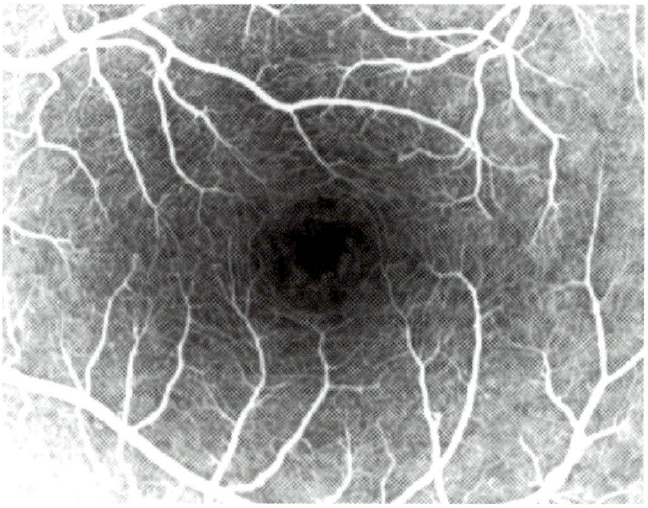

Magnified view of the parafoveal capillary network and foveal avascular zone

RECIRCULATION PHASE

- Begins about 30 seconds after the dye injection.
- Fluorescence within the vessels reduces as lower concentration of fluorescein recirculates.

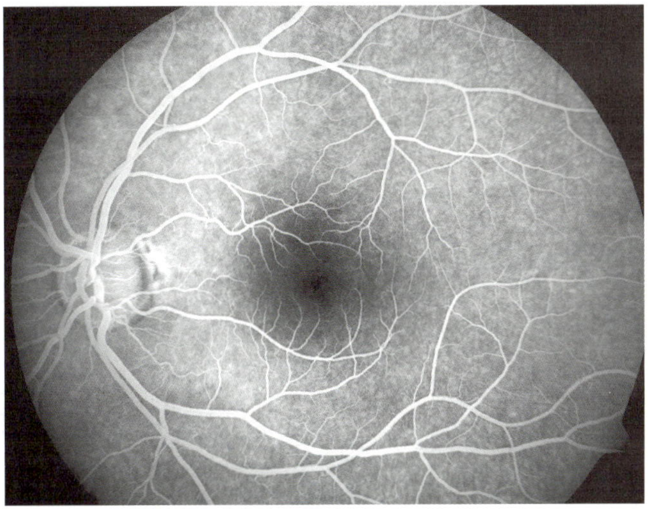

Recirculation phase of the angiogram showing reduced intensity of the dye in the veins

LATE PHASE

- Retinal vessels are empty of the fluorescein dye by 10 minutes after injection.
- Staining of the Bruch's membrane, choroid and sclera result in a diffuse background fluorescence.
- Large choroidal vessels may be seen in silhouette against this background.
- Disc remains hyperfluorescent in late films due to staining.

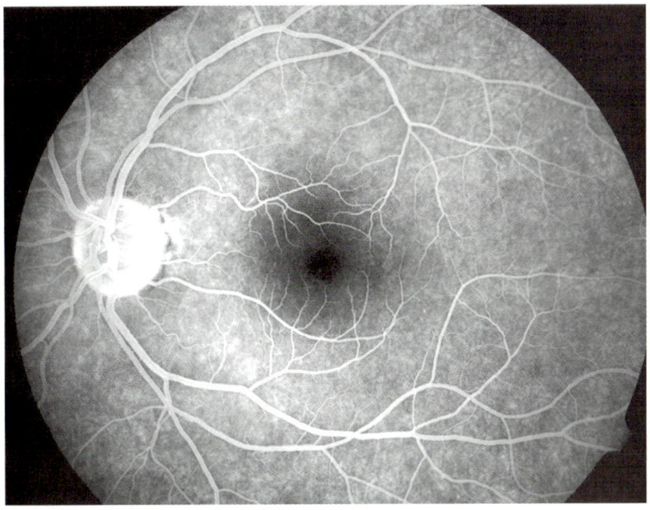

Late phase of the angiogram shows marked reduction in the intensity of the fluorescence throughout the fundus

Time—Arm to choroid	Normal 10-15 seconds	Abnormal > 30 seconds
Complete choroid filling—(From initial appearance of the dye to complete choroidal filling)	3-5 seconds	> 5 seconds
AV transit—(From initial appearance of the dye in the retinal arteriole to complete venous filling)	8-12 seconds	> 15 seconds

NORMAL DISC FLUORESCENCE

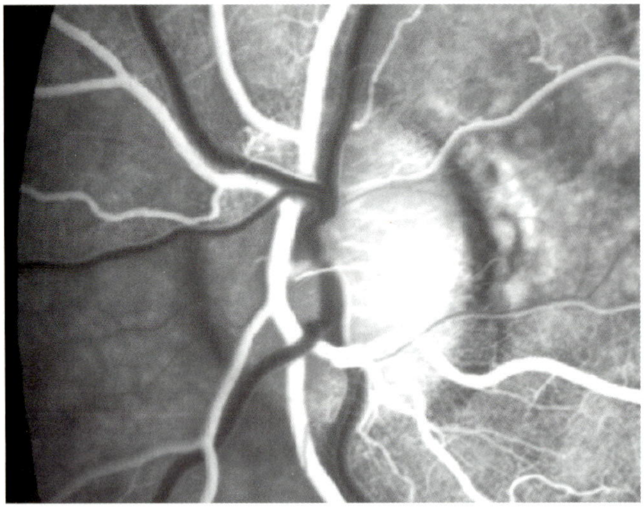

Arterial phase of the angiogram shows a hyperfluorescent disc due to the early filling of the deep and the surface capillary plexus from the posterior ciliary arterial circulation and from branches of the central retinal artery

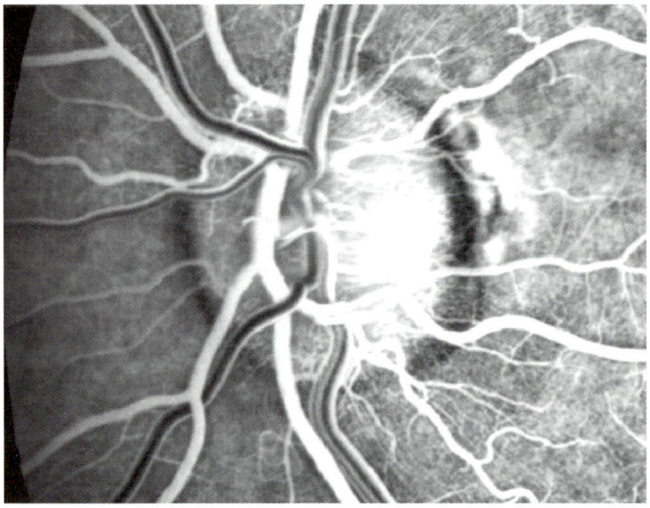

Early arteriovenous phase of the angiogram showing the nasal half of the disc and the adjacent choroid in this case, to be less fluorescent than the temporal half. This is due to the normal sectoral filling of the posterior ciliary arterial circulation

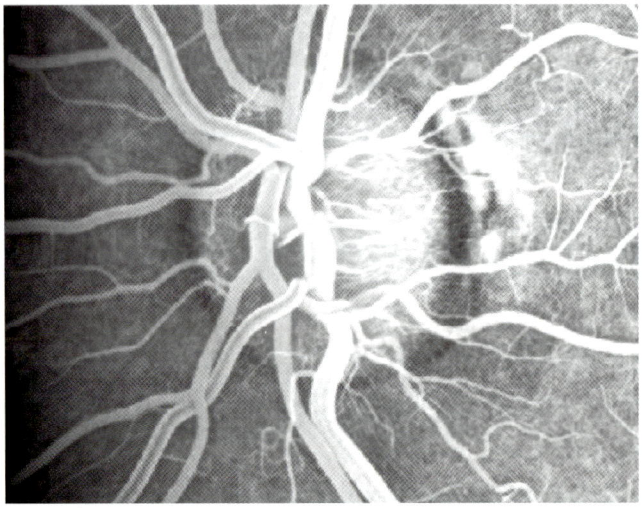

Increased filling of the disc capillaries is seen as the angiogram proceeds. A hypofluorescent zone is seen surrounding the disc, separating it from the choroidal fluorescence. Temporally, additional blocked hypofluorescence is seen due to pigment at the disc margin

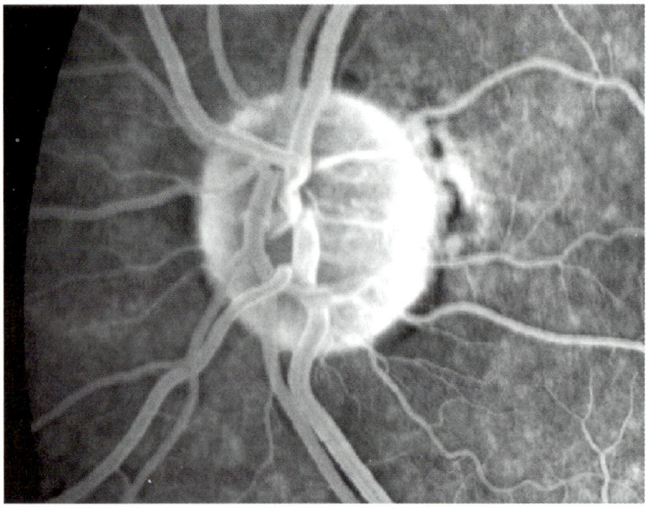

Late hyperfluorescence of the disc is seen. This occurs due to contribution from the deep capillary plexus of the disc, extravasation from the choriocapillaries at the disc margin and from scleral fluorescence at the lamina cribrosa

Chapter 6

Abnormal Fluorescence

HYPOFLUORESCENCE

Blocked Fluorescence

Blocked Retinal and Choroidal Fluorescence

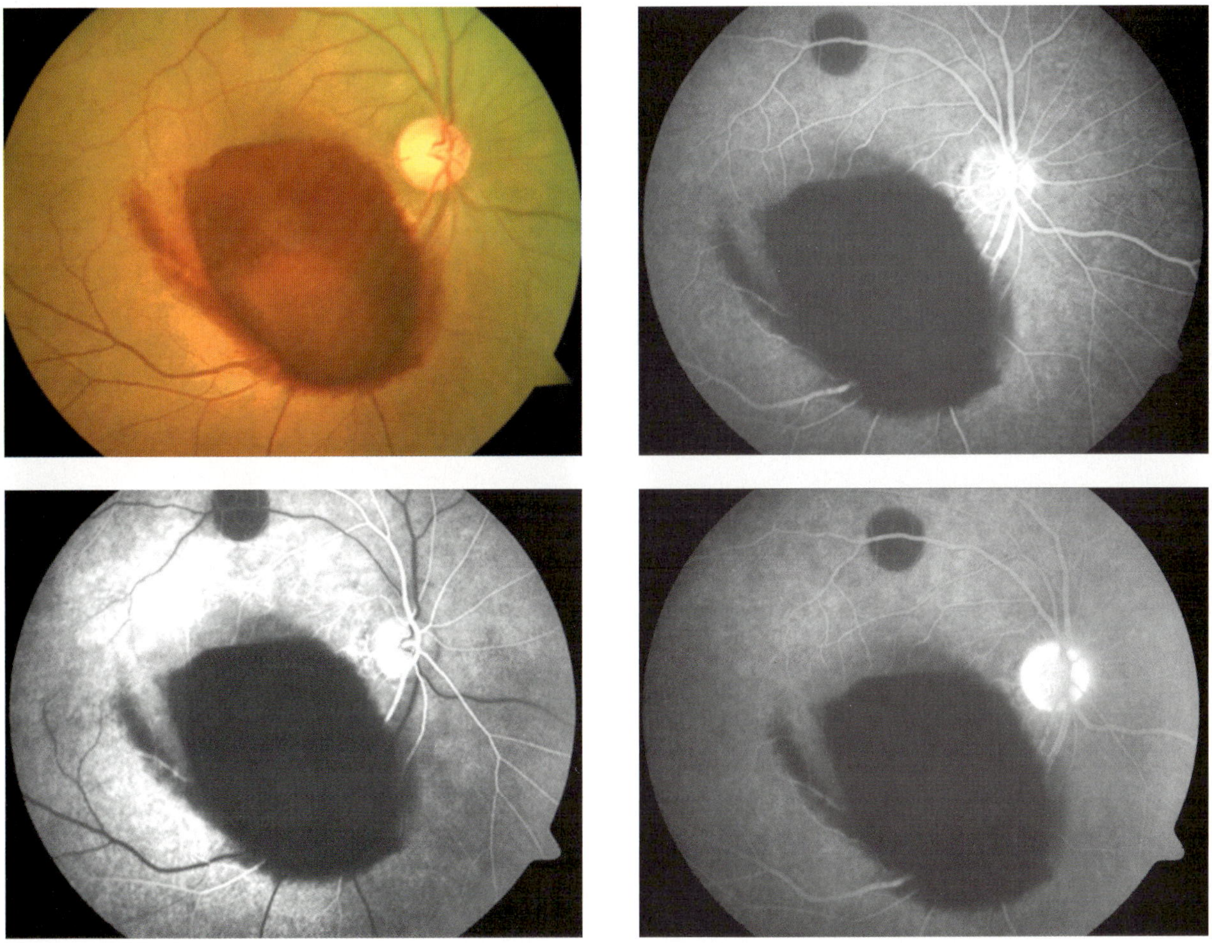

The large subhyaloid hemorrhage in the inferior macula blocks the underlying retinal and choroidal fluorescence through all phases of the angiogram. However, the subretinal hemorrhage along the superotemporal arcade blocks only the underlying choroidal fluorescence

Blocked Choroidal Fluorescence

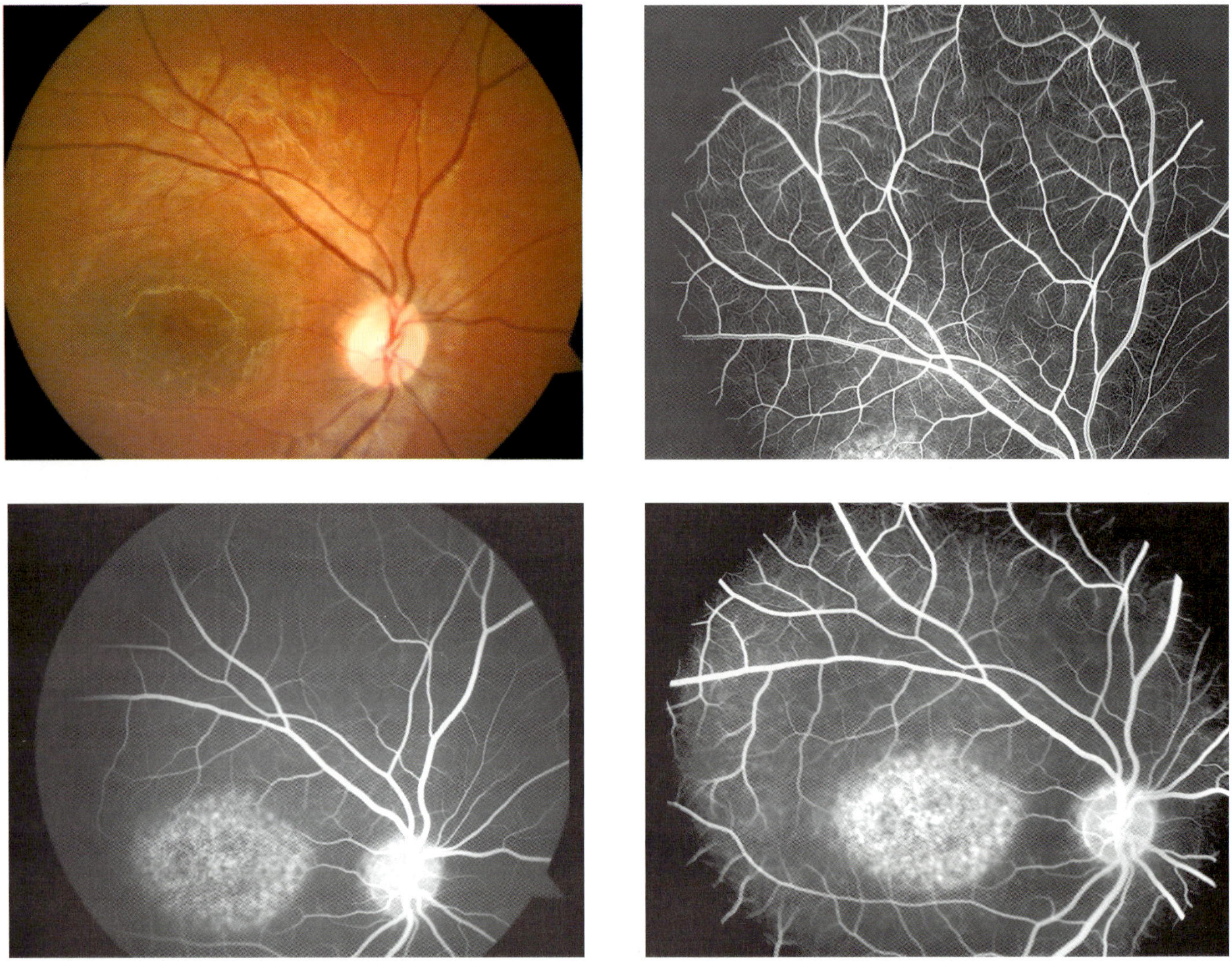

The lipofuscin like material in the retinal pigment epithelium in patients with Stargardt's dystrophy, blocks all the underlying choroidal fluorescence. Choroidal fluorescence is seen only in areas of deficient retinal pigment epithelium at the fovea—an example of transmission or window defect

Blocked Disc Fluorescence

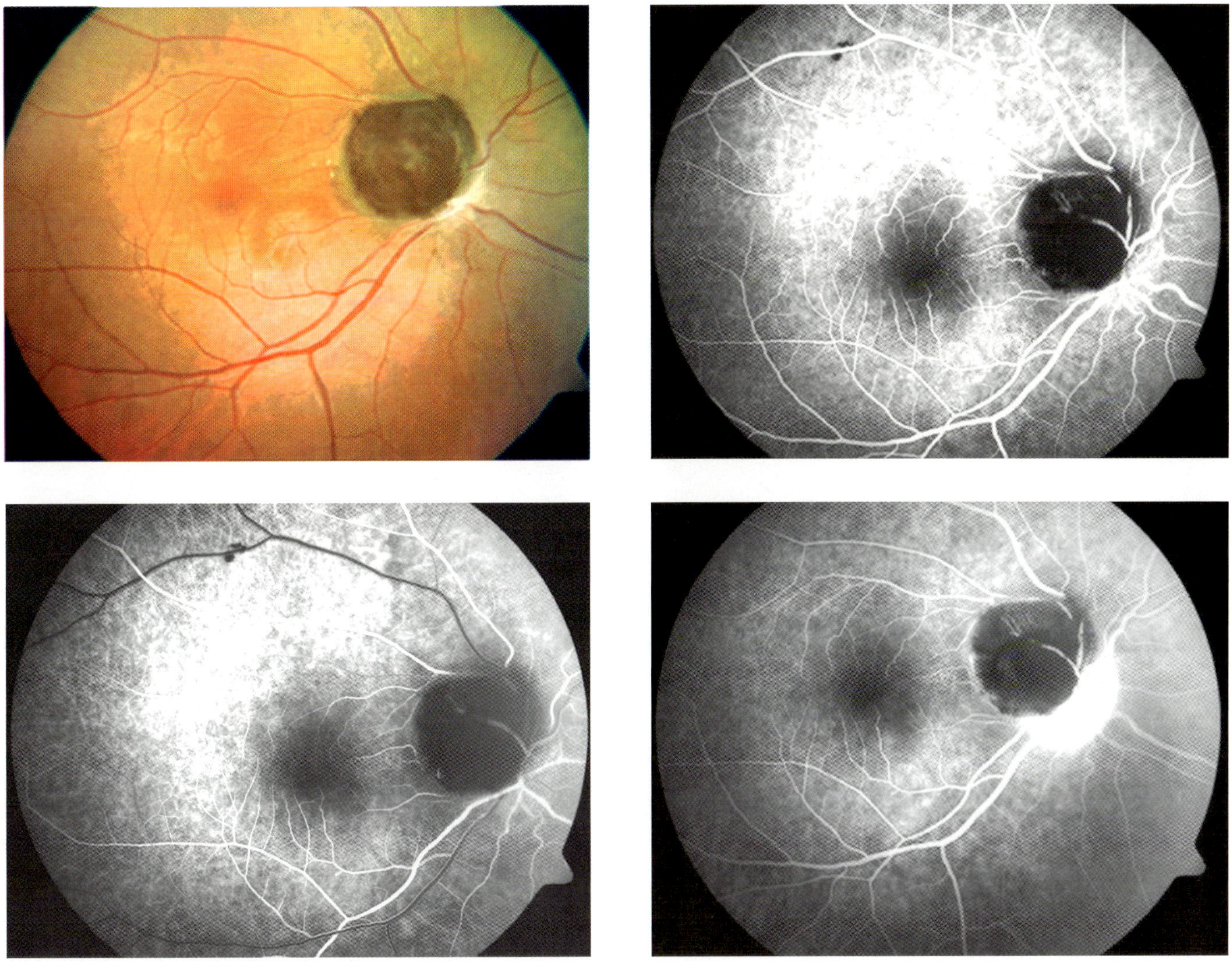

Pigment in the melanocytoma at the disc blocks all the fluorescence emanating from the underlying disc vessels

Vascular Filling Defect

Retinal Vascular Filling Defect

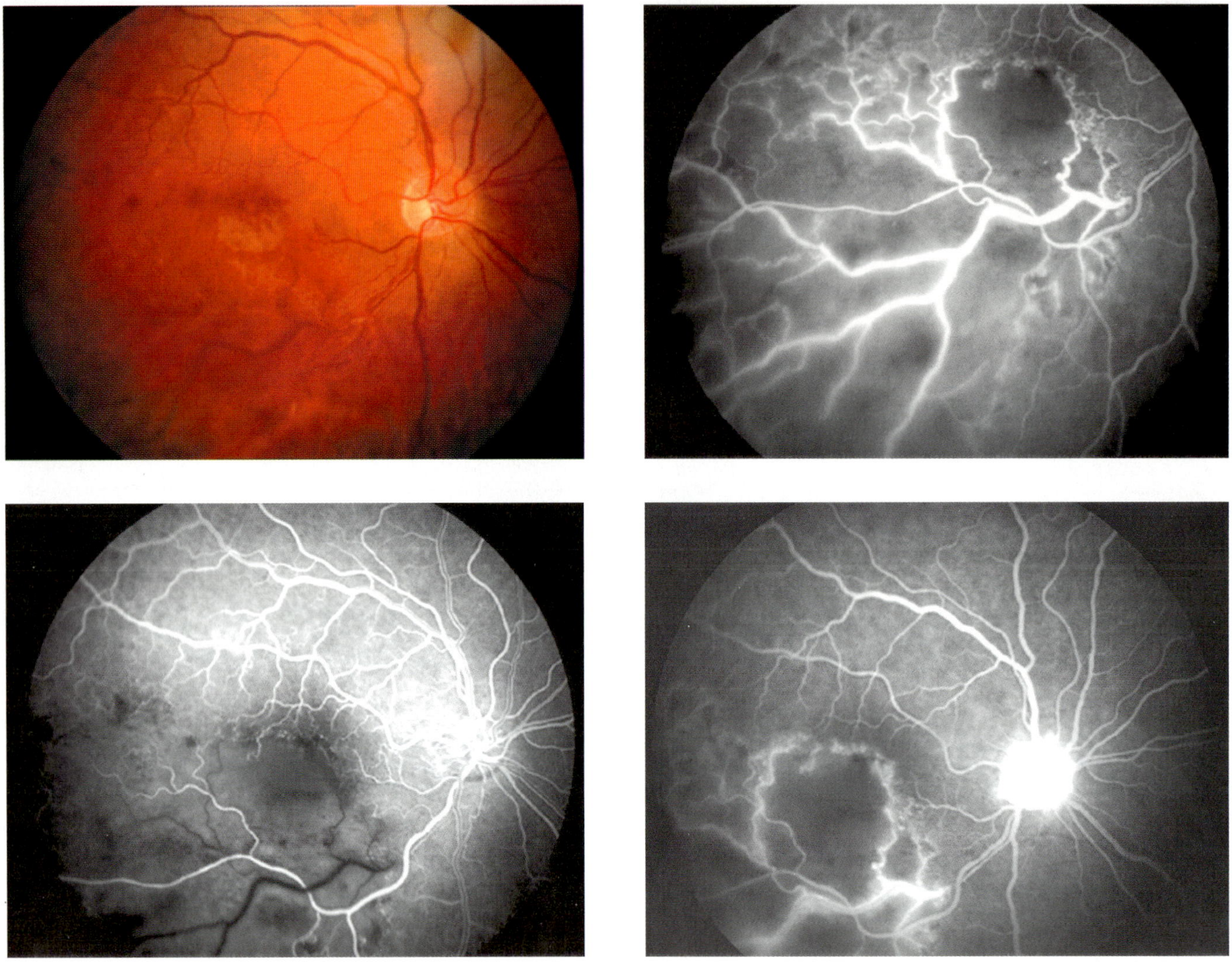

Areas of nonfilling of the retinal vessels due to branch retinal vein occlusion, appear hypofluorescent on the angiogram

Choroidal Vascular Filling Defect

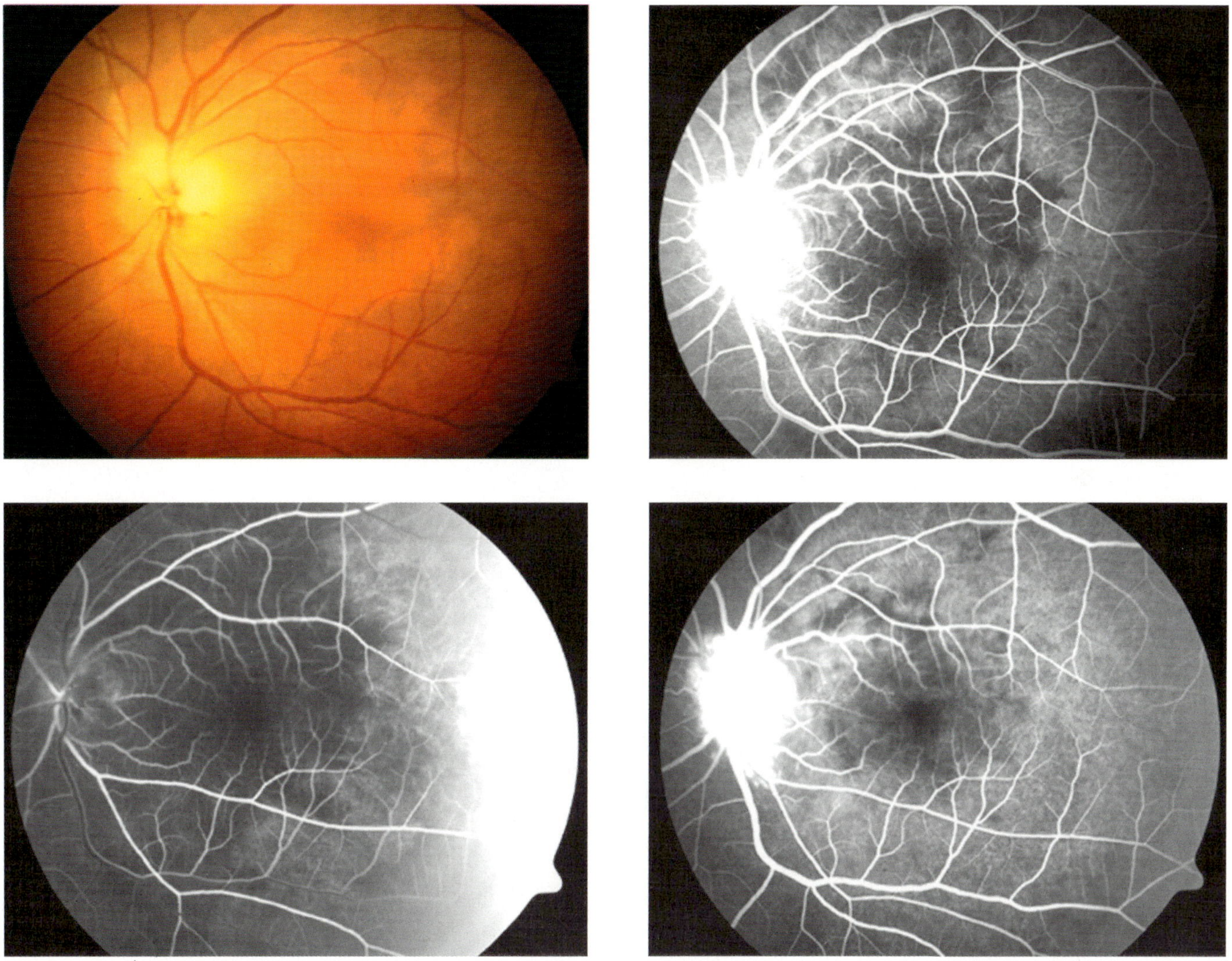

Occlusion of the posterior ciliary artery gives rise to hypofluorescence due to nonfilling of the affected segment of the choroid. Hypofluorescence due to choroidal nonfilling can also occur in conditions like choroideremia where the choriocapillaries are absent

Disc Vascular Filling Defect

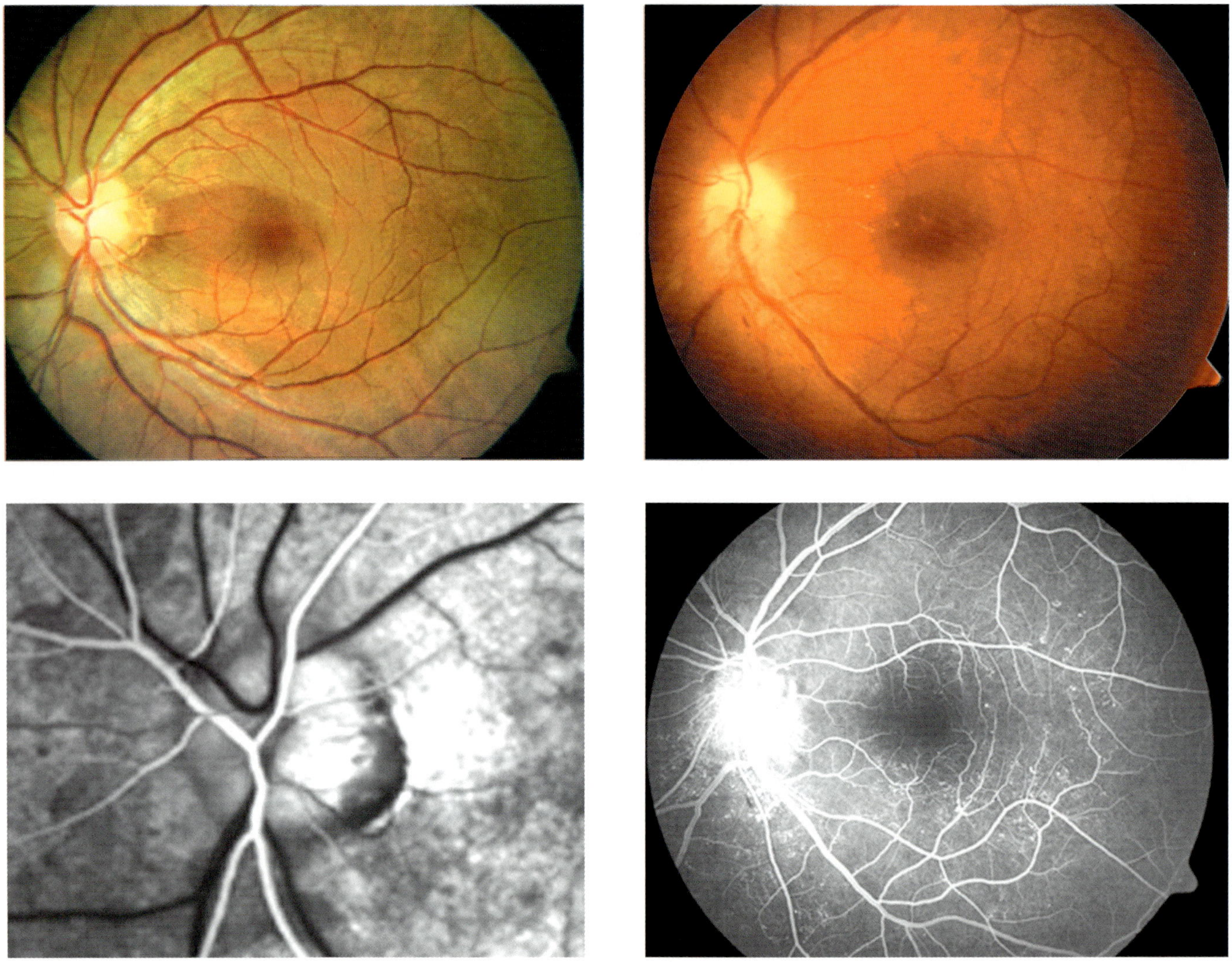

Absence of vessels at the optic nerve head results in absence of filling of superior half of the disc giving rise to hypofluorescence, which is seen in patients with AION

Preinjection Hyperfluorescence

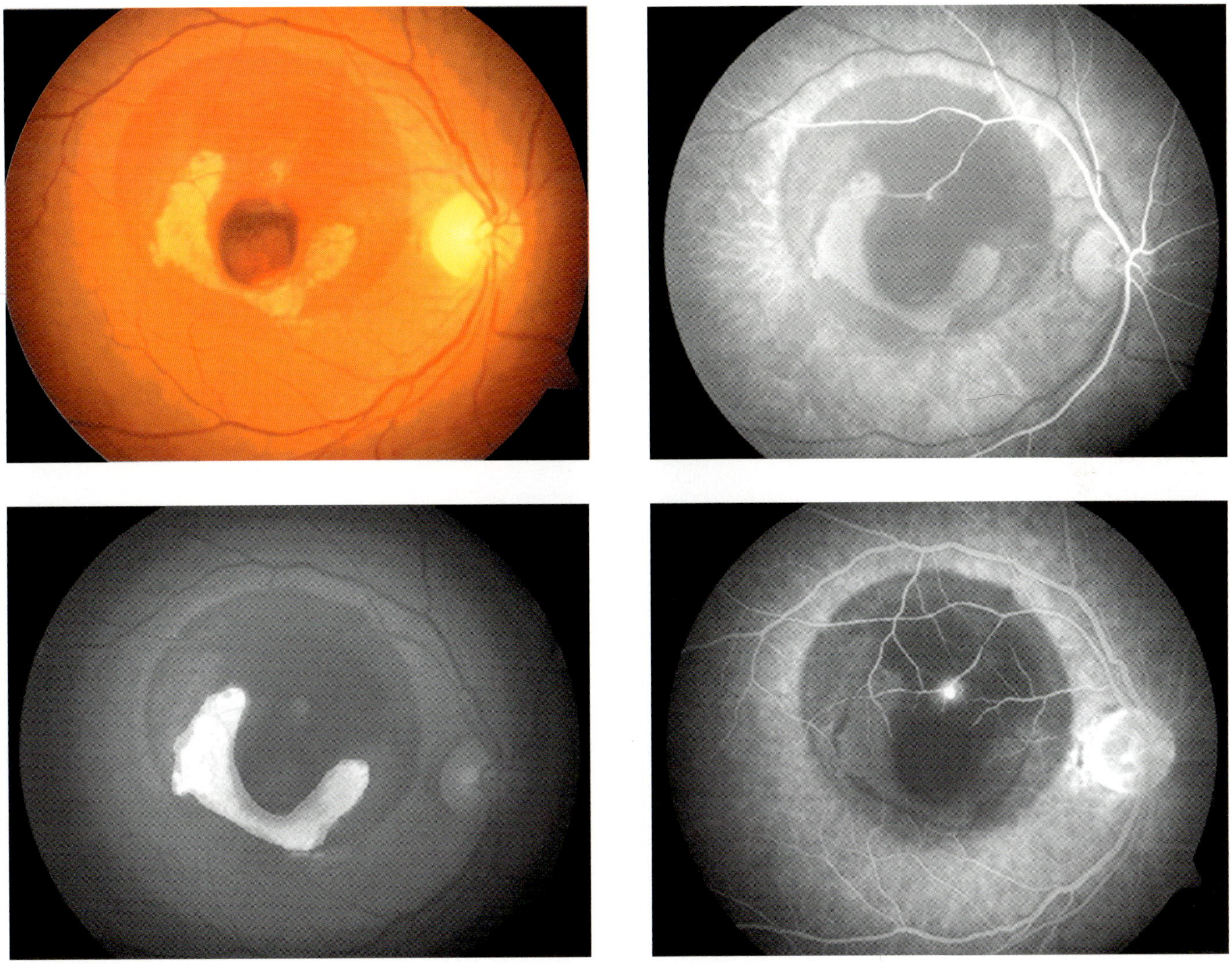

The dehemoglobinized blood reflects sufficient blue light to pass through the barrier filter causing it to appear hyperfluorescent in the preinjection photograph. This can occur despite the filters being well matched. Preinjection hyperfluorescence can be either due to autofluorescence or pseudofluorescence. Autofluorescence is an innate property of certain structures to emit fluorescent light even in the absence of sodium fluorescein. Optic nerve head drusen and astrocytic hamartoma are examples of autofluorescence. Pseudofluorescence occurs due to mismatched barrier and exciter filters

HYPERFLUORESCENCE

Transmitted Fluorescence

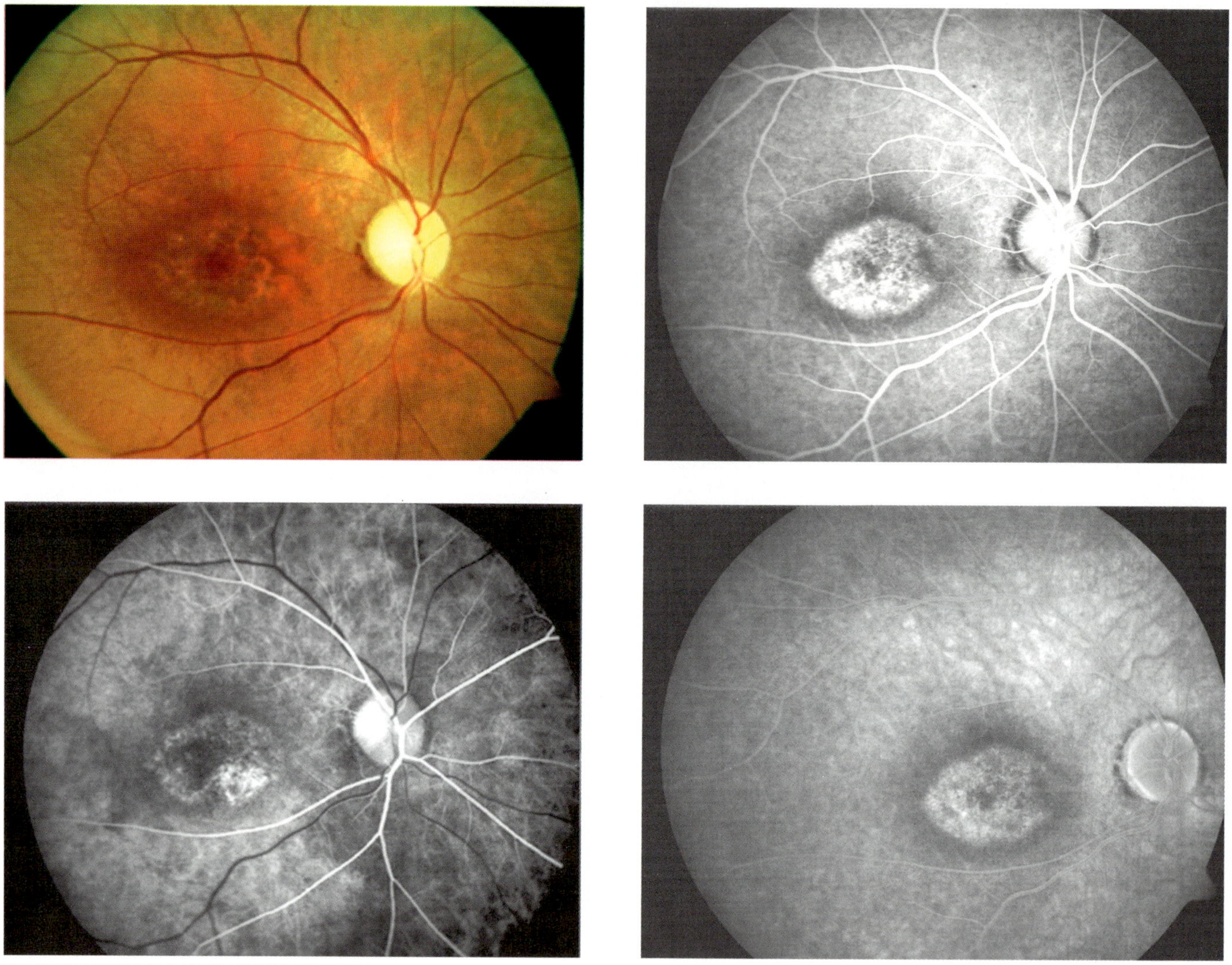

Transmitted fluorescence due to atrophy of the retinal pigment epithelium allowing the underlying choroidal fluorescence to be well seen. Transmitted fluorescence or window defect typically appears in the early choroidal or arterial phase, increases in the arteriovenous phase and fades in the late phase of the angiogram

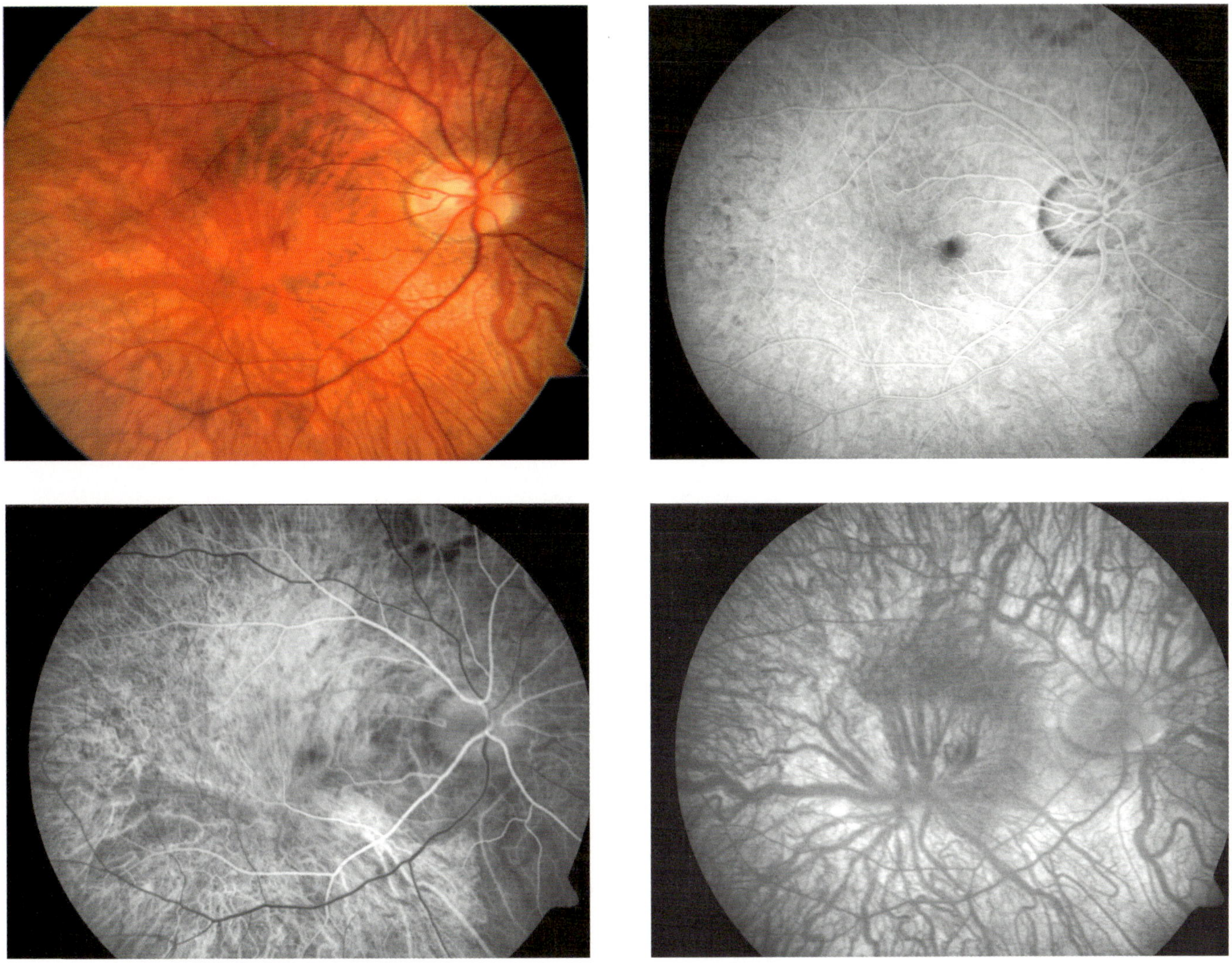

Transmitted fluorescence due to congenital absence of pigment in the retinal pigment epithelium is seen in patients with albinism. In the arteriovenous phase, intense hyperfluorescence is seen from the filling of the choriocapillaries while in the late phase hyperfluorescence occurs due to increased transmission of fluorescence from scleral staining

Hyperfluorescence due to Leakage

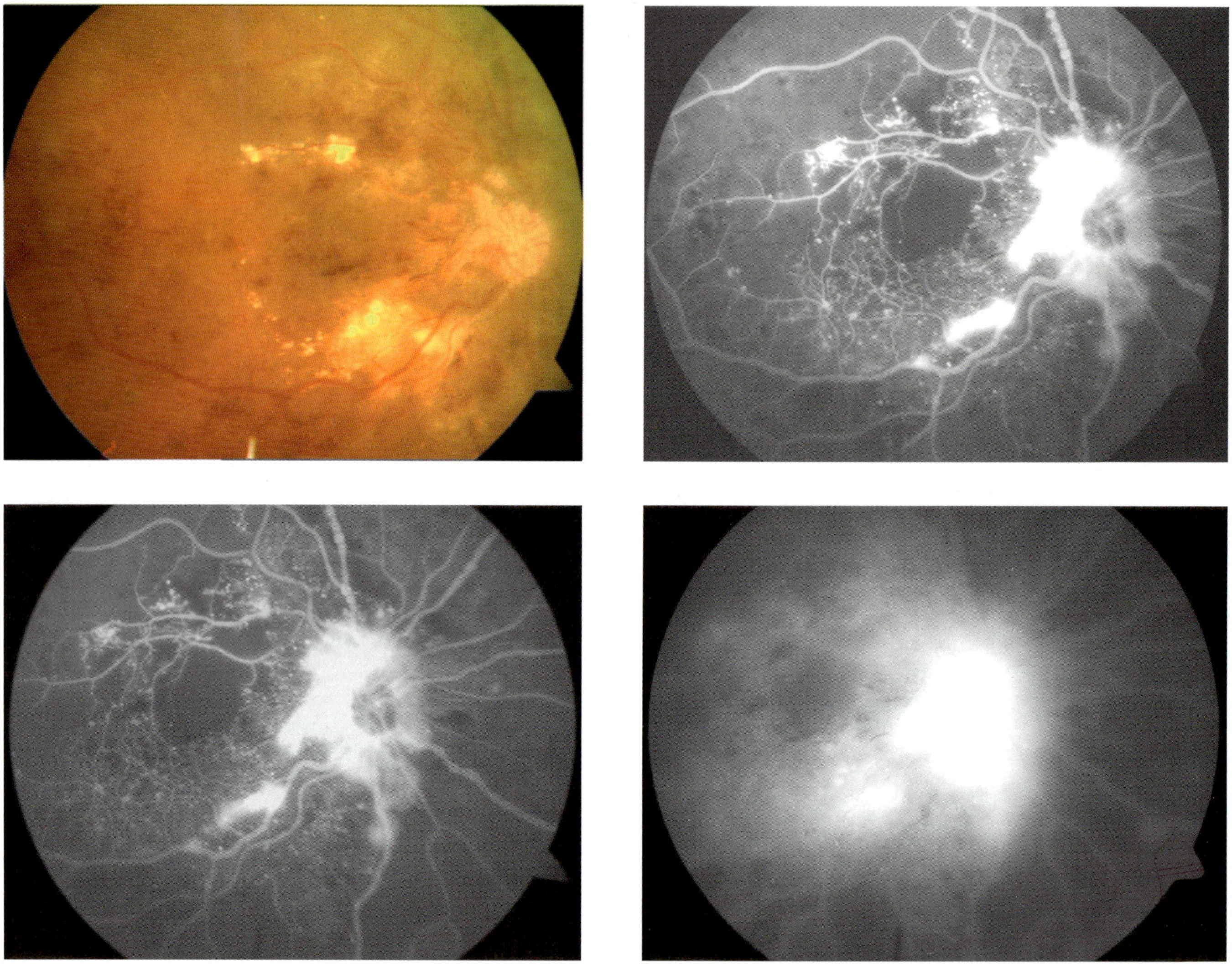

Hyperfluorescence is seen at the disc due to leakage from neovascularization at the disc; the hyperfluorescence (with fuzzy margins) increases in the late phase of the angiogram

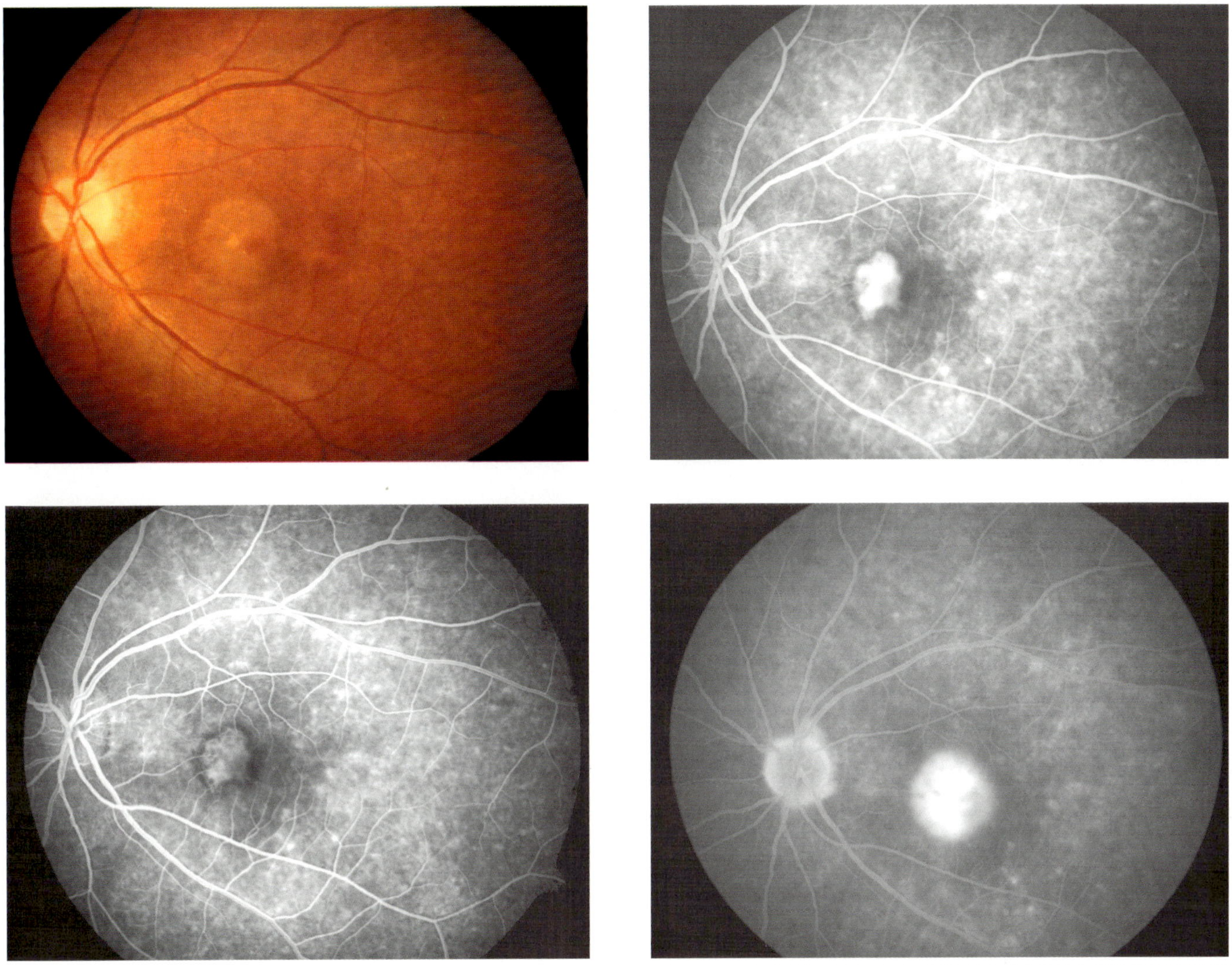

Hyperfluorescence is seen due to presence of neovascularization in the subretinal space. This neovascular membrane increases in hyperfluorescence as the angiogram progresses and is intensely hyperfluorescent in the late films

Hyperfluorescence due to Pooling

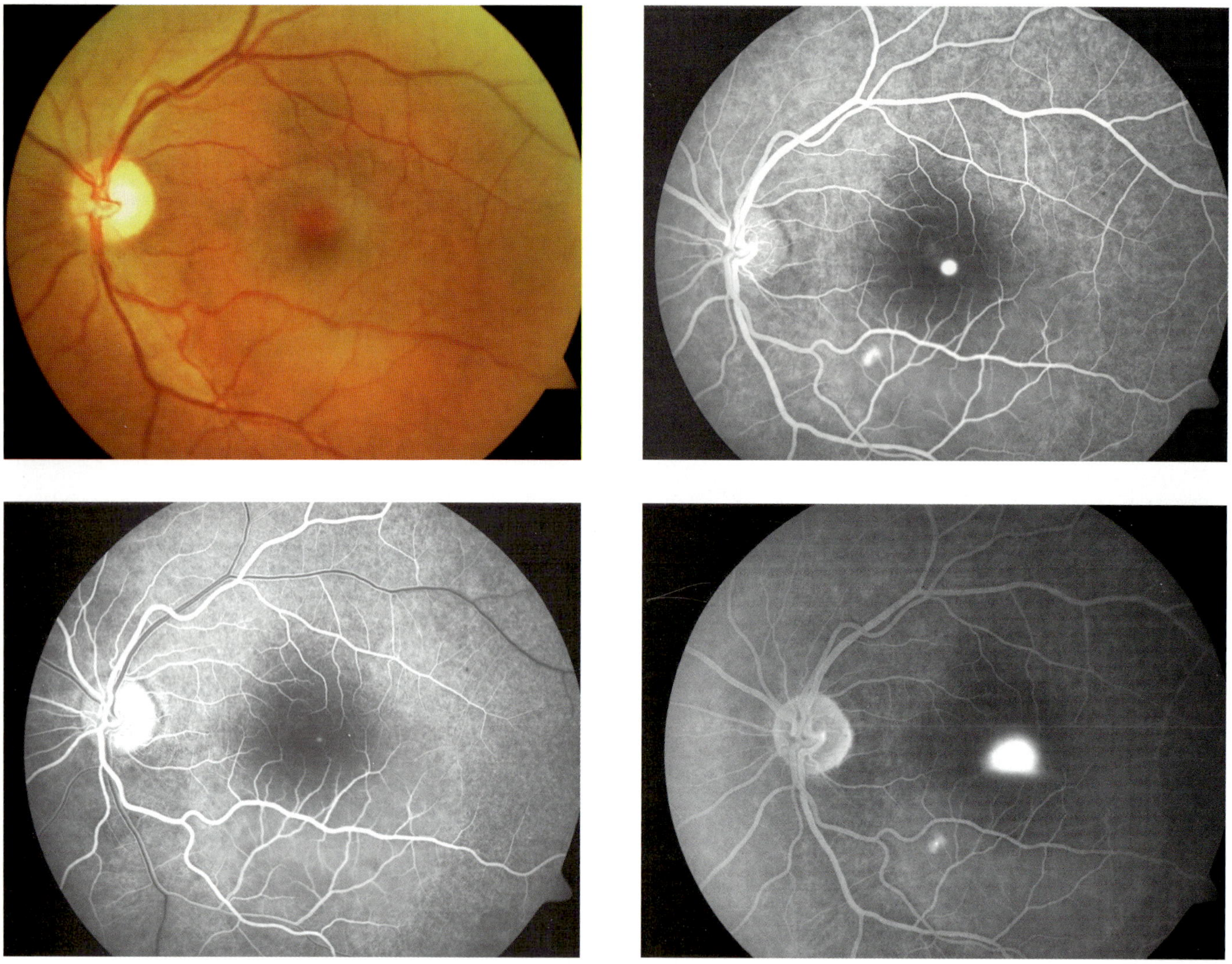

Pooling of the dye in the subretinal space is seen in eyes with central serous retinopathy. Pooling is accumulation of the dye in an anatomical space

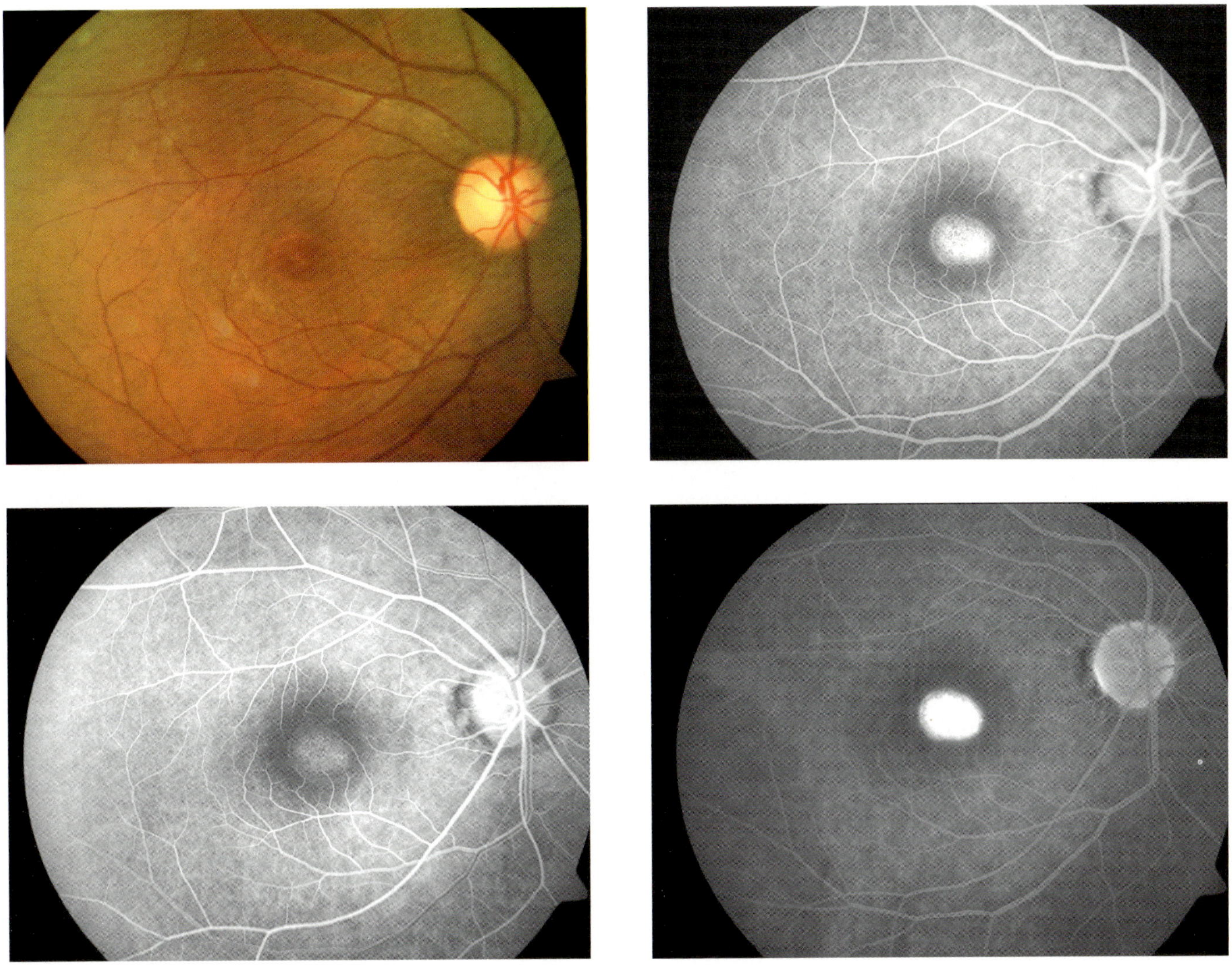

Pooling of the dye in the sub-RPE space is seen in eyes with pigment epithelial detachment

Hyperfluorescence due to Staining

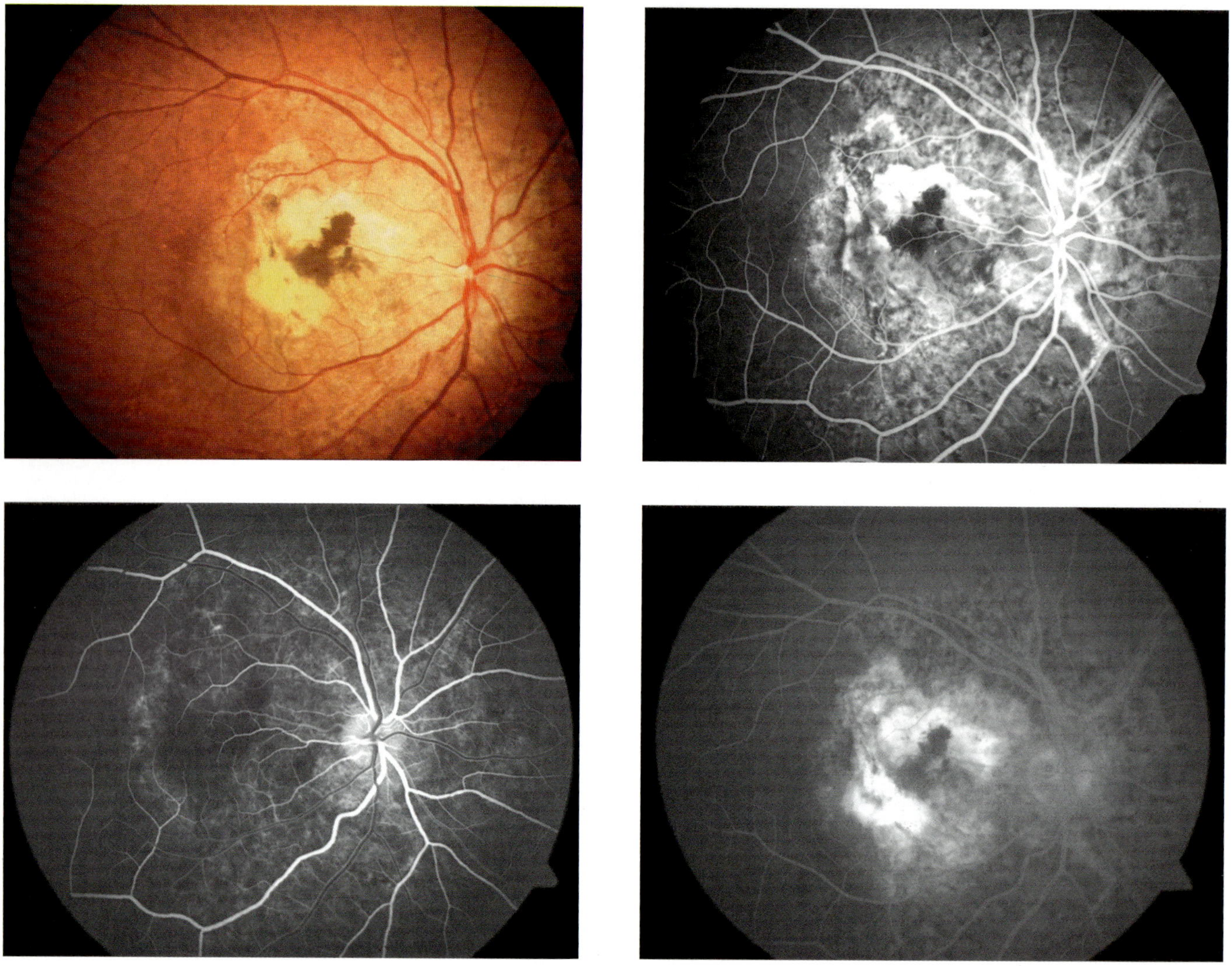

Staining is attachment of the dye molecule to the tissue. It can occur normally in structures like the sclera or in pathological states like staining of the scar as seen in the above case. Unlike leakage, the margins of hyperfluorescence due to staining do not go beyond the scar

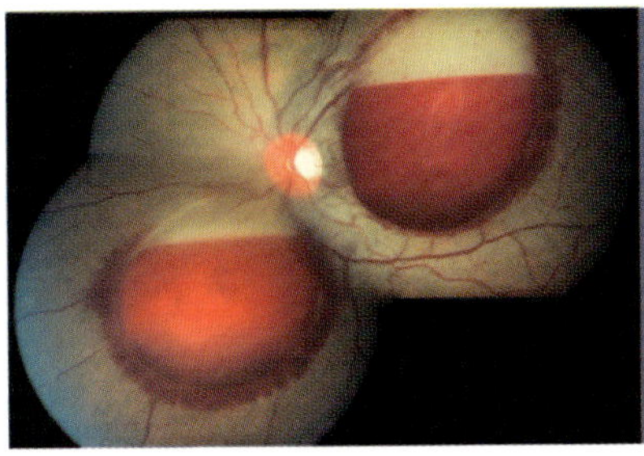

2 Section

Macular Disorders

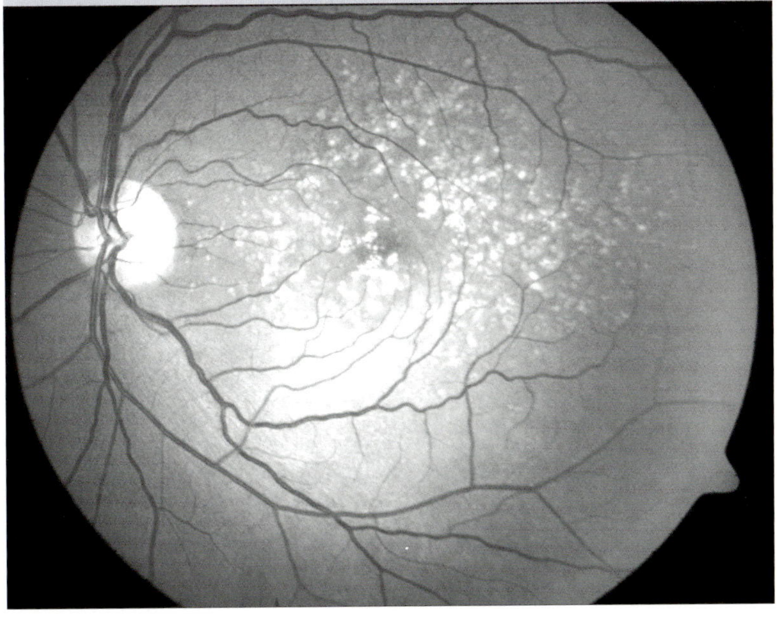

Chapter 7

Drusen

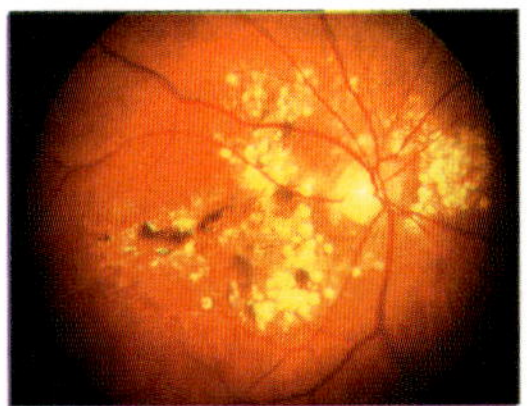

- Hard drusen are generally small, < 63 microns, discrete, flat and yellow-white lesions.
- Soft drusen are larger, usually > 125 microns, softer appearing lesions; they have a tendency to coalesce.
- Basal laminar drusen are innumerable, tiny, round sub-RPE nodules that are better seen on fluorescein angiography than on clinical examination; they occur in a younger age group of patients.
- Radial basal laminar drusen — called as malattia leventinese — are characterized by a radial pattern of innumerable, small elongated drusen. The radial pattern is better seen temporally.

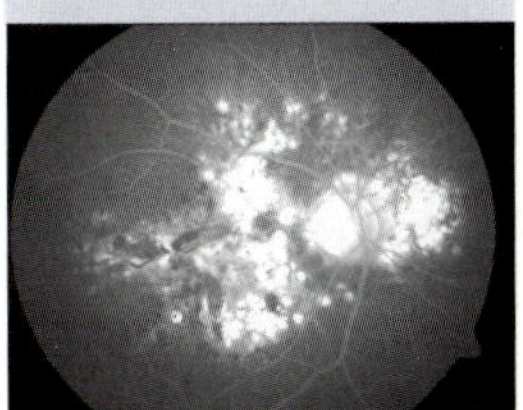

- *Hard drusen:* The RPE atrophy overlying the drusen shows up as window defects in the early phase. The fluorescence fades in the later phase.
- *Soft drusen:* The fluorescein angiographic pattern in soft drusen varies depending on its content. In general, they hyperfluoresce later and either fade or stain in the late phases.
- *Basal laminar drusen:* Innumerable dots of hyperfluorescence seen throughout the posterior pole in the arteriovenous phase give an appearance of a 'starry-sky'. The transmitted fluorescence fades in the late phase.
- *Radial basal laminar drusen:* Transmitted hyperfluorescence corresponding to the radially arranged drusen is seen in the arteriovenous phase. The radial arrangement of the drusen is better seen temporally. Fading of the fluorescence is seen in the late phase.

CASE 1

A 48-year-old male presented with gradual decrease in vision in both the eyes over the past one year. Visual acuity was 6/12; N12 in both eyes.

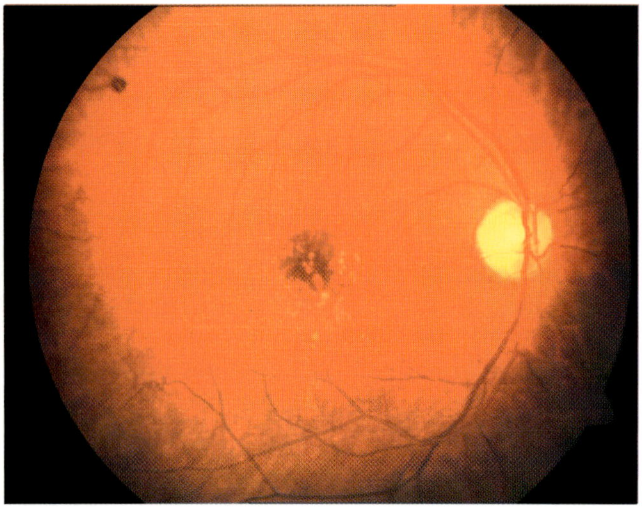

Fundus photograph of the right eye showing multiple discrete drusen at the fovea

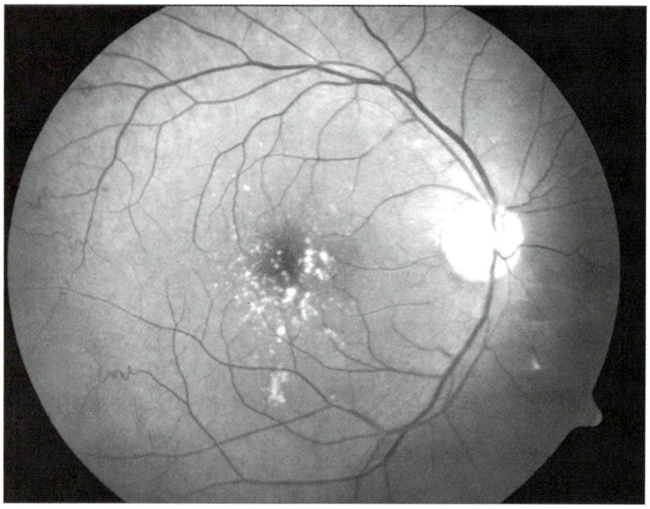

Red free photograph of the right eye showing the drusen

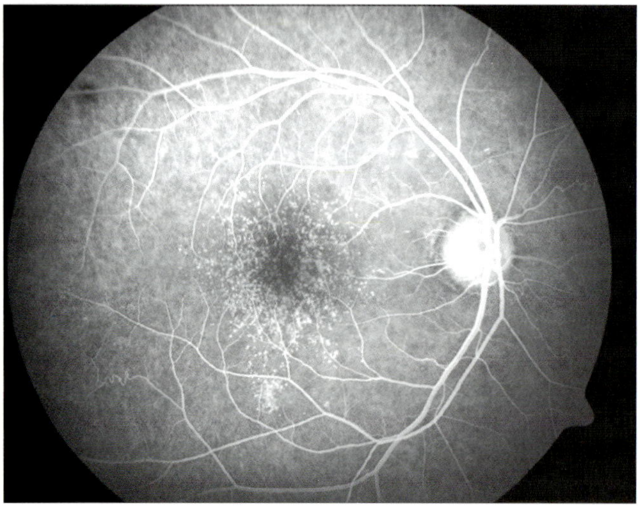

Arteriovenous phase showing discrete early hyperfluorescence corresponding to the drusen location. Note increased number of drusen evident on the angiogram as compared to clinical appearance

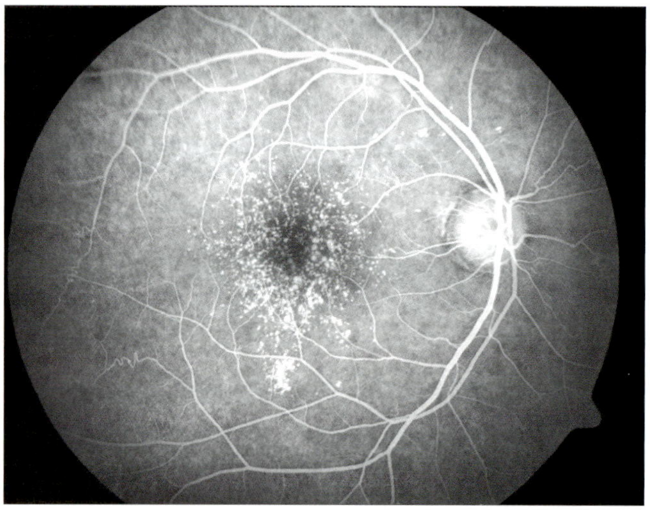

The hyperfluorescence at the drusen has increased in the midarteriovenous phase

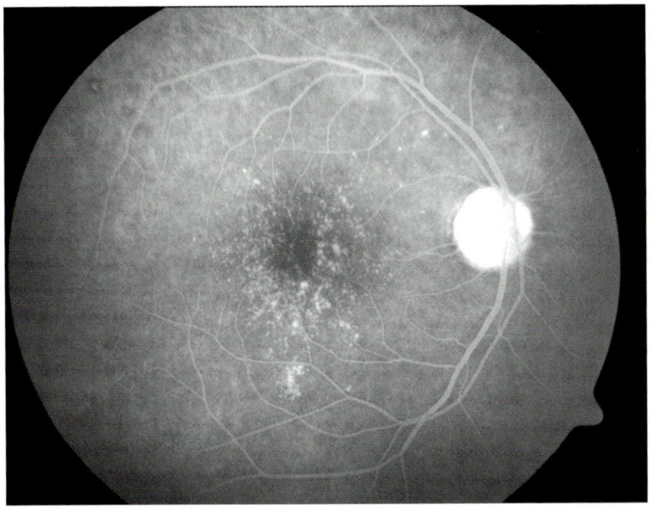

Fading of the hyperfluorescence is seen in the late phase

COMMENT

The RPE atrophy overlying the drusen allows the background choroidal fluorescence to be seen as transmitted hyperfluorescence in the angiogram.

CASE 2

A 49-year-old male presented with history of reduced vision in the right eye of one month duration. Visual acuity was 1/60 in the right eye and 6/6; N6 in the left eye. The right eye had a subfoveal CNVM, and the left eye, drusen at the macula.

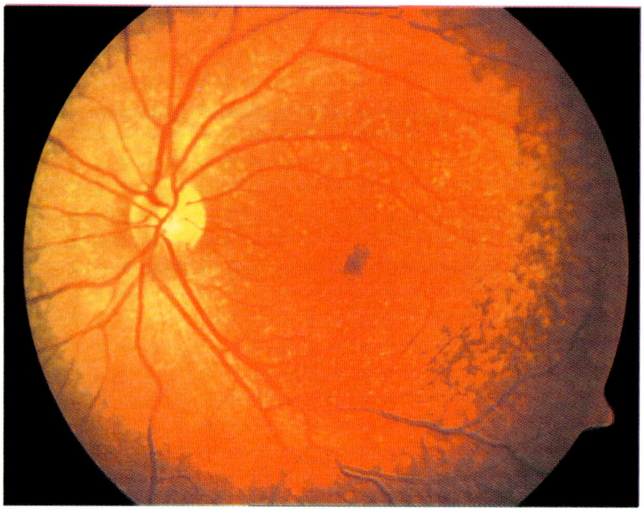

Fundus photograph of the left eye showing innumerable discrete hard drusen scattered throughout the macula

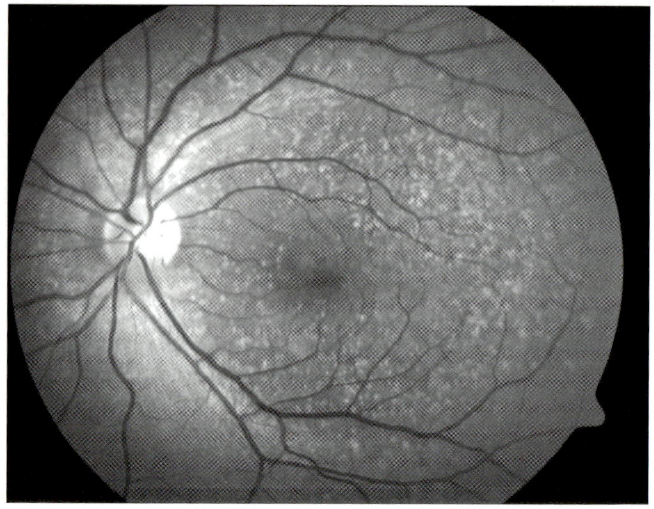

Red free photograph of the left eye showing the drusen

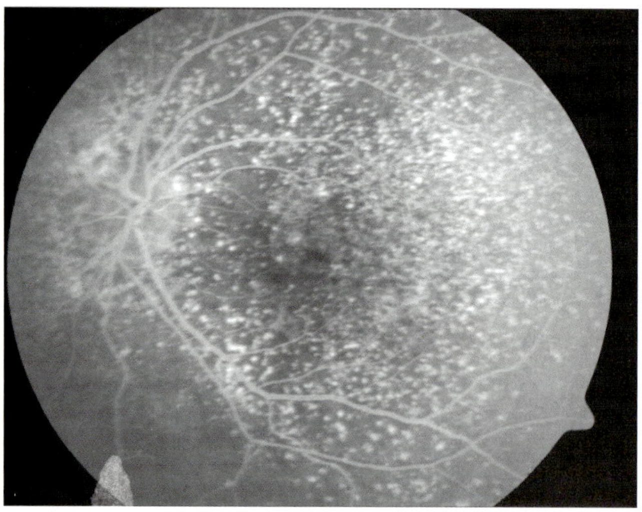

Early hyperfluorescence corresponding to the drusen is seen in the arteriovenous phase

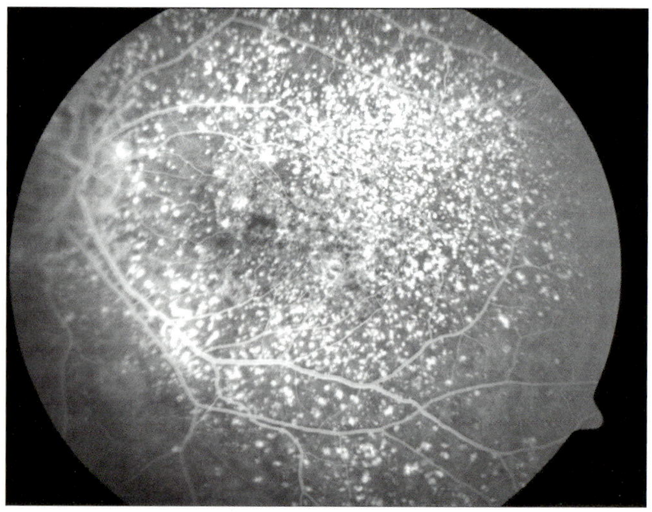

Increased hyperfluorescence is seen in the mid-arteriovenous phase

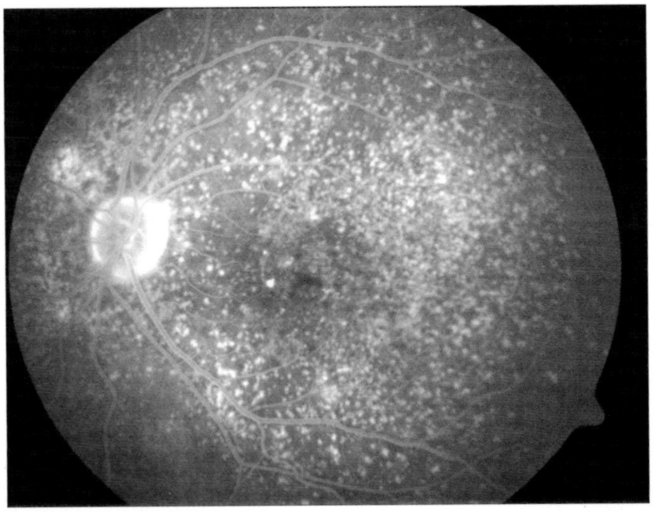

Fading of the hyperfluorescence is seen in the late phase

COMMENT

The hyperfluorescence seen in the angiogram corresponds to the drusen seen clinically.

CASE 3

A 58-year-old female presented with gradual reduction in vision in both the eyes over the last two years; visual acuity was 6/36; N10 in the right eye and 6/6; N6 in the left eye. Central lens changes were noted in the right eye.

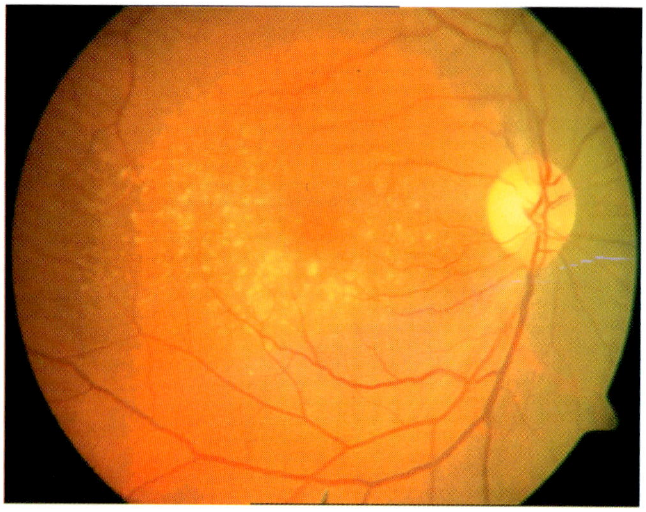

Fundus photograph of the right eye showing multiple discrete hard drusen

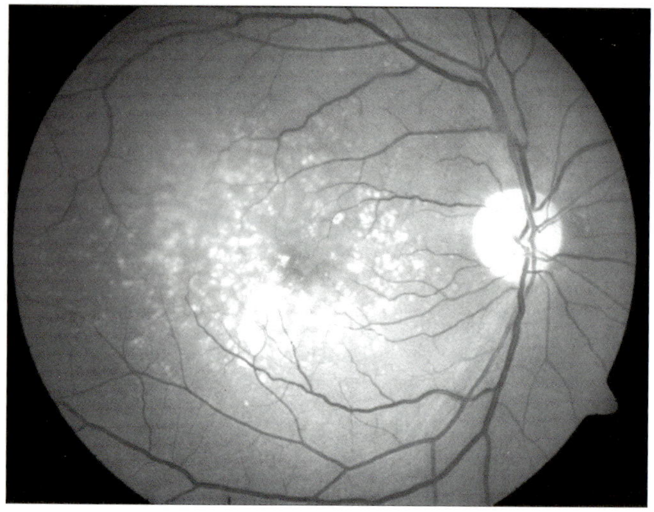

Red free photograph of the right eye

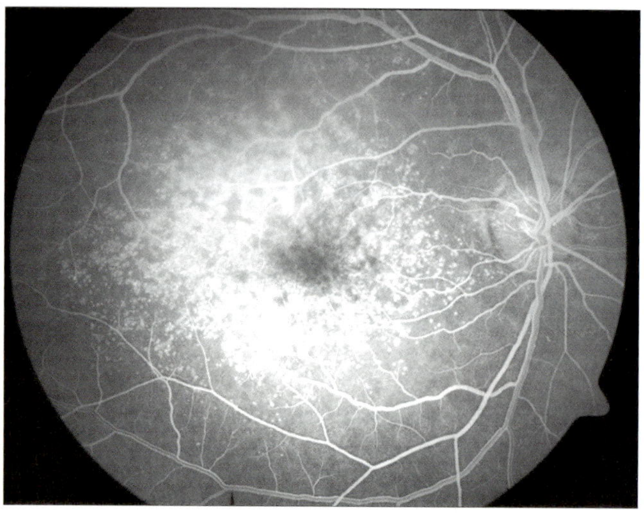

Early hyperfluorescence is seen corresponding to the drusen in the early arteriovenous phase of the angiogram

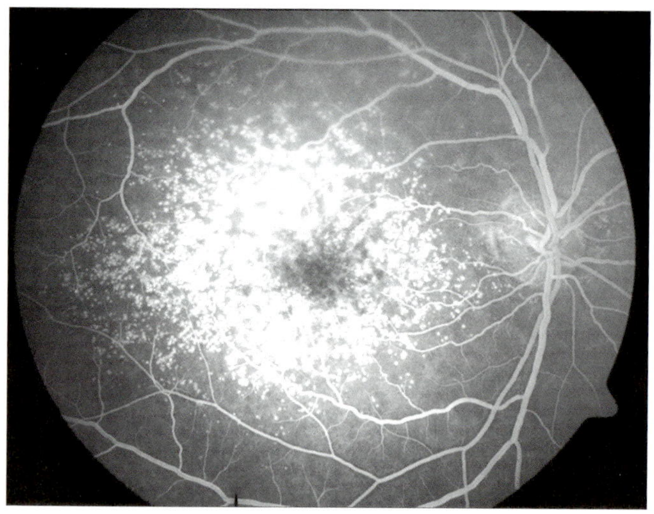

Increased hyperfluorescence is seen in the mid-arteriovenous phase

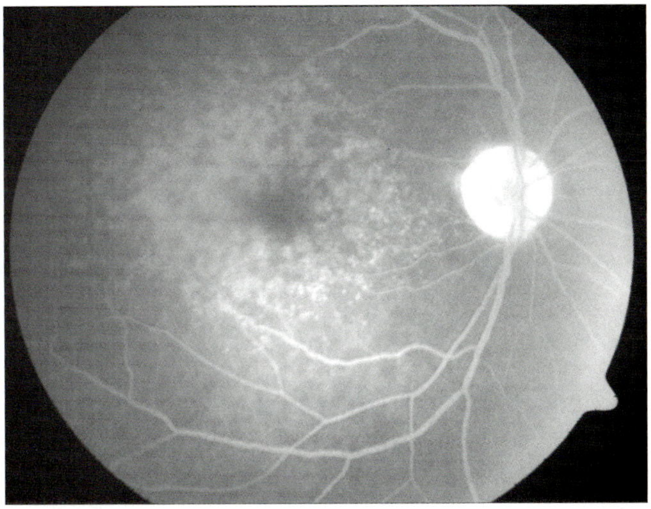

Fading of the hyperfluorescence is seen in the late phase of the angiogram

COMMENT

Hard drusen show early hyperfluorescence which increases in the arteriovenous phase and fades in the late phase of the angiogram.

CASE 3 (*Continued*)

Left Eye of the Patient

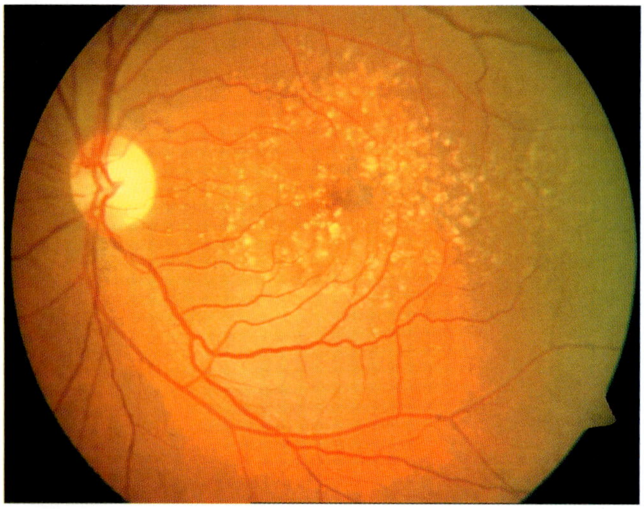

Fundus photograph of the left eye showing multiple discrete hard drusen at the macula

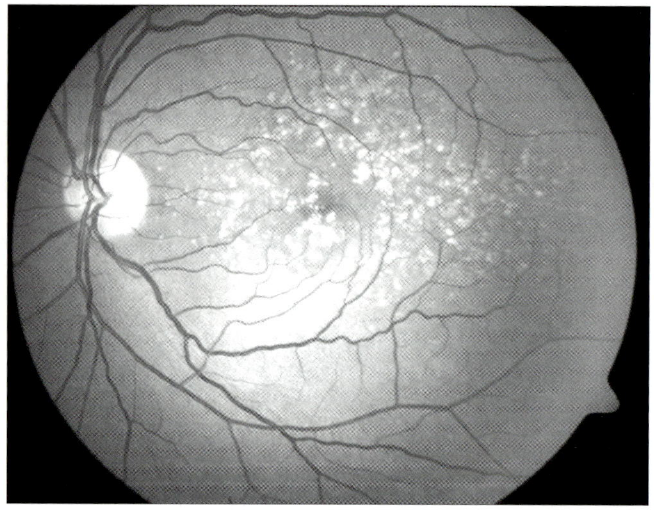

Red free photograph of the left eye

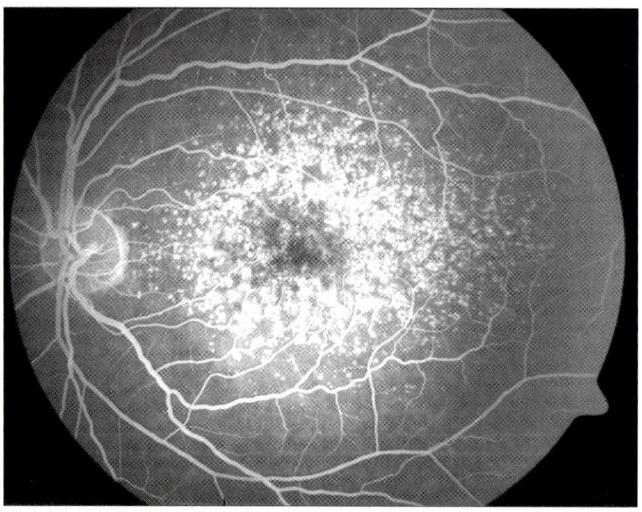

Hyperfluorescence due to transmission defect is noted corresponding to the drusen in the arteriovenous phase of the angiogram

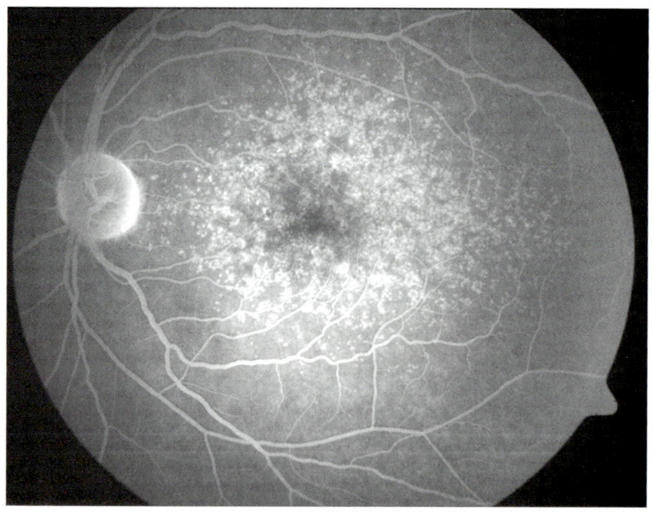

Late phase shows reduction in the intensity of the hyperfluorescence

CASE 4

A 68-year-old male presented with history of mild blurring of vision in the left eye for the last ten days. He gave history of reduced vision in the right eye for the last two years. Visual acuity was 1/60 in the right eye and 6/9; N6 in the left eye. Examination revealed a disciform scar in the right eye and soft drusen in the left eye.

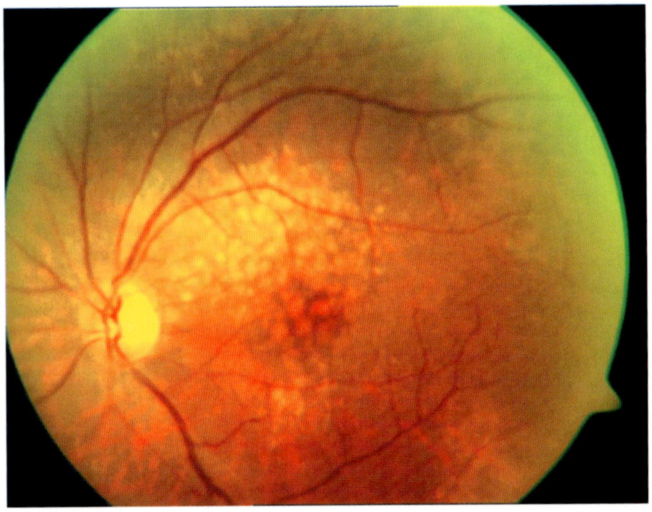

Fundus photograph of the left eye showing multiple large soft drusen in the macula

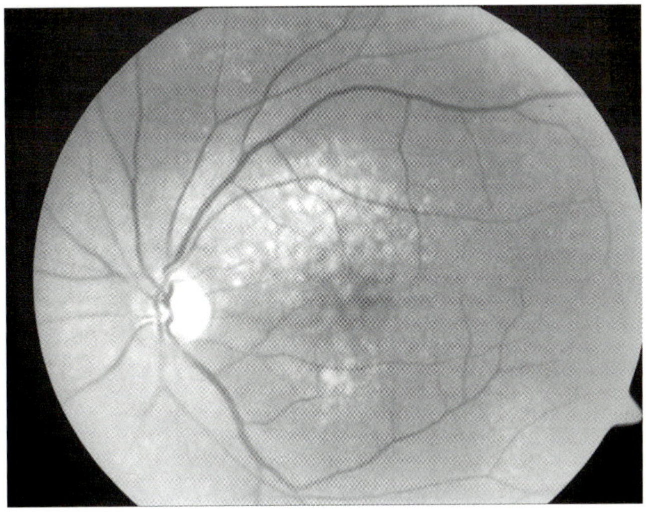

Red free photograph of the left eye

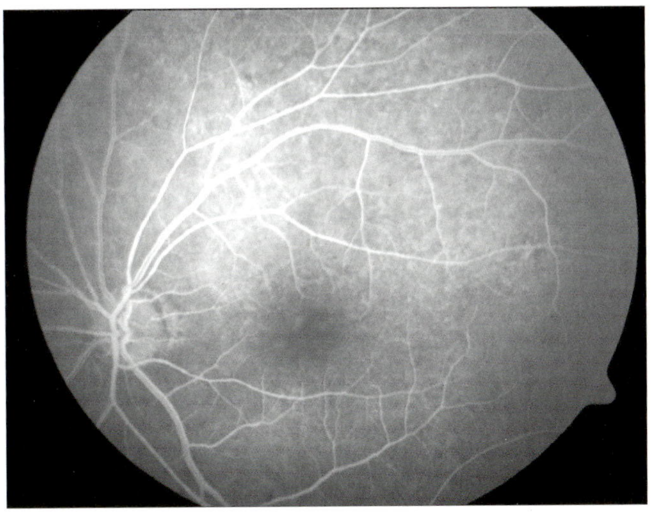

Early arteriovenous phase does not show any hyperfluorescence corresponding to the drusen

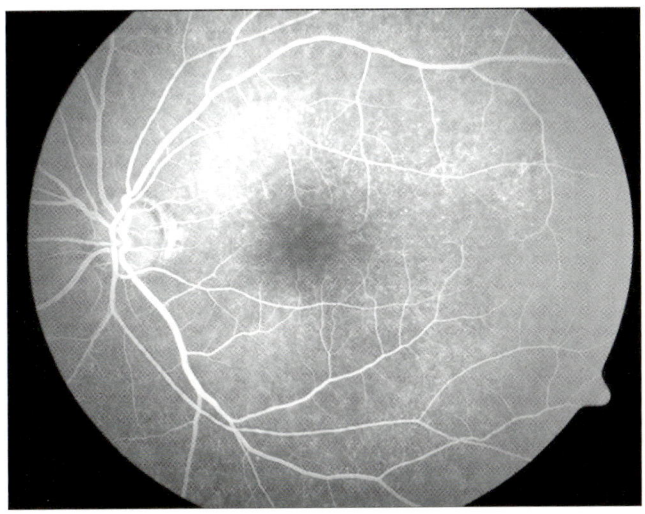

Faint hyperfluorescence is seen around the fovea in the arteriovenous phase. However, the drusen are still not made out

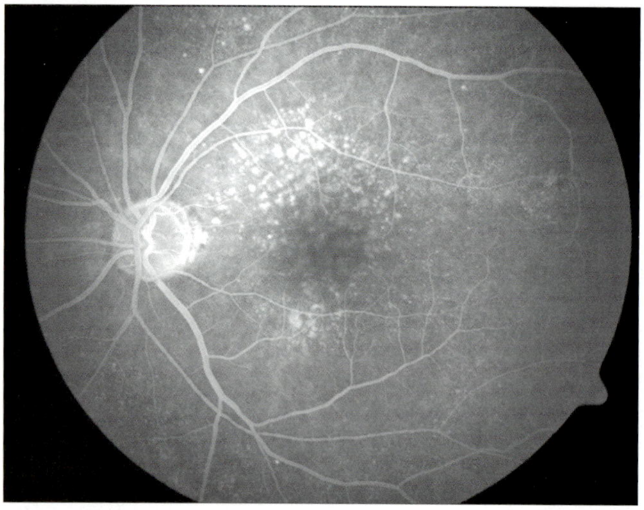

Hyperfluorescence at the drusen is seen only in the late phase of the angiogram

COMMENT

Due to the hydrophobic nature of the soft drusen material, the entry of the dye into the drusen is delayed. Hence, the soft drusen do not show hyperfluorescence until the late stages.

CASE 5

A 56-year-old male presented with metamorphopsia in the left eye for the past four months; visual acuity was 6/9; N6. Fundus examination showed a drusenoid pigment epithelial detachment.

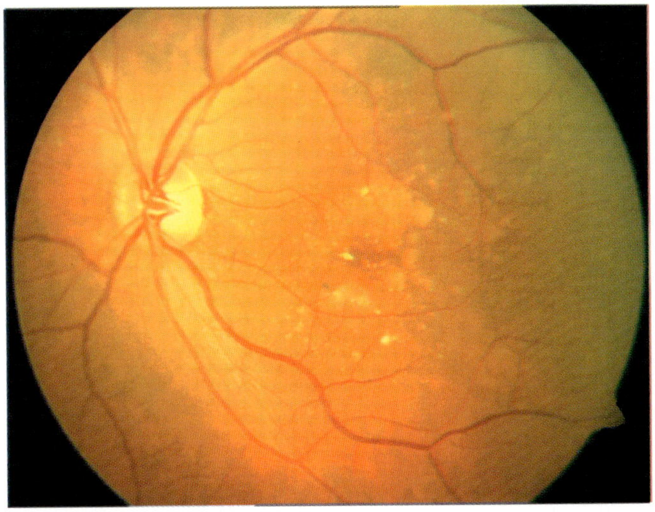

Fundus photograph of the left eye showing two drusenoid RPE detachments superior and inferior to the foveal center. Surrounding drusen are seen. A pigment clump is seen inferonasal to the foveal center

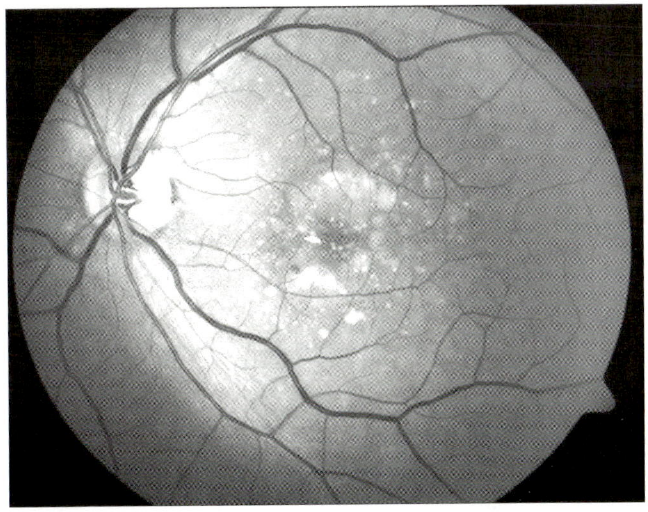

Red free photograph of the left eye

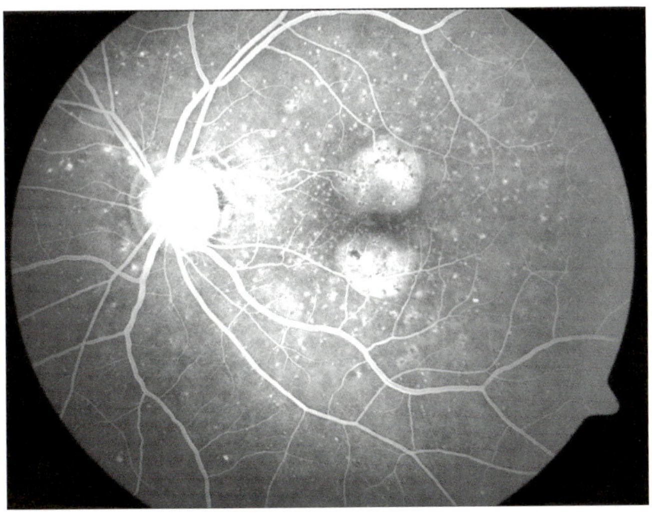

Arteriovenous phase showing filling up of the drusenoid detachments. Blocked hypofluorescence is seen within these due to pigment. Hyperfluorescence is seen in the rest of the macula corresponding to the drusen

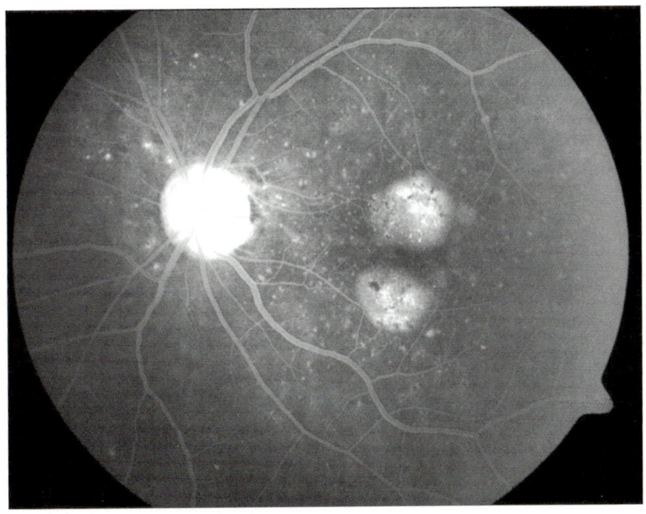

Late phase of the angiogram showing persistent hyperfluorescence at the drusenoid detachment. Hyperfluorescence has faded elsewhere

COMMENT

Confluence of adjacent soft drusen results in a large drusenoid type of pigment epithelial detachment.

BASAL LAMINAR DRUSEN

CASE 6

A 37-year-old female presented with history of noticing a scotoma in the left eye for the past one month; visual acuity was 6/9; N6.

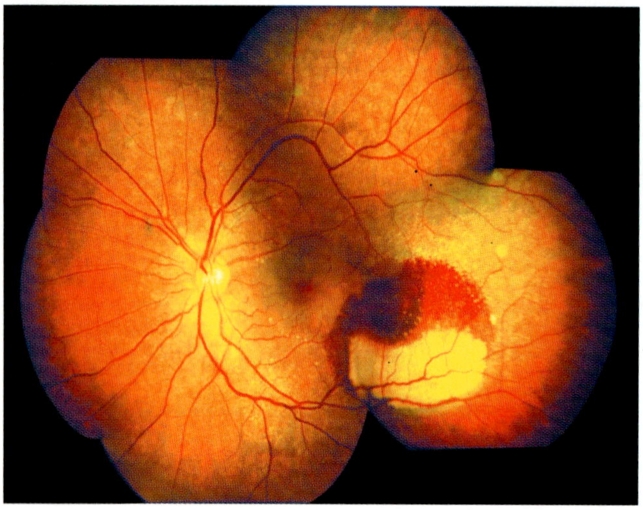

Montage fundus photograph of the left eye showing a mottled appearance at the posterior pole. A large subretinal hemorrhage is seen inferotemporal to the fovea

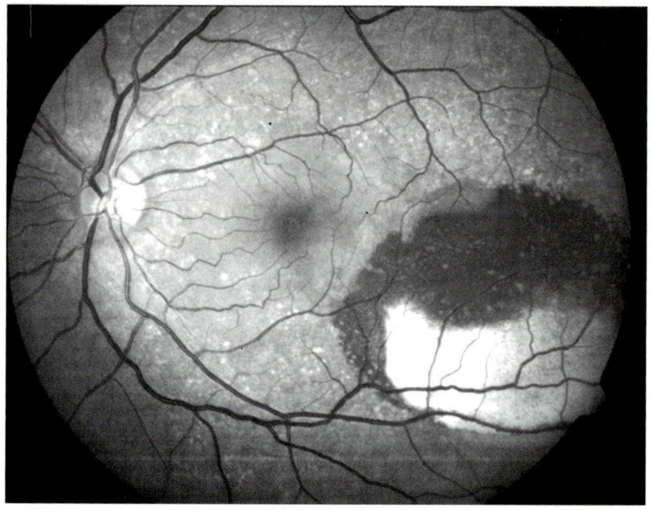

Red free photograph showing few of the subtle drusen. The red and dehemoglobinized subretinal blood are well made out

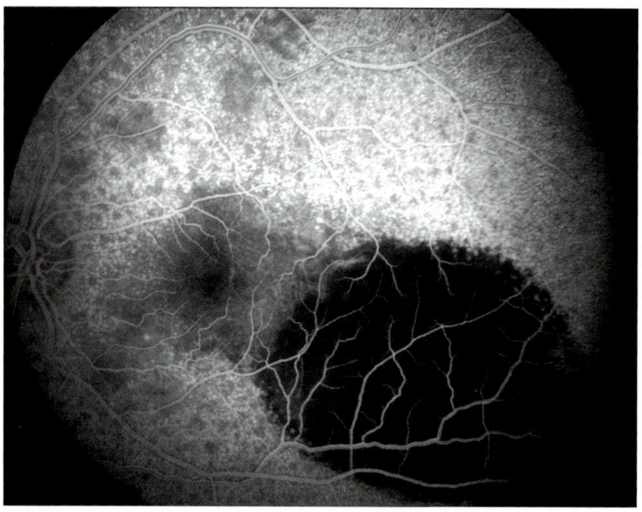

Increased hyperfluorescence in seen in the mid-arteriovenous phase of the angiogram

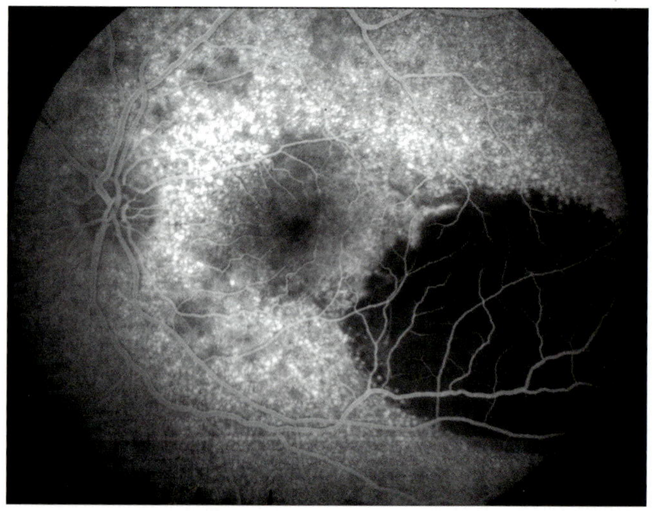

Arteriovenous phase shows the entire posterior pole to be studded with tiny hyperfluorescent dots giving it a 'starry-sky' appearance. Blocked choroidal fluorescence due to the subretinal hemorrhage is seen

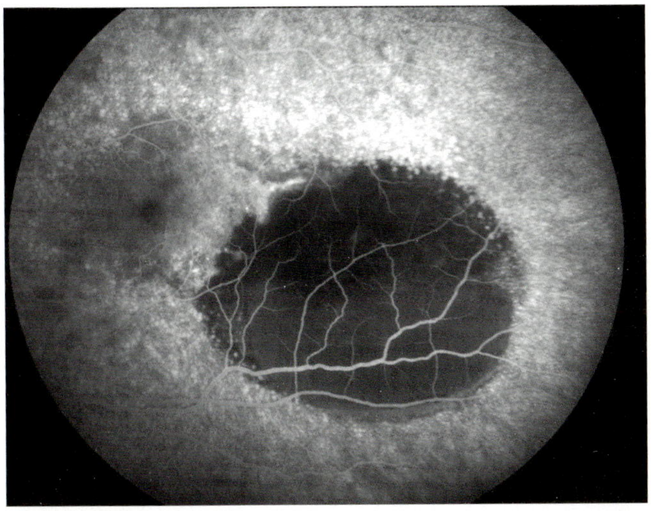

Late phase shows fading of the hyperfluorescence in the area of the basal laminar drusen. Hypofluorescence due to the hemorrhage persists

COMMENT

Basal laminar drusen are better seen on the angiogram than clinically. They appear as innumerable, discrete, tiny, hyperfluorescent dots which gives the angiogram a 'starry sky' appearance.

This patient had an associated spontaneous subretinal hemorrhage which cleared with time. No cause could be found for the hemorrhage.

RADIAL BASAL LAMINAR DRUSEN (MALATTIA LEVENTINESE)

CASE 7

A 34-year-old male presented with reduced vision in both the eyes for the past several years; visual acuity was 6/60; N36 in both eyes.

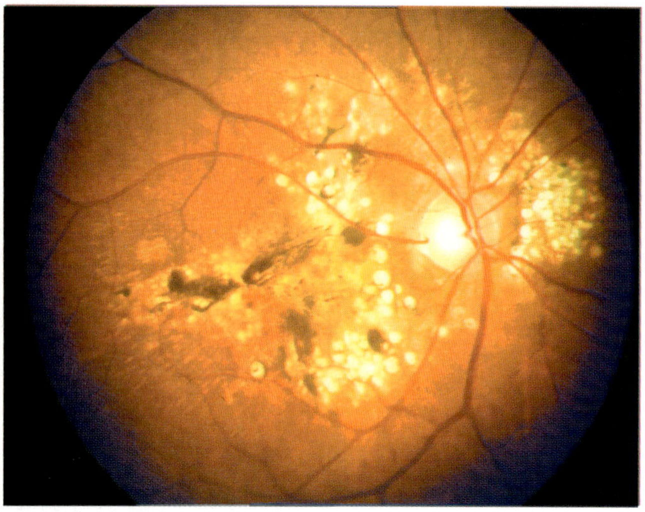

Fundus photograph of the right eye showing a large number of drusen at the posterior pole. Scar with pigmentation is noted at the fovea. The drusen temporally are arranged in a radiating pattern

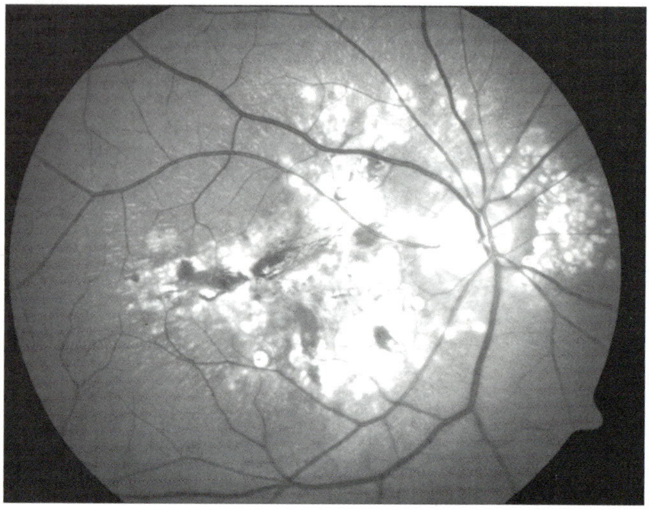

Red free photograph of the right eye. The radial arrangement of the drusen temporally is better seen

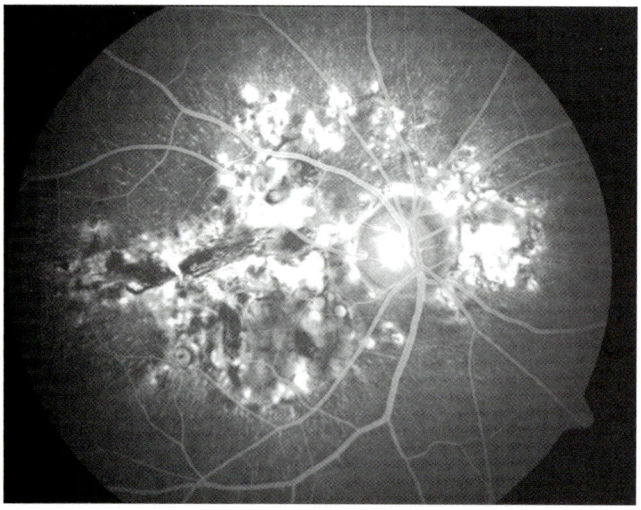

Arteriovenous phase showing the faint radiating lines at the periphery of the lesion. Central blocked fluorescence is seen due to the scar and pigment

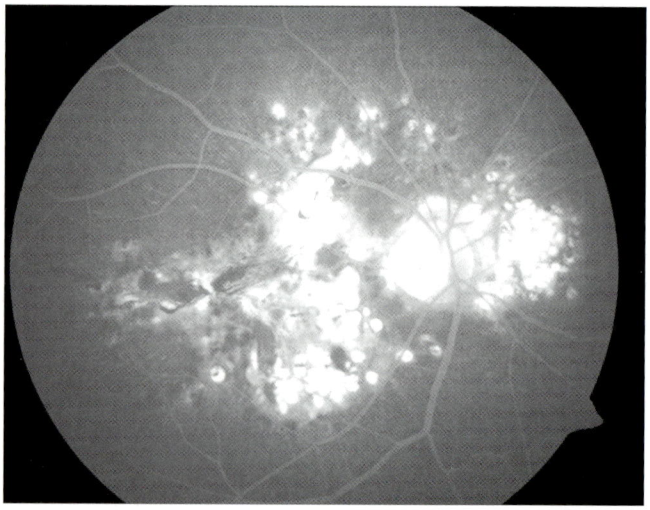

Late phase angiogram showing staining of the drusen

CASE 7 (*Continued*)

Left Eye of the Patient

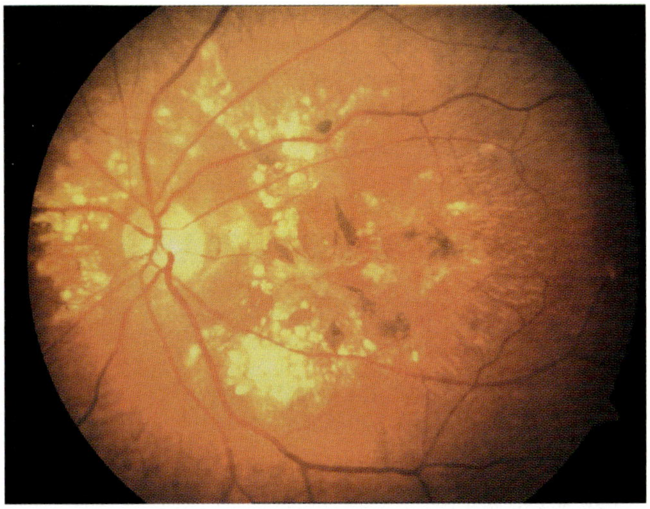

Fundus photograph of the left eye showing similar features as the right eye

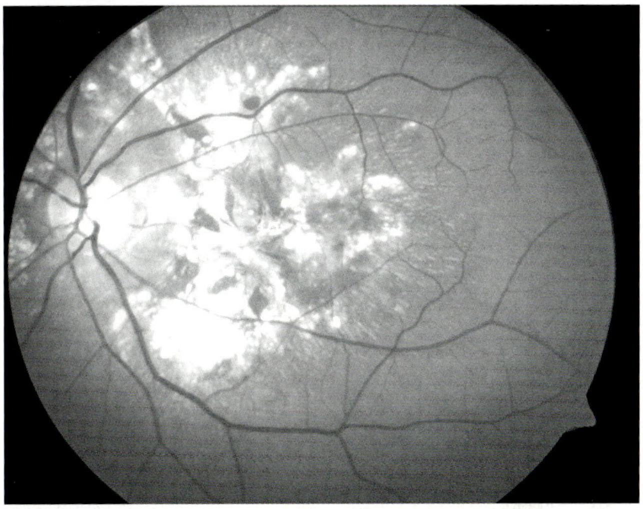

Red free photograph of the left eye

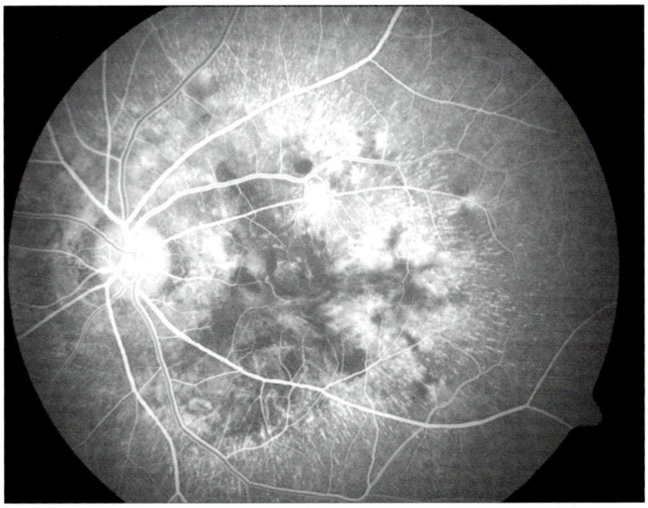

Early arteriovenous phase showing the peripheral radial spokes. Central hypofluorescence due to the scar and pigment is seen

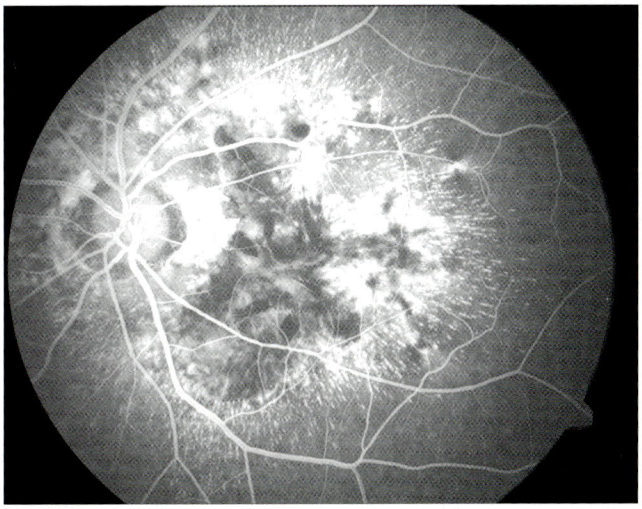

The hyperfluorescence at radial spokes has increased in the midarteriovenous phase

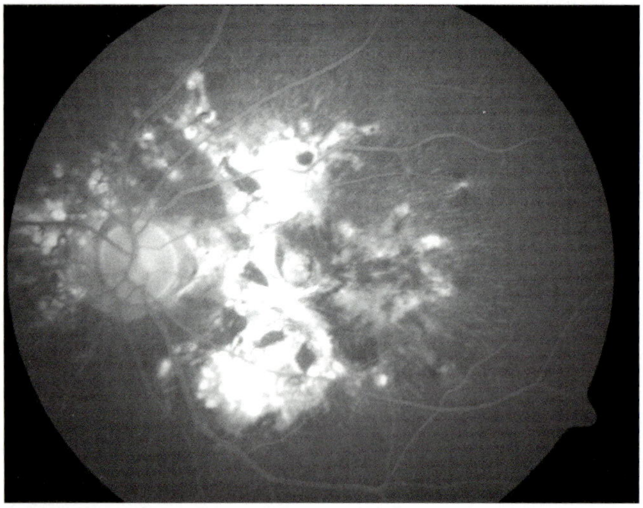

Late phase showing staining of the central scar. The hyperfluorescence at the radial spokes has faded

COMMENT

The typical radiating spoke like pattern of arrangement of drusen is seen more clearly in the temporal macula.

CLINICAL NUGGETS

1. Patients with soft drusen are more likely to develop choroidal neovascular membrane.
2. Amsler grid chart is useful in following patients with drusen.
3. Results from AREDS recommend intake of high levels of antioxidants viz 500 mg of vitamin C, 400 IU of vitamin E, 15 mg of beta carotene, zinc (80 mg of zinc oxide) and copper (2 mg of cupric oxide). It reduces the risk of developing advanced age-related macular degeneration in people with high-risk by about 25 percent over a 6 years period.

   AREDS 2 is studying the role of supplementation of macular xanthophylls (lutein and zeaxanthin) and Omega 3 fatty acids (docosahexaenoic and eicosapentaenoic acid) in the reduction of the risk and rate of progression of age-related macular degeneration.

BIBLIOGRAPHY

1. A Randomized, Placebo-Controlled, Clinical Trial of High-Dose Supplementation with Vitamins C and E, Beta Carotene, and Zinc for Age-Related Macular Degeneration and Vision Loss. AREDS Report No. 8. Age-Related Eye Disease Study Research Group. Arch Ophthalmol. 2001;119:1417-36.
2. Arnold JJ, Quaranta M, Soubrane G, Sarks SH, Coscos G. ICG angiography of drusen. Am J Ophthalmol 1997; 124:344-56.
3. Barendes M, Pauleikhoff D, Chisholm I, C Minassian D, Bird AC. Bilaterality of drusen. BJO 1990;74:180-2.
4. Bressler NM, Bressler SB, Fine SL. Age-related macular degeneration. Surv Ophthalmol 1988;32:375-413.
5. Folk JC. Aging macular degeneration: clinical features of treatable diseases. Ophthalmol 1985;92:594-602.
6. Gass JDM. Stereoscopic atlas of macular diseases. Diagnosis and treatment, Vol 2, 4th edn, CV Mosby. Chapter 3,1997,pp 78-9.
7. Pauleikhoff D, Barondes MJ, Minassian D, et al. Drusen as risk factors in age related macular disease. Am J Ophthalmol 1990;109:38-43.
8. Sarks SH. Drusen and their relationship to senile macular degeneration. Austral J Ophthalmol 1980; 8:117-30.
9. Tanenbaum HL, Eshagian M. Senile disciform degeneration of macula: the other eye—a fluorescein angiographic study. Can J Ophthalmol 1972; 7:280-4.

8

Chapter

Epiretinal Membrane

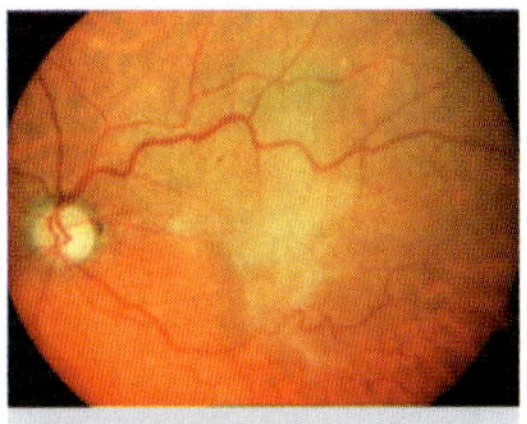

- Epiretinal membranes can be either idiopathic or secondary.
- Secondary causes include retinal vascular occlusions, diabetic retinopathy, following surgical procedures like retinal detachment surgery or cataract surgery, ocular inflammatory conditions and following laser or cryotherapy.
- It varies in severity from very subtle membranes to thick membranes covering the macular region.

Gass Classification

- *Grade 0:* Cellophane maculopathy not associated with any retinal distortion.
- *Grade I:* Crinkled cellophane maculopathy. The wrinkling may be sufficient to provide tortuosity of paramacular vessels pulling them towards the fovea.
- *Grade II:* Macular pucker involving full thickness, may be present along with retinal edema, small retinal hemorrhage, cotton wool spots and infrequently, a localized detachment of the retina.

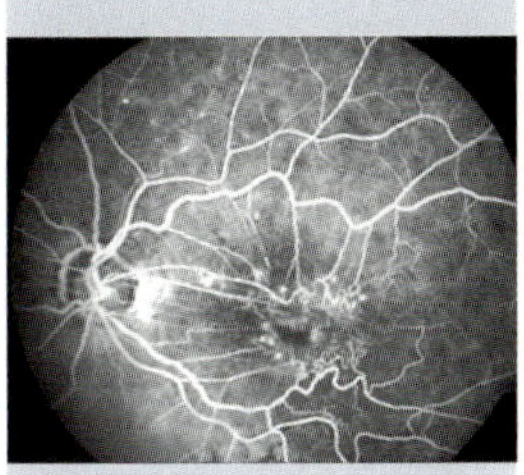

- The vascular tortuosity caused by the epiretinal membranes is very well seen on the fluorescein angiogram.
- The fovea may be displaced and the perifoveal capillary network distorted.
- Varying degree of leakage from the retinal capillaries can be seen in the area of traction.
- Late cystoid changes may be evident.
- In cases of epiretinal membranes secondary to vascular occlusion, the diagnosis is quite evident on the angiogram due to the presence of areas of capillary nonperfusion, microaneurysms or collateral vessels.

CASE 1

A 42-year-old male presented with distortion of vision in the right eye for the past three months; visual acuity was 6/12; N8.

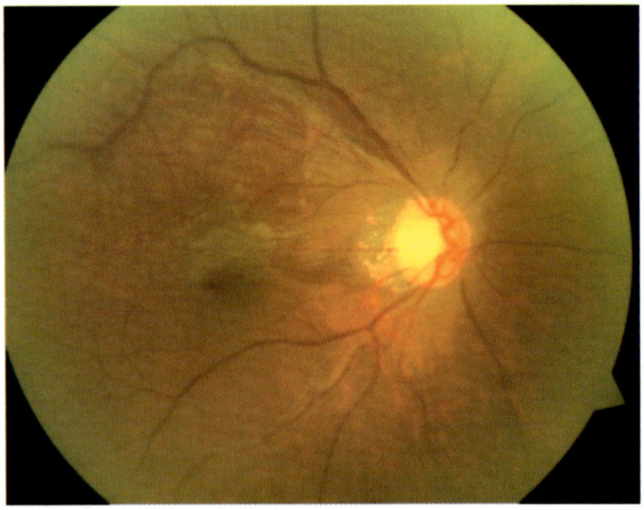

Fundus photograph of the right eye showing an idiopathic epiretinal membrane at the macula

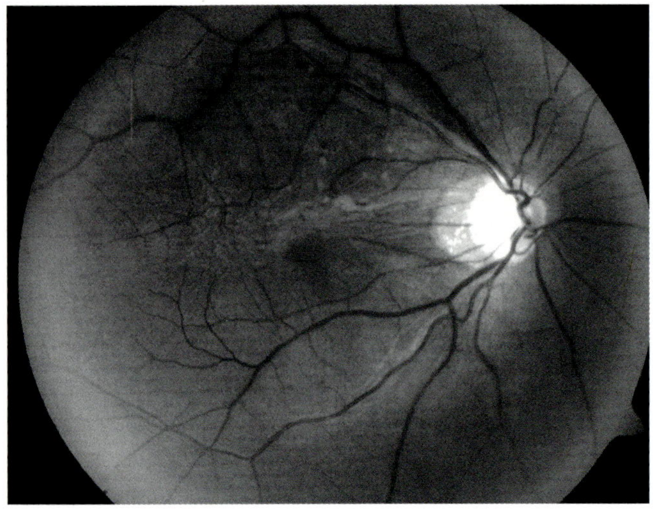

Red free photograph showing the distortion of the macular blood vessels caused by the epiretinal membrane

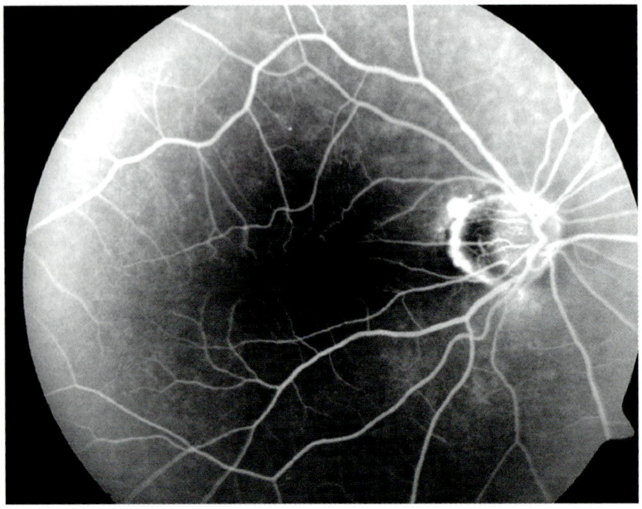

The macular retinal vessels appear distorted in the arteriovenous phase of the angiogram

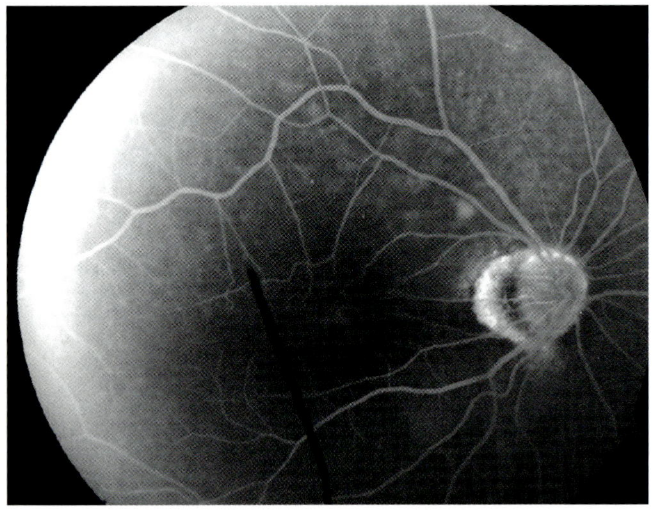

Late phase of the angiogram showing accumulation of the dye at the fovea

COMMENT

Distortion of the macular vessels and late CME are common angiographic findings in cases of epiretinal membrane.

CASE 2

A 74-year-old female (known case of BRVO) presented with history of decreased vision in the left eye for the past one year; visual acuity was 1/60.

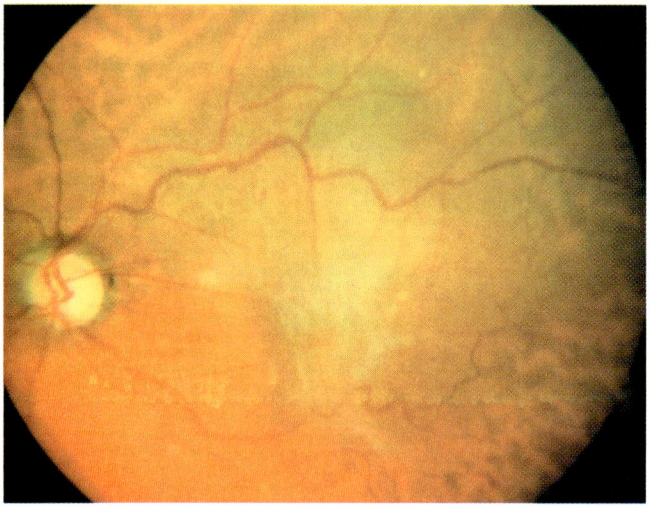

Fundus photograph of the left eye showing a thick epiretinal membrane at the macula

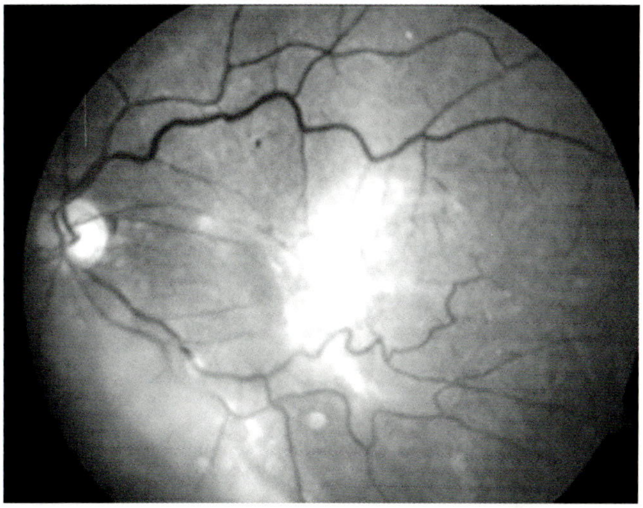

The red free photograph shows the distortion of the vessels at the macula

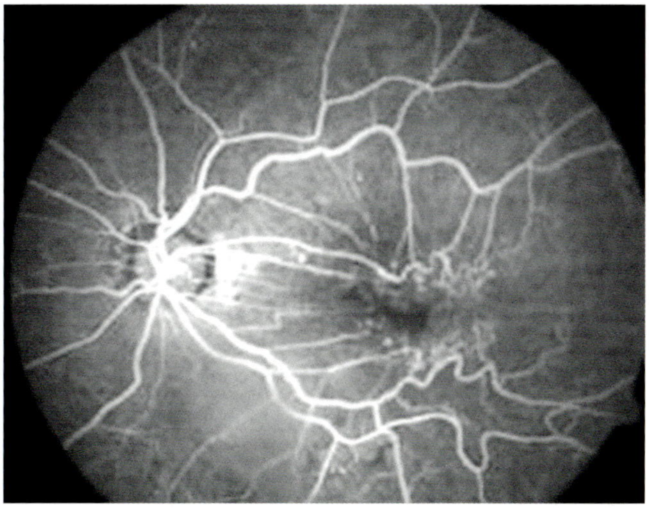

Marked distortion of the retinal vessels is seen. Few hyperfluorescent dots caused by microaneurysms are seen. Areas of capillary nonperfusion are noted in the superior part of the macula

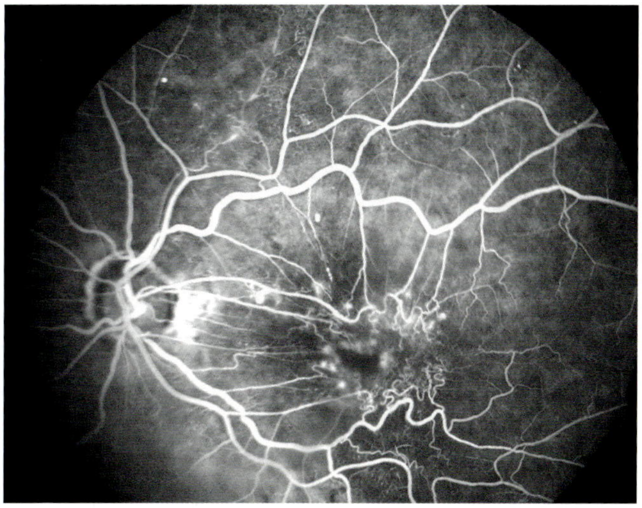

Leakage of dye from the microaneurysms and the tortuous retinal vessels at the fovea are seen

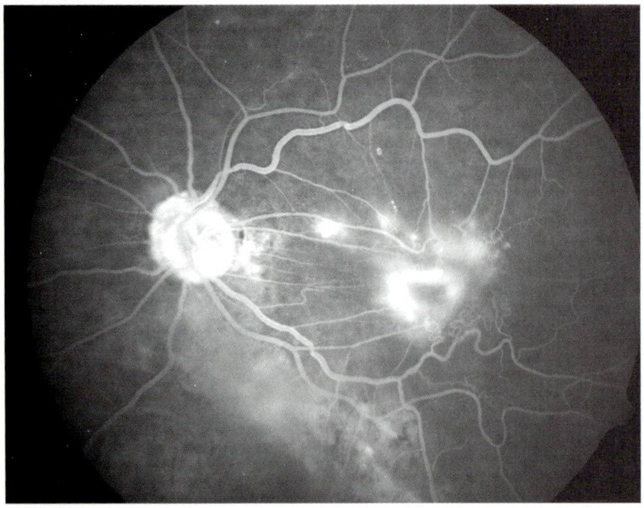

Increased leakage of the dye is seen in the late phase

COMMENT

Fluorescein angiogram is useful to detect underlying vein occlusion in patients presenting with an epiretinal membrane. Microaneurysms and capillary nonperfusion are caused by the vein occlusion.

CLINICAL NUGGETS

1. Use of red free illumination during slit-lamp biomicroscopy facilitates easy recognition of the epiretinal membranes.
2. Superficial retinal hemorrhages and cystoid macular edema can occur in patients with epiretinal membranes.
3. Vitrectomy with surgical removal of the membrane is the treatment of choice for those epiretinal membranes causing visual morbidity.
4. The reduction in visual acuity caused by epiretinal membrane is related to distortion produced in the outer retinal layers and does not depend on the size or degree of transluscency of the membrane.
5. OCT is very useful to image the epiretinal membrane.

BIBLIOGRAPHY

1. Gass JDM. Stereoscopic atlas of macular diagnosis and treatment Vol 2, 4th edition, 1997:938-50.
2. Wise GN. Preretinal macular fibrosis: An analysis of 90 cases. Trans Ophthalmol Soc UK 1972;92:131-40.

Chapter 9

Macular Hole

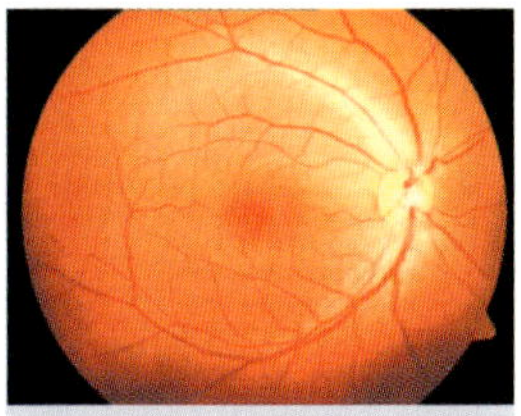

- Various causes of macular hole are idiopathic, trauma, accidental foveal burns with laser, long-standing cystoid macular edema and myopia.
- Idiopathic macular holes are classified as follows: Stages 1A and 1B—Impending macular hole. Stage 2—Small central or eccentric full thickness macular hole. Stage 3—Large full thickness macular hole with no posterior vitreous detachment. Stage 4—Large full thickness macular hole with posterior vitreous detachment.

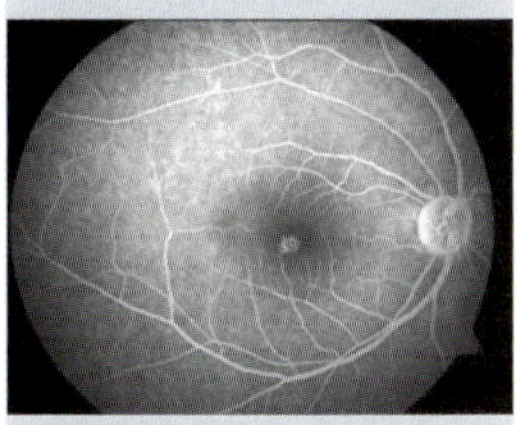

- Fundus fluorescein angiography (FFA) findings depend on the status of the RPE at the base of the macular hole.
- If the RPE is healthy and intact, no change in the normal fluorescence is seen on the angiogram.
- If RPE atrophy has occurred at the base, corresponding hyperfluorescence due to transmission defect is seen in the angiogram; this hyperfluorescence fades in the late films.
- Autofluorescence imaging demonstrates bright fluorescence of macular hole with appearance similar to that obtained by fluorescein angiography. In contrast, macular pseudoholes show no such autofluorescence. Following successful surgical closure, autofluorescence of macular hole is no longer visible. Hence, it is a noninvasive and rapid alternative to fluorescein angiography in the assessment and differential diagnosis of full thickness macular hole.

CASE 1

A 54-year-old female presented with reduced vision in the right eye for the past four months; visual acuity was 6/60; N36.

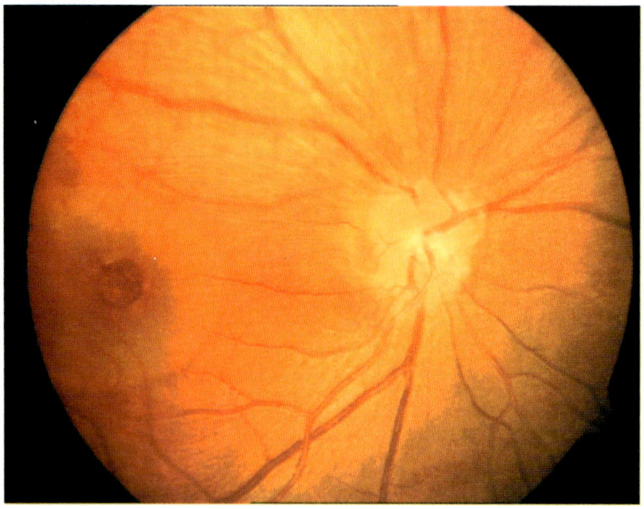

Fundus photograph of the right eye showing a full thickness macular hole at the fovea surrounded by a broad cuff of subretinal fluid

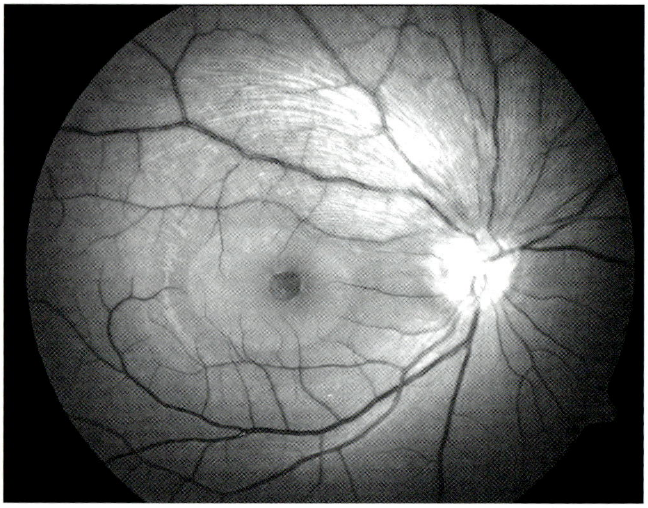

Red free photograph of the right eye

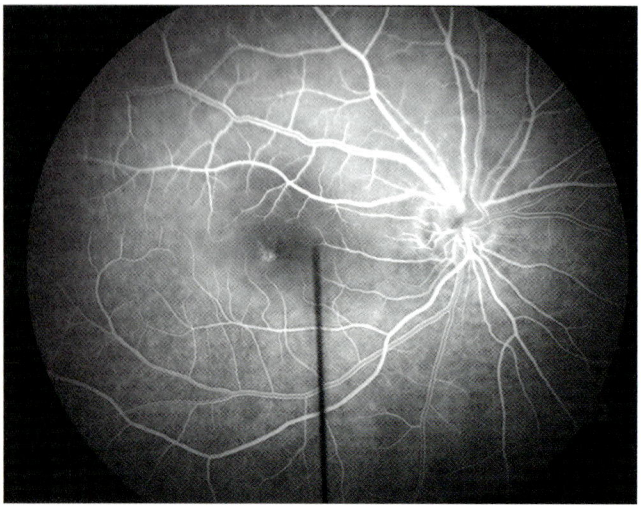

Early arteriovenous phase showing hyperfluorescence due to transmission defect at the base of the macular hole

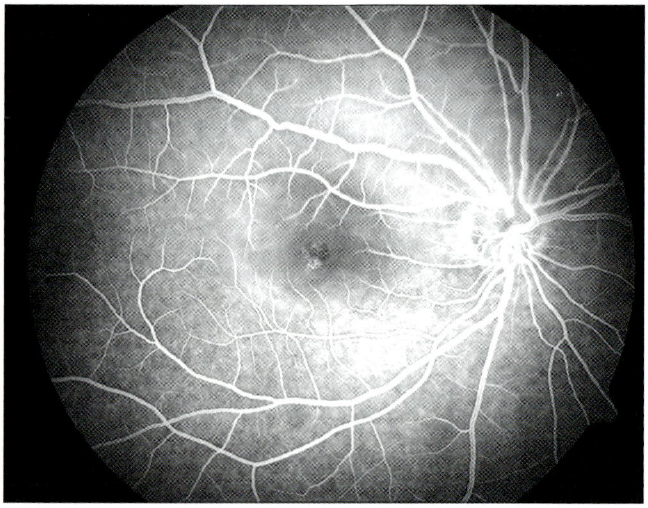

The hyperfluorescence at the macular hole has increased in the arteriovenous phase. The surrounding cuff of subretinal fluid shows a relative hypofluorescence

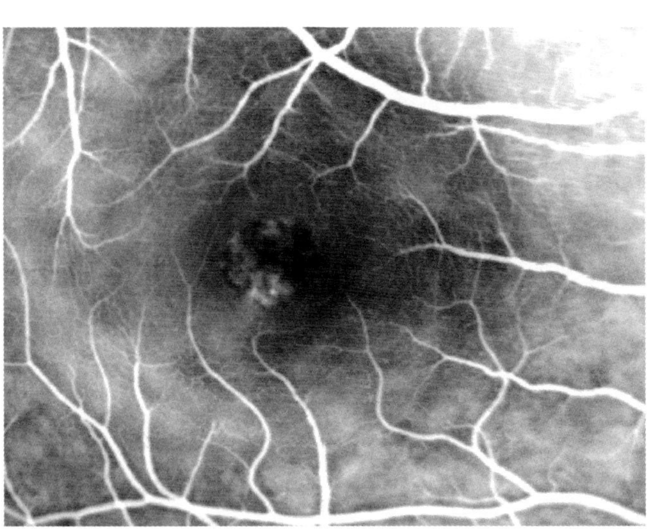

Magnified view of the macular hole showing the hyperfluorescence due to transmission defect at the base of the macular hole

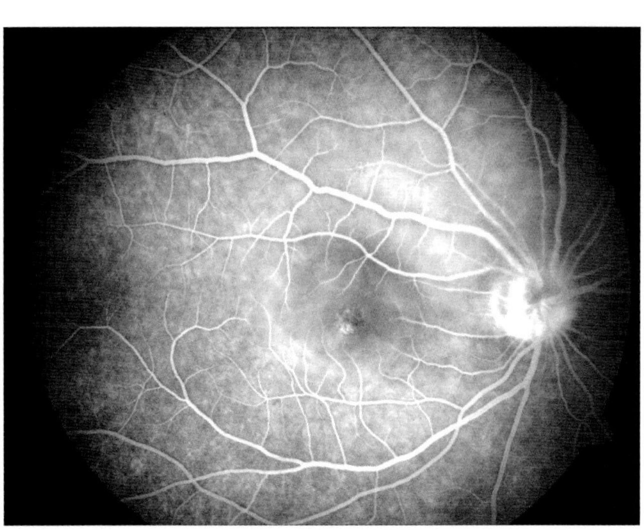

Fading of the hyperfluorescence is seen at the macular hole in the late film

CASE 2

A 36-year-old male presented with history of noticing drop in vision in the right eye following accidental exposure to the laser beam of a range finding device; visual acuity was 6/9; N6. A full thickness macular hole was noted with minimal RPE alteration at the base.

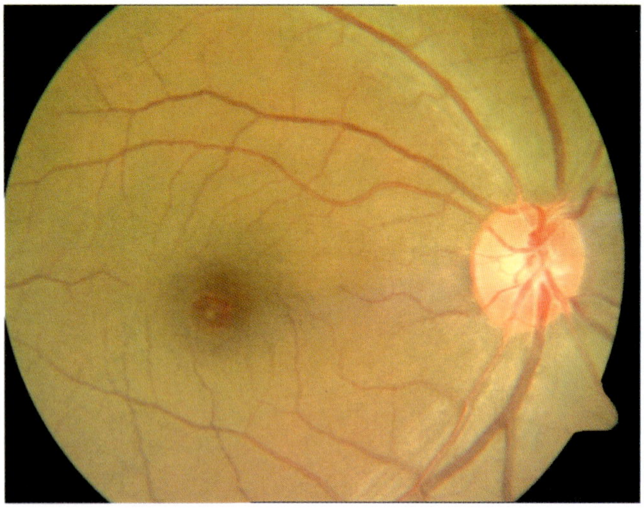

Fundus photograph of the right eye showing the full thickness macular hole

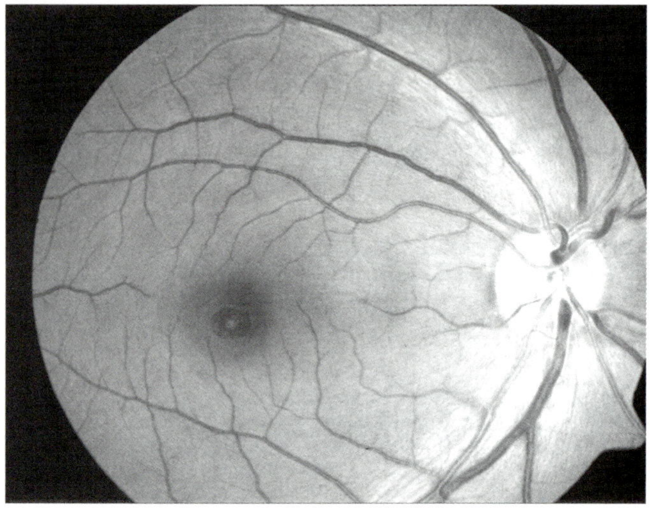

Red free photograph showing some RPE alterations at the base of the macular hole

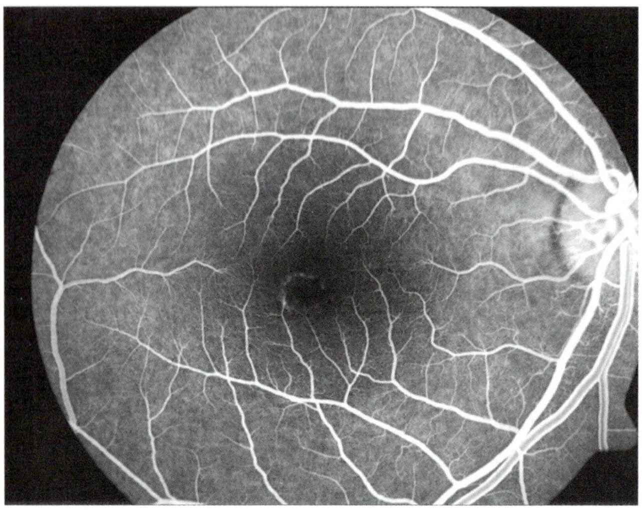

A faint rim of hyperfluorescence is seen at the edge of the macular hole in the early arteriovenous phase

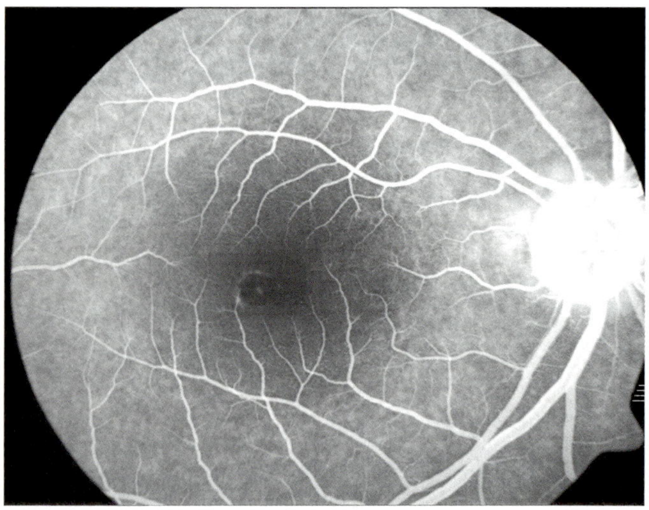

Arteriovenous phase showing increase in the hyperfluorescence at the rim. A faint hyperfluorescence is seen at the base of the macular hole

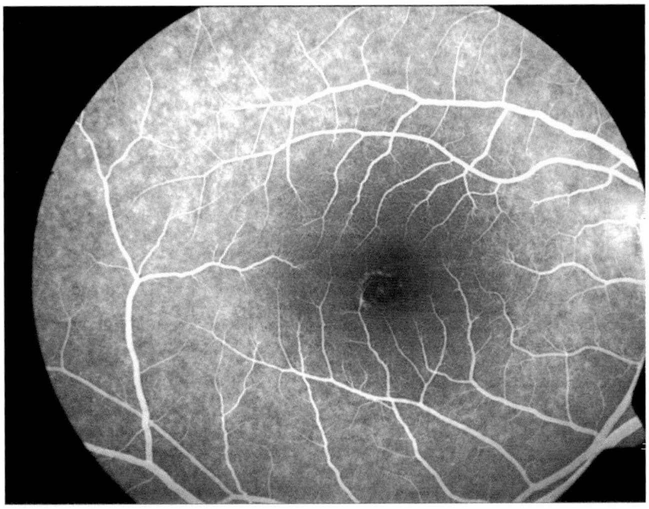

Some fading of the hyperfluorescence is seen in the later part of the angiogram

CASE 2 (*Continued*)

Two months later, the vision had dropped to 6/24; N36. Increased RPE alterations were seen at the base of the macular hole.

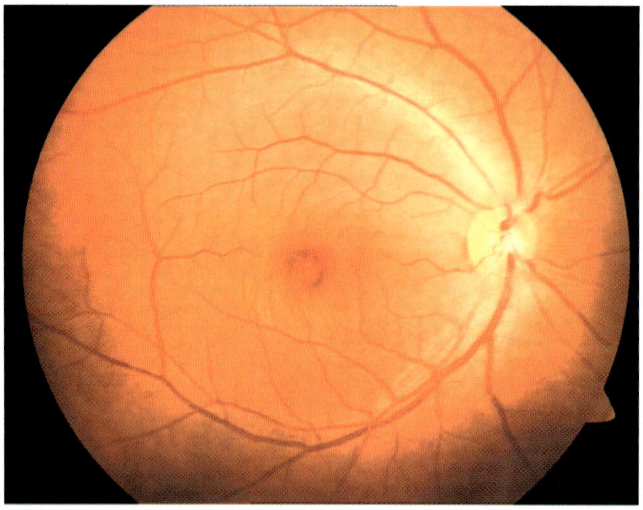

Fundus photograph of the right eye showing the full thickness macular hole with increased RPE alterations at the base

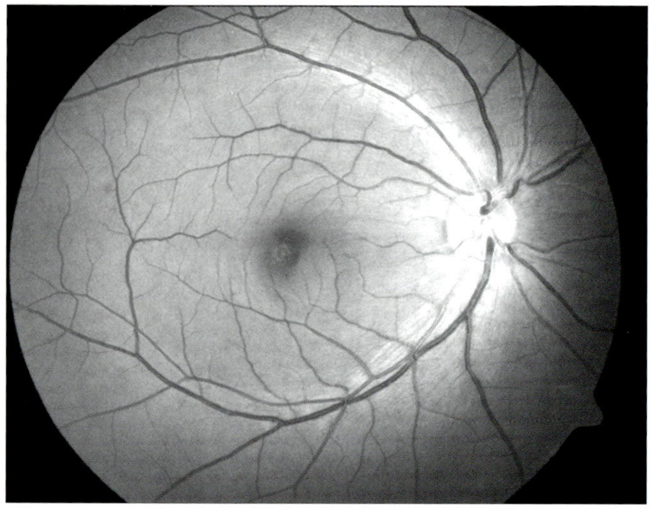

Red free photograph of the right eye

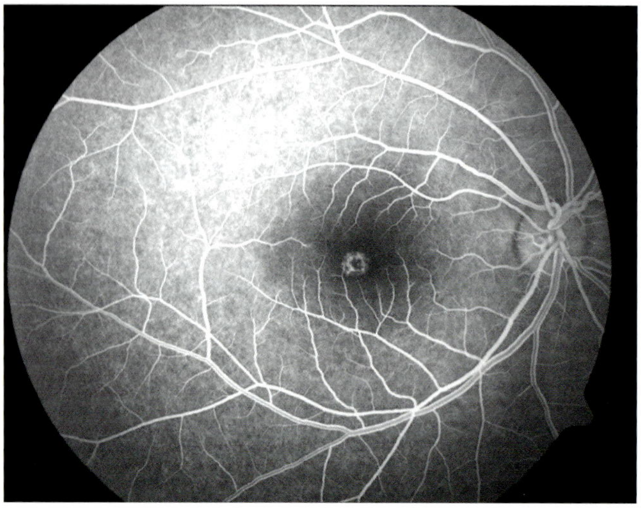

Hyperfluorescence due to transmission effect is seen at the base of the macular hole

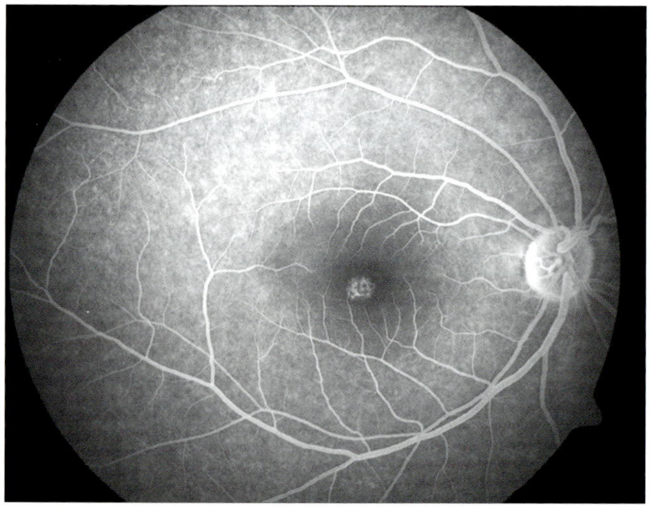

Fading of the transmitted hyperfluorescence is seen in the late phase of the angiogram

COMMENT

The RPE alteration at the base of the macular hole results in 'transmission effect' or 'window defect'.

CLINICAL NUGGETS

1. A positive Watzke Allen sign is seen in 95 percent of eyes with full thickness macular hole.
2. All patients will report a positive laser beam (50 microns) sign.
3. Stage 1 macular holes can regress spontaneously.
4. Vitrectomy with peeling of the internal limiting membrane with gas tamponade is useful in eyes with Stages 2 to 4 macular holes.

BIBLIOGRAPHY

1. Gass JDM. Idiopathic senile macular hole, it's early stages and pathogenesis: Arch Ophthalmol 1988;106: 629-39.
2. Gass JDM. Reappraisal of biomicroscopic classification of stages of development of macular hole: Am J Ophthalmol 1995;119:752-9.
3. Gass JDM. Stereoscopic Atlas of Macular Diseases; Diagnosis and Treatment: Page 922: 4th edition, St.Louis CV Mosby 1997.
4. Gass JDM, Joondeph BC. Observations concerning patients with suspected impending macular holes: Am J Ophthalmol 1990;109:638-46.
5. Von Ruckman A, Fitzke F, Gregor Z. Fundus autofluorescence in patients with macular holes imaged with laser scanning ophthalmoscope. Br J Ophthalmol:1998;82(4): 346-51.

Chapter 10

Myopia

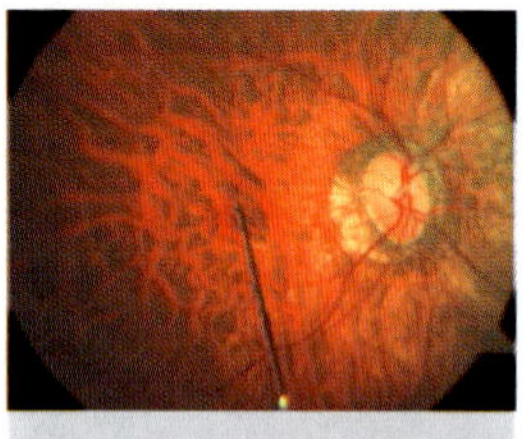

- Degenerative myopia is associated with increased axial length and progressive choroidal degeneration at the posterior pole.
- Tessellated fundus, tilted and oblique optic disc, temporal crescent or myopic conus, breaks in Bruch's membrane (lacquer cracks), atrophy of the RPE and choroid at the posterior pole, and posterior staphyloma are common changes in degenerative myopia.
- Choroidal neovascularization can occur.
- Pathogenesis is not clearly understood and could be due to heredodegenerative factors.

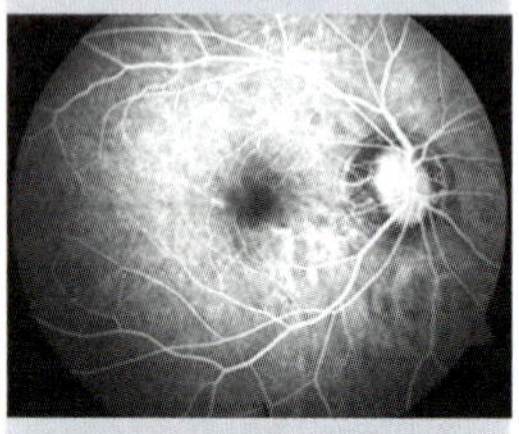

- Lacquer cracks show irregular hyperfluorescence in the early phase of the angiogram. This increases in the arteriovenous phase and fades to some extent in the late phase. They are linear or stellate and may be multiple.
- Large areas of atrophy at the posterior pole may be hypofluorescent in the early stages due to the atrophy of the choriocapillaries. The larger choroidal vessels may be seen through. Scleral staining may be seen in the late phase.

CASE 1

A 53-year-old female presented with history of reduced vision in both the eyes of six months duration. Visual acuity was 6/24; N6 in the right eye and 6/60; N6 in the left eye.

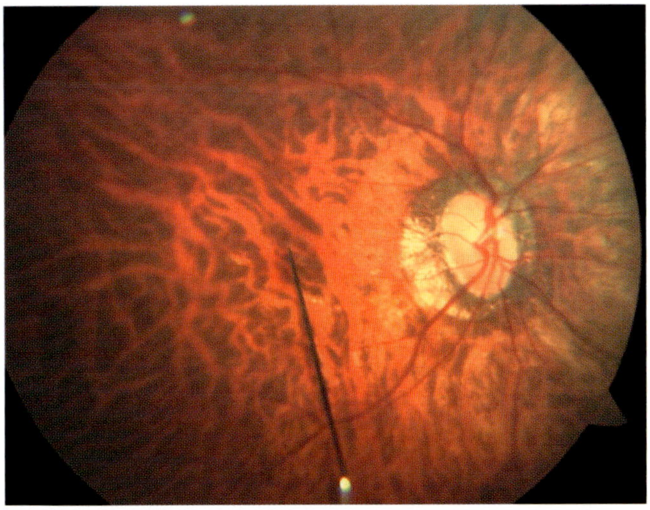

Fundus photograph of the right eye showing a lacquer crack inferior and temporal to the foveal center. Peripapillary atrophy is seen

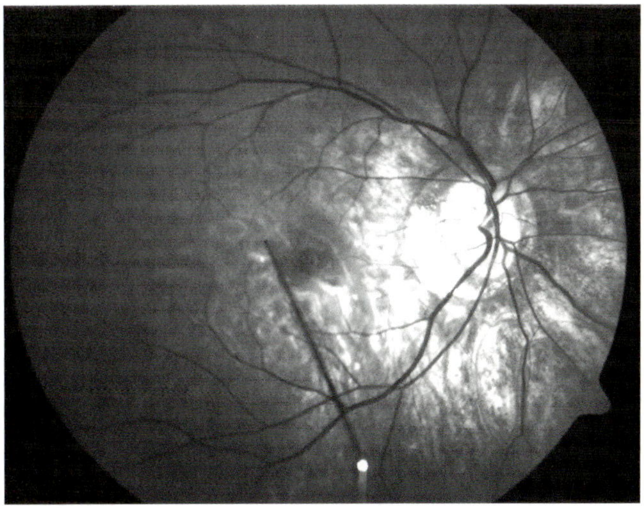

Red free photograph of the right eye

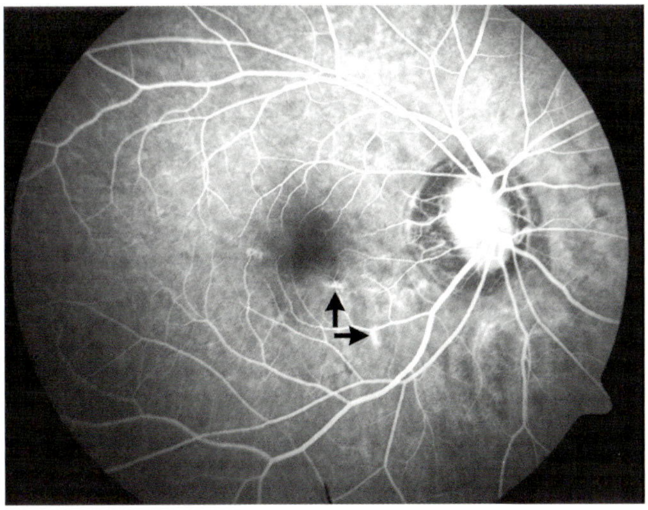

Arteriovenous phase shows hyperfluorescence due to transmission defect in the area of lacquer cracks (arrows)

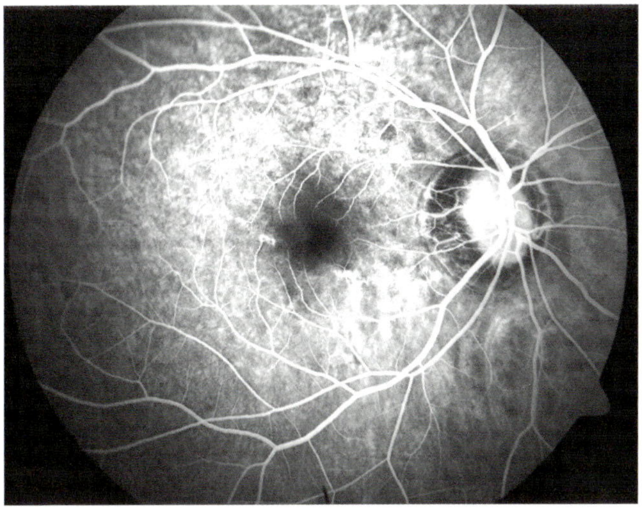

Increased hyperfluorescence is seen at these lesions in the late arteriovenous phase

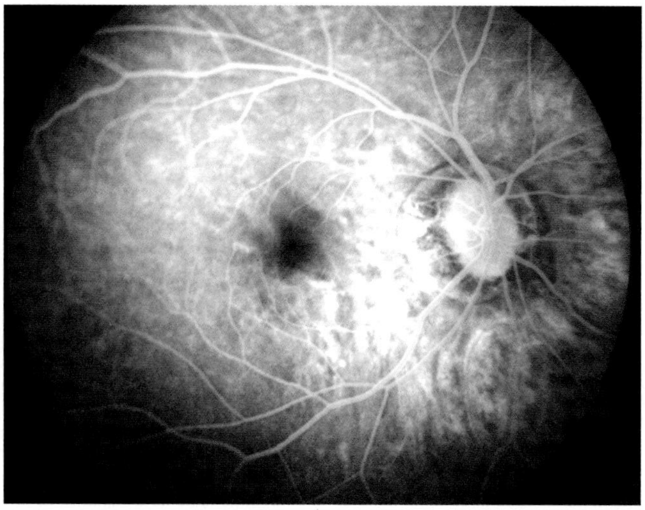

Late phase angiogram shows persistence of the hyperfluorescence at the lacquer cracks

CASE 1 (*Continued*)

Left Eye of the Patient

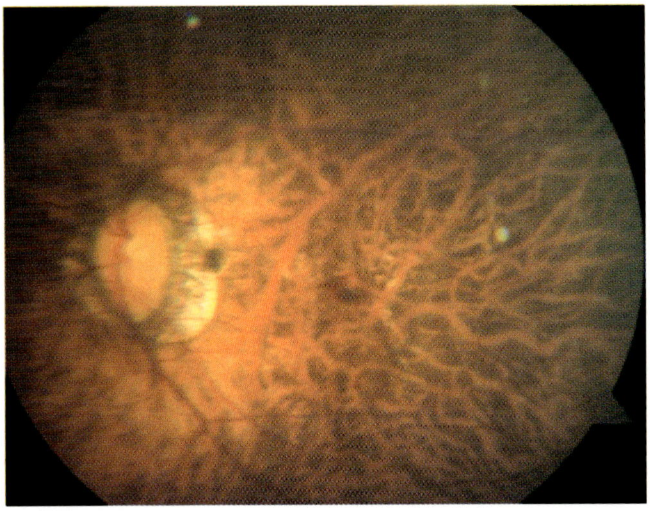

Fundus photograph of the left eye showing the lacquer cracks temporal to the foveal center

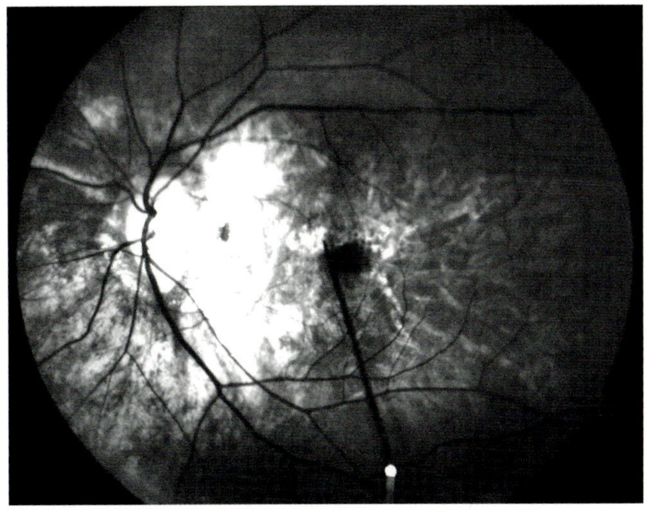

Red free photograph of the left eye

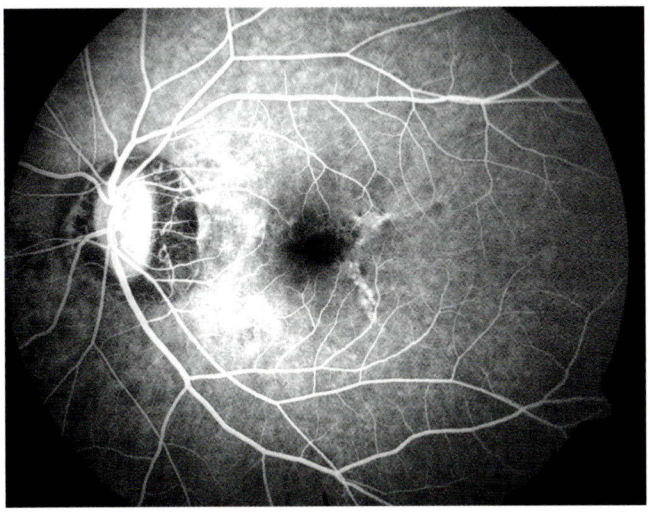

Arteriovenous phase showing hyperfluorescence at the lacquer cracks

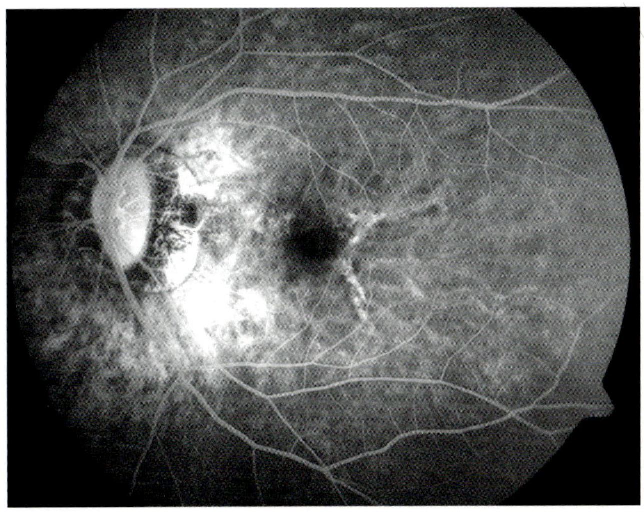

Late phase showing persistence of the hyperfluorescence at the lacquer cracks

COMMENT

Increased visibility of the choroidal fluorescence through the lacquer cracks makes them appear as hyperfluorescent lines.

CASE 2

A 12-year-old girl presented with decreased vision in left eye since a week. Her visual acuity was CF in the right eye (corneal opacity following penetrating trauma) and CF at 2 meters, N<36 in the left eye with –16 Diopter sphere.

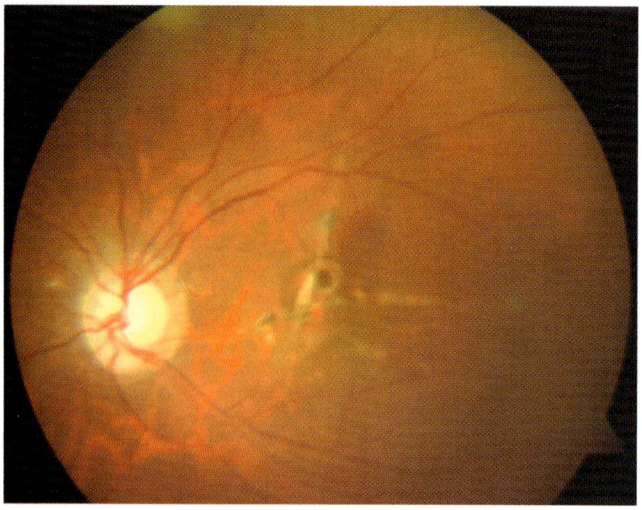

Fundus examination revealed cruciate lacquer cracks running through the fovea with fresh submacular hemorrhage

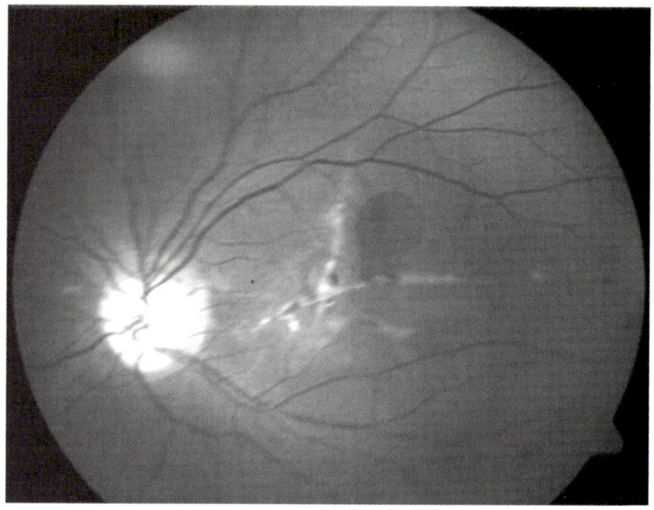

Red free image highlights the lacquer cracks and the dark submacular hemorrhage

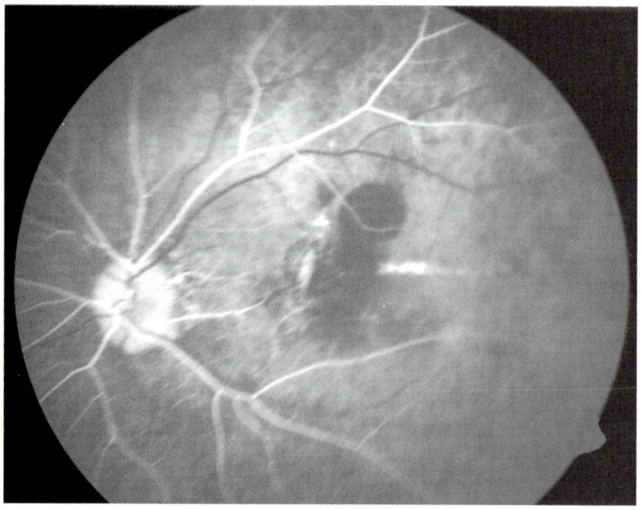

Arterial phase fluorescein angiogram reveals transmitted fluorescence through lacquer cracks and blocked fluorescence due to subretinal hemorrhage

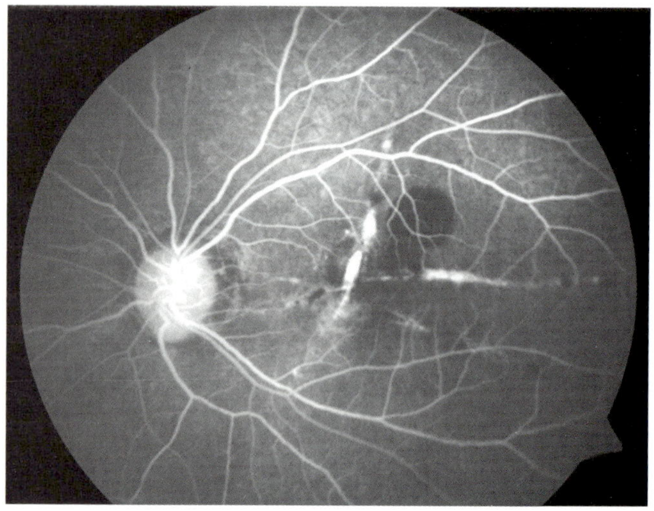

Late A-V phase shows increased hyperfluorescence through the lacquer cracks. The underlying CNV is masked by the subretinal hemorrhage and was picked up by OCT

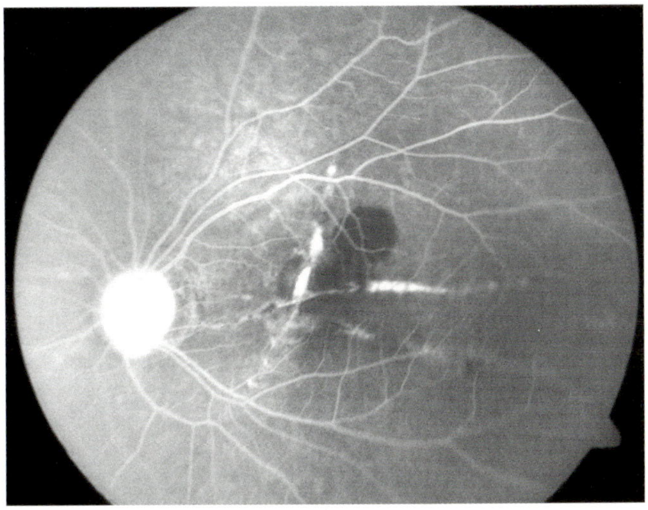

Late phase angiogram reveals staining in the area of lacquer cracks. Blocked fluorescence persists

The patient was treated with intravitreal anti-VEGF agent and followed up after four weeks.

Visit 2

One month post intravitreal anti-VEGF injection, BCVA improved to 6/60; N6 and fundus showed scarred CNVM.

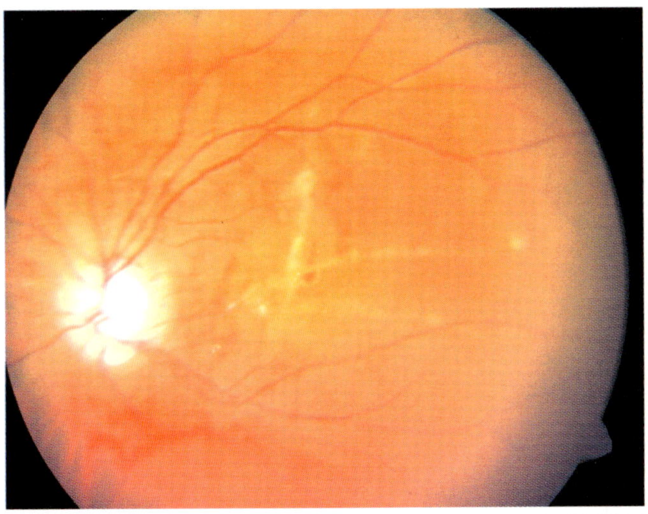

Color fundus photograph of the left eye reveals resolution of the subretinal hemorrhage. The lacquer cracks look more prominent. Yellowish-gray subfoveal lesion is regressed CNV. Clinical findings were confirmed on OCT

CLINICAL NUGGETS

1. Fuchs' spot, which are round or oval areas of subretinal hyperpigmentation, may be sequelae of previous subretinal hemorrhage or choroidal non-vascular membranes.
2. Progressive myopia is characterized by increased axial length with progressive choroidal degeneration in the posterior pole.
3. Spontaneous subretinal hemorrhage can occur at the fovea without any evidence of a neovascular membrane; these usually resolve spontaneously.

BIBLIOGRAPHY

1. Levy JH, Pollock HM, Curtin BJ. The Fuchs' Spot. An ophthalmoscopic and fluorescein angiographic study. Ann Ophthalmol 1977; 9:1433-43.
2. Ohno-Matsui K, Tokoro T. The progression of lacquer cracks in pathologic myopia. Retina 1996; 16(1): 29-37.
3. Quaranta M, Arnold J, Coscas G, Francis C, et al. Indocyanine green angiographic features of pathologic myopia. Am J Ophthalmol 1996; 122:663-71.
4. Spitznas M, Böker T. Idiopathic posterior subretinal neovascularisation (IPSN) is related to myopia. Graefes Arch Clin Exp Ophthalmol. 1991; 229: 536-8.

11 Chapter

Pigment Epithelial Detachment

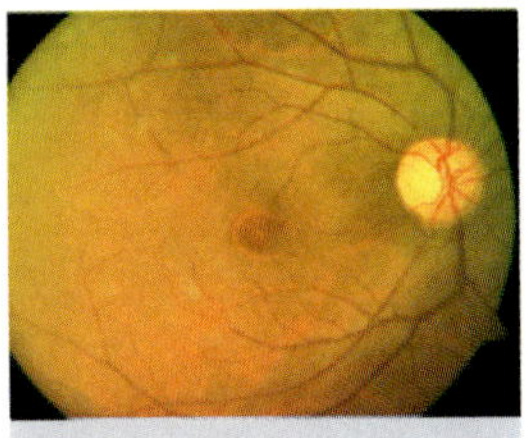

- Retinal pigment epithelial detachment (PED) can occur by itself or in association with central serous chorioretinopathy, age-related macular degeneration or with polypoidal choroidal vasculopathy.
- It can be serous or hemorrhagic depending on the fluid that accumulates under the detached retinal pigment epithelium (RPE).
- PED appears as a well-delineated, blister like round or oval area of RPE detachment, yellow or gray in color. A pink halo is usually seen around the PED
- Serous PEDs are usually around one-fourth disc diameter in size.
- Hemorrhagic PEDs are darker and usually larger in size.
- Long standing PEDs may show pigment migration along their walls.

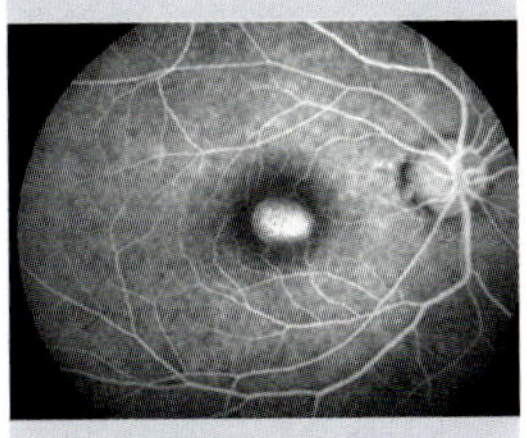

- Serous PED
  - Shows hyperfluorescence in the early phase of the angiogram. The entire extent of the PED is hyperfluorescent.
  - Increase in intensity of the fluorescence is seen as the angiogram progresses due to increased accumulation of the dye. The extent of the lesion remains the same.
  - Late stage shows pooling of the dye. The margins are still well-defined.
  - Irregular blocked fluorescence may be seen within the PED in long-standing cases. This is caused by pigment migration.
- PED associated with age-related macular degeneration
  - PED is slow filling.
  - Presence of an underlying CNVM is indicated by irregular filling of the PED, delayed filling of the PED or notching of the PED.

CASE 1

A 39-year-old male presented with history of decreased vision in the right eye of one year duration; visual acuity was 6/9; N12.

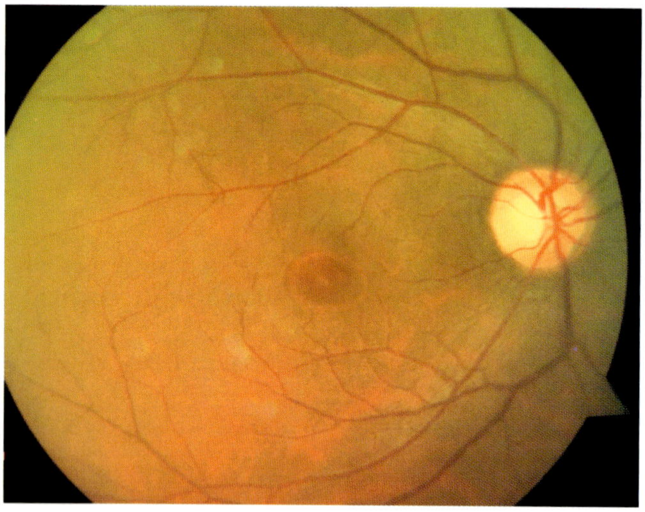

Fundus photograph of the right eye shows a PED at the fovea

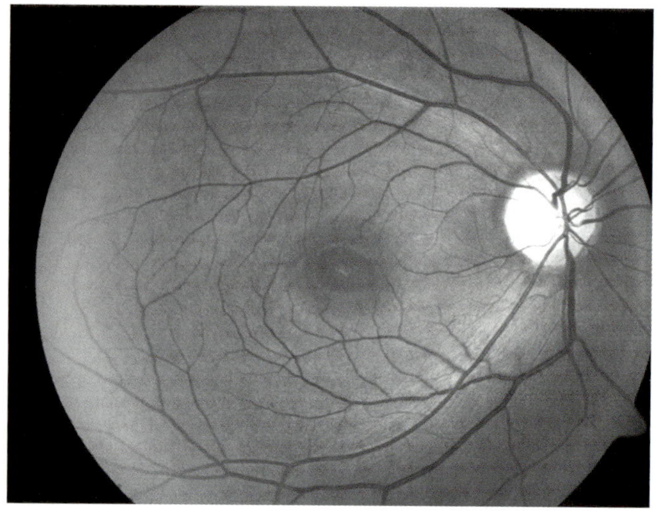

Red free photograph of the right eye

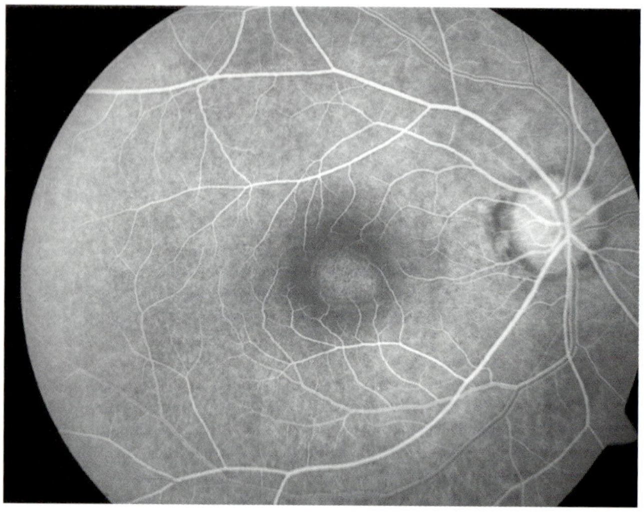

Early arteriovenous phase showing hyperfluorescence at the PED. The margins of the PED are well defined

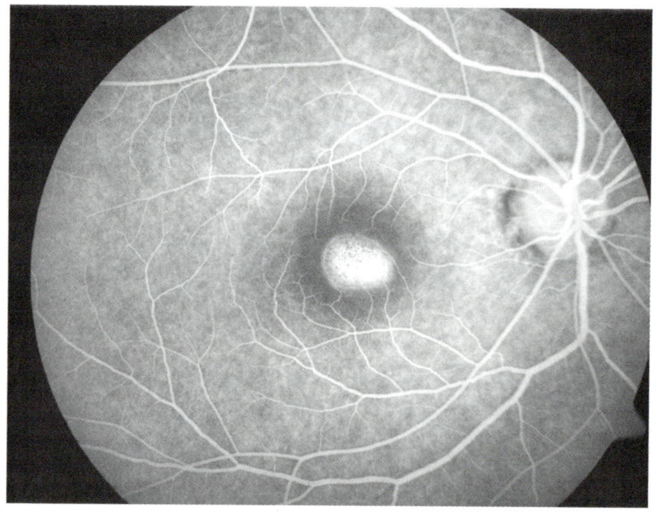

Increase in intensity of hyperfluorescence is seen in the arteriovenous phase. The extent of the lesion remains the same

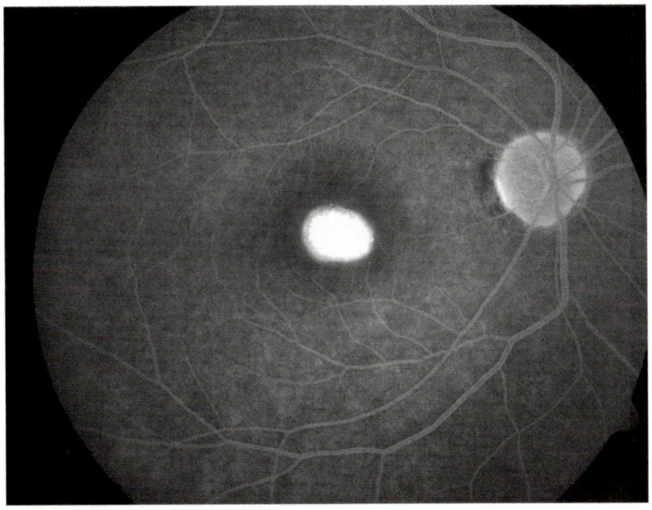

Marked increase in the intensity of the hyperfluorescence is seen within the PED. The margins of the PED remain well defined

COMMENT

PED shows early hyperfluorescence throughout its extent, which increases in intensity as the angiogram progresses. The boundaries of the PED remain well defined.

CASE 2

A 39-year-old male presented with distortion of vision in the right eye for the past one month; visual acuity was 6/6; N6.

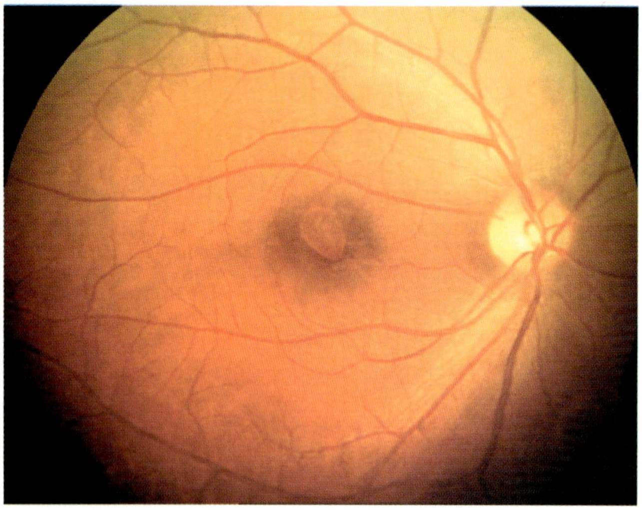

Fundus photograph of the right eye shows a PED at the fovea

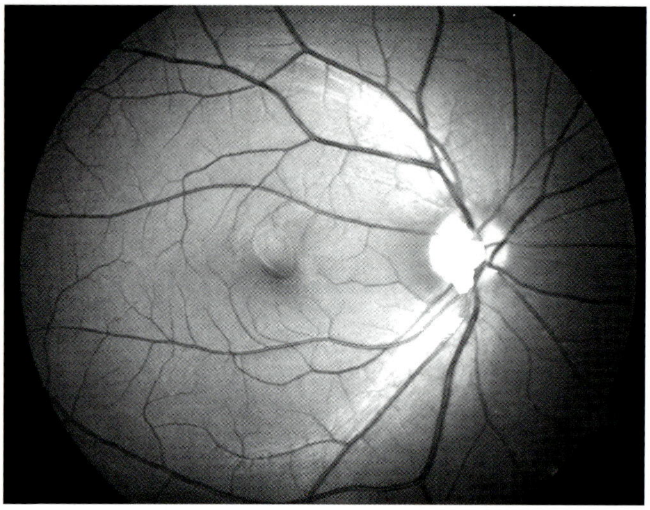

Red free photograph clearly shows the extent of the PED

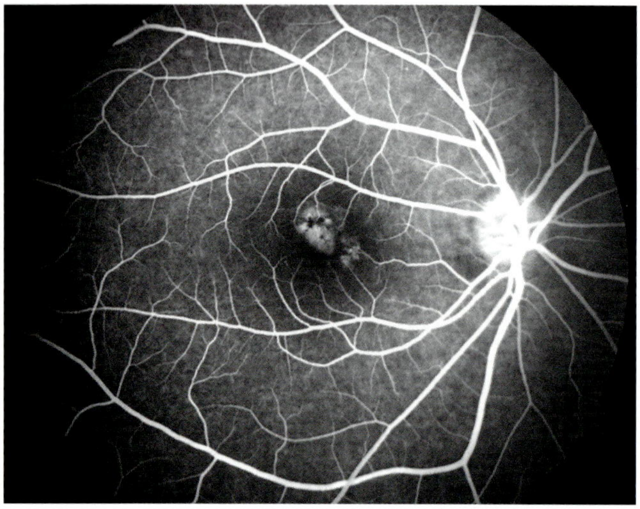

Arteriovenous phase showing hyperfluorescence within the PED. Few patches of blocked fluorescence within this are due to pigment migration along the walls of the PED. Few hyperfluorescent transmission defects are seen inferonasal to the PED

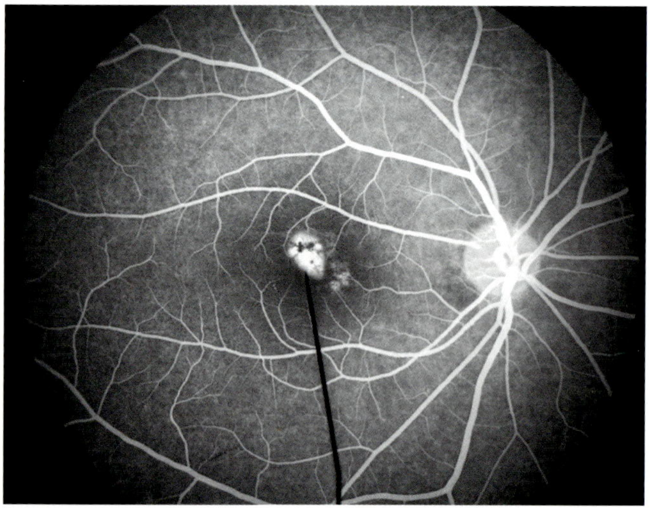

The hyperfluorescence within the PED has increased—consequently the areas of blocked fluorescence are better appreciated

Patient was seen again nine months later. Visual acuity was maintained at 6/6; N6

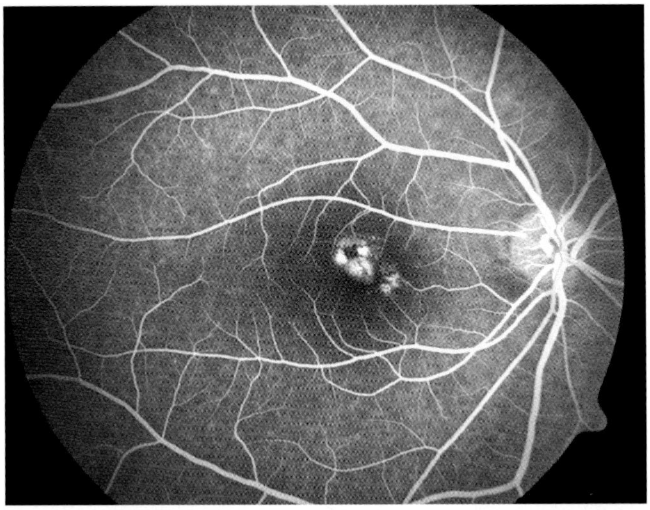

Arteriovenous phase of the same lesion shows a change in the pattern of blocked fluorescence within the PED

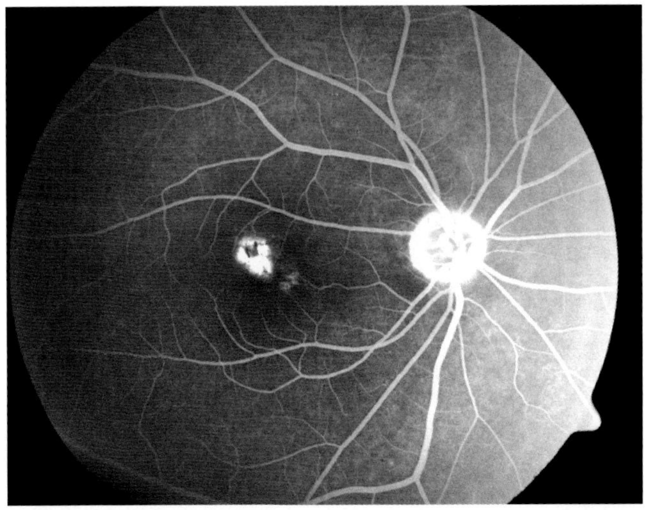

Late phase showing increased intensity of the hyperfluorescence in the PED. The hyperfluorescence inferonasal to the PED has faded indicative of a transmission defect

CASE 3

A 46-year-old male presented with difficulty in near vision in the right eye for the past six months; visual acuity was 6/6; N6.

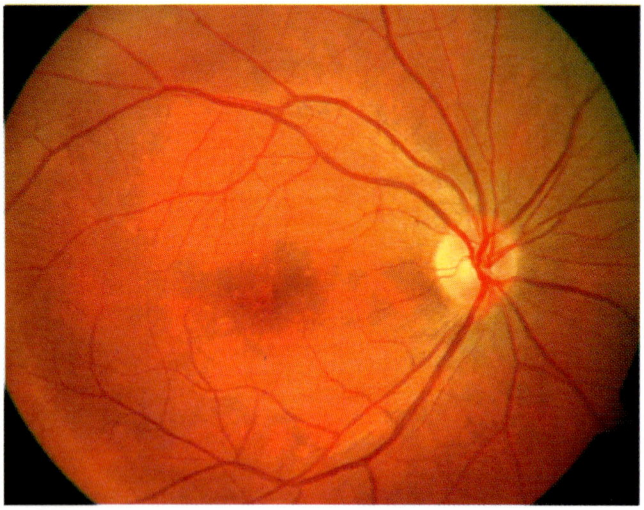

Fundus photograph of the right eye showing a pocket of subretinal fluid superior to the fovea. A few small PEDs are seen inferiorly. A very large PED is seen superotemporally, the lower edge of which is seen in this photograph

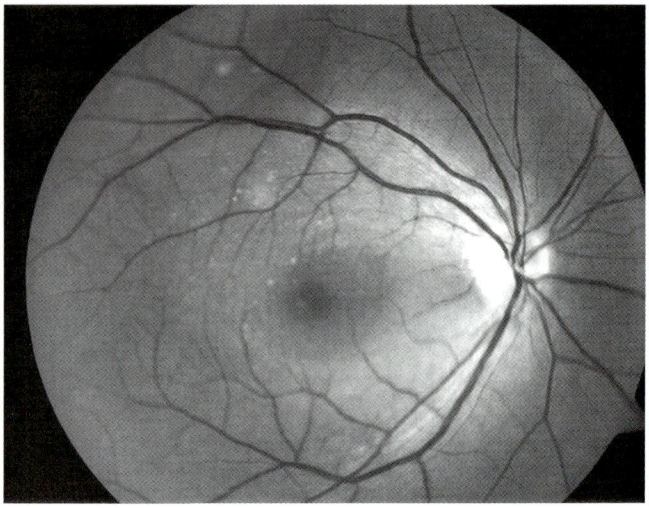

Red free photograph shows the lower edge of the PED in the superotemporal quadrant

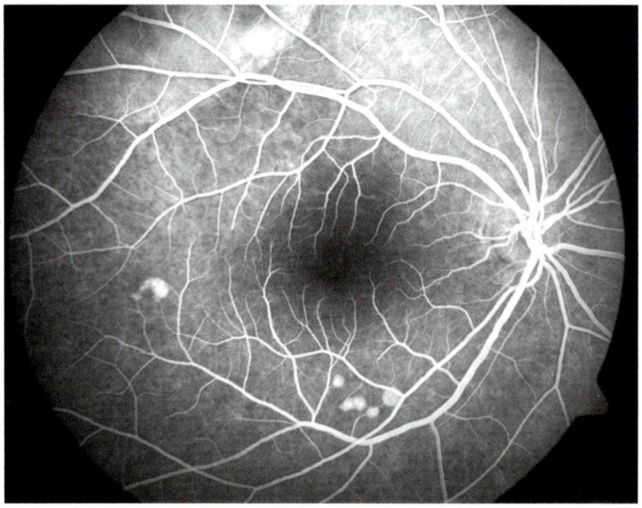

Arteriovenous phase shows filling of the small PEDs in the inferior and temporal part of the macula. Filling of dye is also seen in the lower part of the superotemporal PED

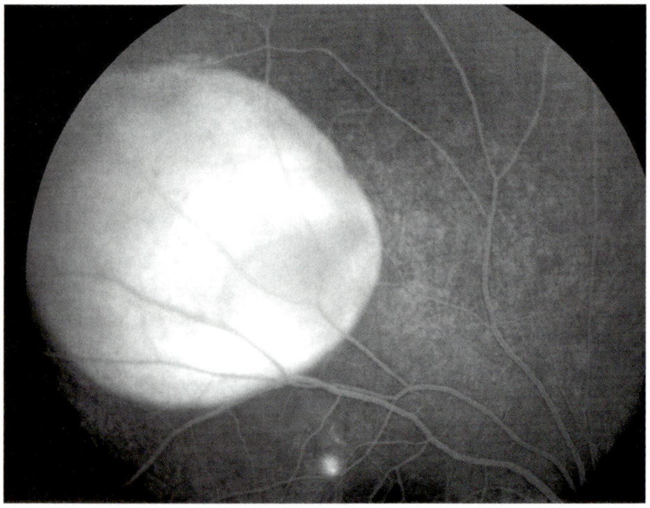

Filling of the large PED is seen. A point leak of dye is seen in the superior part of the macula

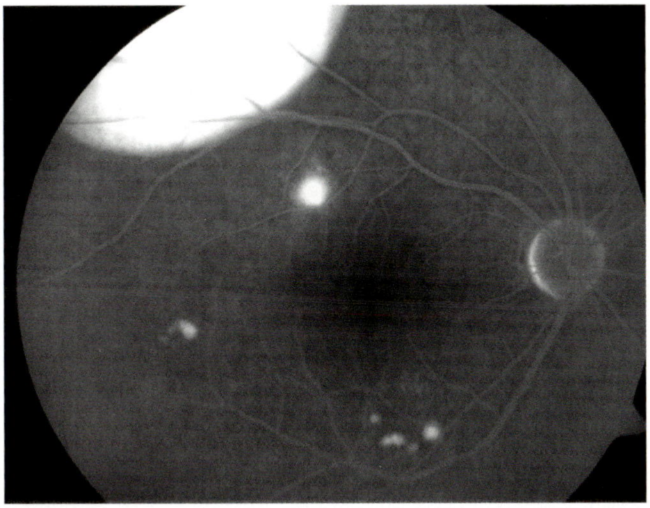

The intensity of hyperfluorescence in the large PED has increased in the late phase. An ink-blot type of central serous chorioretinopathy leak is seen in the superior part of the macula

COMMENT

Large, uniformly filling PEDs are usually found in central serous chorioretinopathy.

CASE 4

A 45-year-old male underwent an ocular examination for complaints of glare and floaters in both the eyes for the past 6 months. Patient was not on any medication and did not have any systemic problem. Visual acuity was 6/5; N6 in both eyes.

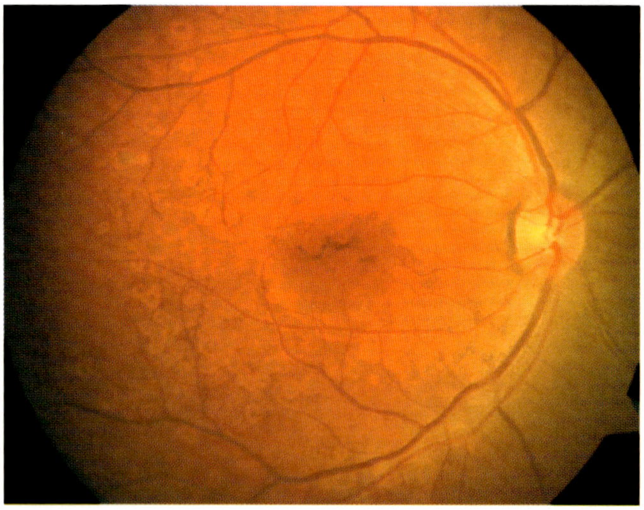

Fundus photograph of the right eye shows innumerable PEDs scattered throughout the posterior pole

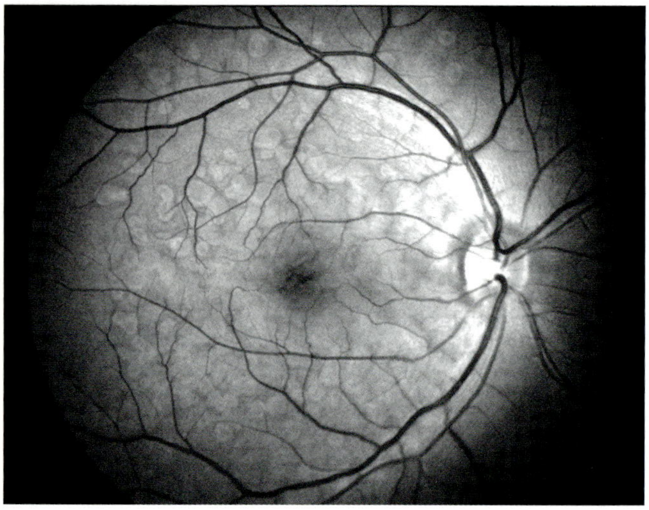

PEDs are well-seen in this red free photograph

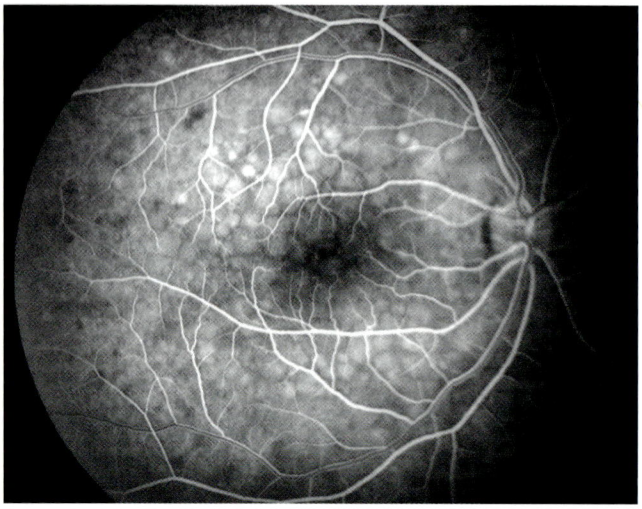

Early arteriovenous phase shows filling of the PEDs

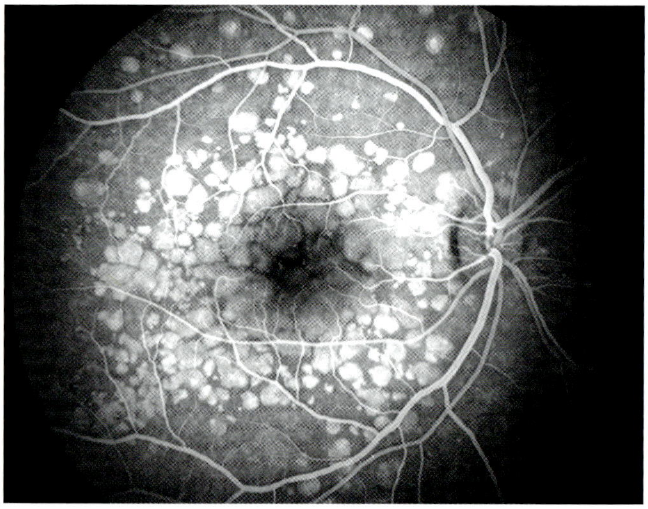

Arteriovenous phase shows increased intensity of the fluorescence within the PEDs

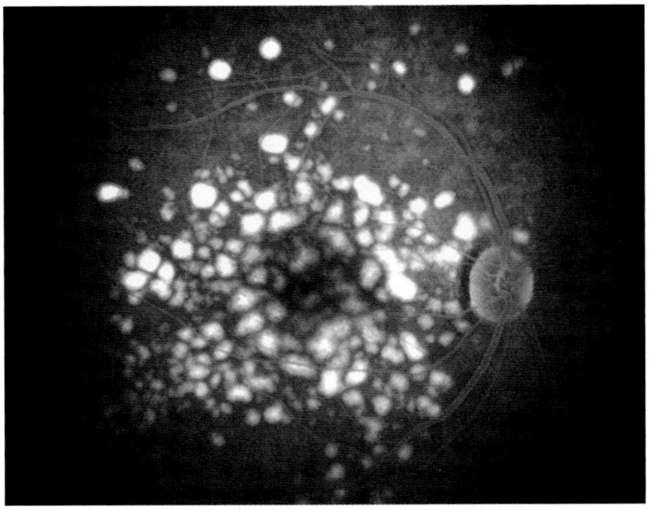

Further increase in the intensity of the dye is seen in the late phase. PEDs are seen even beyond the superior arcade

CASE 4 (*Continued*)

Left Eye of the Patient

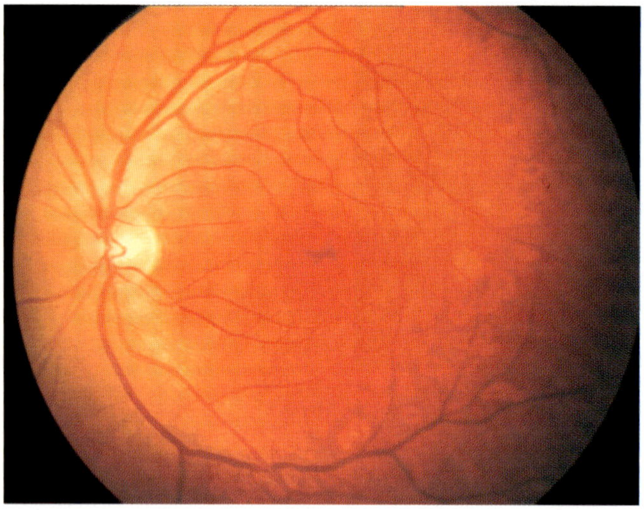

Fundus photograph of the left eye showing the scattered PEDs

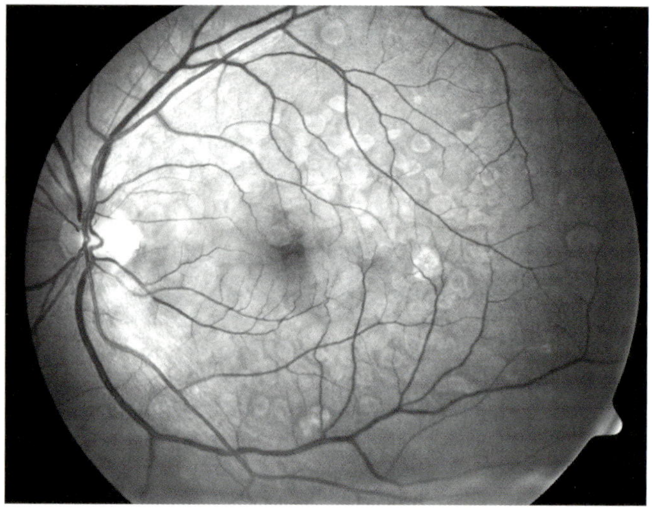

Red free photograph of the left eye

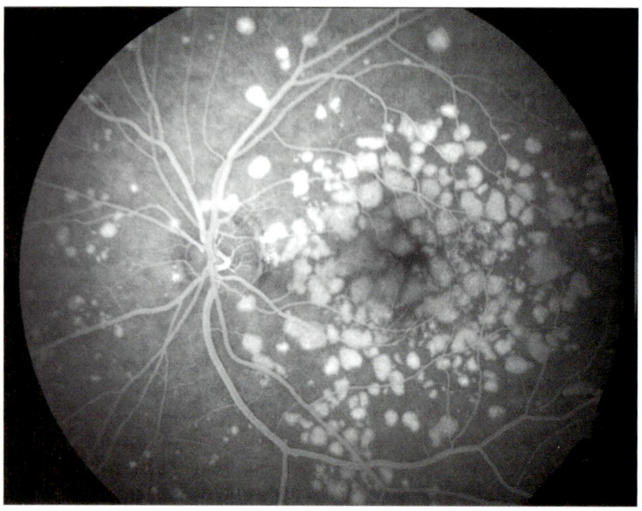

Arteriovenous phase showing dye filling the PEDs, some of which are seen nasal to the disc

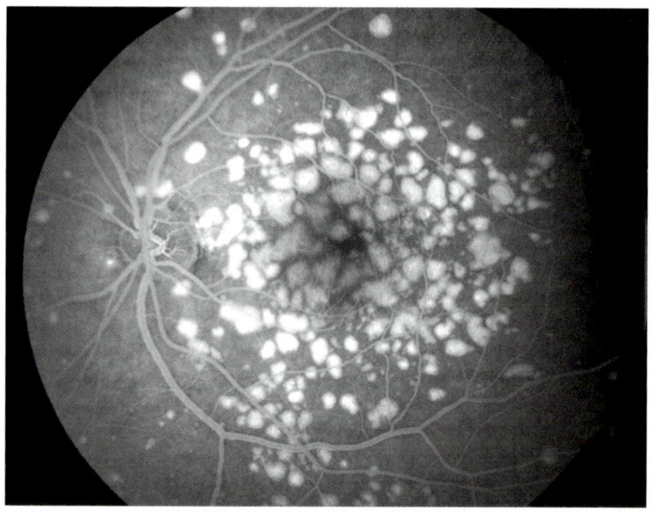

Late phase shows increased intensity of hyper-fluorescence within the PED. The PEDs at the fovea appear less intense than the rest due to masking of its fluorescence by xanthophyll and other macular pigments

COMMENT

This is an unusual case characterized by innumerable serous pigment epithelial detachments concentrated more at the posterior pole. No cause could be found.

CASE 5

A 56-year-old male presented with history of reduced vision in the left eye of three months duration; visual acuity was 6/18; N12.

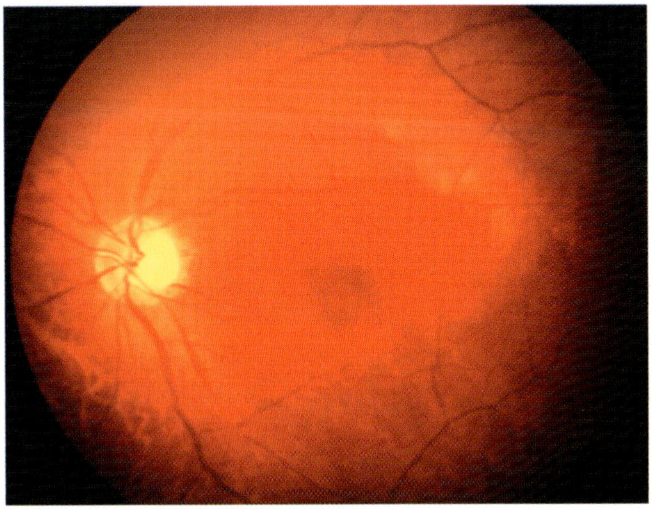

Fundus photograph of the left eye showing a large PED just superior to the fovea. Turbid fluid was noted within the PED

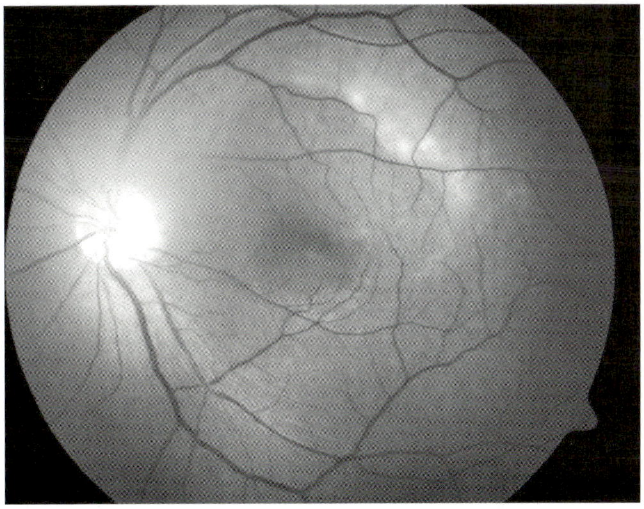

Red free photograph of the left eye highlighting the borders of the PED

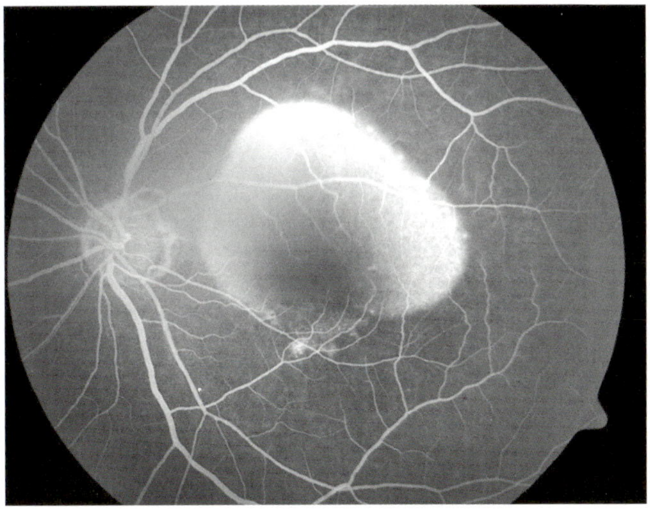

Arteriovenous phase showing filling of the PED. Stippled hyperfluorescence is seen adjacent to the inferior border of the PED. A hyperfluorescent point is seen along its superotemporal border

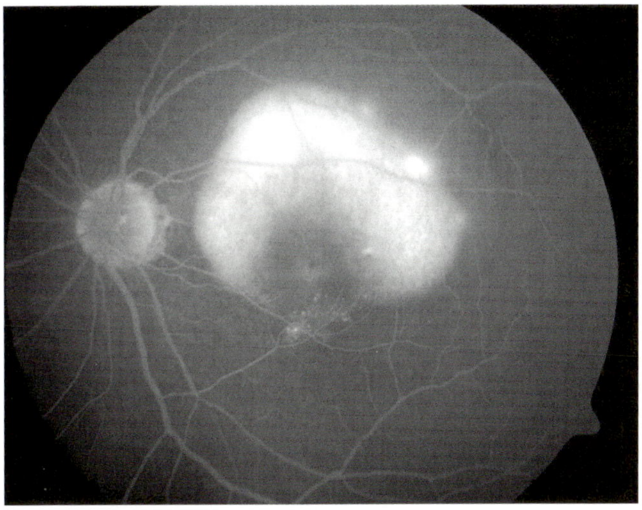

Late phase showing increased filling of the PED. Irregular hyperfluorescence is seen at the fovea. The leak along the superotemporal border has increased

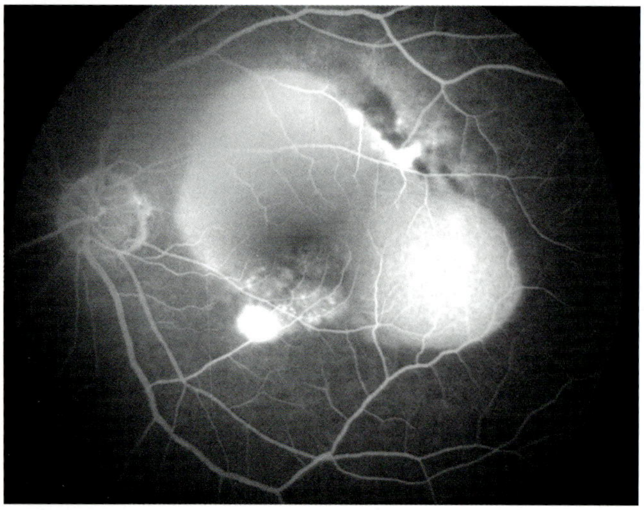

Arteriovenous phase shows a change in the shape and size of the PED two months later. The irregular hyperfluorescence at the fovea has increased causing a notch along the inferior border of the PED. Irregular hyperfluorescence is seen along the superior border

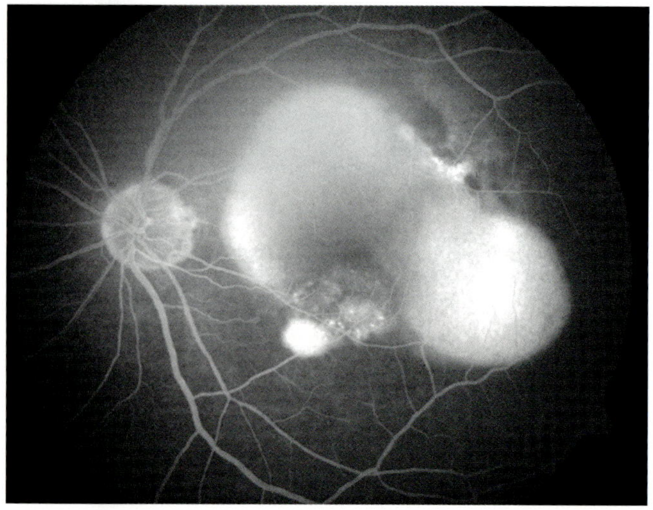

Late phase showing irregular filling of the PED. The stippled hyperfluorescence has increased and become fuzzy at the fovea

COMMENT

Irregularly filling PED and notching of the PED suggests the presence of an underlying neovascular membrane.

CLINICAL NUGGETS

1. Slow filling PEDs, notched PEDs and PEDs with turbid fluid are highly suspicious of an underlying neovascular membrane.
2. Laser photocoagulation at the edge of a PED carries a high-risk of developing a RPE tear.

BIBLIOGRAPHY

1. Bennett SR, Folk JC, Blodi CF, Klugman M. Factors prognostic of visual outcome in patients with subretinal haemorrhage. Am J Ophthalmol 1990;109:33-7.
2. Coscas G, Koenig F, Soubrane G. The pre tear characteristics of pigment epithelial detachments; a study of 40 eyes. Arch Ophthalmol 1990;108:1687-93.
3. Gass JDM. Serous retinal pigment epithelium detachment with a notch; a sign of occult choroidal neovascularisation. Retina 1984;4:205-20.
4. Gass JDM. Stereoscopic atlas of macular diseases (4th edn). Diagnosis and Treatment. Mosby 1997;2:24-6.
5. Nasrallah F, Jalkh AE, Trempe CL, et al. Subretinal haemorrhage in atrophic ARMD. Am J Ophthalmol 1989;107:38-41.

12 Chapter

Age-related Macular Degeneration—Dry Type

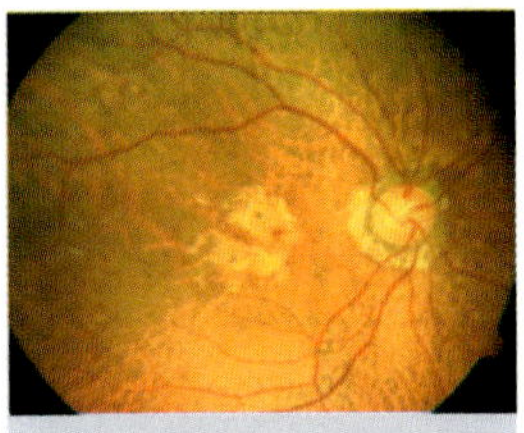

- Dry, atrophic or non-neovascular ARMD is characterized by the presence of drusen, focal hyperpigmentation, RPE degeneration and geographic atrophy of retinal pigment epithelium.

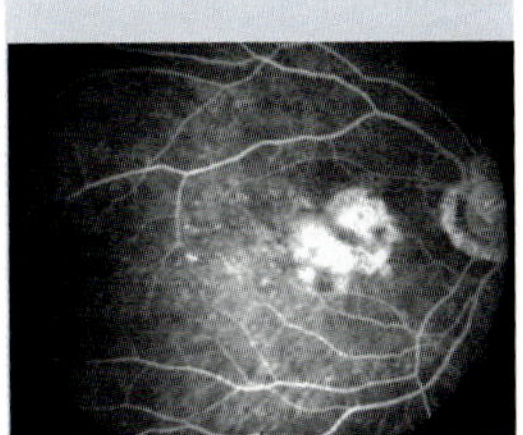

- The angiographic features depend on the type of lesion that is present.
- ***Drusen***
  Hard drusen: These generally show up as window defects in the region of the drusen in the early phases due to atrophy of the overlying retinal pigment epithelium. The fluorescence fades in the late phase of the angiogram.
  Soft drusen: The fluorescein angiographic pattern in soft drusen varies depending on their content. In general, they hyperfluoresce later and either fade or stain in the late phase of angiogram.
- ***Focal hyperpigmentation***
  These areas of focal pigment block the background choroidal fluorescence.
- ***Nongeographic atrophy/RPE degeneration/Incipient atrophy***
  Diffuse stippled hyperfluorescence is noted in the region of pigment mottling at the posterior pole. A pattern of reticular or punctate blockage is seen corresponding to areas of pigment clumps.
- ***Geographic atrophy of the RPE***
  Early hyperfluorescence is noted within the areas of geographic atrophy due to the window defect in the RPE. The choriocapillaris fill slowly within the lesion. However, the choriocapillaris may be entirely absent and filling of the larger choroidal vessels may be easily visualized. The extent of the lesion does not change in the late phases. In the late phase angiogram, hyperfluorescence due to staining of the choroidal tissue and the sclera is seen in the region of the geographic atrophy.

CASE 1

A 58-year-old male presented with history of decreased vision in both eyes over the last one year. Visual acuity was 6/9 in both eyes.

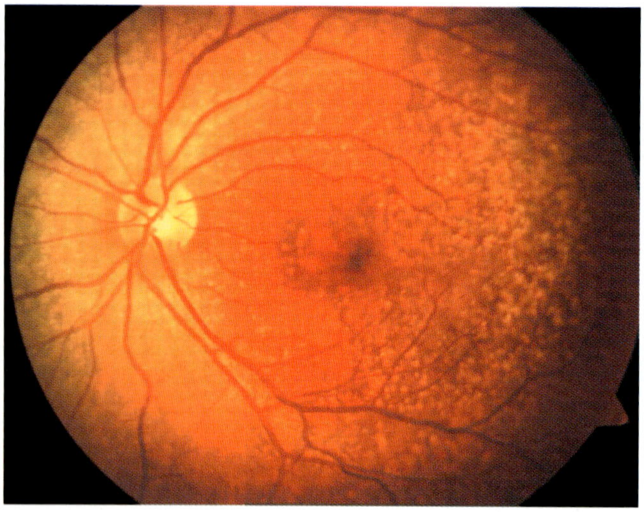

Fundus photograph of the left eye showing innumerable discrete hard drusen scattered throughout the macula and posterior pole

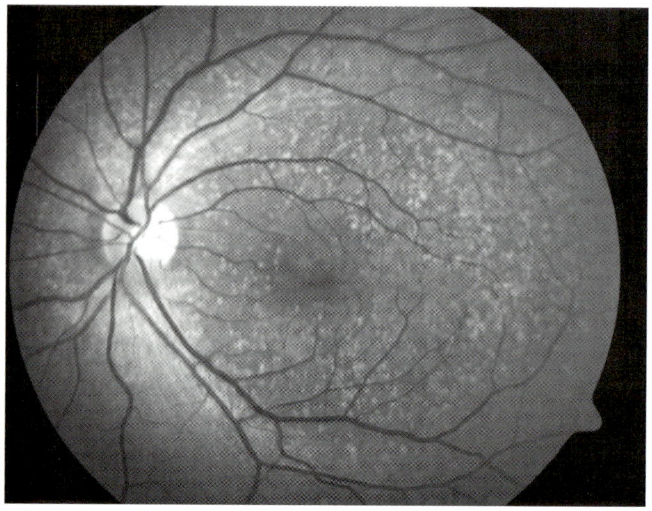

Red free photograph of the left eye showing the drusen

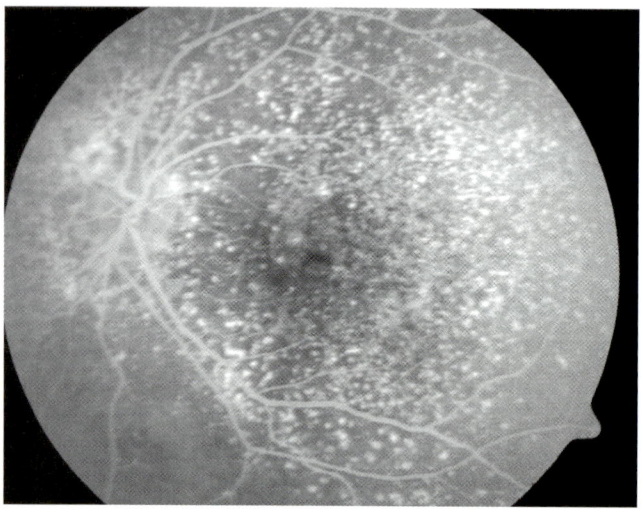

Early discrete, well defined dots of hyperfluorescence corresponding to the drusen are seen in the arteriovenous phase

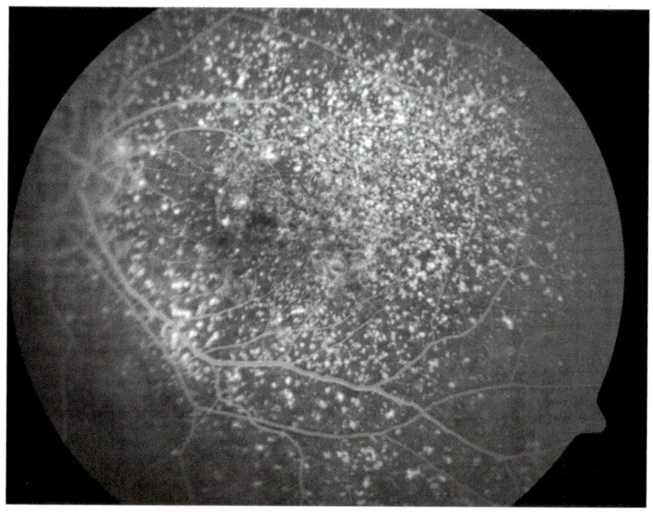

Increased hyperfluorescence is seen over the drusen, in the mid arteriovenous phase

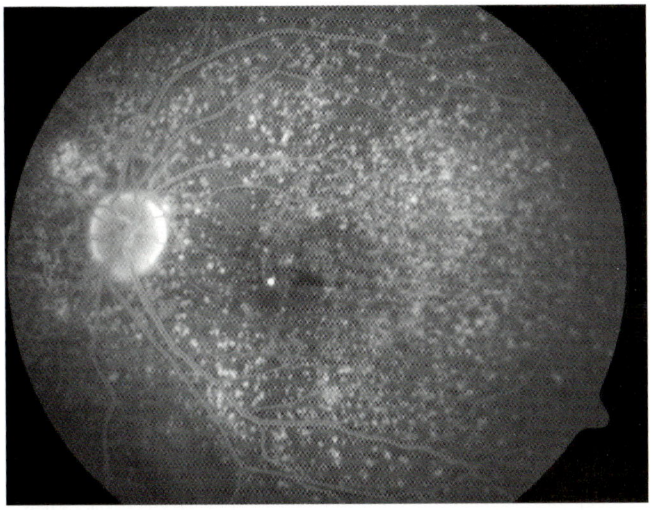

Fading of the hyperfluorescence is seen in the late phase

COMMENT

Hard drusen show early hyperfluorescence which increases in the mid arteriovenous phase and fades in the late phase of the angiogram.

CASE 2

A 68-year-old male presented with history of mild blurring of vision in the left eye for the last ten days. He gave history of reduced vision in the right eye for the last two years. Visual acuity was 1/60 in the right eye and 6/9; N6 in the left eye. Examination revealed a disciform scar in the right eye and soft drusen in the left eye.

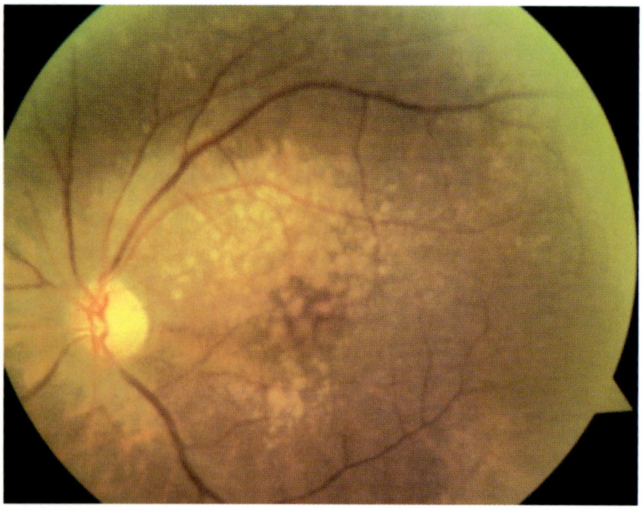

Fundus photograph of the left eye showing multiple large soft drusen in the macula

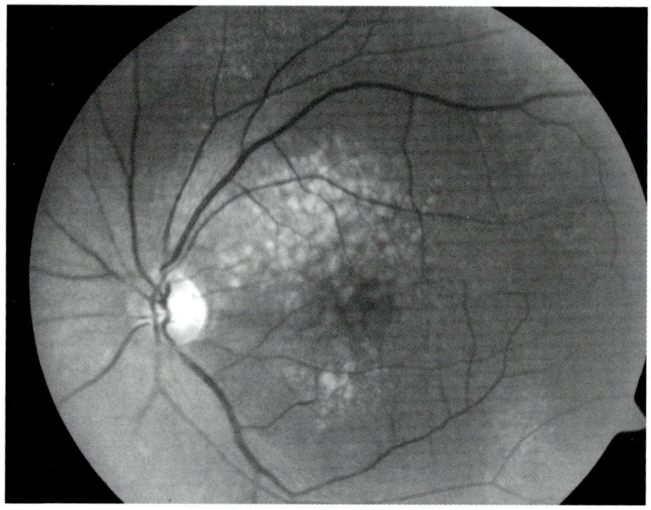

Red free photograph of the left eye delineating the soft drusen

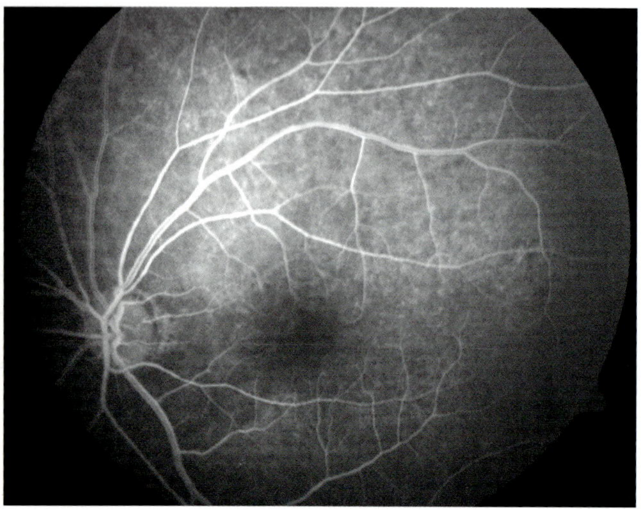

Early arteriovenous phase does not show any hyperfluorescence corresponding to the drusen

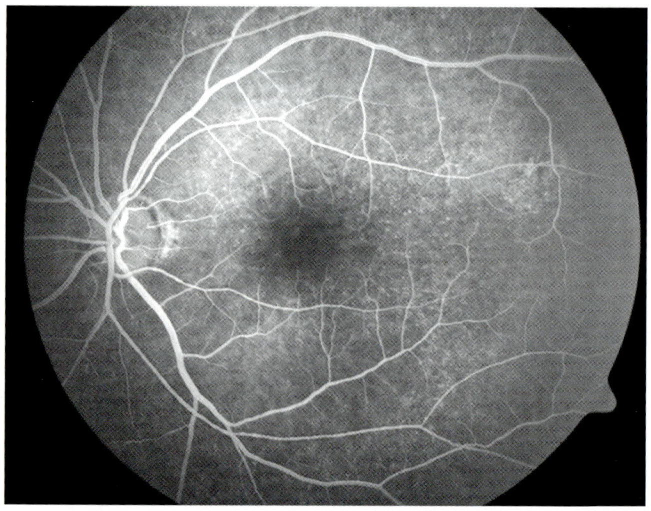

Faint hyperfluorescence in seen around the fovea in the arteriovenous phase. However, the drusen are still not made out

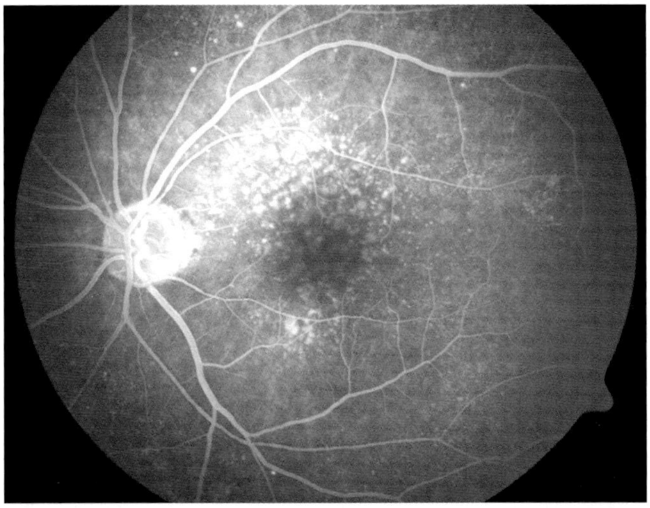

Hyperfluorescence of the soft drusen is seen only in the late phase of the angiogram

COMMENT

Soft drusen show hyperfluorescence only in the later part of the angiogram. They generally stain in the late phase of the angiogram.

CASE 3

A 65-year-old male was found to have age-related macular degeneration in both eyes during an eye examination. Visual acuity was 6/6; N6 in both eyes.

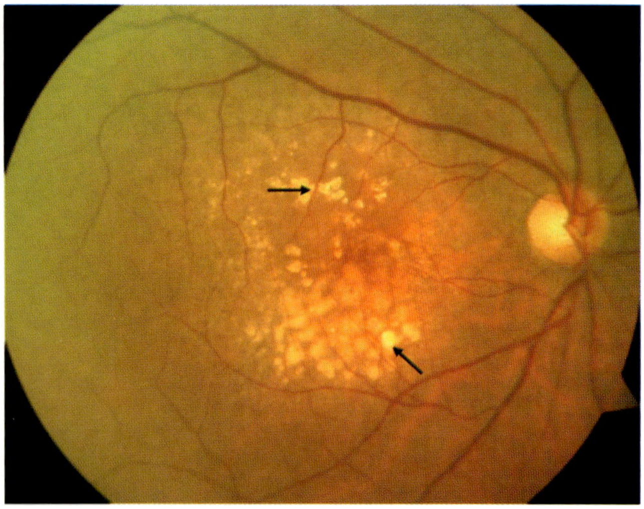

Fundus photograph of the right eye showing large soft drusen. Few calcified drusen are also seen (arrows)

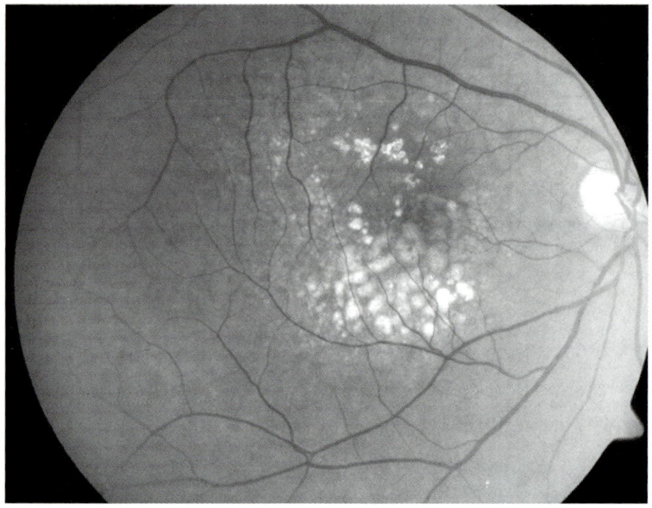

Red free photograph of the right eye

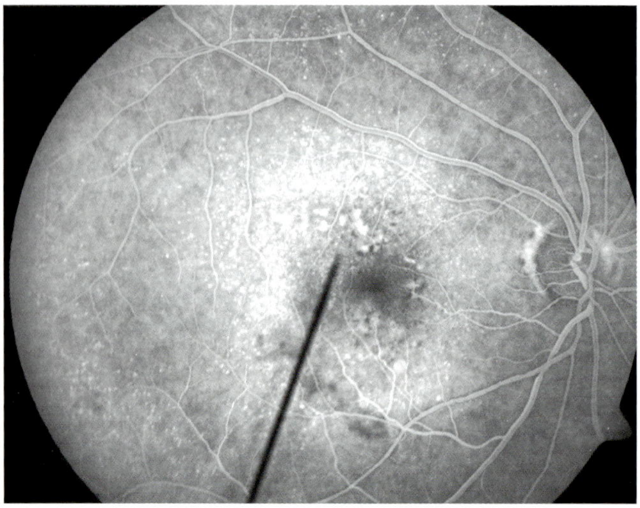

Faint hyperfluorescence is seen at the drusen in early arteriovenous phase

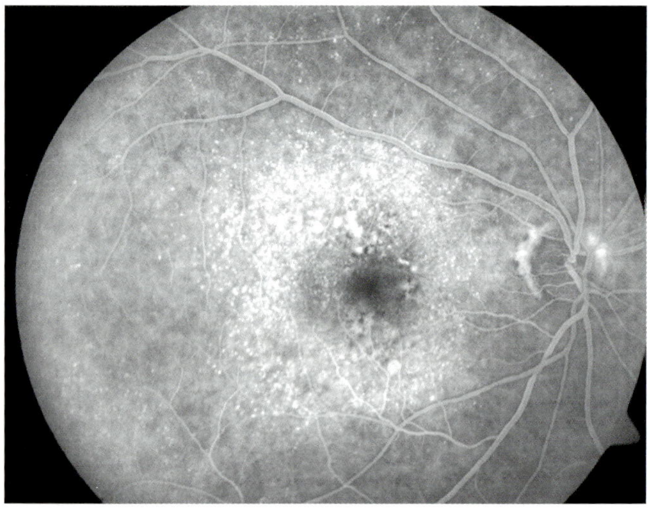

Further increase in the hyperfluorescence is noted as the angiogram progresses

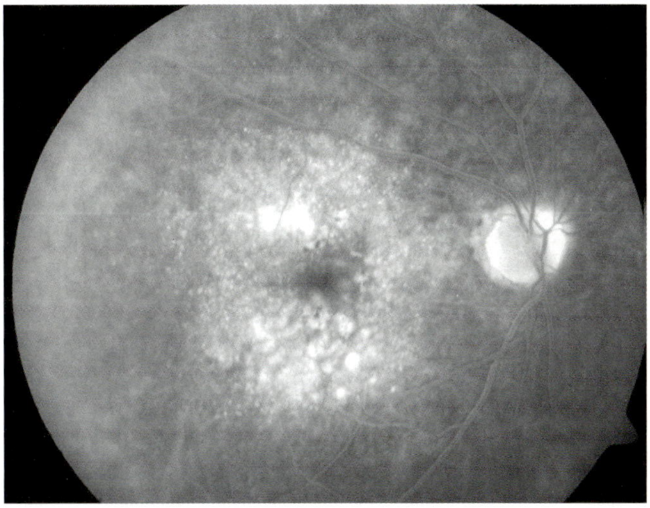

Maximum hyperfluorescence is seen in the late phase due to staining of the soft drusen

COMMENT

The late fluorescence of soft drusen is due to the hydrophobic nature of its content which does not allow easy entry of the dye.

CASE 4

A 66-year-old female presented with history of reduced vision in both eyes for the last three months. Visual acuity was 6/9; N6 in both eyes.

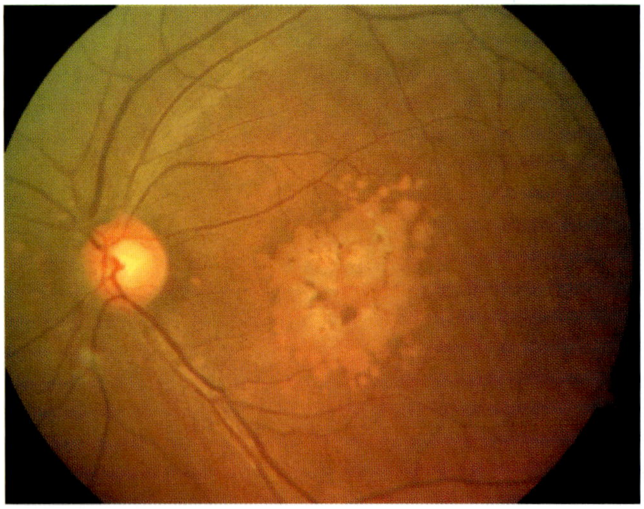

Fundus photograph of the left eye showing a large drusenoid detachment at the fovea. Pigment aggregation can be seen within this detachment. Adjacent large soft drusen are seen

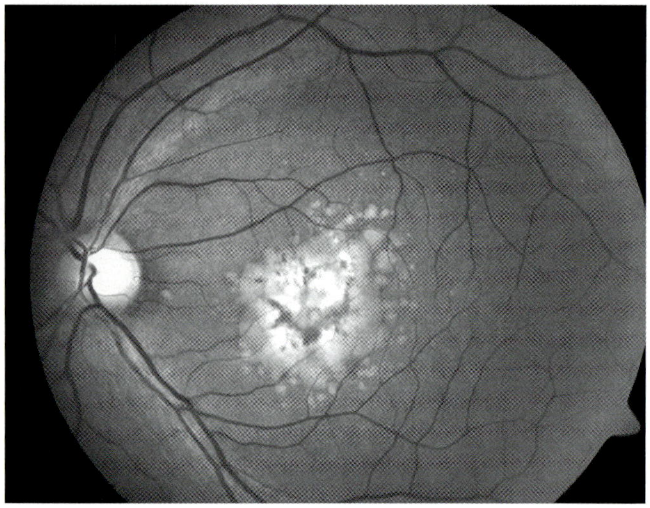

Red free photograph of the left eye. The pigment within the drusenoid detachment is well made out

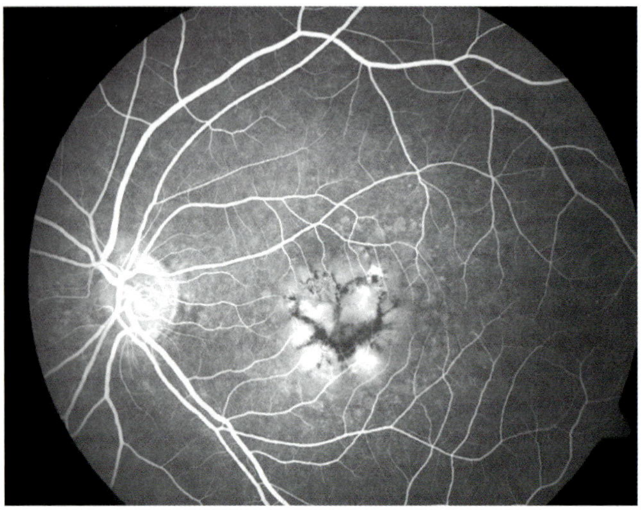

Hyperfluorescence is seen at the drusenoid detachment in the mid arteriovenous phase. Blocked fluorescence is seen due to pigment. The surrounding soft drusen are not very well seen

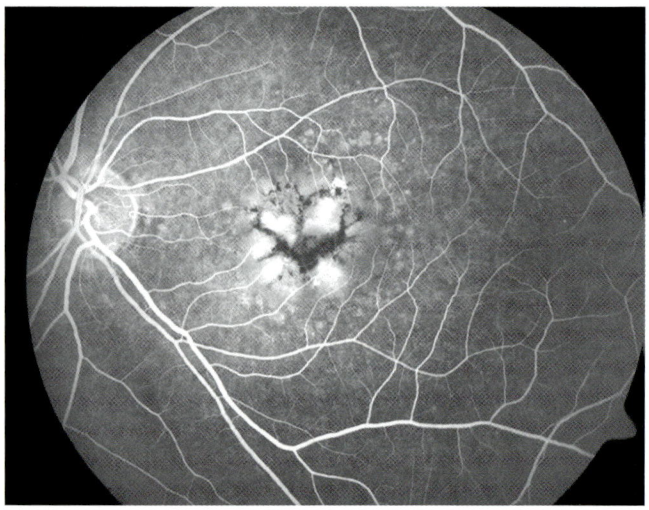

Hyperfluorescence at the drusenoid detachment has increased in the late arteriovenous phase. Faint hyperfluorescence of the surrounding soft drusen can be made out

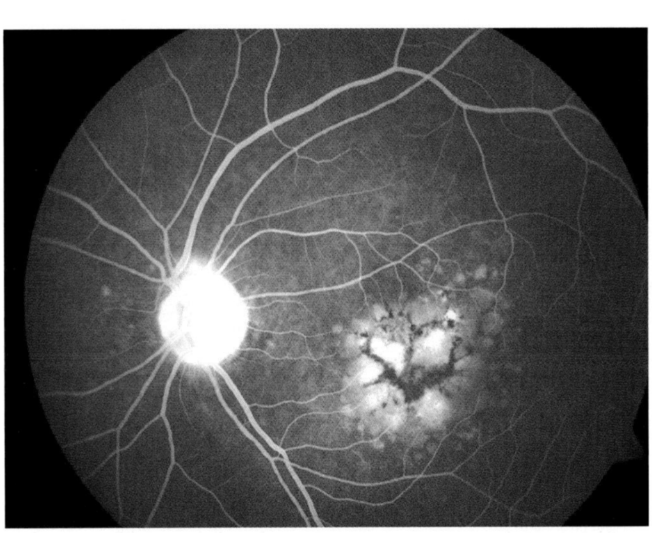

Hyperfluorescence persists at the drusenoid detachment in the late phase of the angiogram. The stained soft drusen are better seen now

COMMENT

Confluence of the soft drusen gives rise to the drusenoid detachment.

CASE 5

An 83-year-old male patient was seen with complaints of decreased vision in the right eye for the past five years. Visual acuity was 6/18; N6 in the right eye and 6/9; N6 in the left eye.

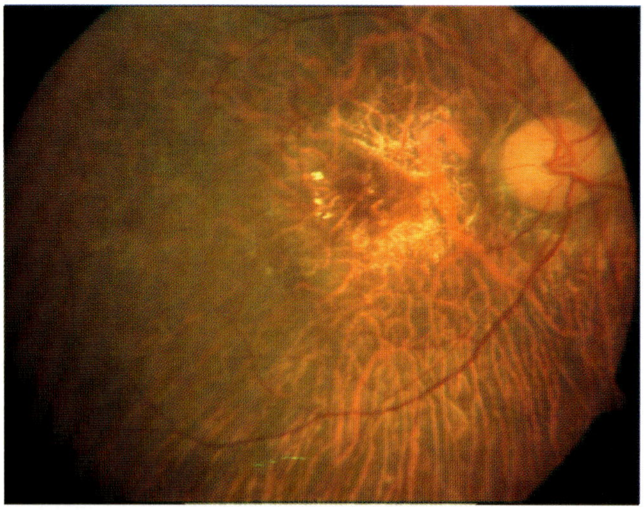

Fundus photograph of the right eye showing large atrophic patches arranged in an annular fashion around the fovea. RPE alteration is noted in the foveal region

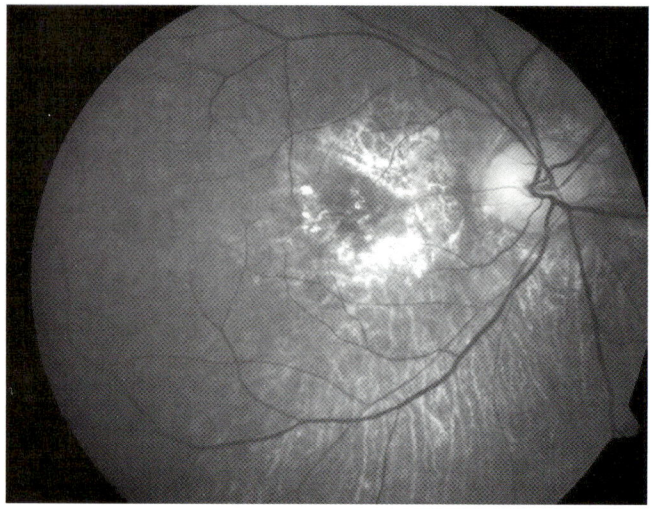

Red free photograph shows well-demarcated atrophic areas with large choroidal vessels

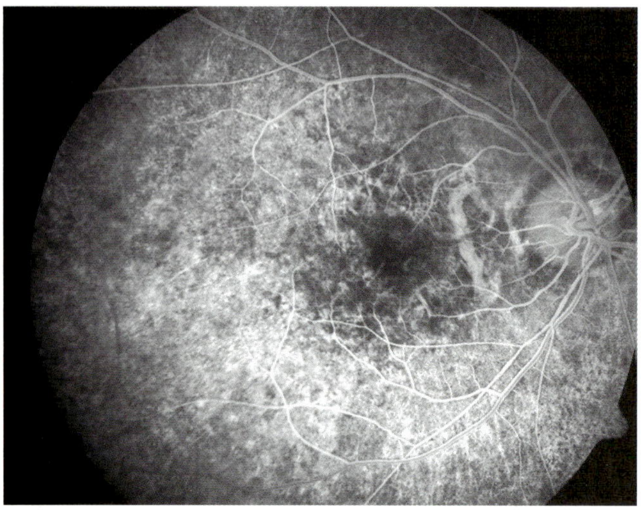

Arteriovenous phase shows relative hypofluorescence in the region of atrophy. The large choroidal vessels are visible. Irregular hyperfluorescence is seen at the rest of the macula

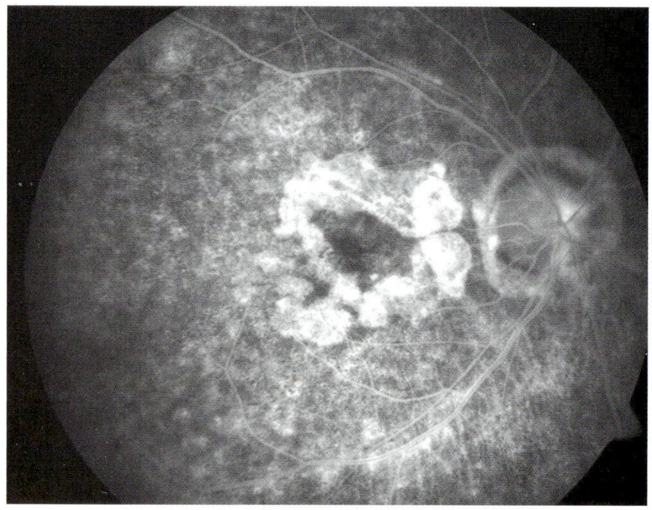

Normal scleral staining is seen through the atrophic areas making them appear hyperfluorescent in the late phase

COMMENT

Early hypofluorescence within an atropic lesion indicates nonfilling of the underlying atrophic choriocapillaris along with atrophy of the RPE.

CASE 6

A 74-year-old male patient presented with history of poor vision in both eyes for the past three years. Visual acuity was 1/60 in both eyes.

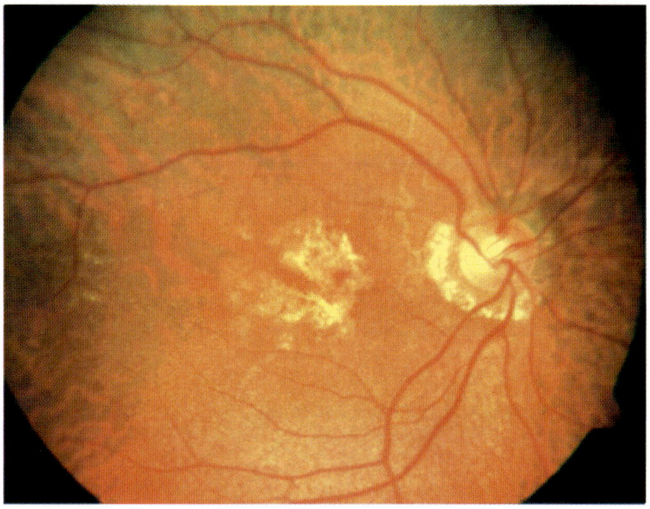

Fundus photograph of the right eye showing a large well demarcated atrophic patch in the foveal region. A horizontal band of preserved RPE is seen at the center

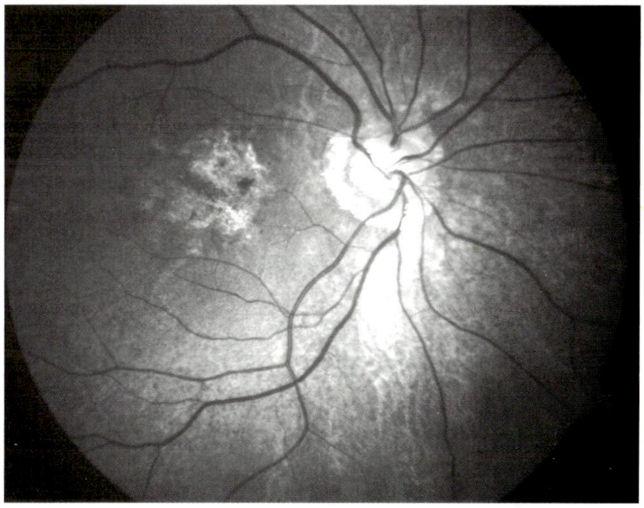

Red free photograph highlights these findings. Peripapillary atrophy is seen

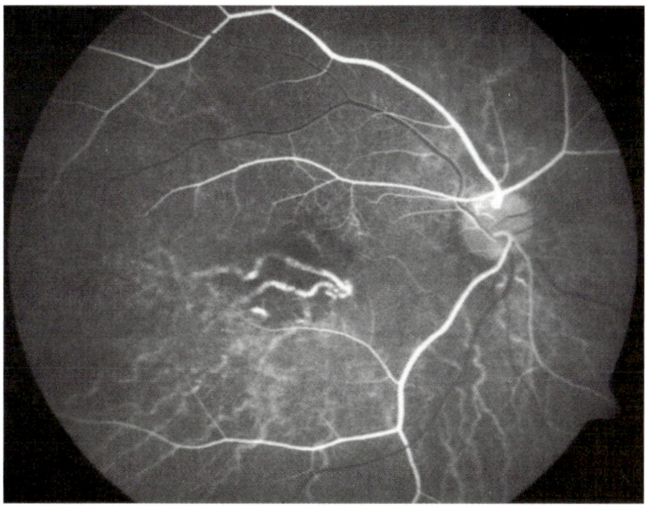

Arterial phase shows hypofluorescence in the region of atrophy indicating absence of choriocapillaris. Large choroidal vessels are seen within the atrophic area

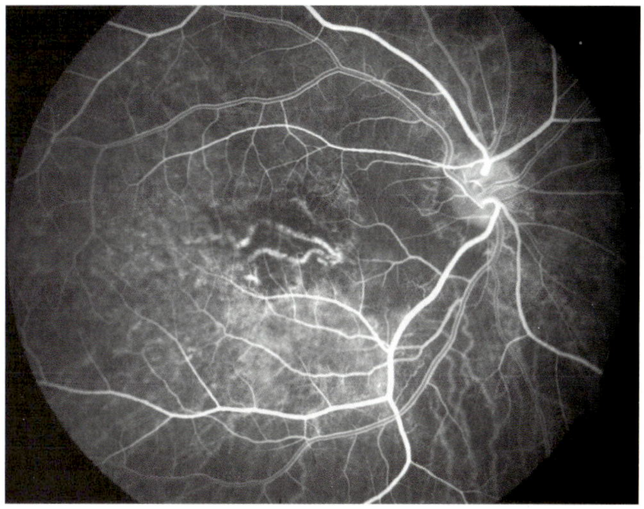

The hypofluorescence is well made out in the area of atrophy as the choriocapillaris fill up elsewhere. Irregular hyperfluorescence is noted temporally

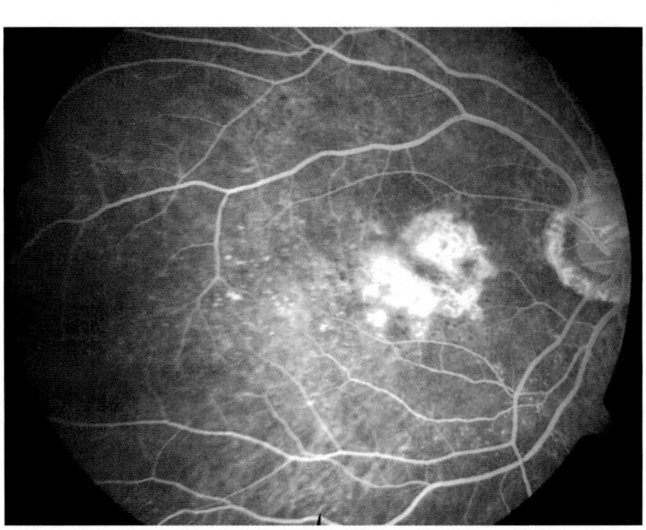

The atrophic area appears hyperfluorescent in the late films due to the increased visibility of the normal scleral staining. The horizontal band of preserved RPE blocks the background fluorescence

CASE 6 (*Continued*)

Left Eye of the Patient

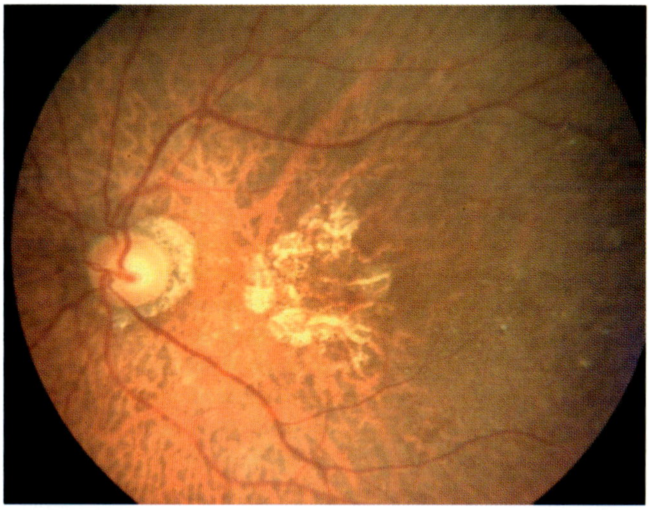

Fundus photograph of the left eye showing multiple discrete atrophic patches around the foveal center

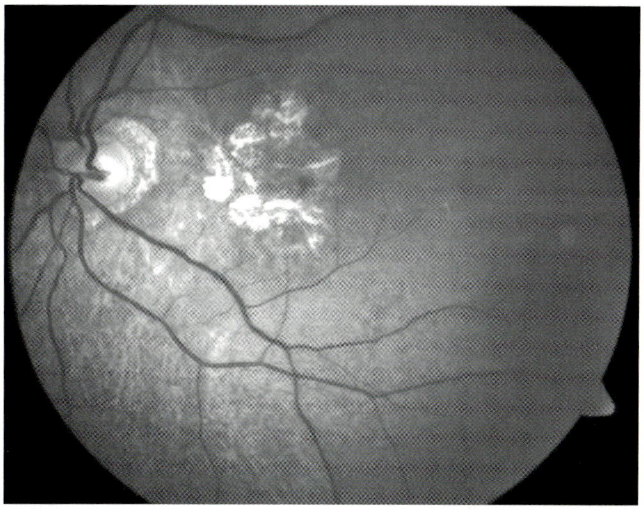

Red free photograph shows well-demarcated atrophic patches

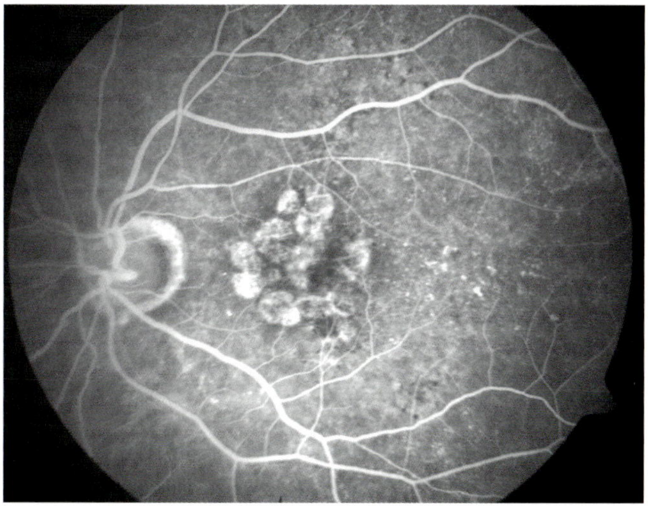

The atrophic patches appear hyperfluorescent in the arteriovenous phase due to transmission window defect indicating preservation of the underlying choriocapillaris

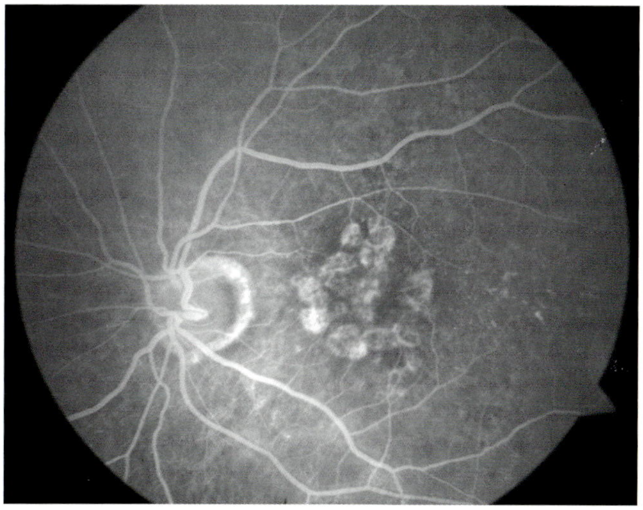

Some fading of the hyperfluorescence in the atrophic area is seen in the late phase

COMMENT

Early hyperfluorescence in the region of RPE atrophy indicates the filling of the underlying choriocapillaris which has not atrophied along with the RPE.

CASE 7

A 62-year-old male presented with history of reduced vision in the left eye of one year duration. He was asymptomatic in the right left eye. Visual acuity was 6/6; N6 in the right eye and 6/60; N36 in the left eye. A cicatrized CNVM was seen in left eye.

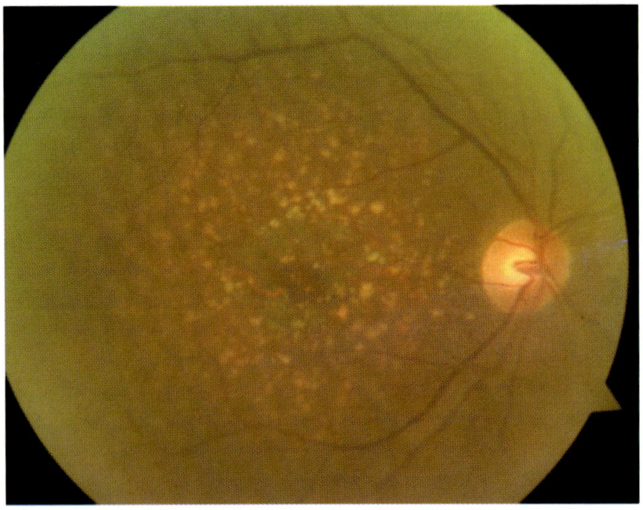

Fundus photograph of the right eye showing atrophic patches arranged in an annular fashion around the fovea. Regressing drusen are seen scattered throughout the macula

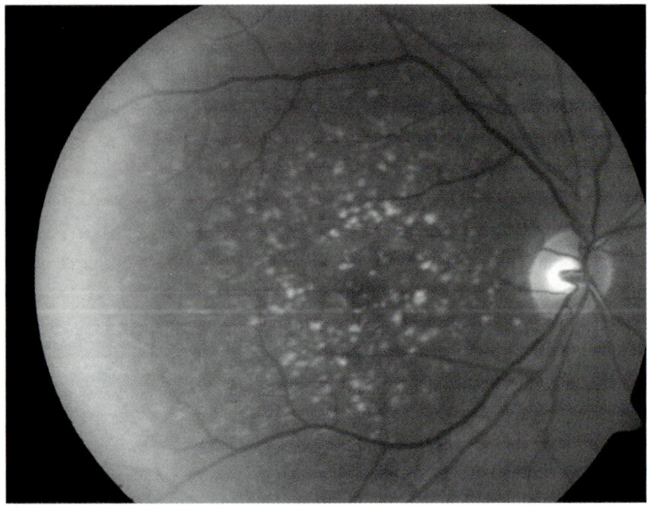

These features are well-made out in the red free photograph

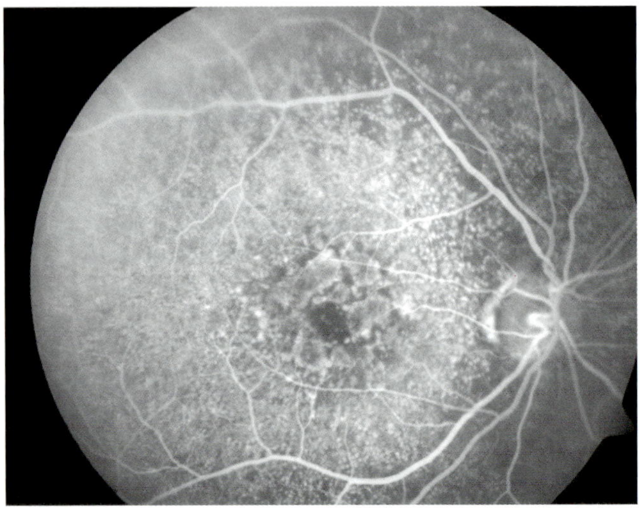

Hyperfluorescence is seen in the region of the atrophy. Irregular stippled hyperfluorescence is seen at the rest of the macula

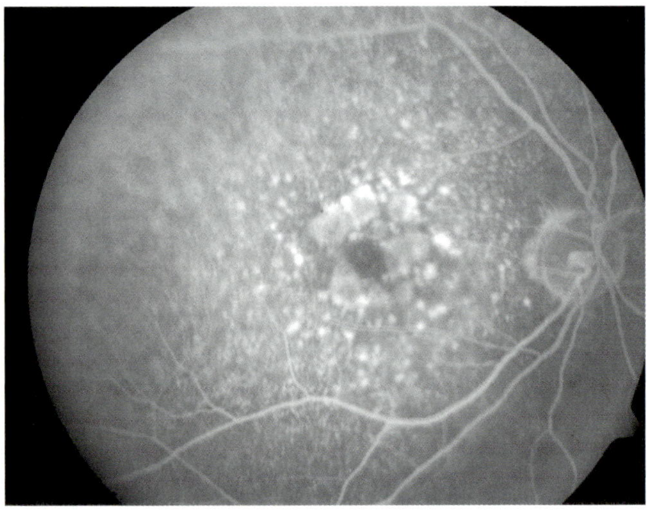

The hyperfluorescence has increased in the region of RPE atrophy. Discrete hyperfluorescence is noted at the sites of the drusen

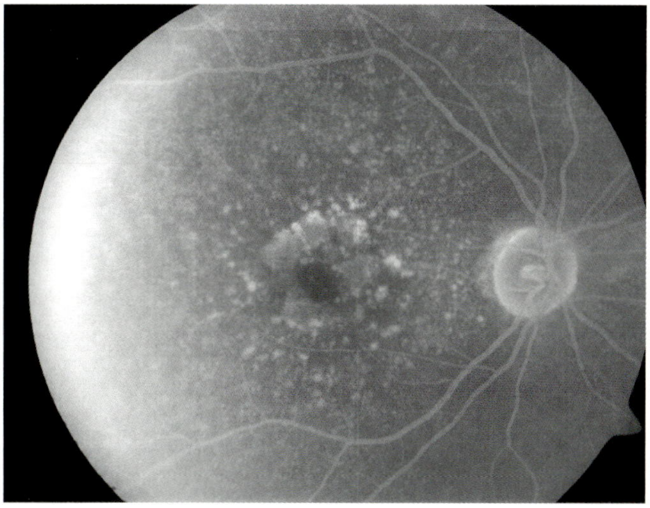

Fading of the hyperfluorescence is seen in the late phase

COMMENT

The foveal center is usually involved late in the course of development of geographic atrophy.

CLINICAL NUGGETS

1. The AREDS and LAST study have shown the beneficial effect of micronutrients in non-neovascular ARMD.
2. Eyes with focal hyperpigmentation are more prone for development of choroidal neovascular membranes.
3. Choroidal neovascularization rarely develops in areas of geographic atrophy.

BIBLIOGRAPHY

1. Barendes M, Pauleikhoff D, Chisholm I, C Minassian D, Bird AC. Bilaterality of drusen. BJO 1990;74:180-2.
2. Bird AC, Bressler NM, Bressler SB, et al. An international classification and grading system for age-related maculopathy and age related macular degeneration. Surv Ophthalmol 1995;39:367-76.
3. Bressler NM, Bressler SB, Fine SL. Age-related macular degeneration. Surv Ophthalmol 1988;32:375-413.
4. Koenig F, Saubrane G, Coscas G. Angiographic aspect of senile macular degeneration. Jap Journal of Ophthalmol 1989;33:57-65.
5. Richer S, Stiles W, Statkute L, Pulido J, Frankowski J, Rudy D, Pei K, Tsipursky M, Nyland J. Double-masked, placebo-controlled, randomized trial of lutein and antioxidant supplementation in the intervention of atrophic age-related macular degeneration: the Veterans LAST study (Lutein Antioxidant Supplementation Trial). Optometry 2004;75(4):216-30.
6. Tanenbaum HL, Eshagian M. Senile disciform degeneration of macula : the other eye—a fluorescein angiographic study: Can J Ophthalmol 1972;7:280-4.

13

Chapter

Age-related Macular Degeneration—Wet Type

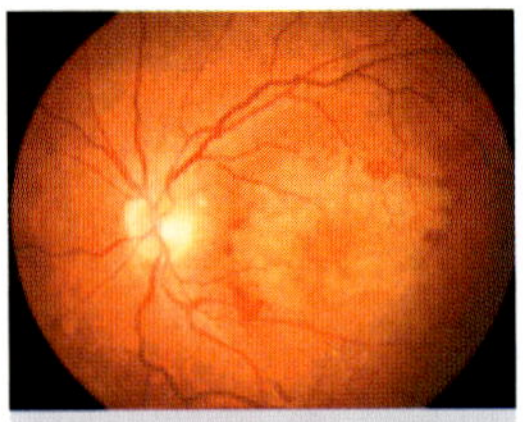

- Characterized by the development of choroidal neovascular membrane (CNVM).
- Clinically there is presence of subretinal fluid, subretinal or sub-RPE hemorrhage and lipid exudation; more often a gray subretinal neovascular membrane is seen at the macula.

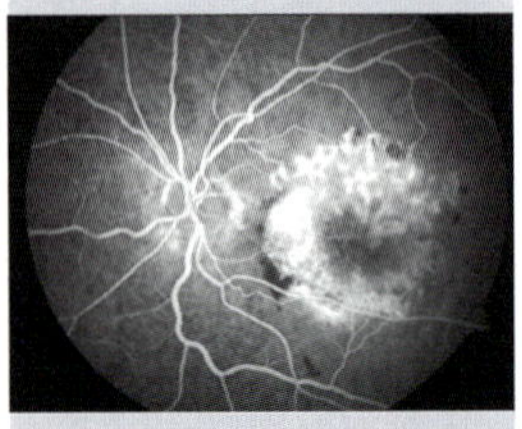

Three basic angiographic patterns of wet ARMD have been described:

1. Classic CNV shows up in the early phase as a bright, well demarcated area of hyperfluorescence which increases in intensity and extent in the mid and late films due to progressive leakage of dye, which obscures the boundaries of the CNV. Occasionally, the actual vascular network may be seen in the early phase.
2. Occult CNV includes two fluorescein angiographic patterns.
   a. Fibrovascular PED. This is seen as a speckled hyperfluorescence within 1 to 2 minutes of dye injection with persistence of staining or leakage of the fluorescein dye in the late phase. This could be well demarcated or poorly demarcated.
   b. Late leakage of undetermined source. This consists of areas of leakage of dye at the level of the RPE in the late phases of the angiogram. It does not correspond to an area of CNV or a fibrovascular PED to account for the leakage.
3. Retinal Angiomatous Proliferans (RAP)

CASE 1

A 62-year-old male presented with distortion of vision in the right eye of one week duration. Visual acuity was 6/9; N8 in the right eye and 6/60; N36 in the left eye. A cicatrized CNVM was noted in the left eye.

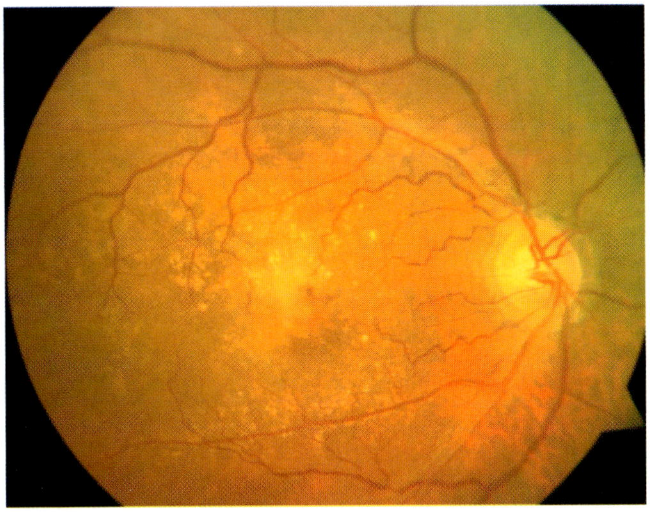

Fundus photograph of the right eye showing drusen at the macula. An area of subretinal whitening with adjacent speck of hemorrhage and hard exudate is seen superotemporal to the fovea

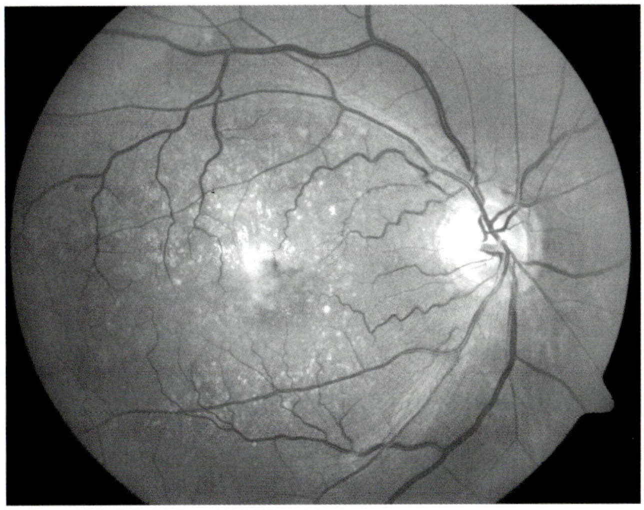

Red free photograph showing the changes superotemporal to the foveal center

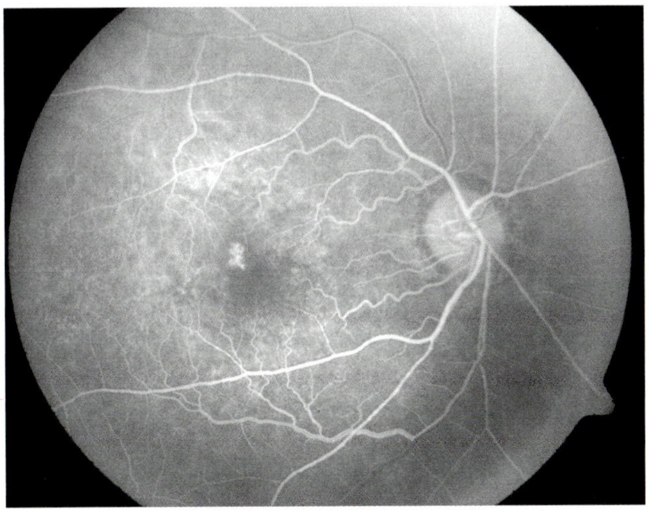

Early arteriovenous phase of the angiogram showing a well defined vascular network suggestive of a classic CNVM. Irregular hyperfluorescence due to window transmission defect of drusen is seen surrounding the fovea

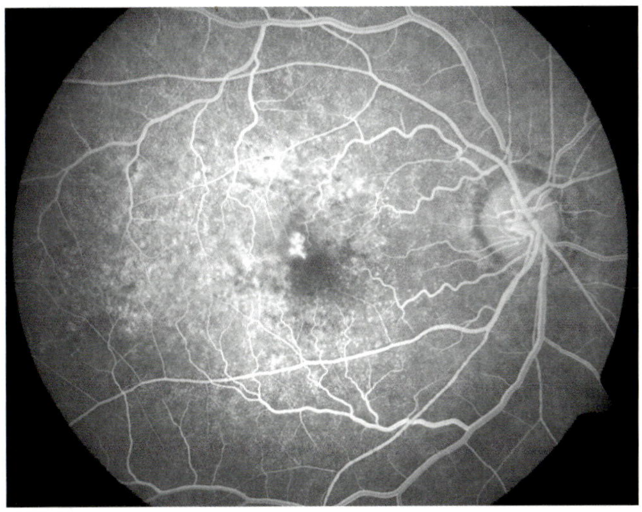

Arteriovenous phase showing increased hyperfluorescence of the CNVM. Hyperfluorescence due to drusen in the surrounding area has also increased

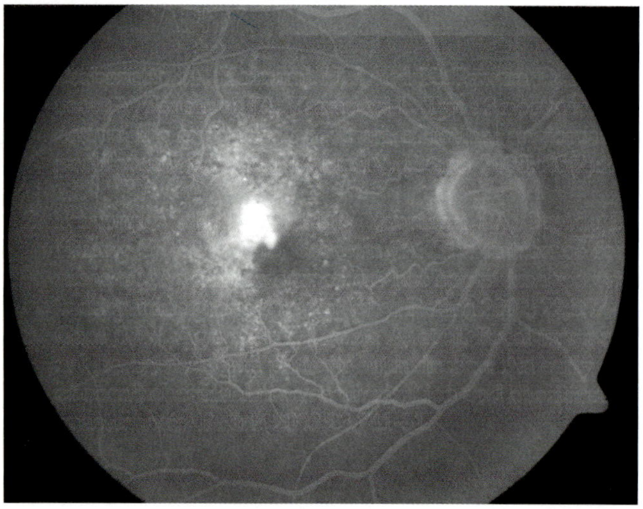

Increased hyperfluorescence with a fuzzy margin is seen in the late phase. The transmitted hyperfluorescence in the rest of the macula has faded

COMMENT

A small juxtafoveal, classic CNVM is seen in this case. The vessels constituting the CNVM are made out in the early phase. Dye leakage from these vessels blurs out its details in the late phase of the angiogram.

CASE 2

A 57-year-old male presented with reduced vision in the right eye for the past ten days. Visual acuity was 6/18; N12 in the right eye.

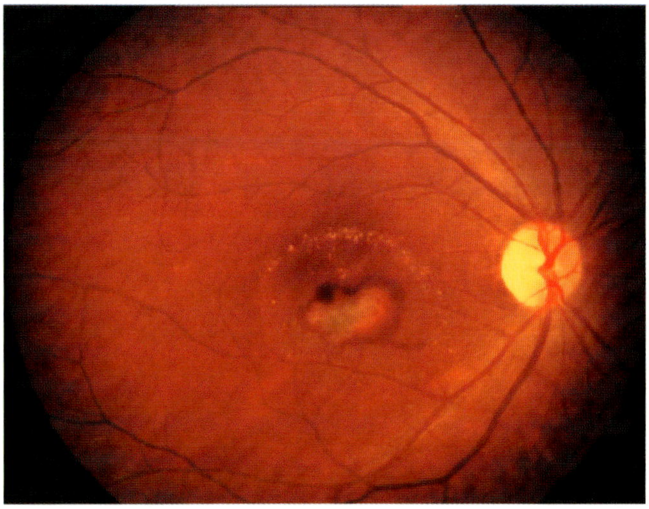

Fundus photograph of the right eye showing a juxtafoveal membrane with surrounding rim of subretinal hemorrhage. Subretinal fluid and hard exudates are also seen

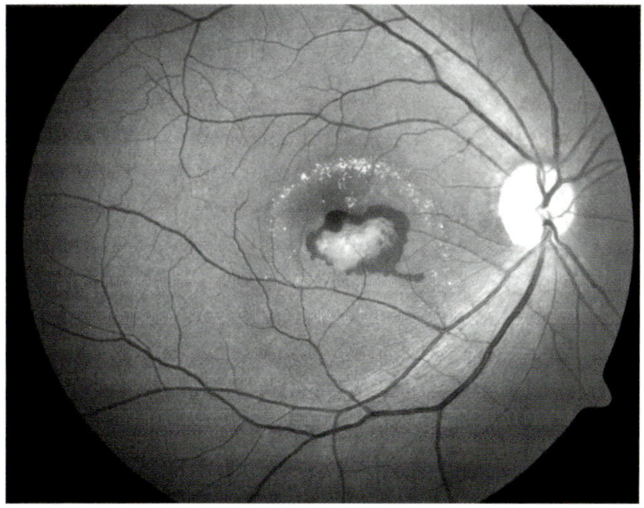

Red free photograph shows the CNVM and the subretinal hemorrhage

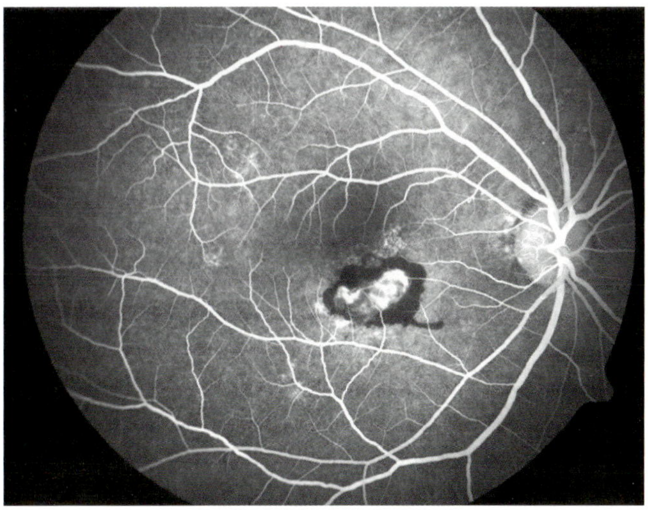

Arteriovenous phase shows filling up of the juxtafoveal classic CNVM. Surrounding blocked choroidal fluorescence due to the subretinal blood is seen

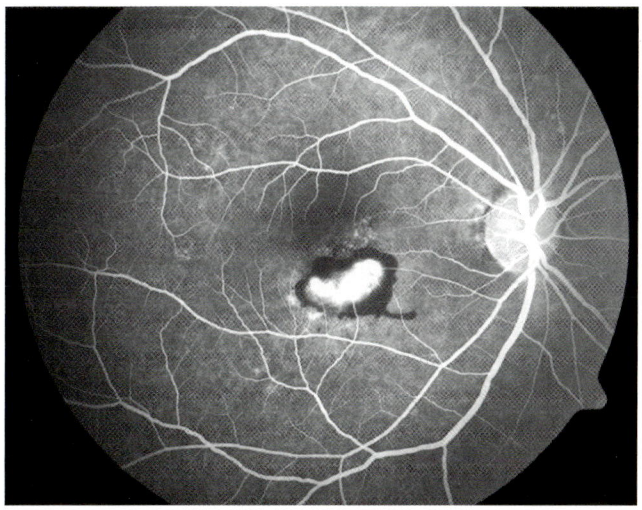

Leakage of dye from the new vessels obscures the details of the CNVM

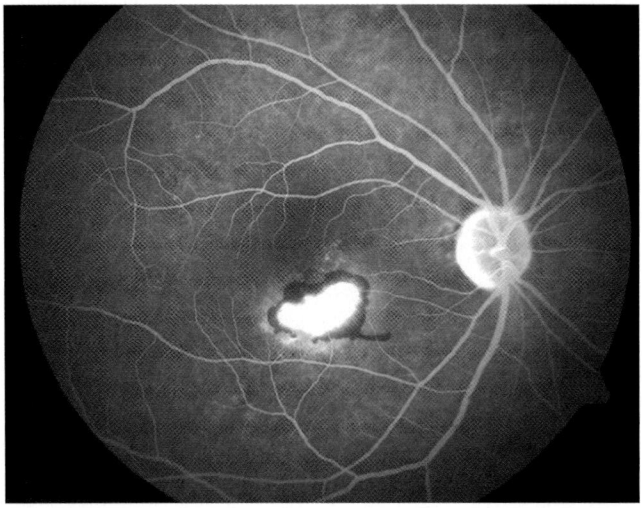

Intense hyperfluorescence of the CNVM is seen in the late phase

COMMENT

A large classic juxtafoveal membrane with surrounding rim of subretinal hemorrhage is seen. When treating this CNVM with laser, it is necessary to include the rim of hemorrhage in the treatment.

CASE 2 (*Continued*)

Argon laser photocoagulation was done to the juxtafoveal CNVM. One month later the visual acuity in the right eye was 6/9; N8.

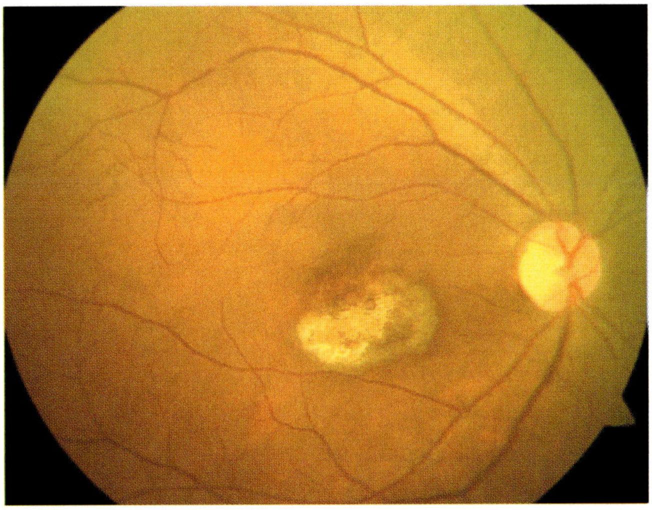

Laser photocoagulation scar is seen inferior to the foveal center. No subretinal fluid, hard exudate or hemorrhage is seen

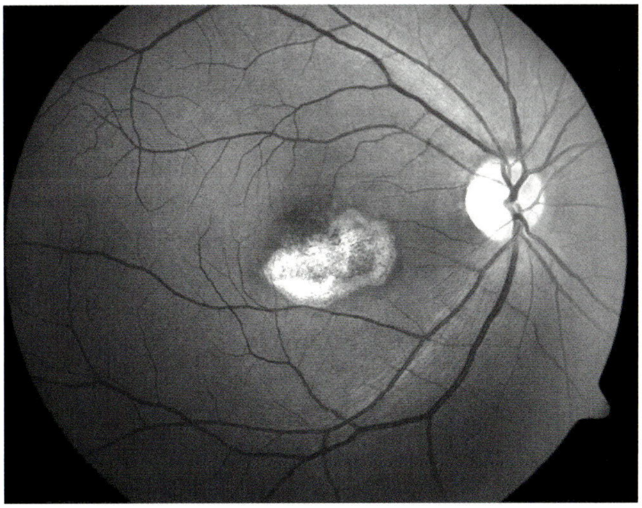

Red free photograph of the right eye

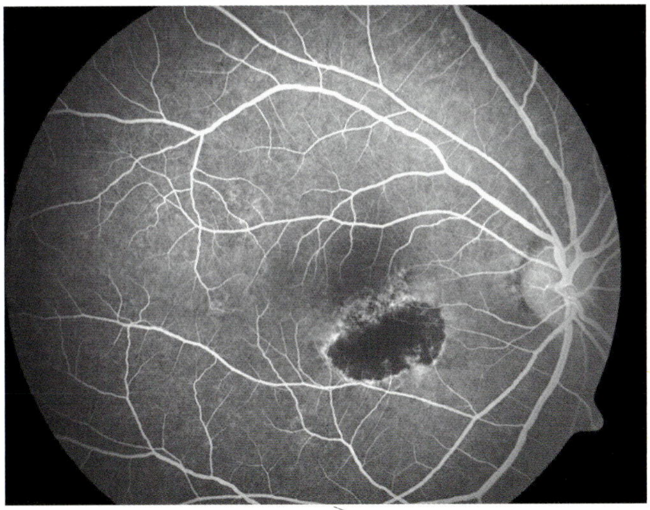

Hypofluorescence with a rim of hyperfluorescence is seen at the laser scar in the arteriovenous phase

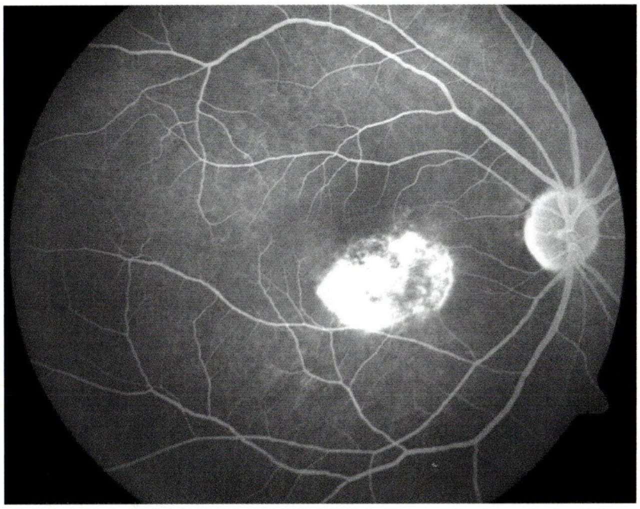

Late staining of the scar is seen. Note that the margins are well defined and the hyperfluorescence has not extended beyond the lesion boundary

COMMENT

Following laser photocoagulation of the CNVM, hyperfluorescence within the center of the laser scar which does not extend beyond the margins of the scar in the late phase, is generally not considered as recurrence of the membrane.

CASE 3

A 63-year-old male presented with distortion of vision in the right eye of two weeks duration. Visual acuity was 6/6; N6.

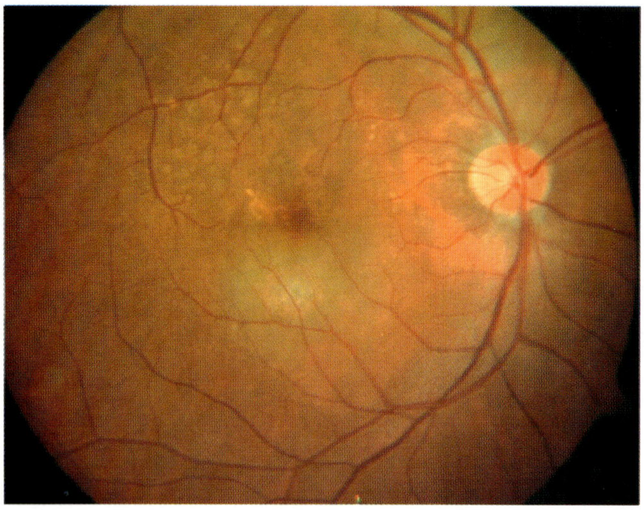

Fundus photograph of the right eye showing a CNVM inferior to the foveal center. Soft drusen are seen in the superior macula

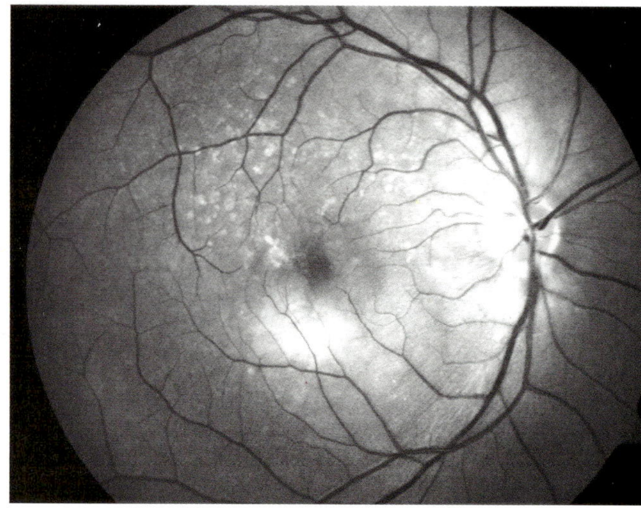

Red free photograph showing the CNVM and the drusen

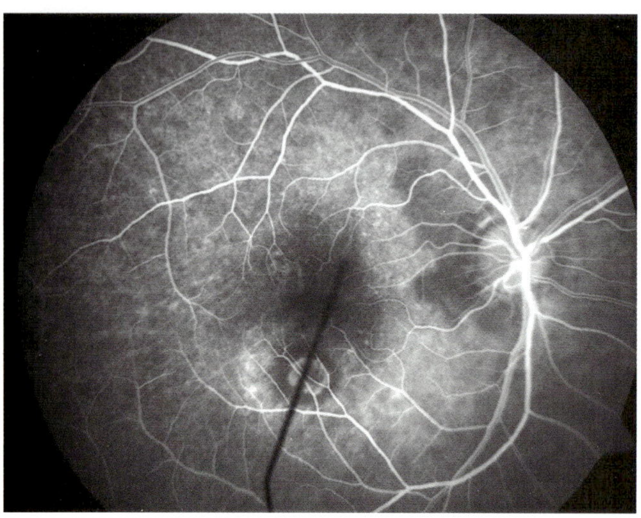

Early arteriovenous phase of the angiogram showing the filling up of the extrafoveal, classic CNVM

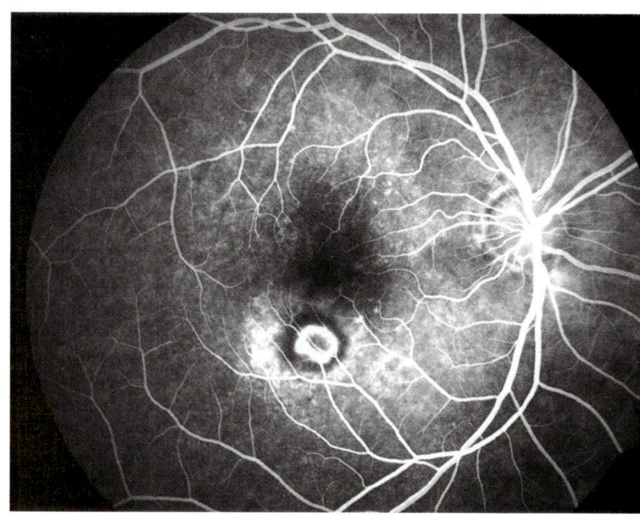

Increased hyperfluorescence is seen in the mid arteriovenous phase of the angiogram. Note the rim of hypofluorescence surrounding the CNVM

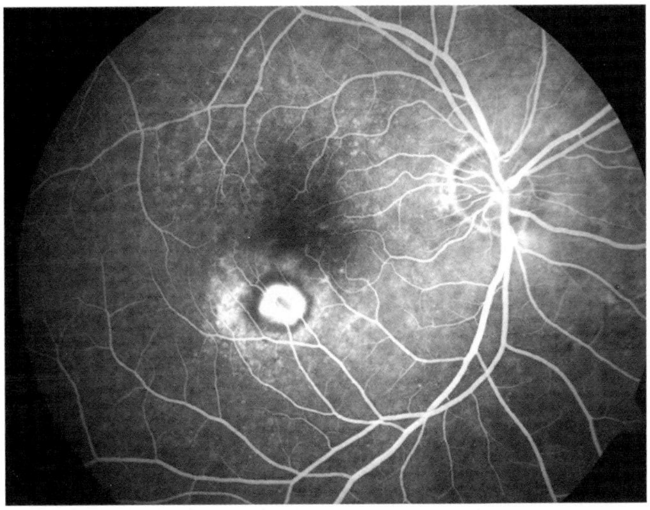

Intense hyperfluorescence is seen at the CNVM in the late phase. The soft drusen shows only minimal staining even in the late films

CASE 3 (*Continued*)

Argon laser photocoagulation was done to the extrafoveal CNVM. Patient was lost to follow-up and presented only six months later with reduced vision in the right eye. Visual acuity was 6/24; N18.

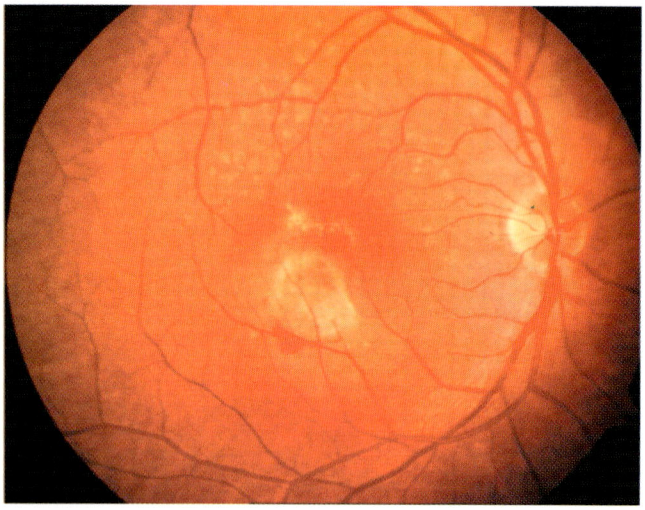

Fundus photograph of the right eye showing the laser scar inferior to the foveal center with a subretinal hemorrhage along its lower edge. The foveal edge of the scar appears heaped up

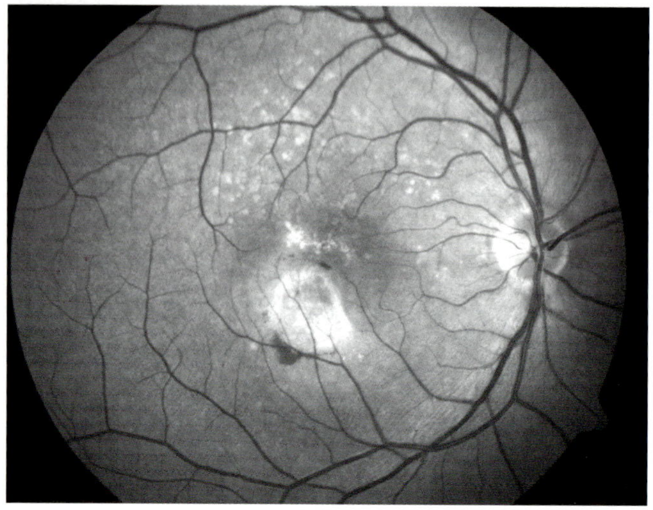

Red free photograph of the right eye

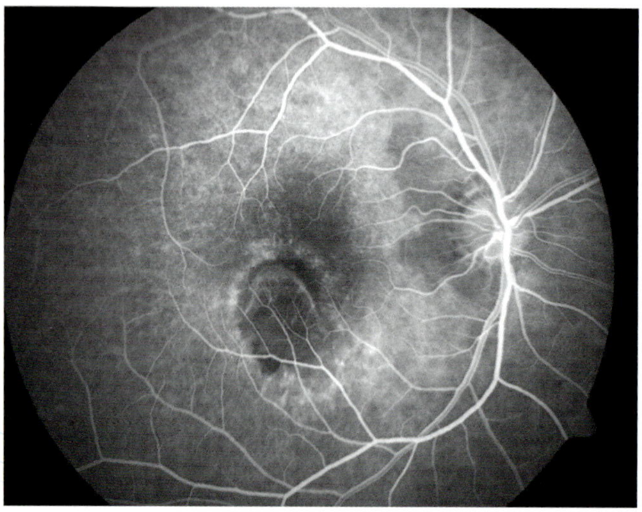

Hyperfluorescence is seen at the superior edge of the scar. A vascular network suggestive of a recurrent CNVM can be made out in this hyperfluorescent area

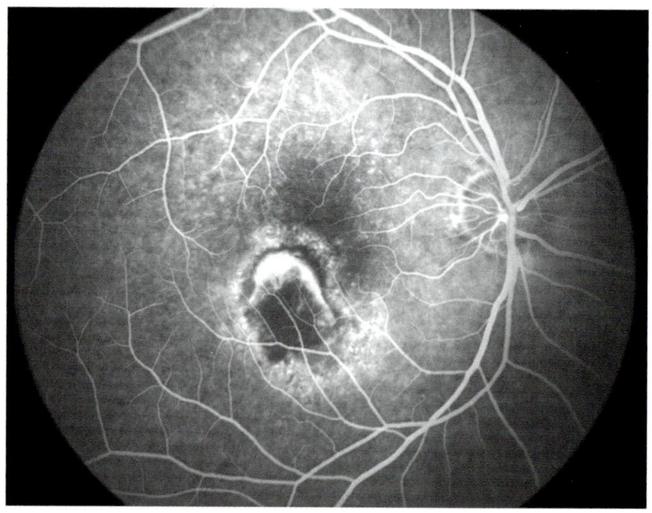

Leakage of dye causes increased hyperfluorescence of the recurrent membrane in the arteriovenous phase

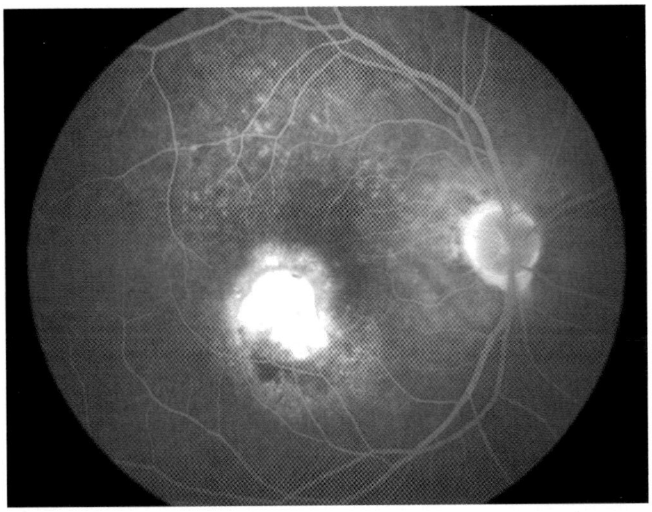

Intense hyperfluorescence with fuzzy margins is seen at the recurrent CNVM in the late phase. Staining of the inferior laser scar is seen

COMMENT

Following laser photocoagulation of the CNVM, hyperfluorescence with leakage in the later phase of the angiogram, occurring at the periphery of the laser scar is generally considered as recurrence of the CNVM.

CASE 4

A 60-year-old male presented with a history of metamorphopsia in the right eye for the past one month. Left eye had poor vision since one year. Visual acuity was 6/9; N6 in the right eye and 1/60 in the left eye. A disciform scar was noted in the left eye.

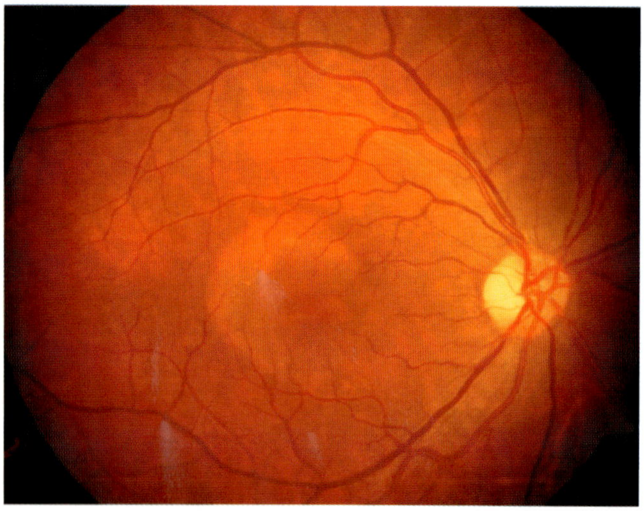

Fundus photograph of the right eye showing a pigment epithelial detachment at the fovea

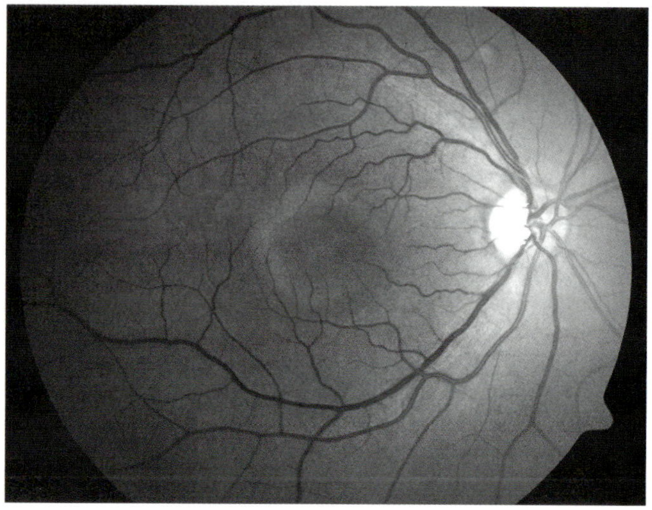

Red free photograph of the right eye shows the PED

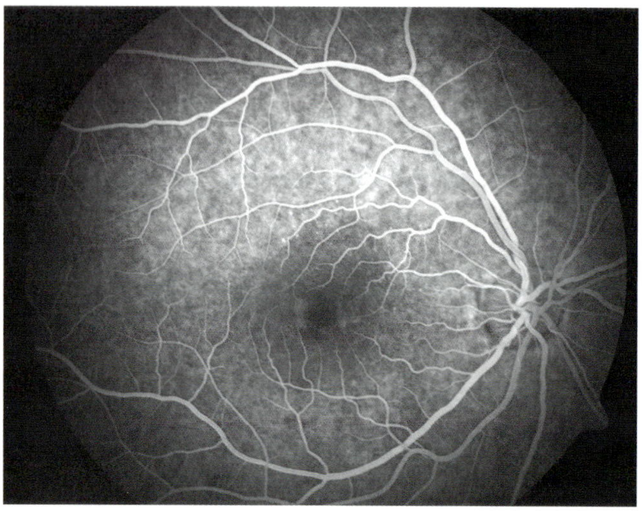

Mid arteriovenous phase showing only faint hyperfluorescence in the parafoveal region

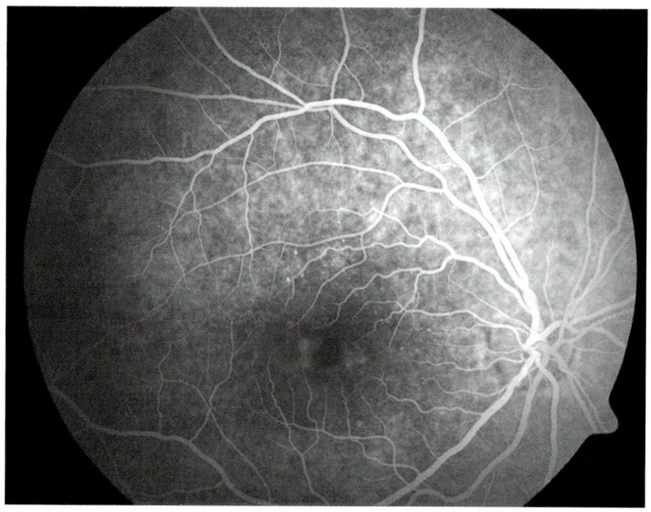

The hyperfluorescence in the center has marginally increased in the late arteriovenous phase. No subretinal vascular network is seen

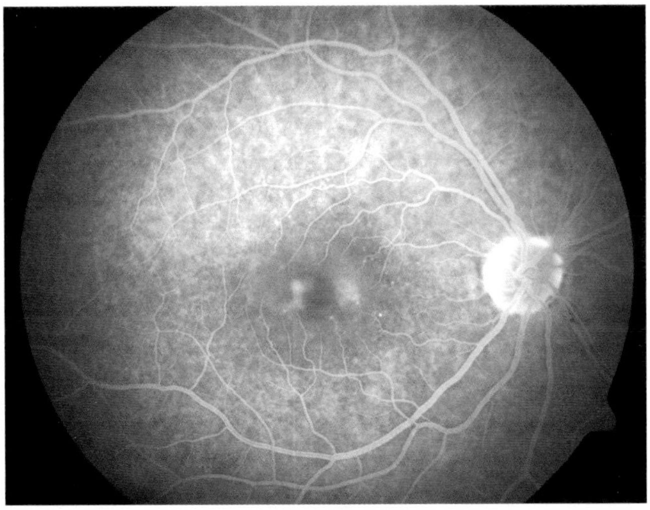

Late phase showing minimal fuzzy hyperfluorescence in the parafoveal region

CASE 4 (*Continued*)

Three months later, visual acuity in the right eye had dropped to 6/24; N36.

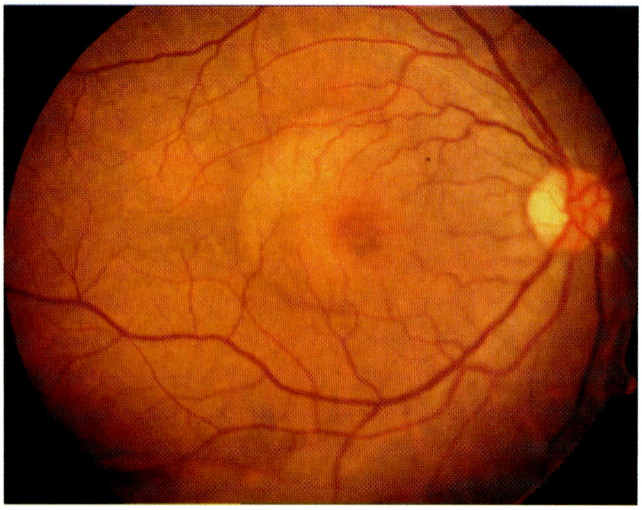

Fundus photograph of the right eye showing a PED at the fovea. Hemorrhage is seen at the foveal center. Note the increase in the size of the PED

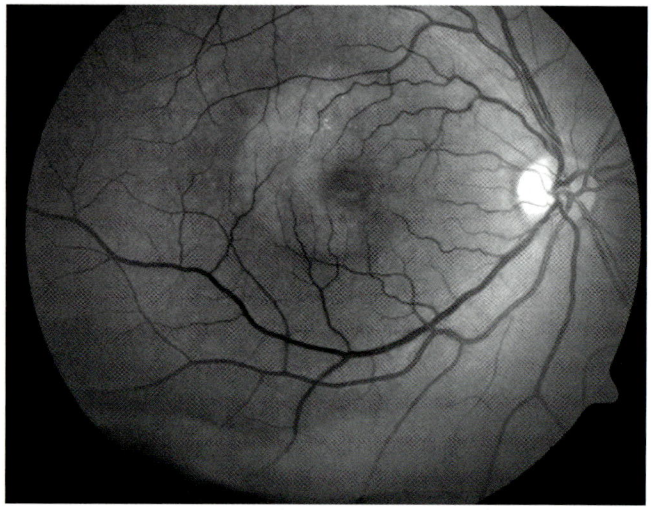

Red free photograph of the right eye

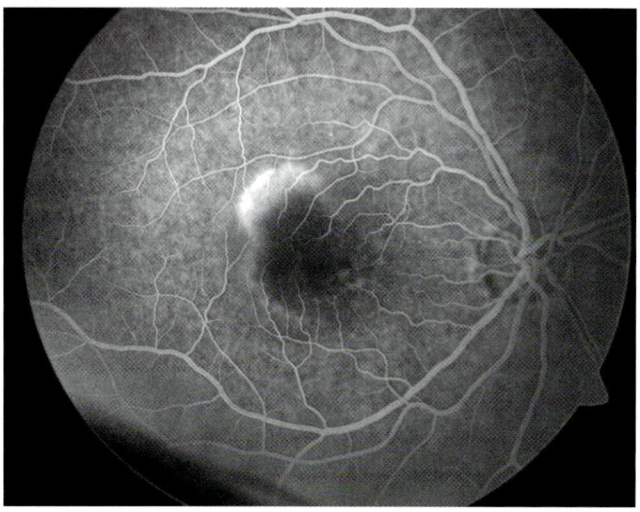

Mid arteriovenous phase shows filling of the upper part of the PED. Faint irregular hyperfluorescence is seen in the rest of the area of PED

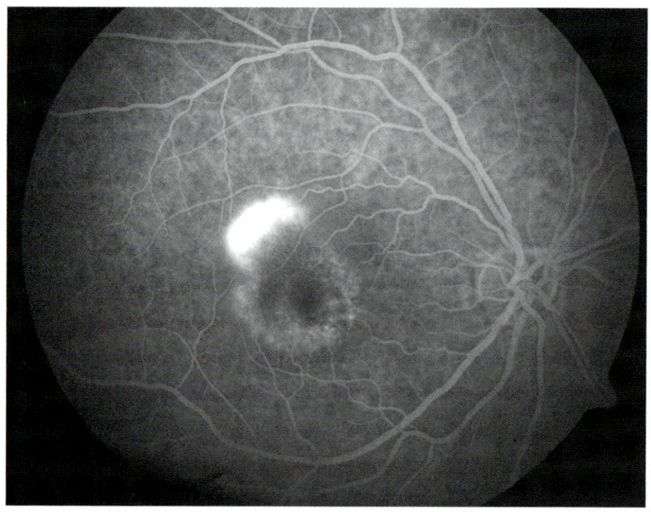

The stippled hyperfluorescence in the lower part of the PED has increased. Increased filling of the superior part of the PED is seen

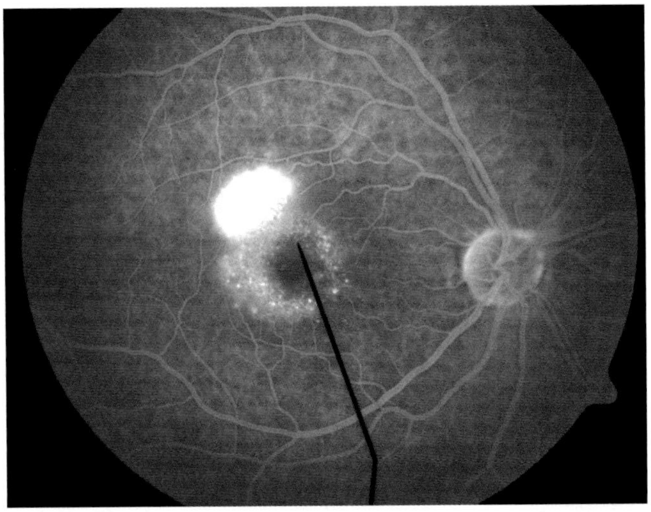

Late phase shows increased stippled hyperfluorescence around the fovea suggestive of an occult CNVM. Pooling of the dye is noted superiorly

COMMENT

A slow filling PED is highly suspicious of an occult CNVM.

CASE 5

A 68-year-old male presented with a history of reduced vision in the left eye of one month duration. Visual acuity was 6/24; N18 in the right eye and 6/9; N6 in the left eye. Soft drusen with RPE alterations were seen at the fovea in the right eye.

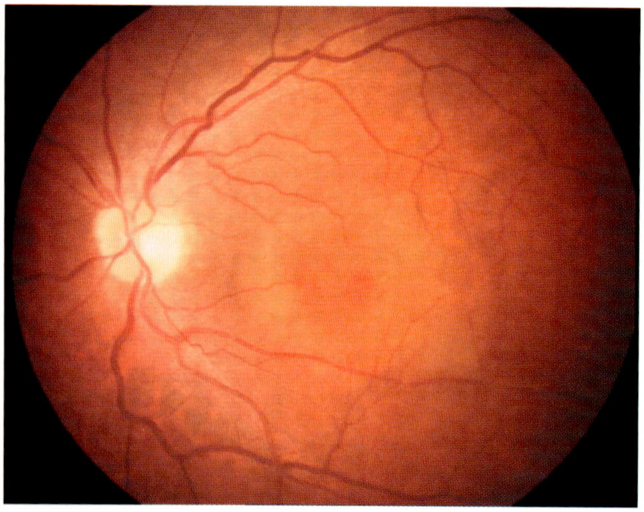

Fundus photograph of the left eye showing a large solid appearing PED at the macula. The center of the PED appears depressed

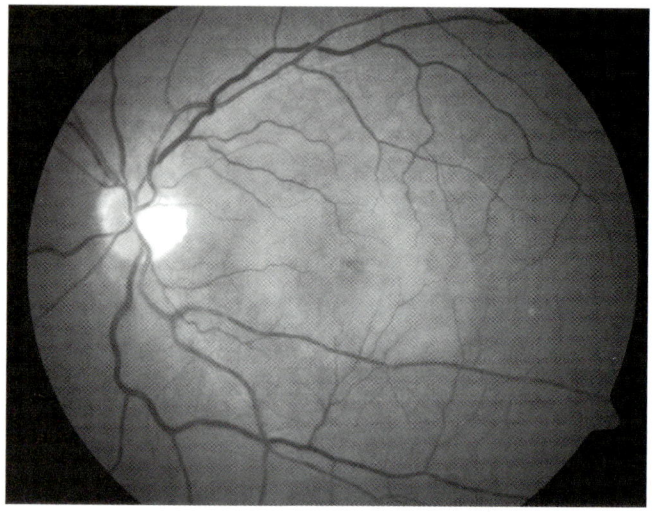

Red free photograph of the left eye. A speck of hemorrhage is noted at the center

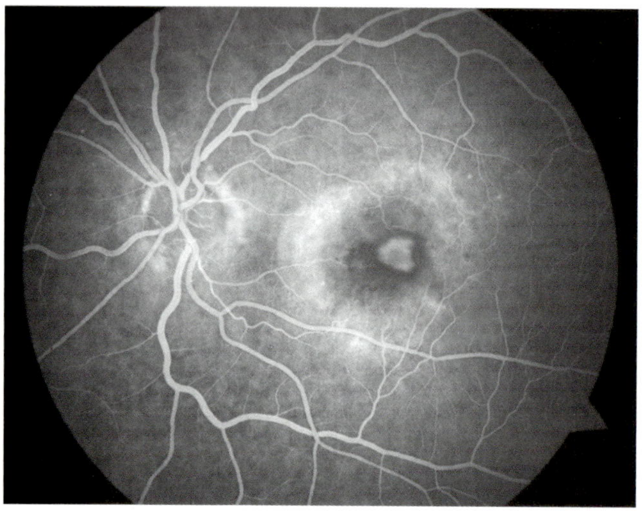

Arteriovenous phase showing hyperfluorescence throughout the extent of the lesion. Central hyperfluorescence due to a small classic membrane is seen

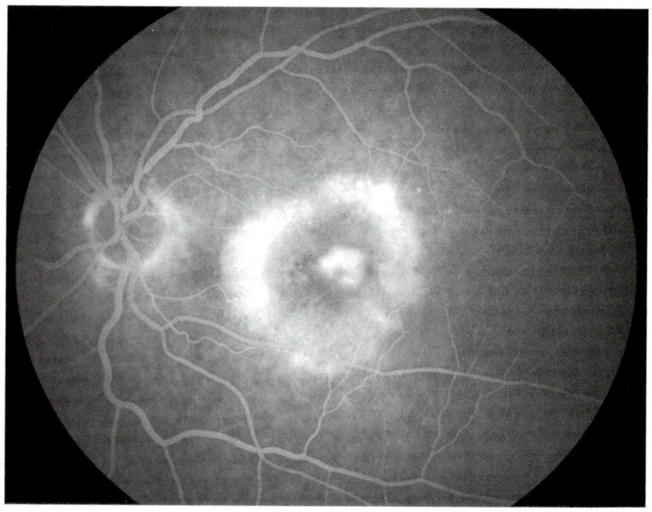

Overall hyperfluorescence throughout the lesion has increased. The intensity of fluorescence at the central classic membrane has also increased

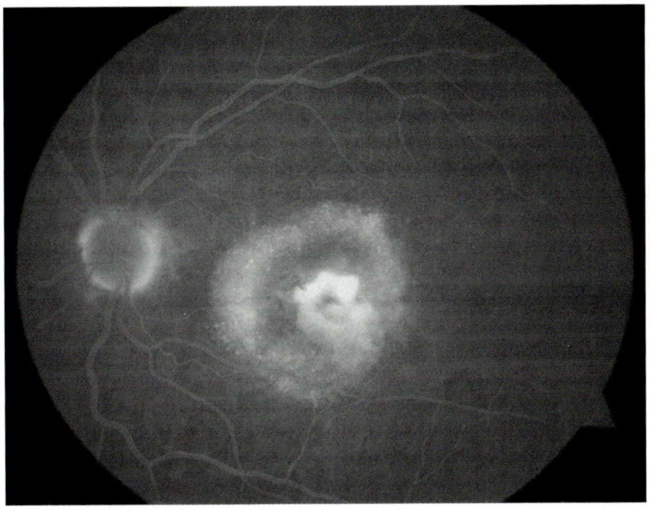

Late phase angiogram showing fuzzy hyperfluorescence centrally. Stippled hyperfluorescence due to filling of the rest of the PED is seen suggestive of a large occult CNVM

COMMENT

Patient is having a large occult membrane with a small classic component which is less that fifty percent of the entire lesion. This is a minimally classic CNVM.

CASE 5 (*Continued*)

Three months later, visual acuity was 6/18; N18.

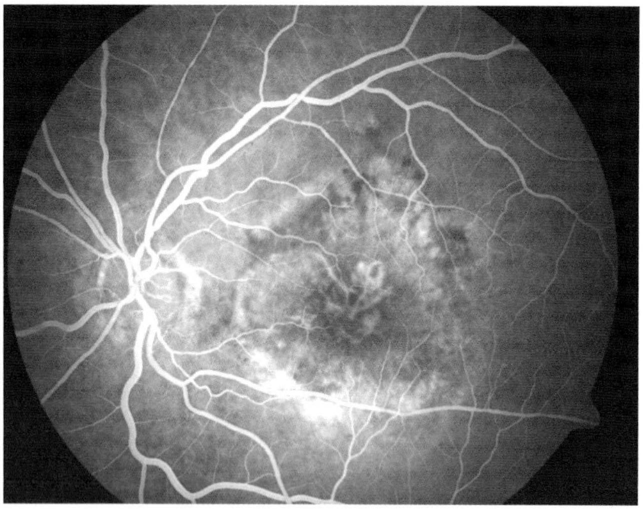

Arteriovenous phase showing increase in the size of the central classic membrane

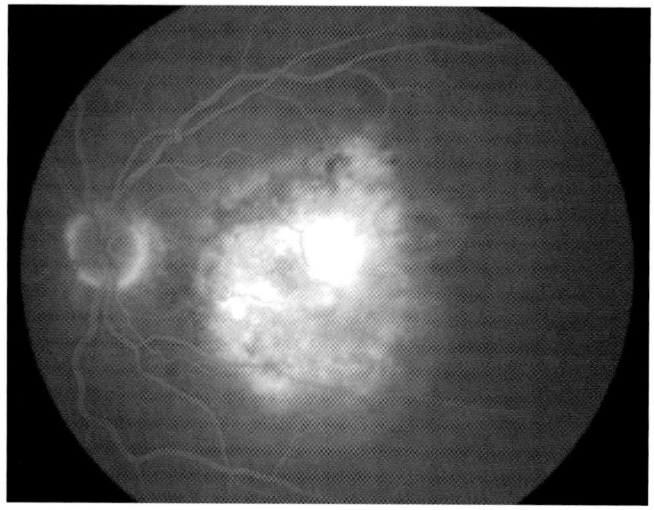

Late phase showing increased intensity of hyperfluorescence

Three months later, visual acuity was maintained.

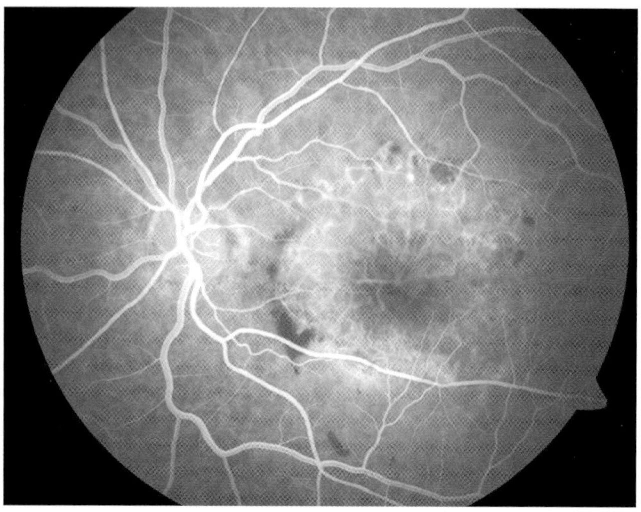

Further increase in the size of the classic membrane is seen. The vessels of the CNVM is very well made out

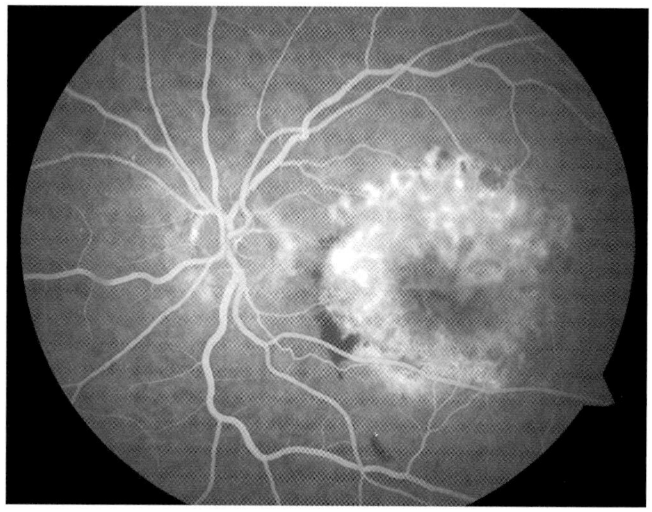

Leakage of the dye from the neovascular vessels is seen

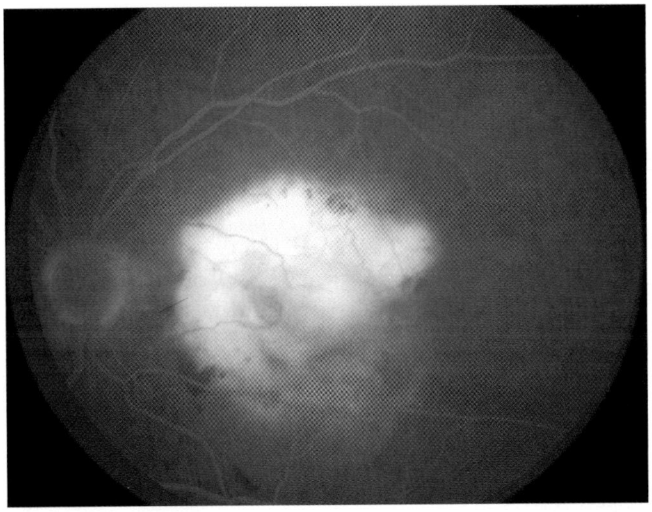

Intense hyperfluorescence is seen in the late phase due to staining of the neovascular tissue and due to pooling of the dye in the subretinal space

COMMENT

The classic part of the CNVM has increased and now, constitutes more than fifty percent of the entire lesion. This is a predominantly classic membrane.

CASE 6

A 73-year-old male patient presented with a history of reduced vision in both eyes for the past two years. Visual acuity was 1/60 in the right eye and 6/24; N36 in the left eye. Both eyes showed changes of wet type of age related macular degeneration.

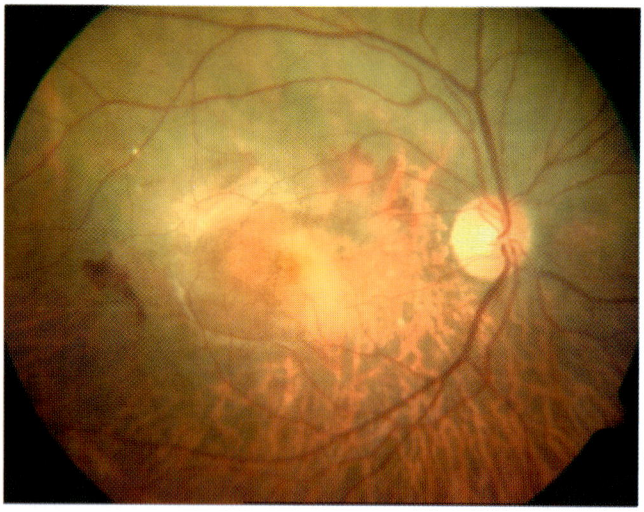

Fundus photograph of the right eye showing a large scarred CNVM at the macula

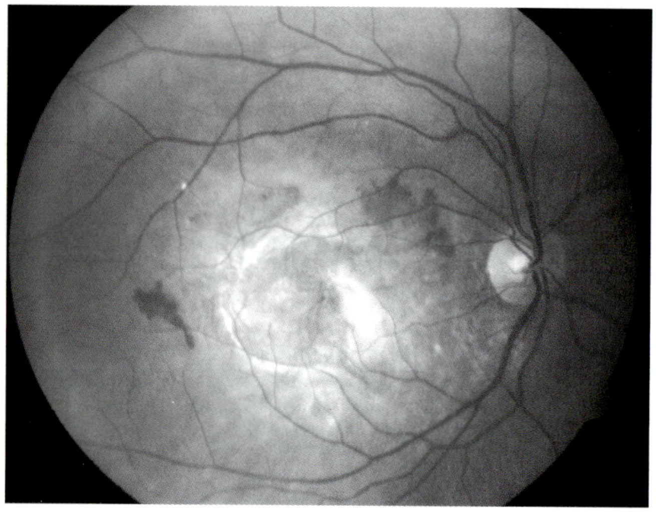

Red free photograph of the right eye

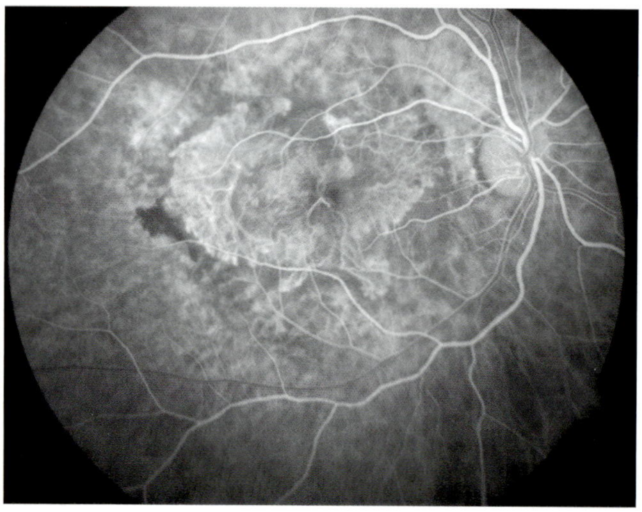

Early arteriovenous phase shows the large network of vessels of the choroidal neovascular membrane

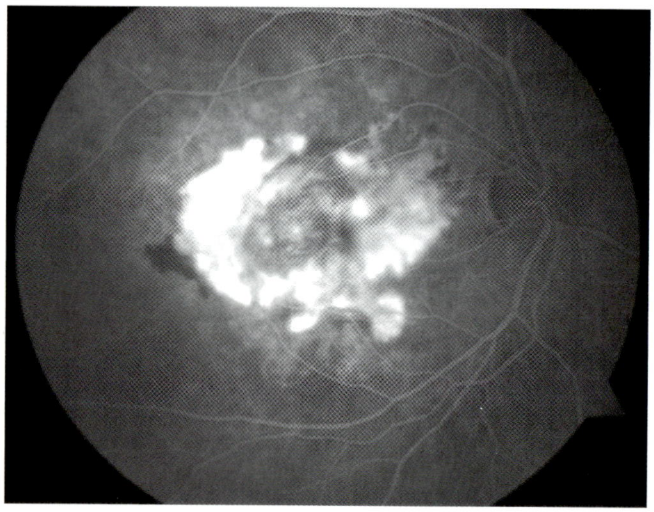

Late arteriovenous phase of the angiogram showing leakage of the dye from the edge of the CVNM

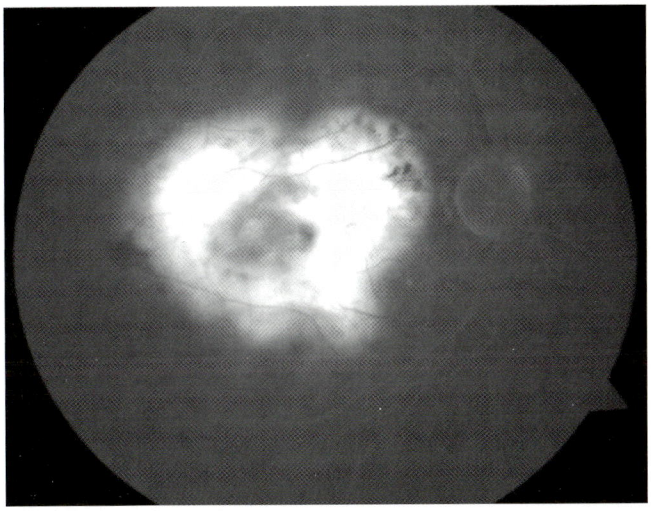

Intense hyperfluorescence is seen in the late phase due to staining of the tissue and due to leakage and pooling of the dye in the subretinal space

COMMENT

Patient has a scarring CNVM with some activity still noted on the angiogram. The vascular network of the CNVM is well-made out even in the mid arteriovenous phase indicating less leakage from the new vessels.

CASE 7

A 75-year-old gentleman presented with diminution of vision in the left eye since two months. BCVA was 6/7.5; N6 in the right eye and 6/18; N6 in the left eye. Clinical examination revealed an occult CNV with subretinal fluid in the left eye. Clinical findings were confirmed on fundus fluorescein angiography and OCT.

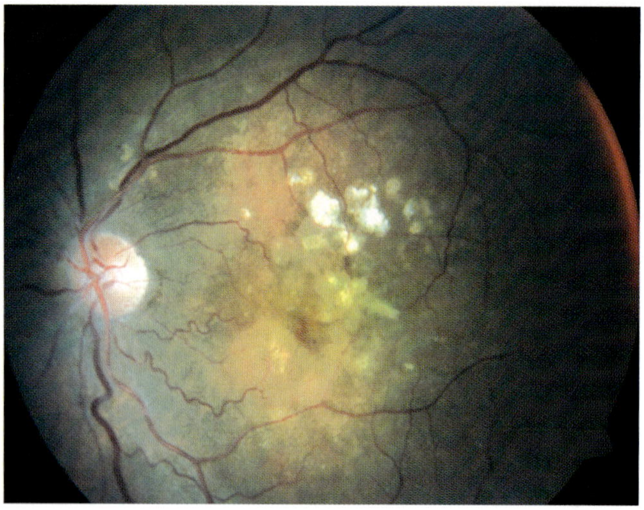

Color fundus photo of the left eye reveals multiple large calcific drusen superior to the fovea, hard drusen close to the fovea and soft drusen inferior to the fovea. Subretinal fluid could be seen involving the fovea and inferior to it

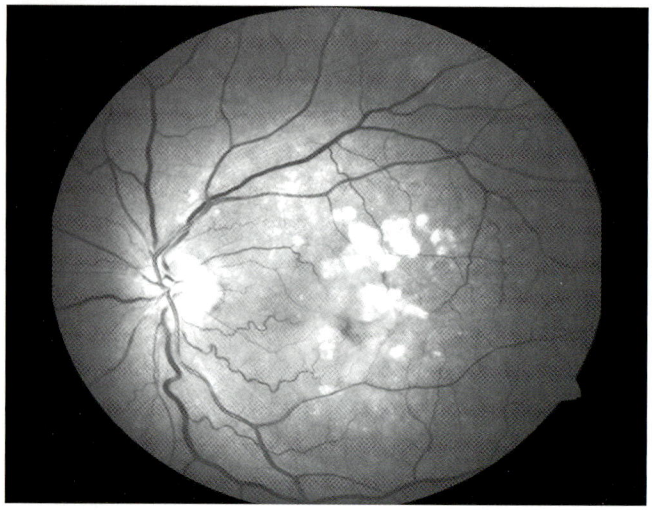

Red free photograph of the left eye highlights the multiple drusen

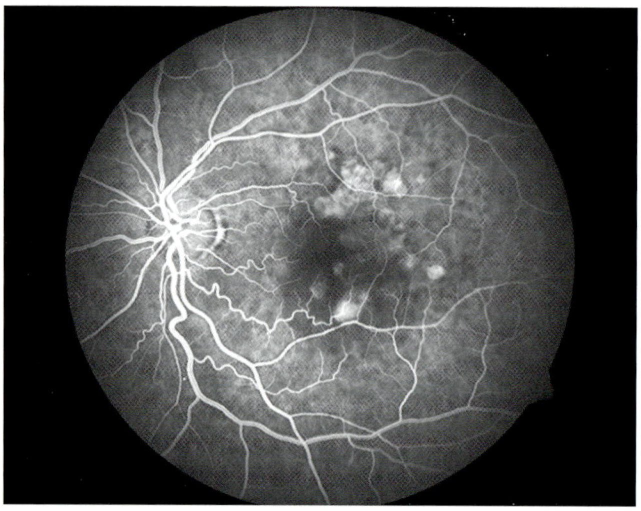

Hyperfluorescence in the mid-AV phase corresponds to the staining of the drusen

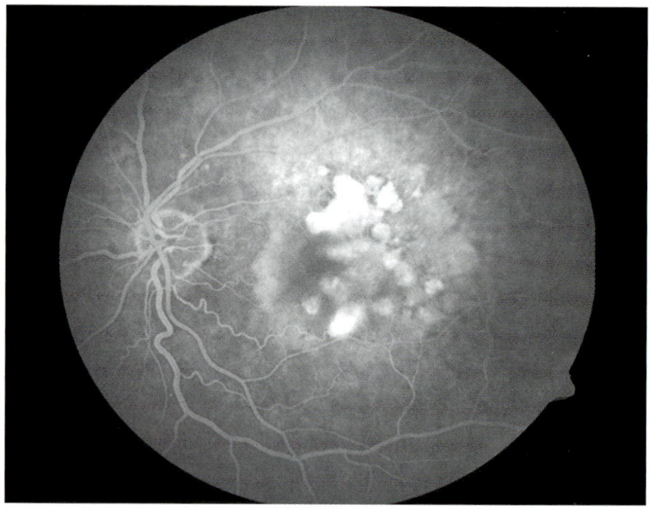

Late AV phase reveals increase in hyperfluorescence due to staining of drusen. There is increased fuzziness noted inferior to the fovea suggestive of late leakage

CASE 7 (*Continued*)

Patient underwent 2 intravitreal injections of bevacizumab in the left eye at one-monthly intervals. Vision stabilized at 6/12; N6 after the second injection.

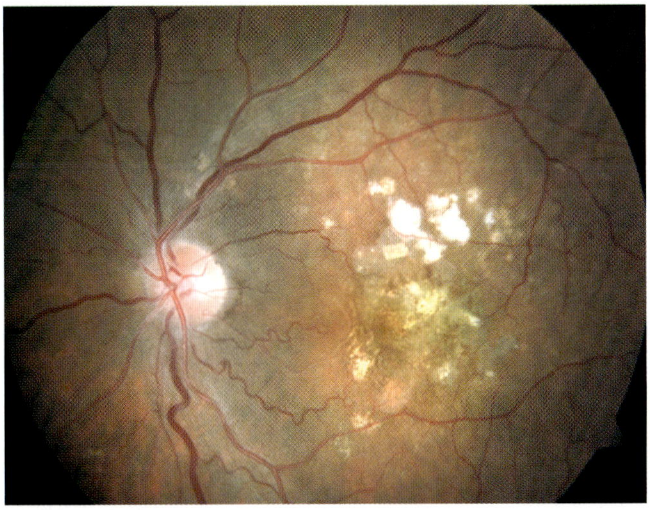

Color fundus photo of the left eye reveals resolution of subretinal fluid

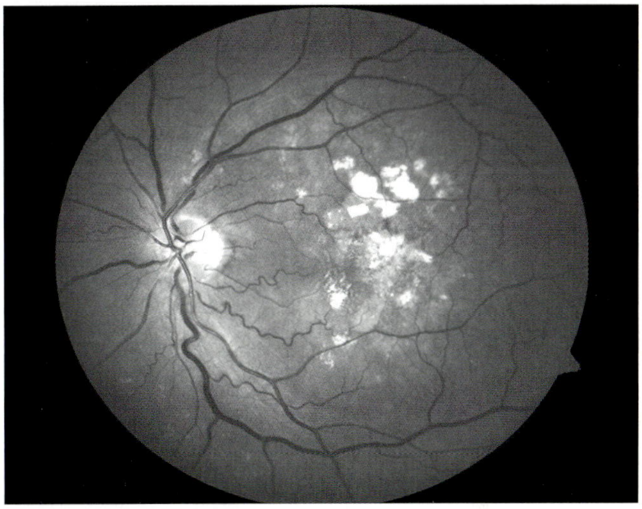

Red free photograph of the left eye

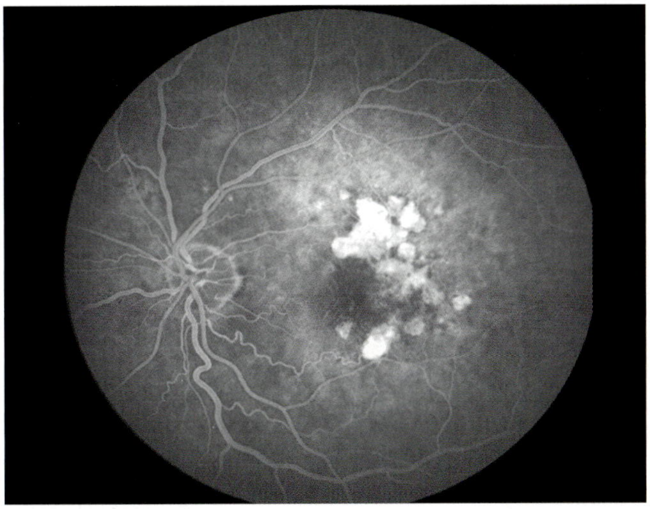

Hyperfluorescence in the mid-AV phase corresponds to the staining of the drusen

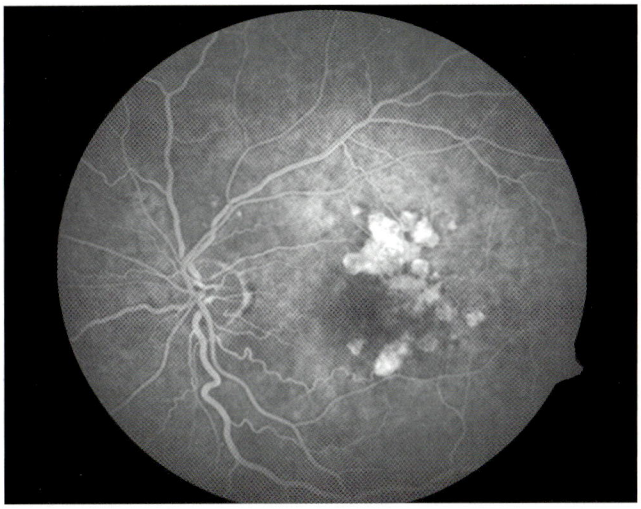

Late AV phase reveals absence of fuzziness previously noted inferior to the fovea. Staining of the drusen can be made out

COMMENT

ANCHOR trial included 423 patients with predominantly *classic* age-related CNVM and found that monthly injections of Ranibizumab (Lucentis) for 2 years was beneficial over PDT alone in preserving vision in more than 90% eyes and improving vision in 40% eyes.

MARINA trial included 716 patients with predominantly *occult* age-related CNVM and found that monthly injections of Ranibizumab (Lucentis) for 2 years was beneficial over sham in preserving vision in more than 90% eyes and improving vision in 30% eyes at 2 years follow-up.

FOCUS trial included 162 patients with predominantly *classic* age-related CNVM and found that combination of PDT followed by monthly injections of Ranibizumab (Lucentis) for 2 years was beneficial over PDT alone in preserving vision in more than 90% eyes and improving vision in 25% eyes.

PIER trial included 184 patients with or without *classic* age-related CNVM and found that monthly injections of Ranibizumab (Lucentis) for 3 months followed by 3 monthly injections for 2 years was beneficial over sham in preserving vision in more than 90% eyes and improving vision in approximately 10% eyes at 2 years follow-up.

PrONTO trial (Prospective OCT Imaging of Patient with Neovascular AMD Treated with intraocular Lucentis) included 40 eyes with subfoveal CNVM and found that initial monthly injections of Ranibizumab for 3 months followed by retreatment on the basis of fixed criteria (variable dosing regimen) lead to maintenance of vision in 90% eyes and improved vision in 40% eyes after 2 years.

CLINICAL NUGGETS

1. Photodynamic therapy can be considered for classic, predominantly classic and fully occult choroidal neovascular membranes.
2. Transpupillary thermotherapy can be a treatment option for occult choroidal neovascular membranes.
3. Newer treatment modalities being tried for ARMD include use of antiangiogenic factors and steroids.
4. The mainstay of treatment is antivascular endothelial growth factor (anti-VEGF) antibodies.
5. Strategies for treatment include pharmacologic monotherapy, combination photodynamic therapy (PDT) and anti-VEGF agents or PDT monotherapy.
6. Preferred treatment regimens include 'treat and extend' or 'loading dose and PRN'.

BIBLIOGRAPHY

1. Abraham P, Yue H, Wilson L. Randomized, double-masked, sham-controlled trial of ranibizumab for neovascular age-related macular degeneration: PIER study 2 years. Am J Ophthalmol 2010; 150: 315-324.e1
2. Antoszyk AN, Tuomi L, Chung CY, Singh A. FOCUS Study Group. Ranibizumab combined with verteporfin photodynamic therapy in neovascular age-related macular degeneration (FOCUS): 2 years results. Am J Ophthalmol 2008; 145: 862-74.
3. Bird AC, Bressler NM, Bressler SB, et al. An international classification and grading system for age-related maculopathy and age-related macular degeneration. Surv Ophthalmol 1995;39:367-76.
4. Bressler NM, Bressler SB, Fine SL. Age related macular degeneration. Surv Ophthalmol 1988;32:375-413.
5. Bressler SB, Bressler NM, Fine SL, et al. Natural course of choroidal neovascular membranes within the foveal avascular zone in senile macular degeneration. Am J Ophthalmol 1982;93:157-63.
6. Brown DM, Michels M, Kaiser PK, Heier JS, Sy JP, Ianchulev T. ANCHOR Study Group. Ranibizumab versus verteporfin photodynamic therapy for neovascular age-related macular degeneration: Two-year results of the ANCHOR study. Ophthalmol. 2009; 116: 57-65.e5
7. Lalwani GA, Rosenfeld PJ, Fung AE, Dubovy SR, Michels S, Feuer W, et al. A variable-dosing regimen with intravitreal ranibizumab for neovascular age-related macular degeneration: 2 years of the PrONTO Study. Am J Ophthalmol 2009; 148: 43-58.e1

8. MPS Group: Argon laser photocoagulation for senile macular degeneration: results of a randomized clinical trial. Arch Ophthalmol 1982;100:912-8.
9. MPS Group: Persistent and recurrent neovascularisation after krypton laser photocoagulation for neovascular lesions of ocular histoplasmosis. Arch Ophthalmol 1989;107:344.
10. MPS Group: Subfoveal neovascular lesions in age-related macular degenerations. Guidelines for evaluation and treatment in the macular photocoagulation study. Arch Ophthalmol 1991;109:1242.
11. MPS Group: Visual outcome after laser photocoagulation for subfoveal choroidal neovascularisation secondary to age-related macular degeneration: the influence of initial lesion size and initial visual acuity. Arch Ophthalmol 1994;112:480-88.
12. Rishi P, Sen PR, Shroff D, Chhablani J. Combined photodynamic therapy and intravitreal ranibizumab as primary treatment for choroidal neovascularization associated with age-related macular degeneration in an Indian patient. Indian J Ophthalmol 2008; 56(5): 438-9.
13. Rosenfeld PJ, Brown DM, Heier JS, et al. MARINA Study Group. Ranibizumab for neovascular age-related macular degeneration. N Engl J Med 2006; 355:1419-31.
14. Sylus SO, Bressler NM, Maguire MG, Sacheat AP, Bressler SB. Detecting recurrent choroidal neovascularisation: comparison of clinical exam with and without fundus fluorescein angiography. Arch Ophthalmol 1994;111:1561-6.

Chapter 14

Retinal Angiomatous Proliferans

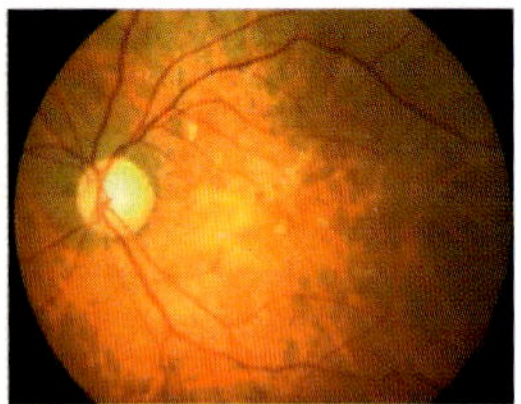

- Retinal angiomatous proliferans (RAP) is a newly recognized disorder in patients with age-related macular degeneration
- Patients tend to be older and more commonly white
- Among patients previously diagnosed as exudative AMD, RAP may represent 8 to 22% of newly diagnosed cases and up to 25% of occult or minimally classic
- The initial lesion itself is always extrafoveal presumably because of the foveal capillary-free zone
- It is designated as Type 3 neovascularization
- It may have a rapidly progressive natural course leading to significant functional loss of vision
- Yannuzzi et al have proposed a three-stage evolution of these lesions. The proposed origin of RAP is supposed to be from intraretinal neovascularization
- *Stage I:* Intraretinal neovascularization (IRN).
- *Stage II:* Subretinal neovascularization with retinoretinal anastomosis with PED.
- *Stage III:* Choroidal neovascularization with vascularized PED and retinochoroidal anastomosis (RCA).

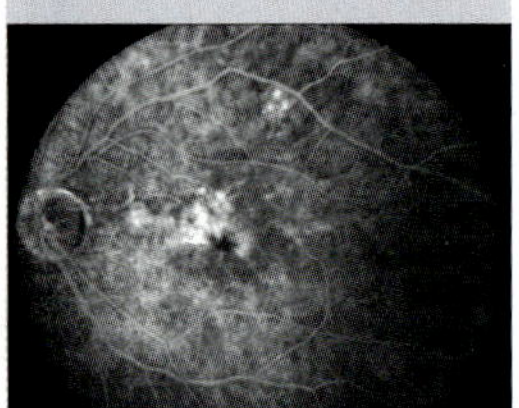

- *Stage I:* Fluorescein angiogram shows focal area of intraretinal staining with indistinct borders corresponding to the IRN and surrounding intraretinal edema
- *Stage II:* Fluorescein angiogram shows indistinct zone of staining within and beneath the retina, hyperfluorescence due to pooling into a serous PED, blockage of fluorescence corresponding to an intraretinal hemorrhage and thereby resembles occult CNV
- *Stage III:* Fluorescein angiogram shows leakage from the CNV and staining of the surrounding PED. (Picture resembling occult CNV).

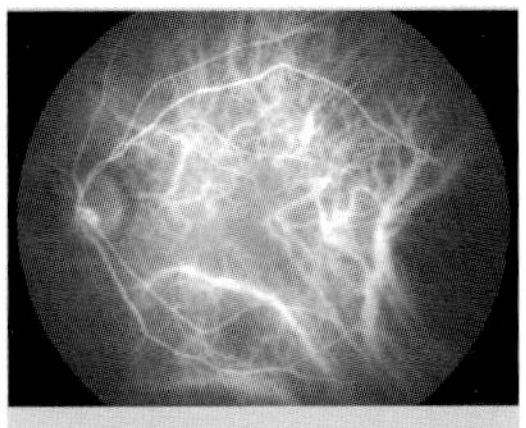

ICG-A shows neovascularization arising from retinal capillaries and dilation of retinal vessels.

- *Stage I:* ICG angiography shows dilatation of retinal vessels and a focal area of intense hyperfluorescence within the retina, or a hot spot at the site of the IRN
- *Stage II:* Indocyanine green angiography shows a distinct focal area of intense hyperfluorescence ("hot spot") corresponding to intraretinal neovascularization. Also may show anastomoses with retinal vessels. The hot spot can be seen in the hypofluorescence of a serous PED
- *Stage III:* ICG-A is very useful for detecting RCA. Best imaged during the mid and late phases of the ICG angiography when they become increasingly hyperfluorescent as dye leaks intraretinally. Unlike polypoidal CNV, RAP usually does not exhibit a washout of dye in the late-phase ICG study.

  High speed ICG can also show the direction of blood flow

  Rouvas et al recently has described 5 different patterns of RAP on basis of ICG namely focal, irregular, circular, multimodal and combined hyperfluorescence.

STAGE 1—RETINAL ANGIOMATOUS PROLIFERANS

CASE 1

A 75-year-old man presented with defective vision in both eyes since the last 8 months. His BCVA was 6/60; N10 in right eye and 6/24; N8 in left eye. Evaluation showed chronic CME in the right eye with RPE changes and subfoveal CNVM in the left.

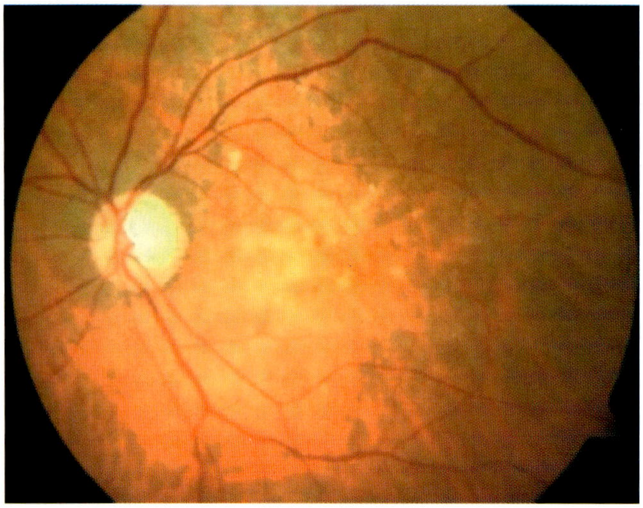

Color fundus photograph of left eye shows a retinal vessel dipping into retina superonasal to fovea with intraretinal hemorrhage at this point. Retinal edema is seen at macula

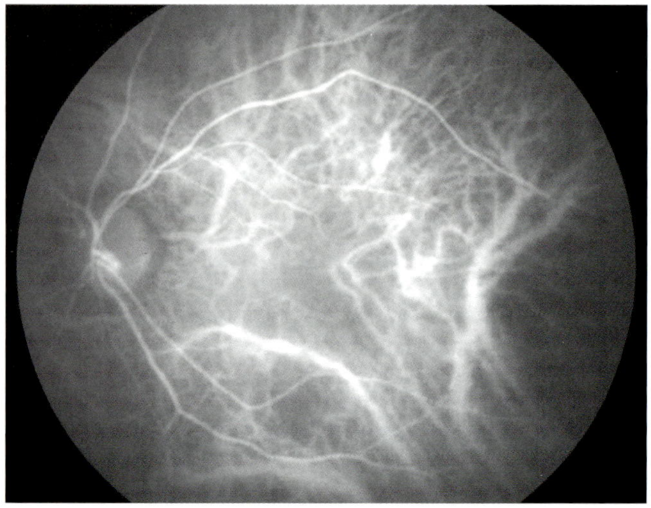

Indocyanine green angiography shows area of hyperfluorescence in the area of the lesion

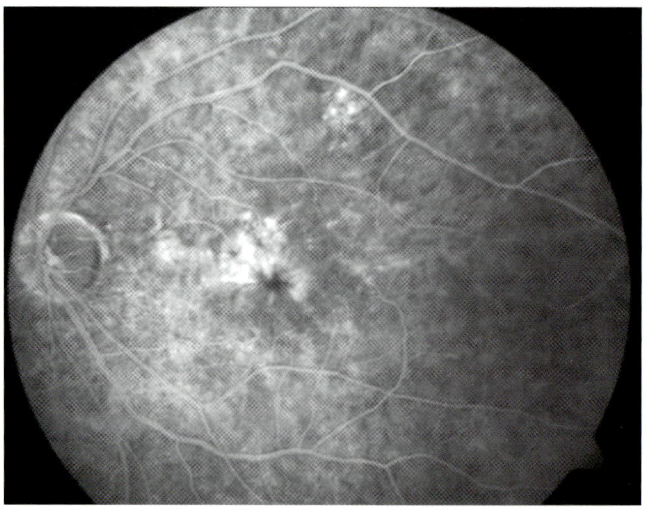

Fluorescein angiography late phase shows the dipping retinal vessel with hyperfluorescence around it with presence of cystoid macular edema

STAGE 2—RETINAL ANGIOMATOUS PROLIFERANS

CASE 1

Right eye of the same patient as described above.

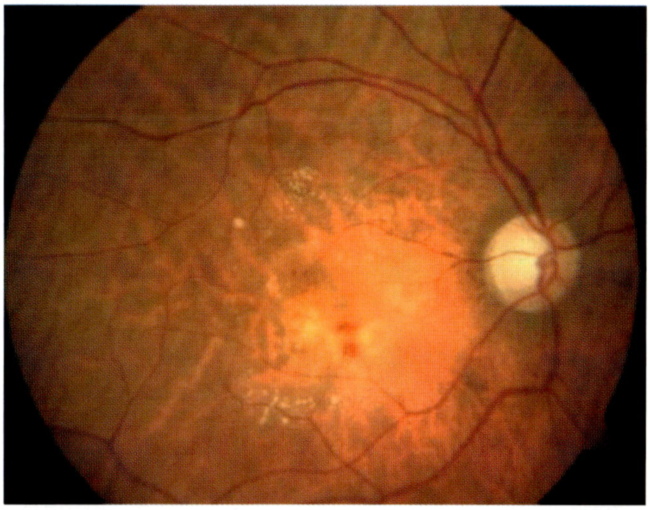

Color fundus photo of right eye shows a retinal vessel dipping into retina superonasal to fovea with intraretinal hemorrhage at this point. Intraretinal hemorrhages seen inferonasal to fovea. Retinal edema is seen at the macula. Localized hard exudates are seen around the lesion

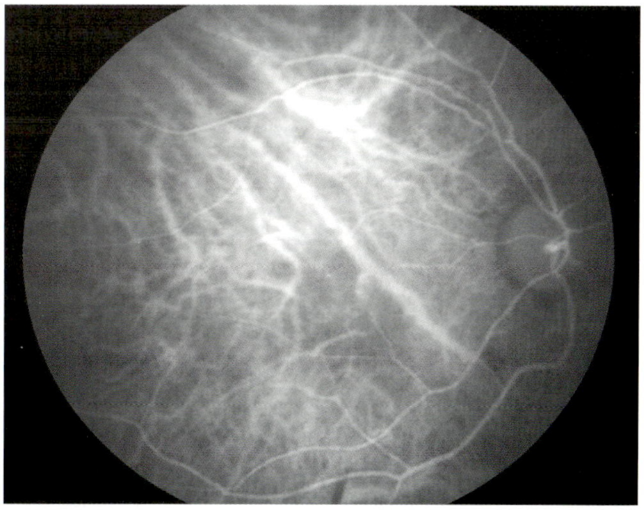

Indocyanine green angiography shows retinal vessel anastomosis and a spot of hyperfluorescence at the site of lesion

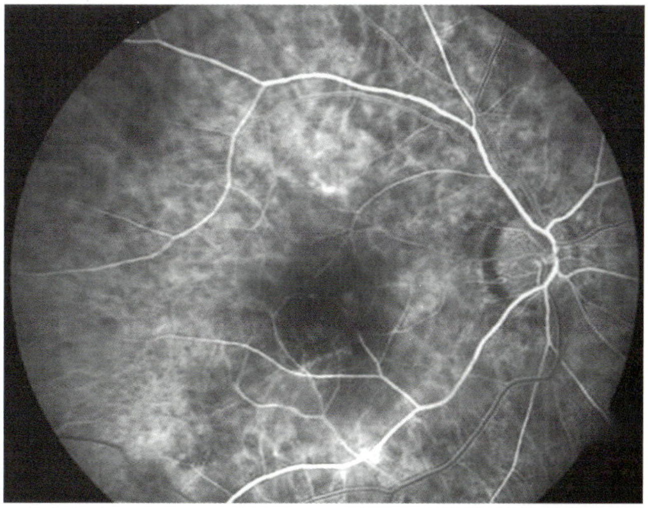

Fluorescein angiography early phase shows dilated retinal capillaries inferonasal to fovea with anastomosis of retinal vessels nasal to fovea

STAGE 3—RETINAL ANGIOMATOUS PROLIFERANS

CASE 1

A 54-year-old lady presented with defective vision in both eyes since 1 year. At presentation, her BCVA was 6/24; N12 in the right eye and 6/60; N36 in the left. Clinical evaluation revealed CNVM in both eyes that were confirmed on FFA. The patient underwent PDT in both eyes.

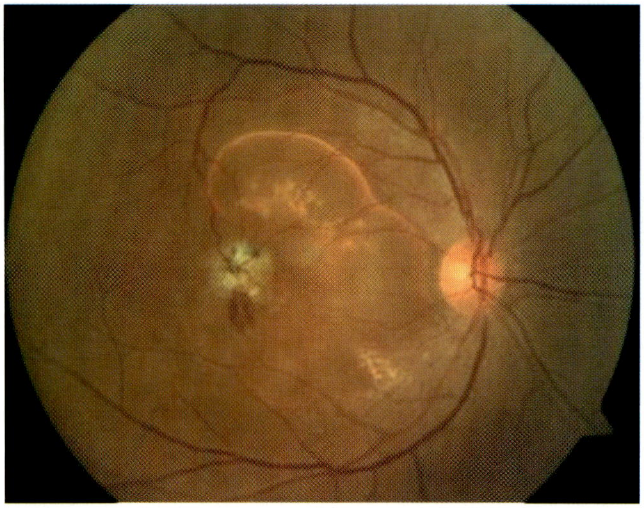

Color fundus photograph of right eye shows CNV temporal to fovea with retinal vessel dipping into the center with a large serous pigment epithelial detachment adjacent to it. A superficial retinal hemorrhage is seen inferior to CNV and at the site of CNV

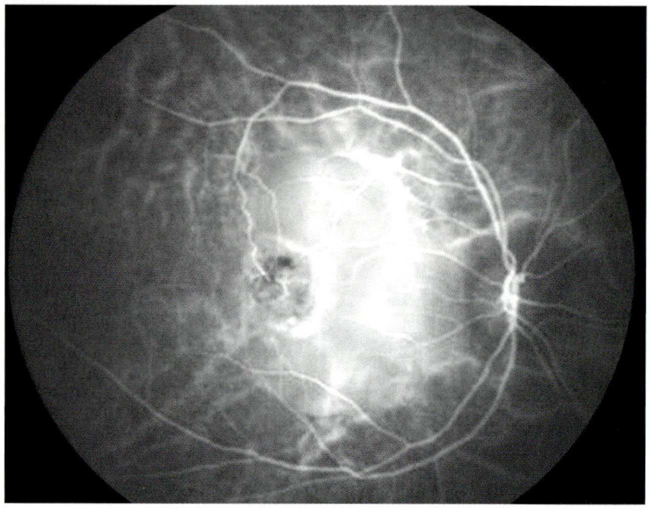

Indocyanine green angiography shows hyperfluorescence of pigment epithelial detachment and retinochoroidal anastomosis in the area of CNV

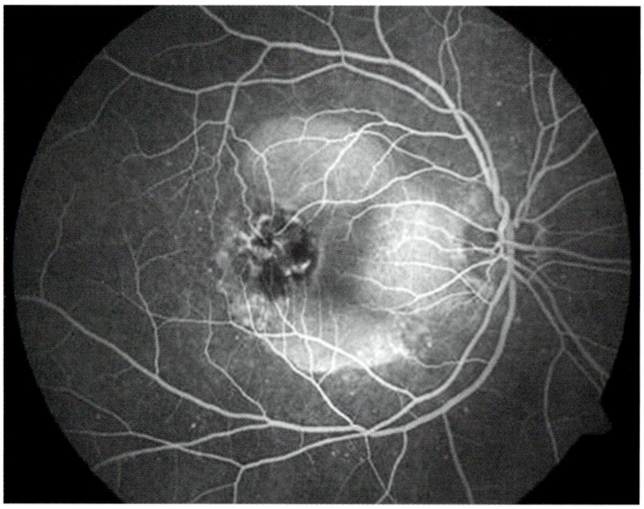

Fluorescein angiography arteriovenous phase shows dipping retinal vessel with hyperfluorescence around it due to CNV with uniform hyperfluorescence of pigment epithelial detachment. Blocked fluorescence from the hemorrhage component is seen inferior to CNV

NATURAL COURSE OF RETINAL ANGIOMATOUS PROLIFERANS (RAP)

CASE 1

This is the same 75-year-old gentleman as described above in Stage 1 RAP, who presented with visual acuity of 6/60; N10 in the right eye. The patient did not undergo any treatment and was reviewed one year after the initial visit.

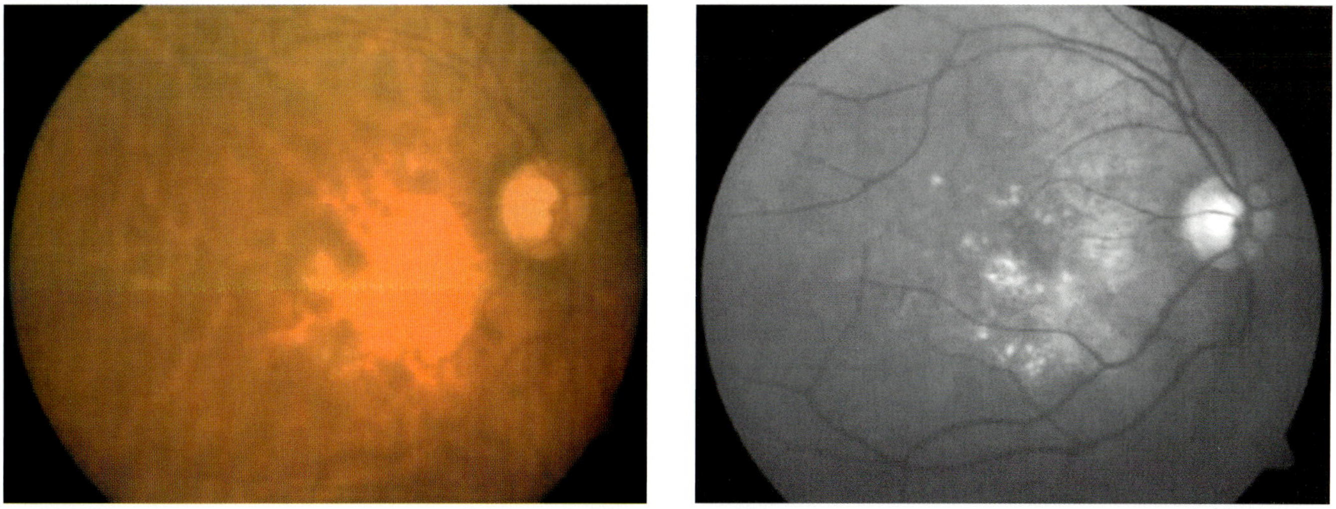

Color fundus photograph and red free photograph of right eye shows RPE alterations mainly inferior to the fovea

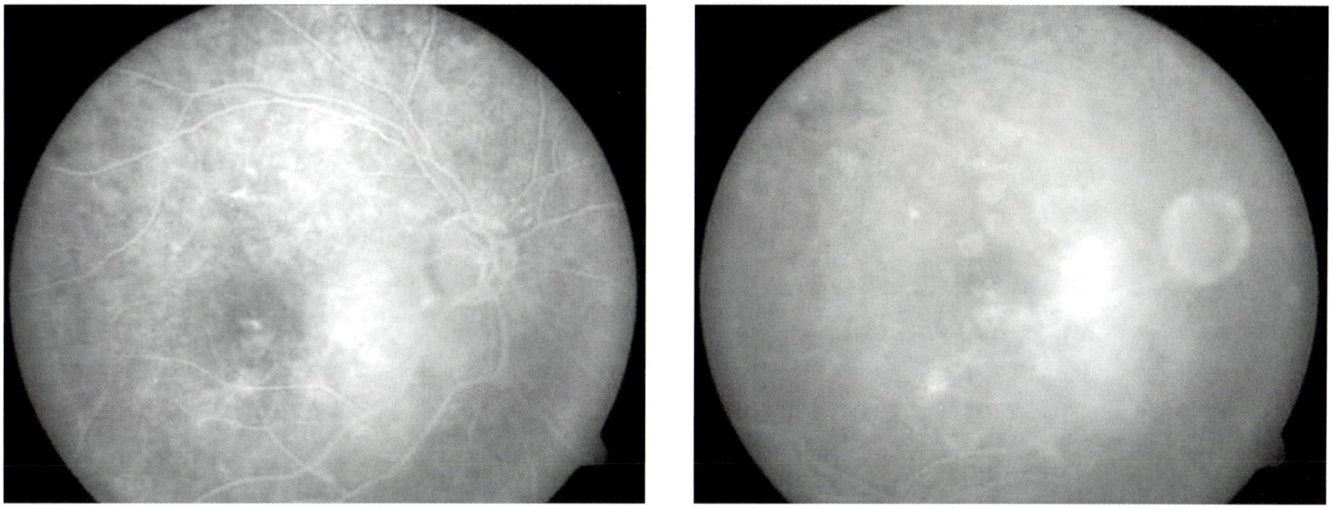

Fluorescein angiography in late phase shows area of hyperfluorescence inferior to fovea with indistinct borders

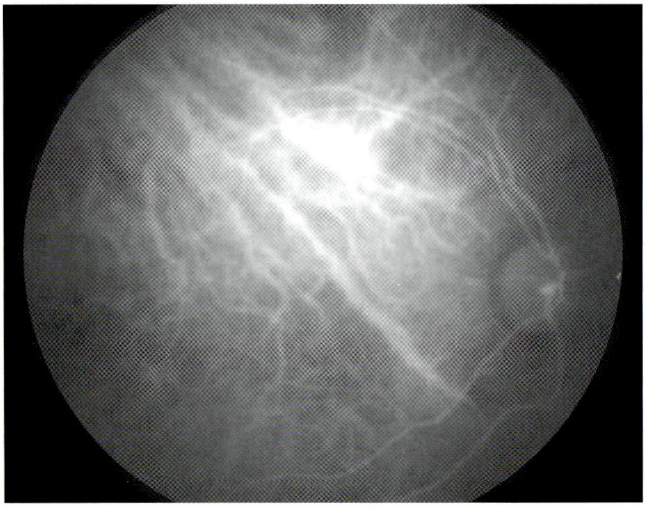

Indocyanine green angiography appears normal

1 year later

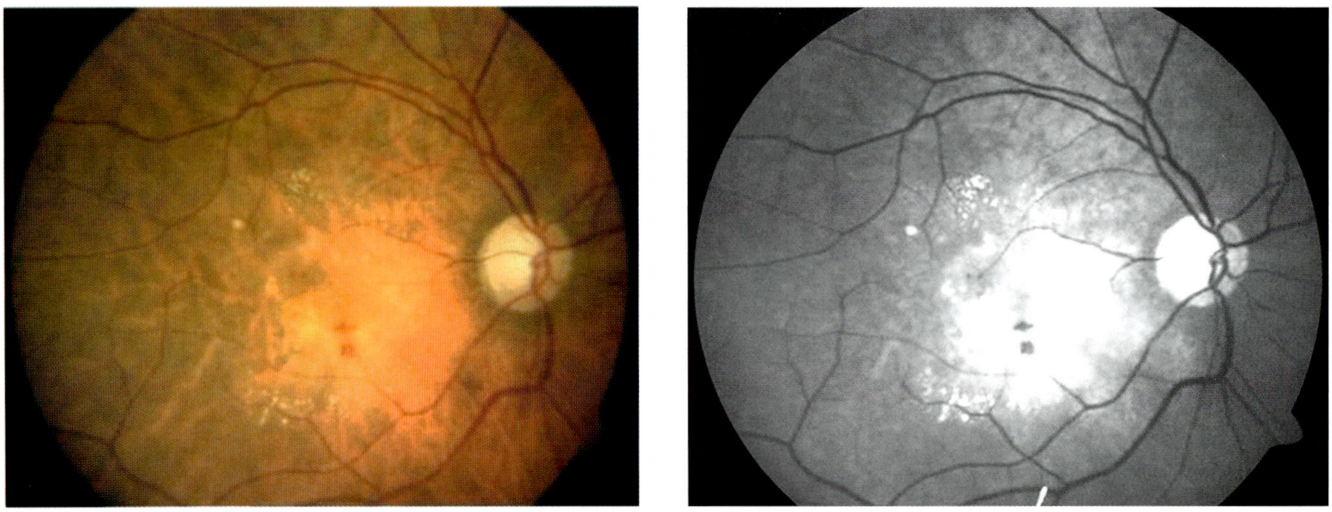

Color fundus and red free photograph of right eye shows a retinal vessel dipping into the retina superonasal to the fovea with intraretinal hemorrhage at this point. Superficial retinal hemorrhages also seen inferonasal to the fovea. Retinal edema is seen at macula. Localized hard exudates are seen around the lesion

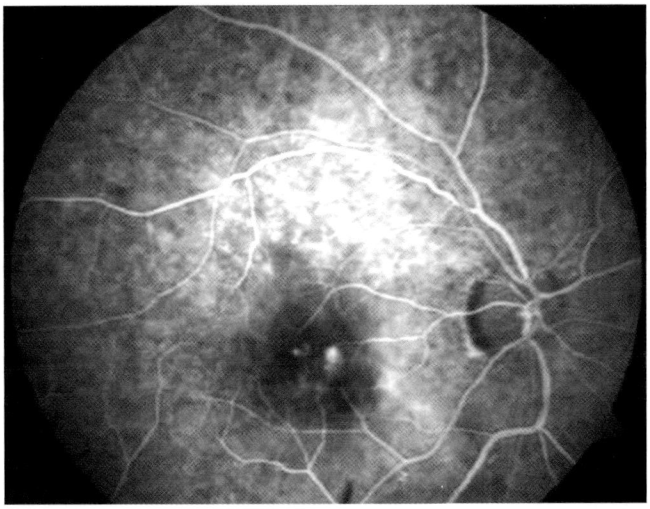

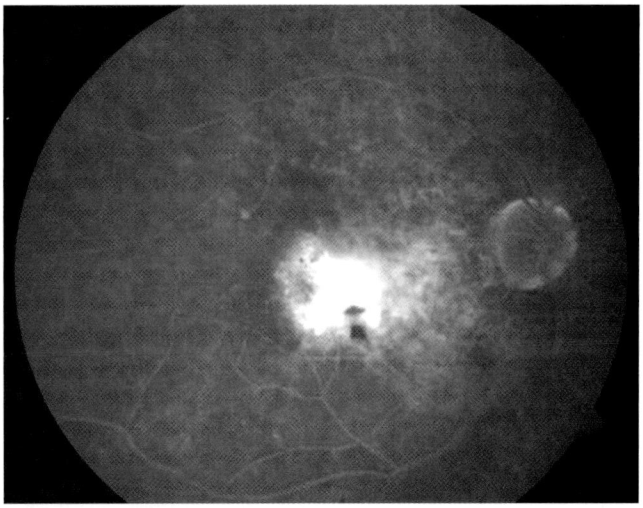

Fluorescein angiography early phase shows dilated retinal capillaries inferonasal to fovea with retinal vessel dipping in retina nasal to fovea with hyperfluorescence at the site of dipping. Late phase shows intense hyperfluorescence due to leak from CNV and cystoid macular edema with blocked fluorescence from hemorrhage

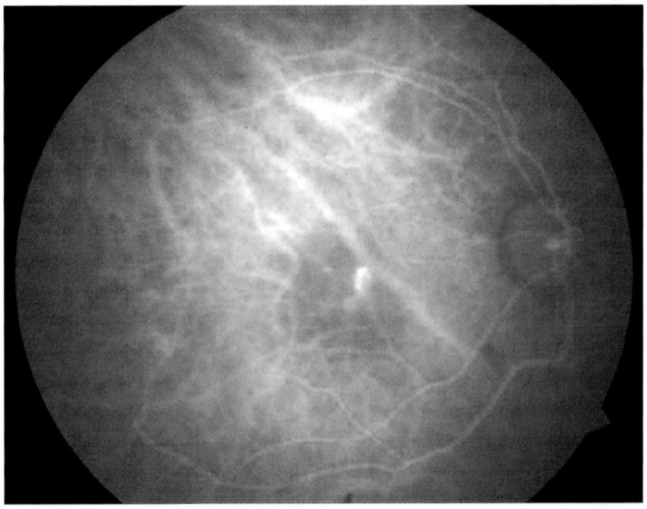

Indocyanine green angiography in late phase shows hyperfluorescent spot (hot spot) at site of lesion

CLINICAL SUSPICION OF RETINAL ANGIOMATOUS PROLIFERANS (RAP)

CASE 1

This patient is a 65-year-old gentleman, who presented with sudden visual blurring in his left eye since 4 months. His BCVA at presentation was 6/60; N36 in the left eye and 6/6; N6 in the right eye. Clinical evaluation and imaging revealed subfoveal active CNV in the left eye associated with RAP lesion.

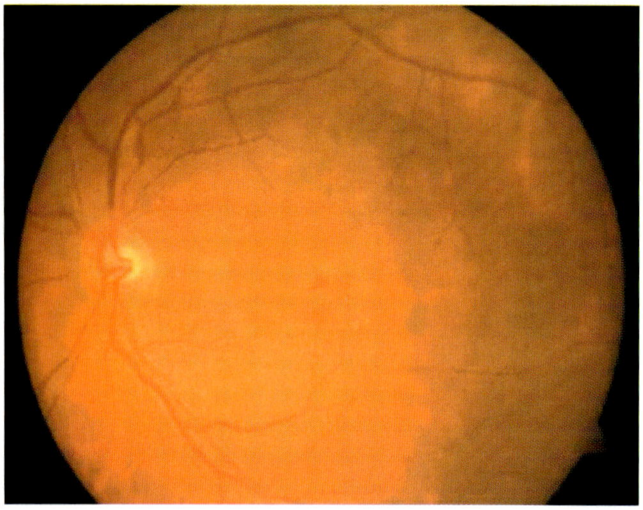

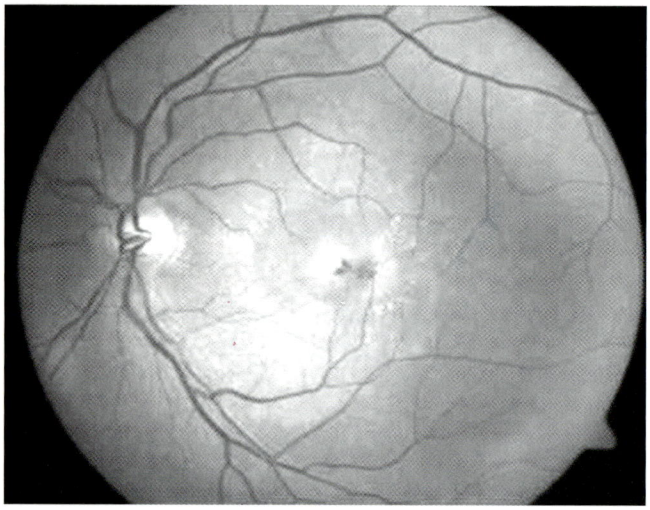

Color fundus and red free photograph of left eye shows serous pigment epithelial detachment at fovea with intraretinal hemorrhages and retinal vessels dipping in the lesion

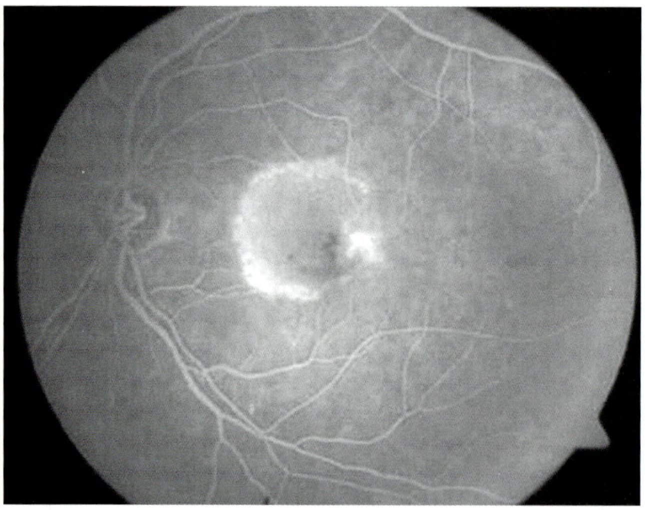

Fluorescein angiogram late phase shows hyperfluorescence from pigment epithelial detachment with blocked fluorescence from hemorrhage component of lesion at the edge of the pigment epithelial detachment

CASE 2

The left eye of the same 54-year-old lady as described above in Stage 3 RAP lesion. At presentation, her BCVA was 6/24; N12 in right eye and 6/60; N36 in the left eye. She underwent PDT in both eyes.

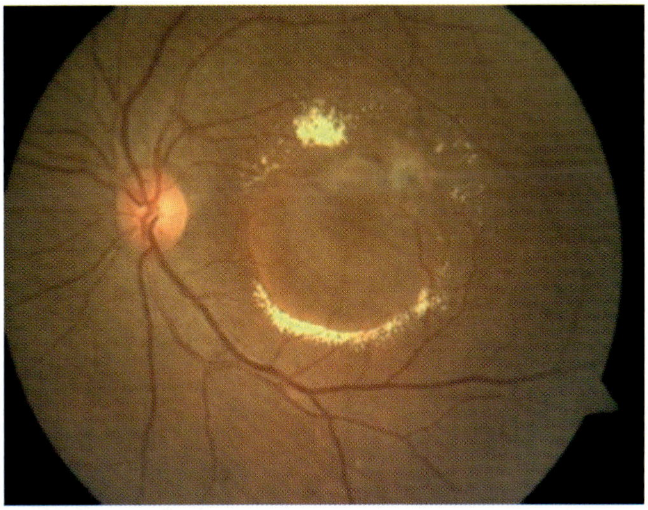

Color fundus photograph of the left eye shows large serous pigment epithelial detachment with CNV adjacent to PED superotemporal to fovea. Hard exudates are seen at the margins of pigment epithelial detachment. Superficial retinal hemorrhage is seen at the site of CNV

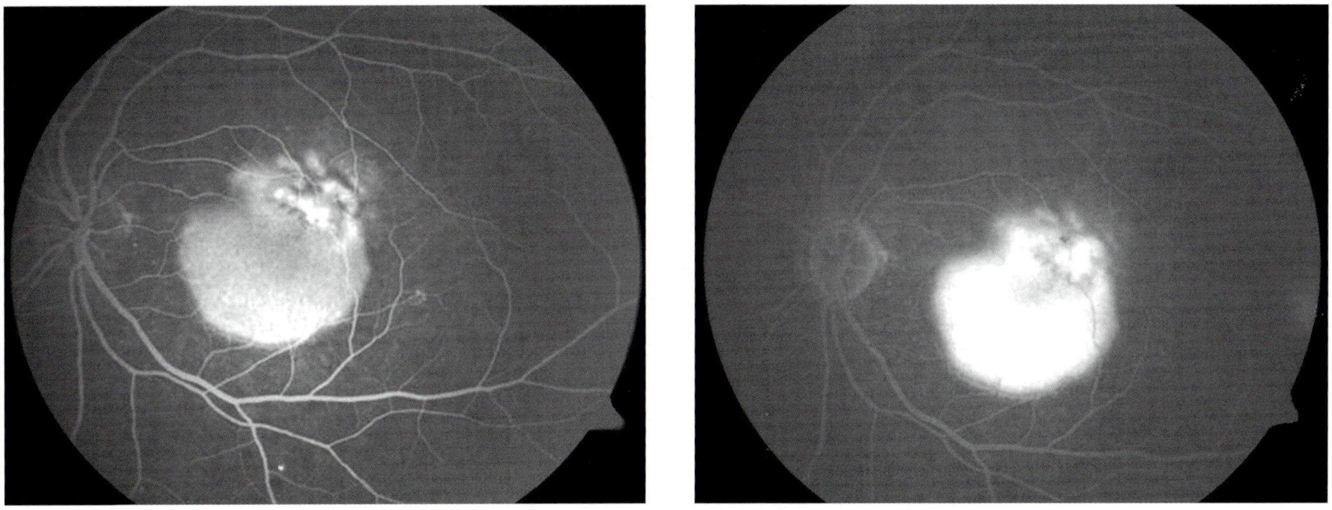

Fluorescein angiography in arteriovenous phase shows uniform hyperfluorescence of pigment epithelial detachment. Filling of CNV can be seen at this phase with increasing hyperfluorescence and fuzziness of borders at late phase due to leakage. Late phase shows pooling of the dye in pigment epithelial detachment

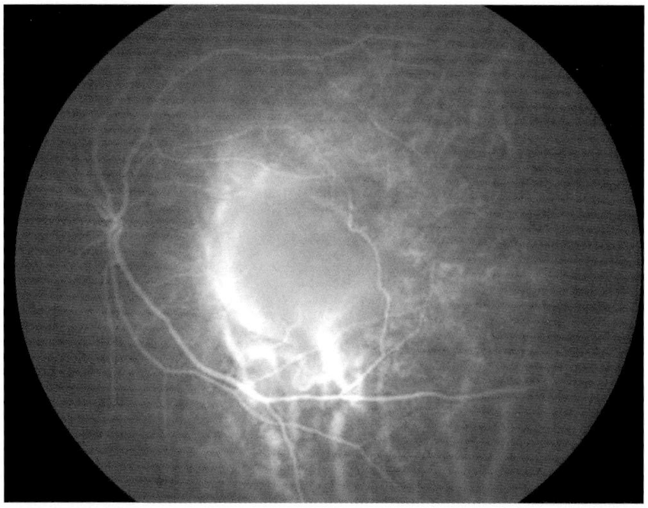

Indocyanine green angiography shows hyperfluorescence of pigment epithelial detachment with retinal vessel anastomosis in the area of CNV

CASE 3

This 76-year-old lady presented with poor vision in right eye, noticed since one week. Her BCVA was 2/60; N18 in right eye and 6/9; N6 in the left. Clinical evaluation revealed subfoveal CNVM with RAP lesion. Clinical findings were confirmed on FFA, OCT and ICG.

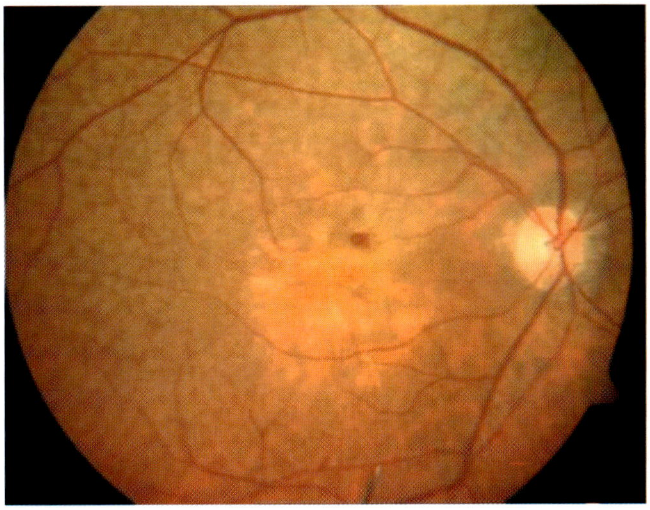

Color fundus photograph of right eye shows a retinal vessel dipping into retina superonasal to fovea with intraretinal hemorrhage at this point. Retinal edema is seen at macula

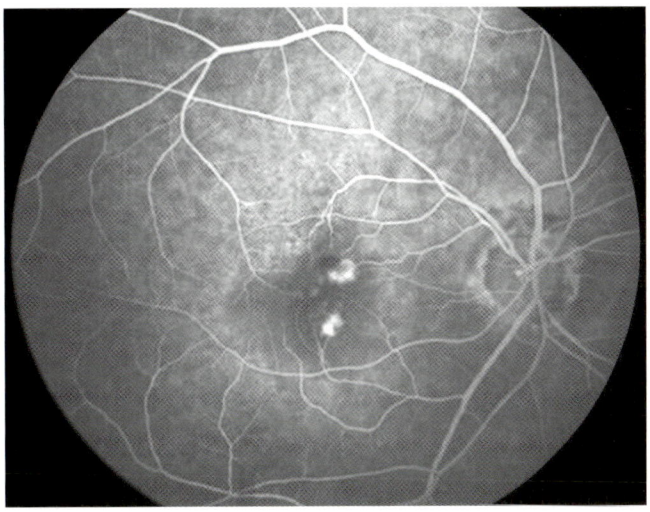

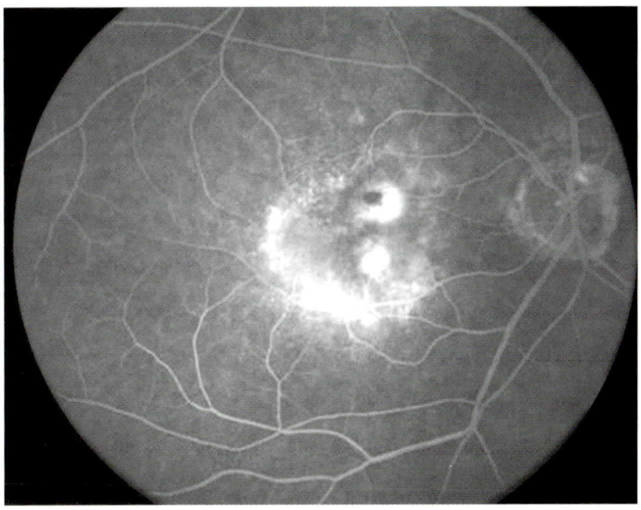

Fluorescein angiography shows the dipping retinal vessel with hyperfluorescence around it. Also hyperfluorescence is seen inferior to fovea. Late phase shows increase in hyperfluorescence with fuzziness of borders suggestive of leakage. Blocked fluorescence is seen due to the hemorrhage. Area of hyperfluorescence around the lesion is seen due to retinal edema

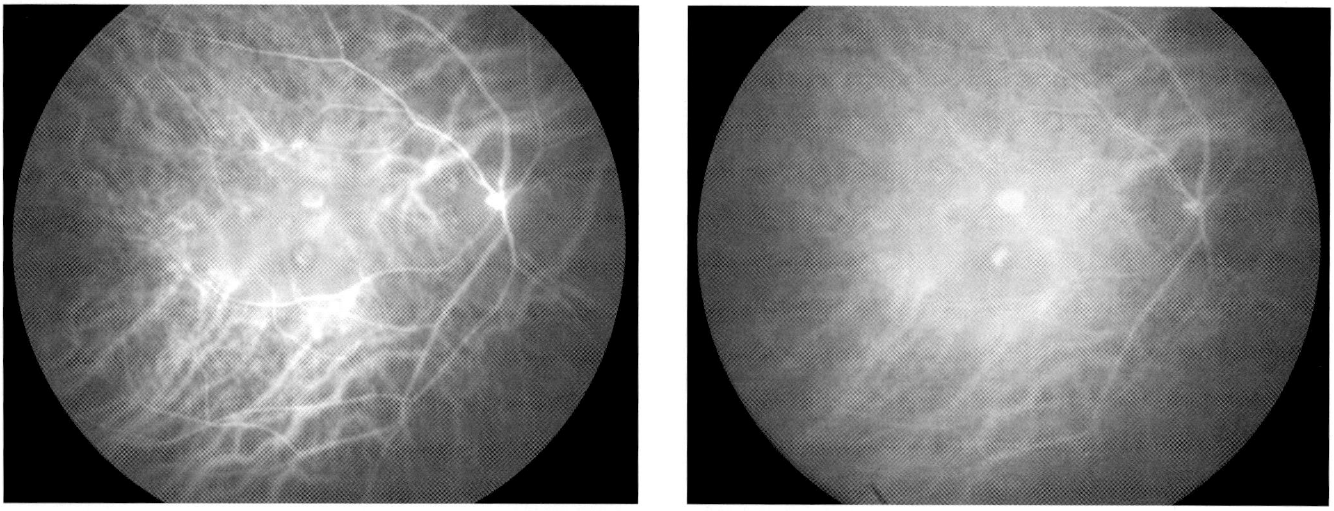

Indocyanine green angiography shows 2 spots of hyperfluorescence in the area of the lesion persisting in late phase (Hot spot)

CASE 4

This 77-year-old lady presented with a gradual diminution of vision in both eyes since 2 to 3 years. Her BCVA at presentation was 6/60; N36 in right eye and 6/9; N12 in the left. Fundus evaluation revealed the presence of foveal RAP lesion with PED and CME that was confirmed on FFA.

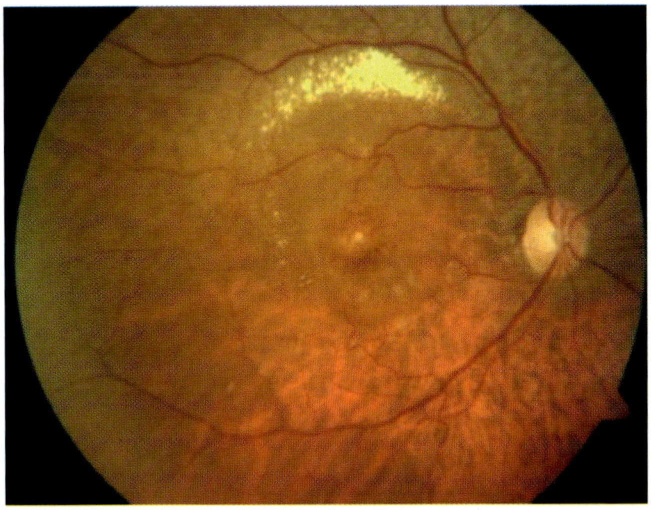

Color fundus photograph of the right eye shows large serous pigment epithelial detachment with subfoveal CNV with retinal vessel dipping in the lesion superonasally. Hard exudates are seen superiorly at margins of pigment epithelial detachment. Superficial retinal hemorrhage is seen at the site of CNV along with dilated retinal capillaries

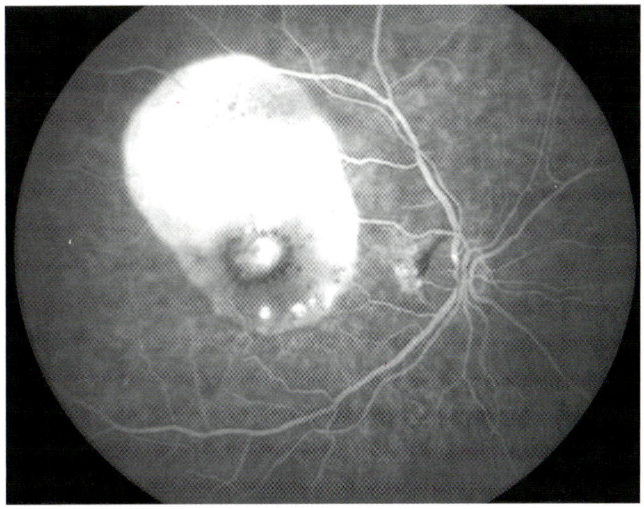

Fluorescein angiography shows hyperfluorescence due to pooling in the pigment epithelial detachment. Hyperfluorescence is also seen due to filling of the CNV; surrounded by blocked fluorescence due to hemorrhages with retinal vessel dipping into it

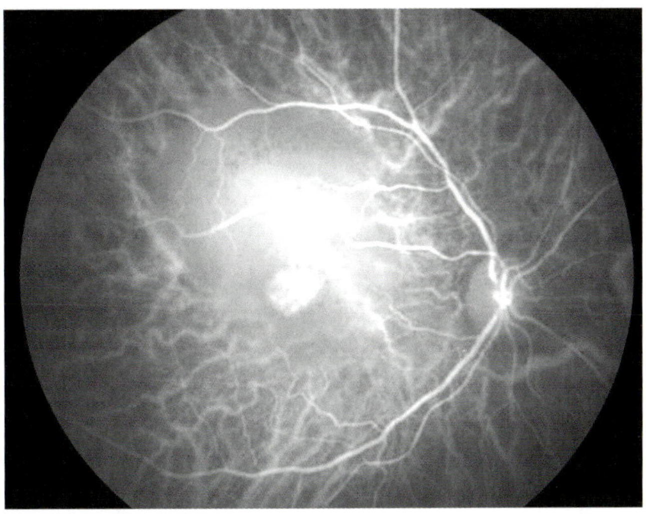

Indocyanine green angiography shows hyperfluorescence of the pigment epithelial detachment and hyperfluorescence in the area of lesion with retinal vessel dipping

BIBLIOGRAPHY

1. Barbazetto IA, Koizumi H, Laud K, Ferrara D, Matsumoto Y, Sorenson JA, Yannuzzi L. Type 3 neovascularization: the expanded spectrum of retinal angiomatous proliferans. Freund KB, Ho IV, Retina 2008; 28(2):201-11.
2. Fernandes LH, Freund KB, Yannuzzi LA, Spaide RF, Huang SJ, Slakter JS, Soreson JA. The nature of focal areas of hyperfluorescence or 'hot spots' imaged with indocyanine green angiography. Retina 2002; 22:557-68.
3. Gass JDM, Agarwal A, Lavina A, et al. Focal inner retinal hemorrhages in patients with drusen: An early sign of occult choroidal neovascularization and chorioretinal anastomosis. Retina 2003;23:741-51.
4. Rouvas AA, Papakostas TD, Ntouraki A, Douvali M, Vergados I, Ladas ID. Angiographic and OCT features of retinal angiomatous proliferans. Eye (Lond) 2010; 24(11):1633-42.
5. Yannuzzi LA, Freund KB, Takahashi BS. Review of retinal angiomatous proliferans or type 3 neovascularization. Retina. 2008; 28(3):375-84.
6. Yannuzzi LA, Freund KB, Takahashi BS. Review of retinal angiomatous proliferans or type 3 neovascularization. Retina. 2008; 28(3):375-84.
7. Yannuzzi LA, Negrao S, Iida T, et al. Retinal angiomatous proliferans in age related Macular degeneration. Retina 2001;21:416-34.

15

Chapter

Polypoidal Choroidal Vasculopathy

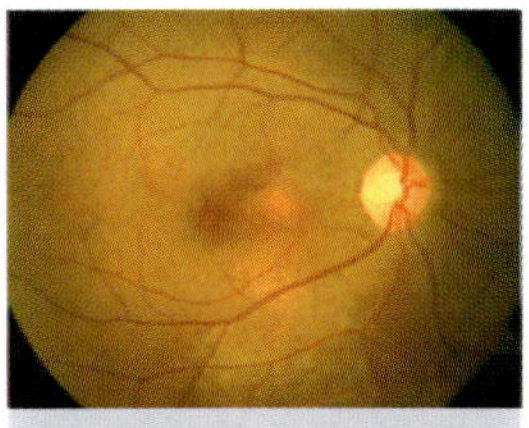

- The lesion in polypoidal choroidal vasculopathy (PCV) arises from the inner choroidal plexus and consists of a network of choroidal vessels which terminate in spheroidal, polyp-like lesions.
- Clinically, the polyps are seen as orange-red subretinal nodules.
- Patients usually present with hemorrhagic pigment epithelial detachments associated with hard exudates.

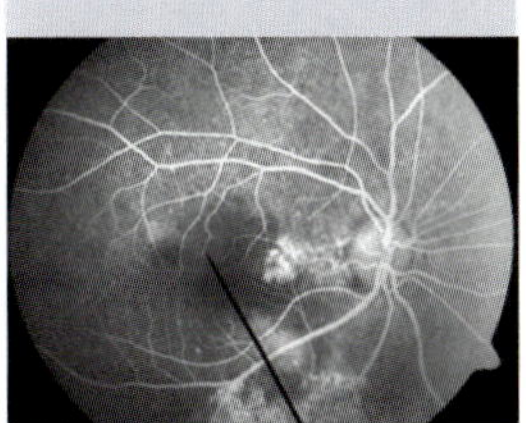

- Fluorescein angiogram shows areas of stippled hyperfluorescence in the region of the polyps which increases in intensity and may become fuzzy in the late films.
- Occasionally, polyps may be seen in the fluorescein angiogram.

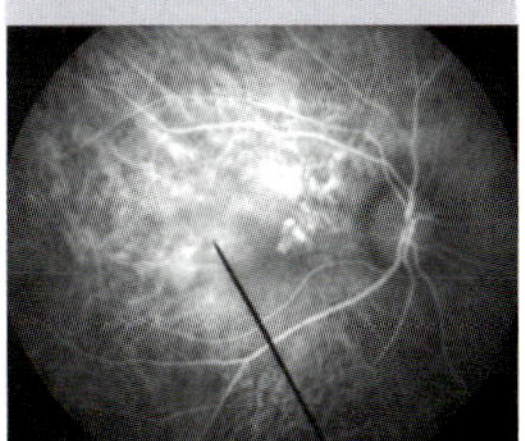

- ICG angiogram is essential for detecting the choroidal network of vessels and the polyps.
- Polyps may not be seen in the early phase of the ICG.
- In the midphase they are seen to appear usually in clusters at the termination of the choroidal network of vessels. Occasionally the polyp may be solitary and large.
- Late phase angiogram shows either a washout of the dye from the polyp with staining of its walls or may show retention of the dye within the polyp with leakage into the surrounding tissue.

CASE 1

A 64-year-old male presented with hazy vision in the left eye for the past six months; visual acuity was 6/12; N8.

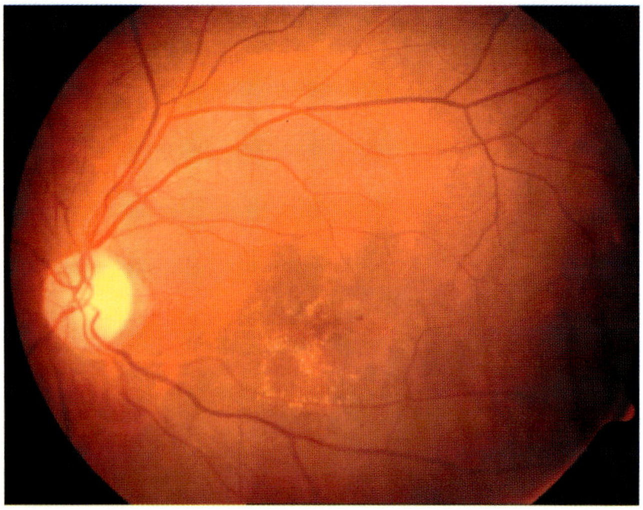

Fundus photograph of the left eye showing orange-red subretinal lesion inferior and inferotemporal to the foveal center. Associated minimal hard exudates are also seen

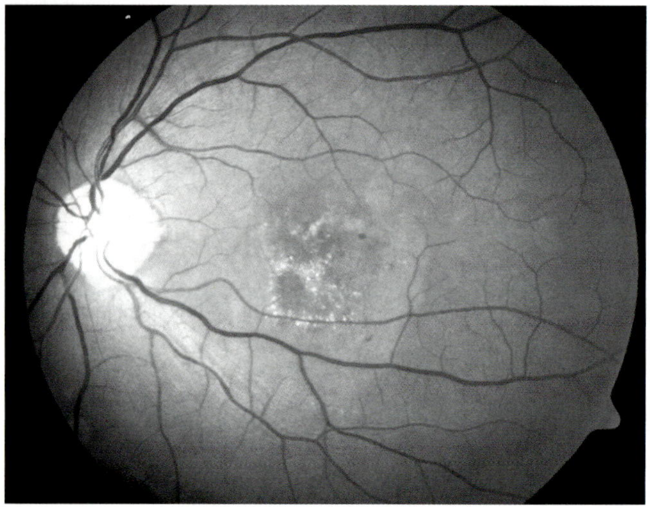

Red free photograph of the left eye

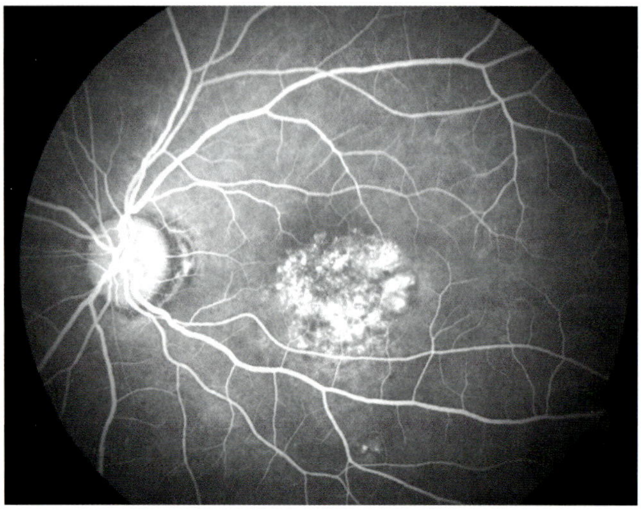

Arteriovenous phase shows a stippled hyperfluorescence at the fovea. Small polyp like lesions can be made out temporally

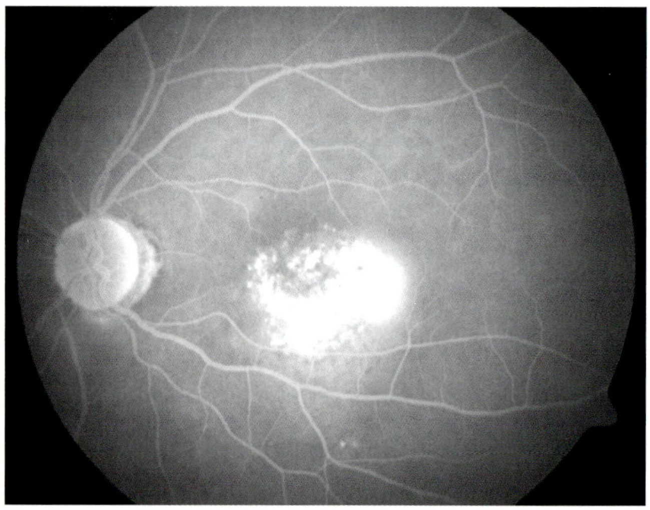

Late phase shows increased fuzzy hyperfluorescence especially temporally indicative of leakage of dye from the polyps

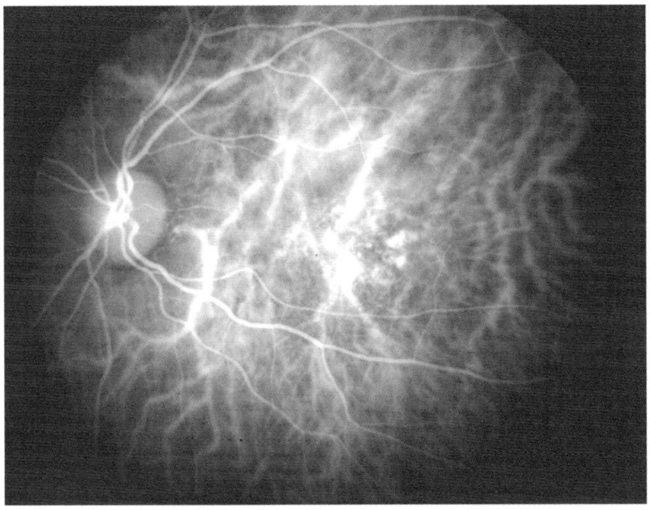

Midphase ICG angiography shows a small central network of choroidal vessels terminating as polyps at the periphery. The temporal polyps are more prominent

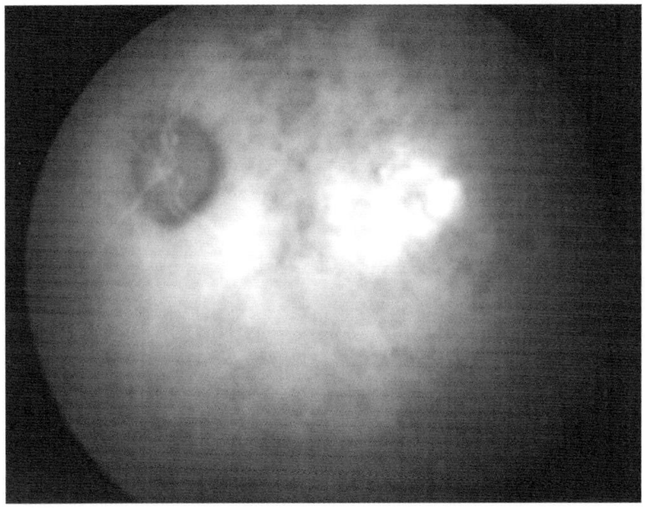

Late phase ICG angiogram showing some leakage of the dye from the temporal polyps

CASE 2

A 62-year-old male presented with reduced vision in the left eye for the past two months; visual acuity was 6/9; N8.

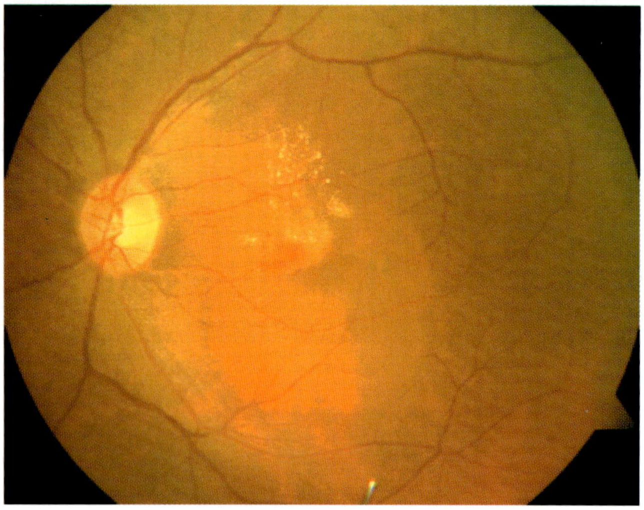

Fundus photograph of the left eye showing orange-red subretinal lesion just nasal to the foveal center. A pocket of subretinal fluid is noted in the inferior macula. Hard exudates are seen superiorly

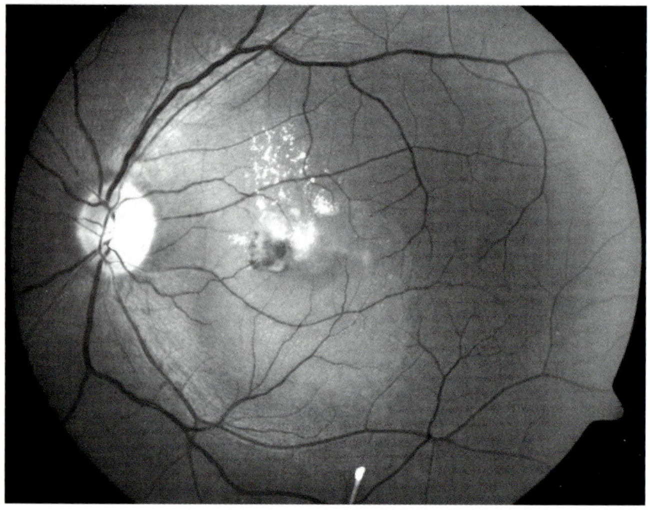

Red free photograph of the left eye

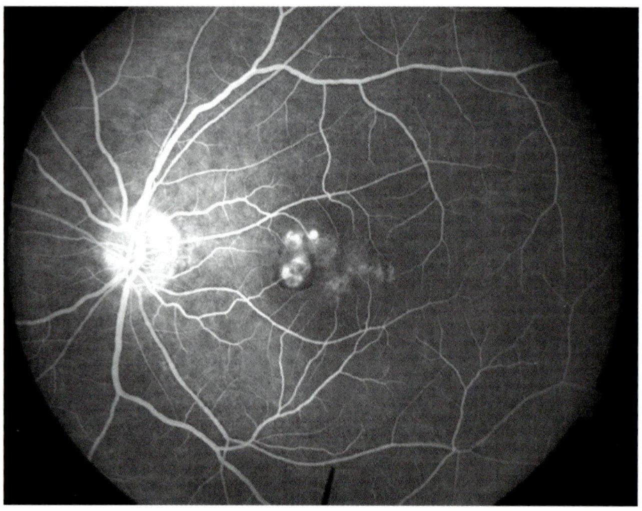

Arteriovenous phase showing hyperfluorescent spots at the fovea

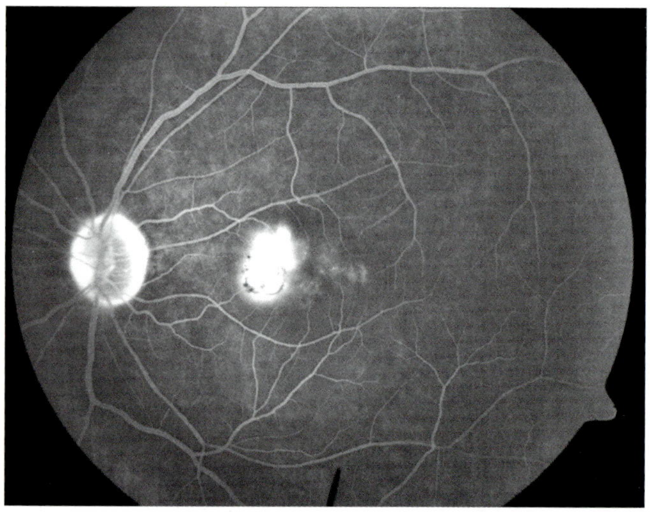

Late phase shows increased intensity of the hyperfluorescent spots with leakage of the dye into the surrounding tissue

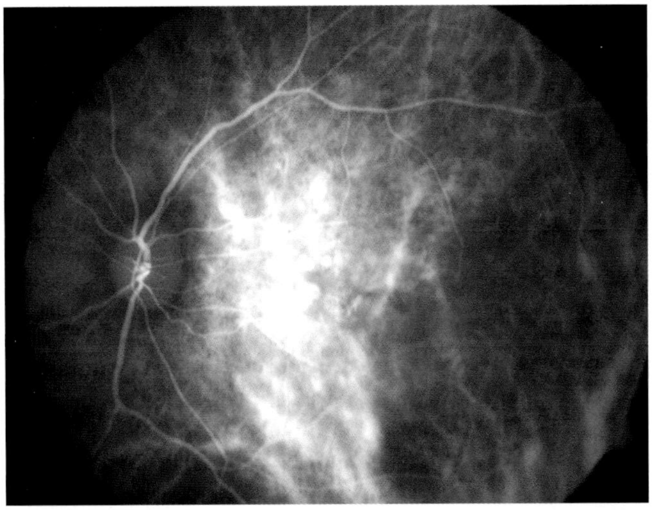

Midphase ICG shows a cluster of polyps. The network of choroidal vessels is not made out. The polyps roughly correspond to the hyperfluorescent spots seen on the fluorescein angiogram

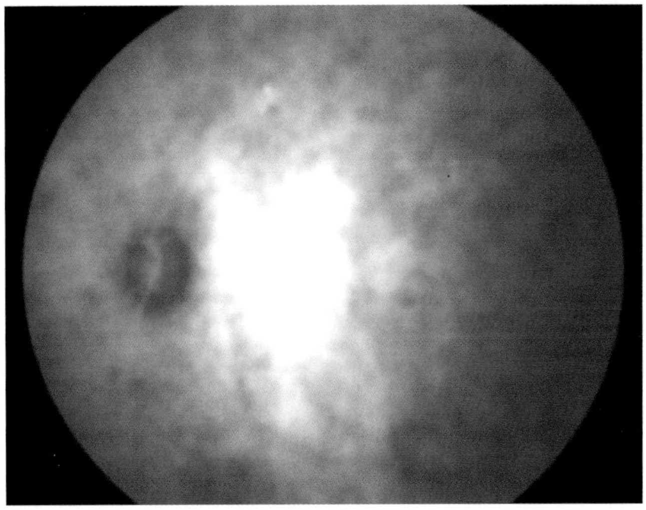

Late phase ICG picture shows retention of the dye within the polyps with minimal leakage through its walls

CASE 3

A 44-year-old male presented with sudden decrease in the vision in right eye for the past fifteen days; visual acuity was 6/24; N12.

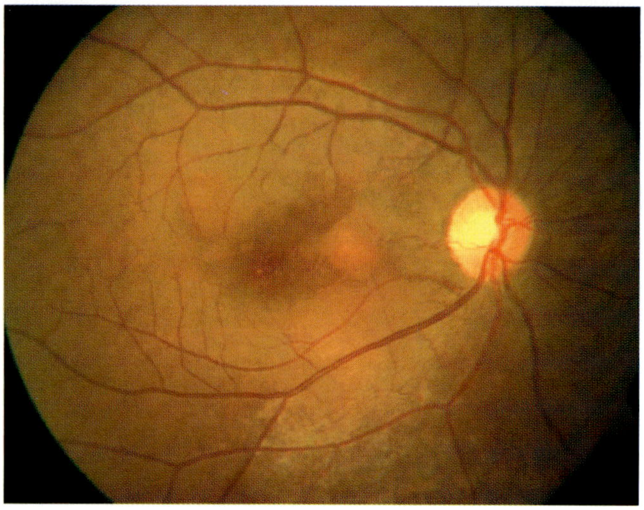

Fundus photograph of the right eye showing orange subretinal nodule with adjacent subretinal hemorrhage. RPE alterations are noted inferiorly

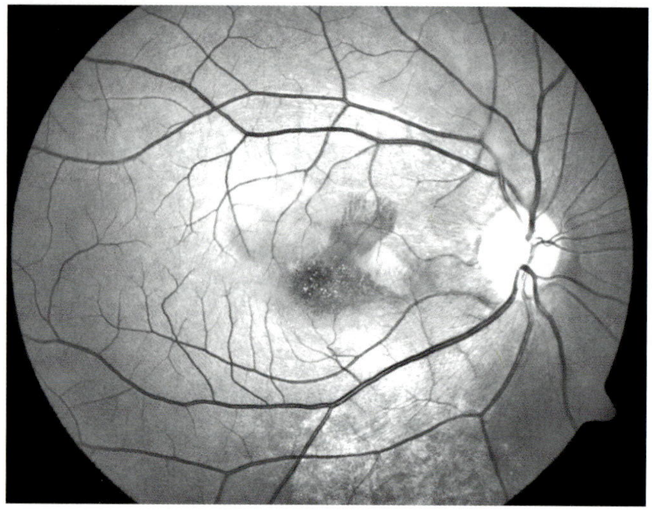

Red free photograph of the right eye. The inferior RPE alterations are well seen

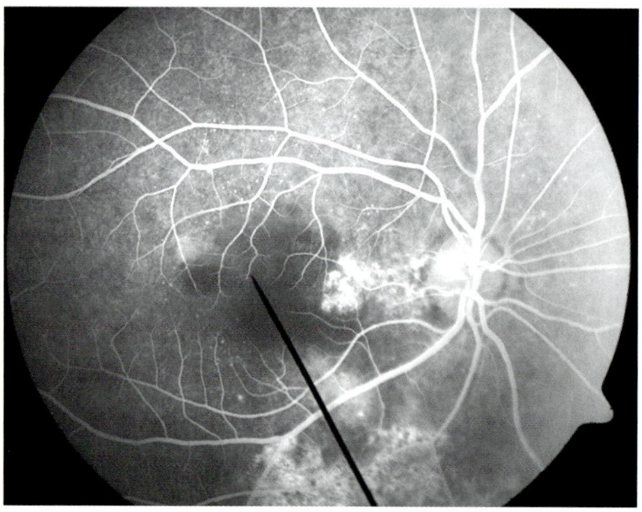

Arteriovenous phase shows a stippled hyperfluorescence nasal to the fovea. Blocked choroidal fluorescence due to hemorrhage is noted at the fovea with ill-defined hyperfluorescence noted temporal to it

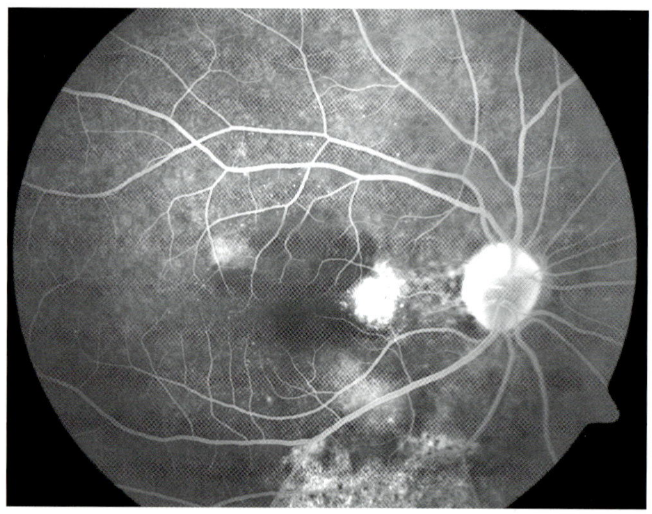

Intense fuzzy hyperfluorescence is seen nasal to the fovea. Faint hyperfluorescence is seen in the temporal macula. Transmitted hyperfluorescence is noted inferiorly

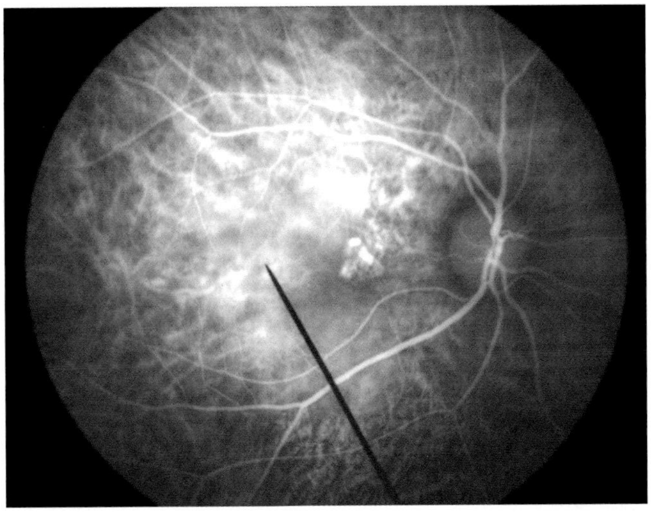

Midphase ICG shows a network of choroidal vessels temporal to the disc terminating into polyps nasal to the fovea

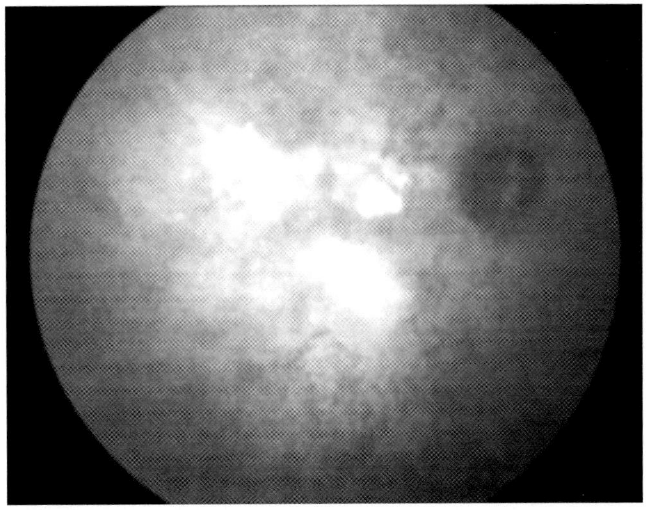

The polyps nasal to the fovea have emptied with staining of their walls seen in the late phase of ICG angiogram. Some dye retention is seen in the temporal macula probably in small polyps which are not well seen in the earlier phases of the angiogram

CASE 4

A 60-year-old female came for a routine eye examination; visual acuity was 6/6; N6 in both eyes.

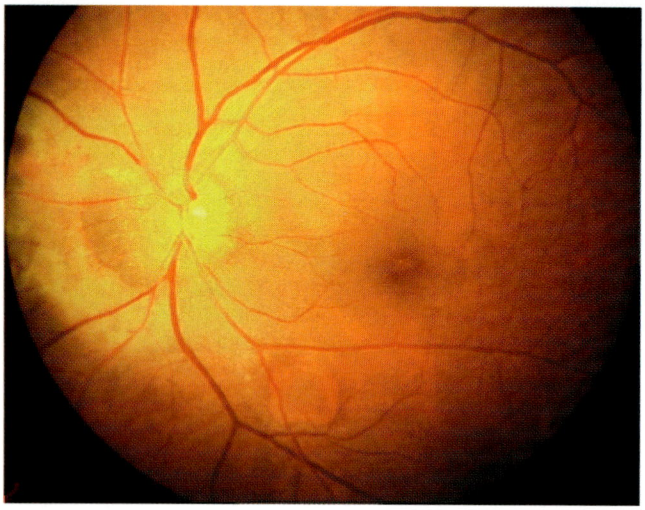

Fundus photograph of the left eye showing a partially hemorrhagic PED nasal to the disc. A serous PED is seen along the inferotemporal arcade

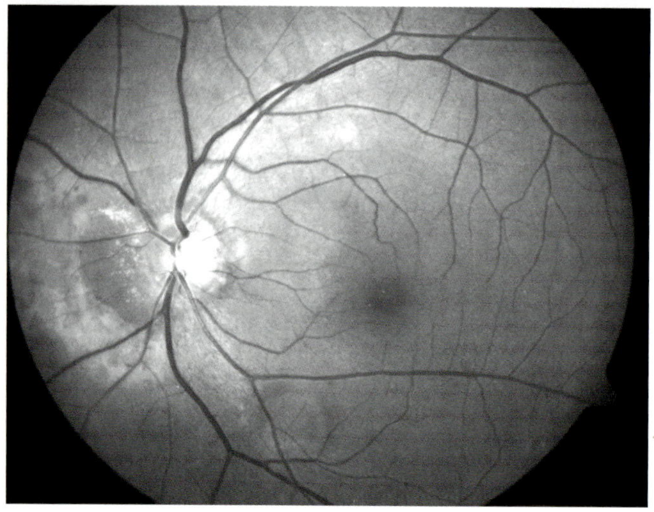

Red free photograph of the left eye

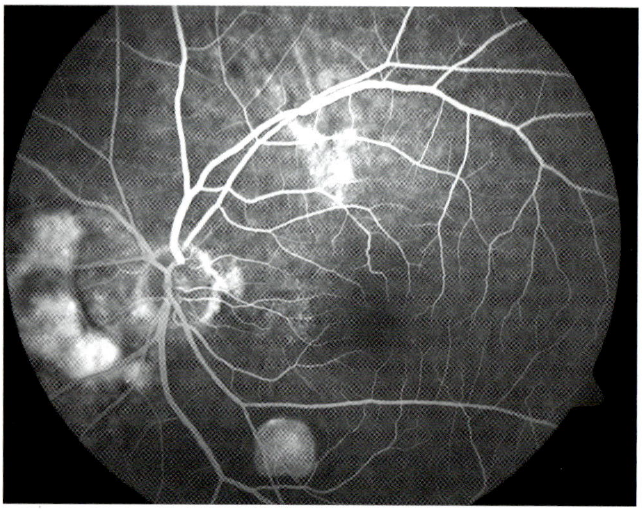

Arteriovenous phase shows filling of the PED inferotemporal to the disc. Filling of nasal PED is also seen with some blocked fluorescence due to hemorrhage seen adjacent to the disc

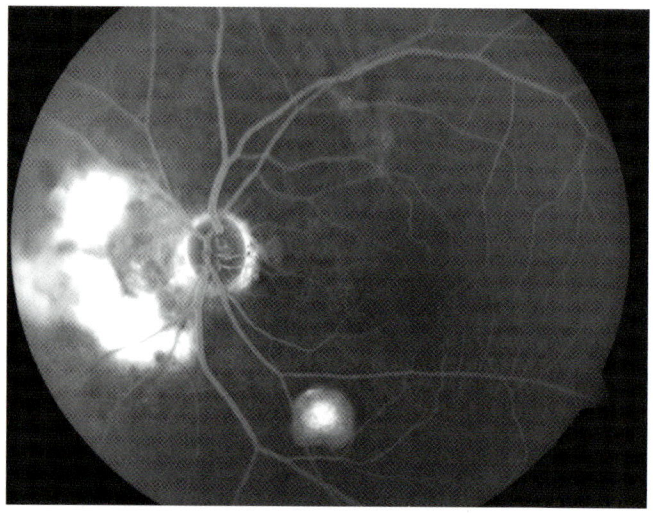

Late phase shows increased intensity of hyperfluorescence with fuzzy margins nasal to the disc

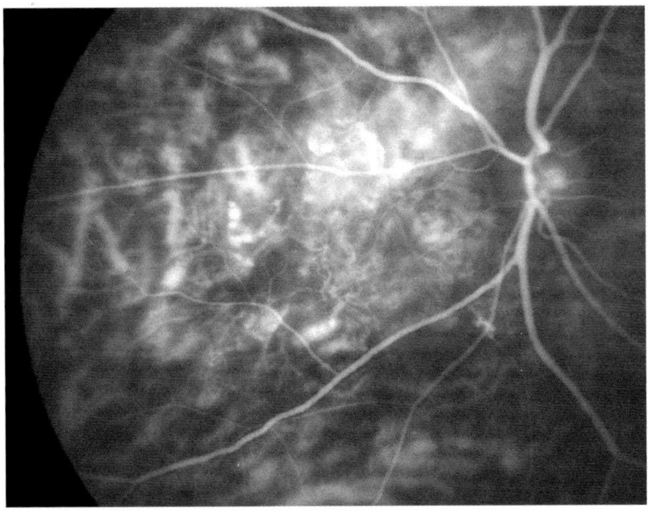

Midphase ICG angiogram showing a large network of choroidal vessels ending in clusters of polyps

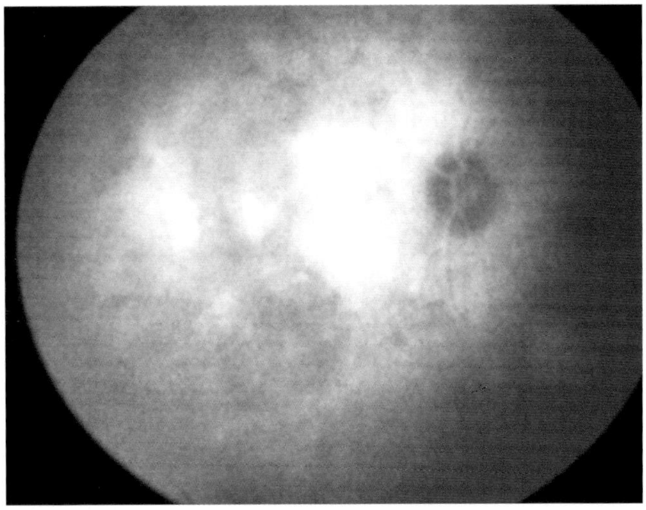

Very minimal leakage of the dye from the polyps is seen in the late phase of the ICG angiogram

CASE 5

A 64-year-old male presented with reduced vision in the right eye for the past one year; visual acuity was 6/9; N8.

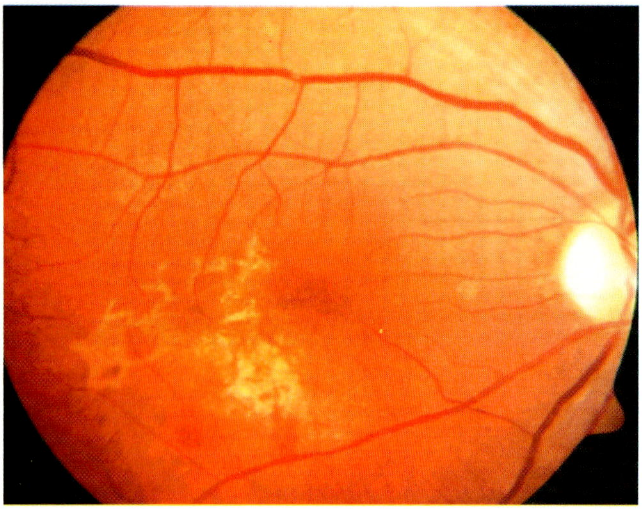

Fundus photograph of the right eye showing RPE alterations and scarring in the temporal macula. An orange-red subretinal nodule is seen in the inferotemporal macula

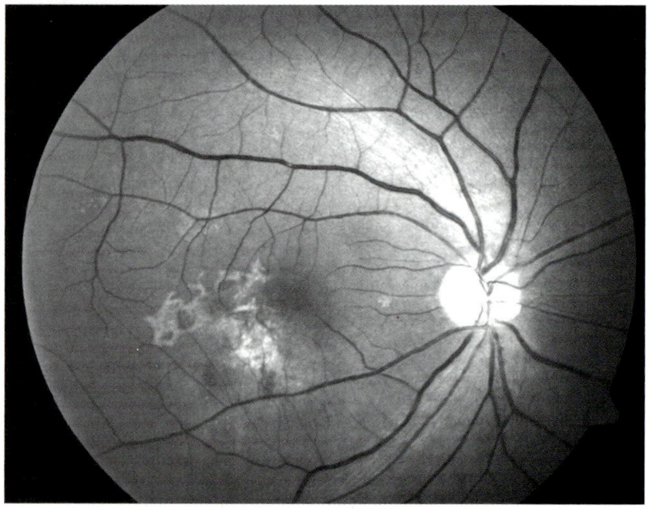

Red free photograph of the right eye showing the dark subretinal nodule in the inferotemporal macula

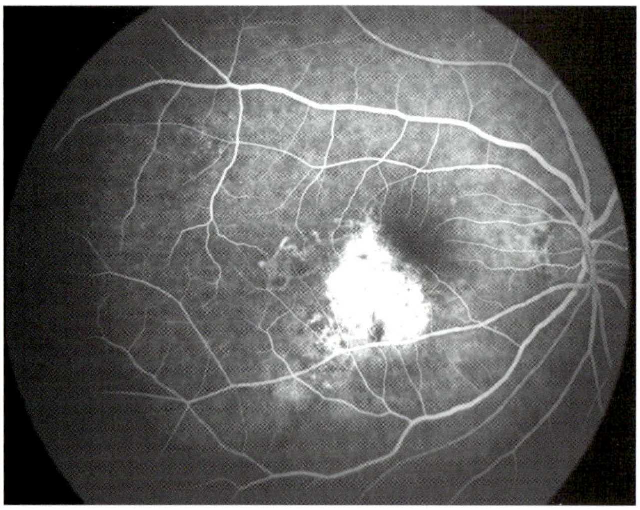

Arteriovenous phase shows hyperfluorescence in the region of the RPE alteration and scarring. Faint irregular hyperfluorescence is noted at the site of the subretinal nodule

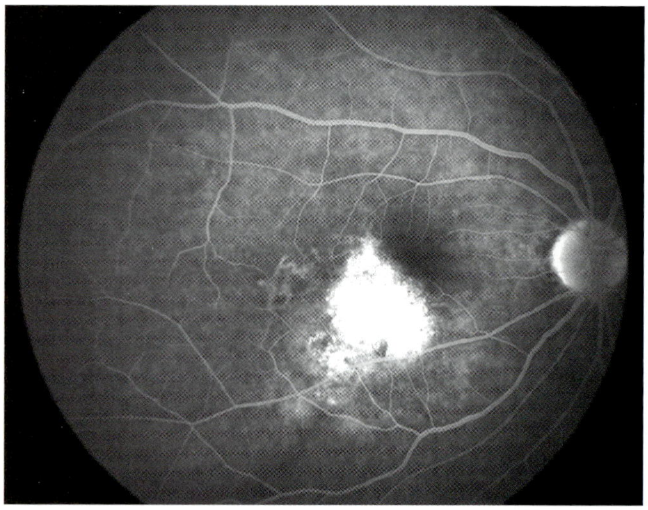

Late phase shows staining of the scar. Very minimal increase of fluorescence is noted at the site of the nodule

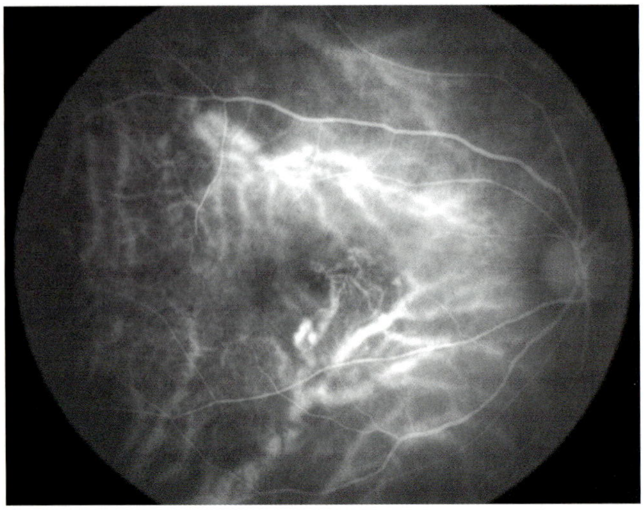

Midphase ICG angiogram showing a small cluster of polyps in the inferotemporal macula. A fine network of choroidal vessels is made out nasal to the polyps

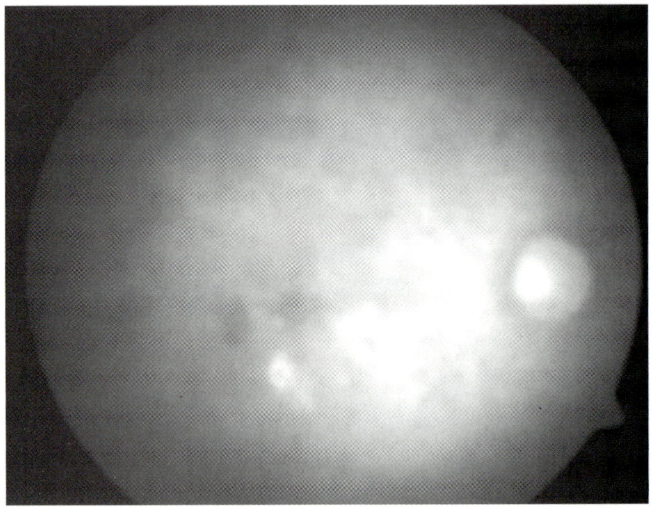

Late phase of the ICG shows staining of the walls of the polyps

CLINICAL NUGGETS

1. Indocyanine green angiography is essential for diagnosing polypoidal choroidal vasculopathy.
2. Subretinal orange nodules and hemorrhagic PEDs are common findings in eyes with polypoidal choroidal vasculopathy.
3. Photodynamic therapy is an established modality of treatment for polypoidal choroidal vasculopathy.
4. Anti-VEGF agents have a limited role in the treatment of polypoidal choroidal vasculopathy.

BIBLIOGRAPHY

1. Ciardella AP, Donsoff IM, Yannuzzi LA. Polypoidal choroidal vasculopathy. Ophthalmol Clin North Am 2002;15(4):537-54.
2. Moorthy RS, Lyon AT, Rabb MF, Spaide RF, Yannuzzi LA, Jampol LM. Idiopathic polypoidal choroidal vasculopathy of the macula. Ophthalmology, 1946.
3. Uyama M, Wada M, Nagai Y, Matsubara T, Matsunaga H, Fukushima I, Takahashi K, Matsumura M. Polypoidal choroidal vasculopathy: natural history. Am J Ophthalmol 2002;133(5):639-48.
4. Yannuzzi LA, Sorenson J, Spaide RF, Lipson B. Idiopathic polypoidal choroidal vasculopathy (IPCV). Retina 1990; 10(1):1-8.

Chapter 16

Choroidal Neovascular Membranes (Other than ARMD)

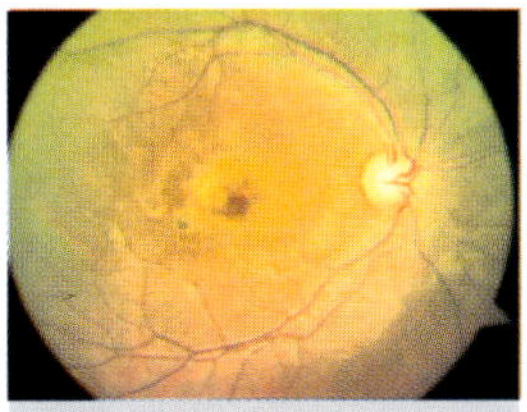

- Any pathologic process that disturbs the retinal pigment epithelium and the Bruch's membrane can lead to the development of a choroidal neovascular membrane.
- Causes include:
  - Idiopathic
  - Myopic
  - Postinflammatory
  - Angioid streaks
  - Choroidal rupture
  - Hereditary dystrophies
  - Choroidal osteoma, etc.

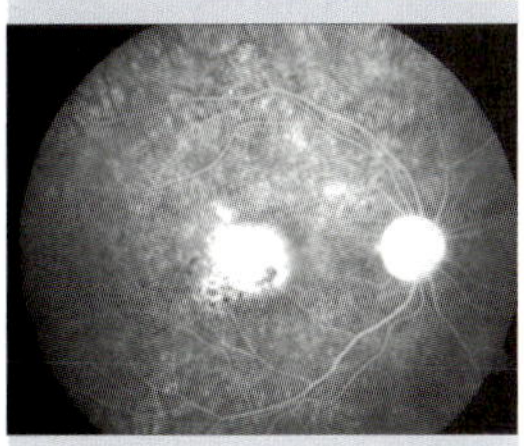

IDIOPATHIC CNVM

- Usually a classic membrane showing a lacy network of vessels in the early phase with leakage in the later phase of the angiogram.
- Could be either extrafoveal, juxtafoveal or subfoveal.

MYOPIC CNVM

- Usually occurs at the lacquer cracks.
- Small in size and close to the foveal center.
- Shows early hyperfluorescence with late staining. Leakage of dye is minimal.

POSTINFLAMMATORY CNVM

- Usually a classic membrane showing early lacy pattern of hyperfluorescence with late leakage.
- Arises from the edge of the choroiditis patch.

MYOPIC CNVM

CASE 1

A 34-year-old myope, presented with sudden drop in vision in the right eye of one week duration. Visual acuity was 6/12; N8.

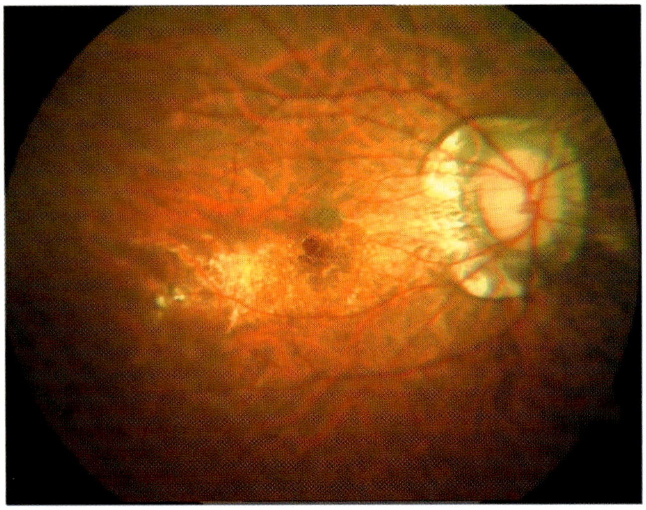

Fundus photograph of the right eye showing a small gray membrane just superior to the foveal center

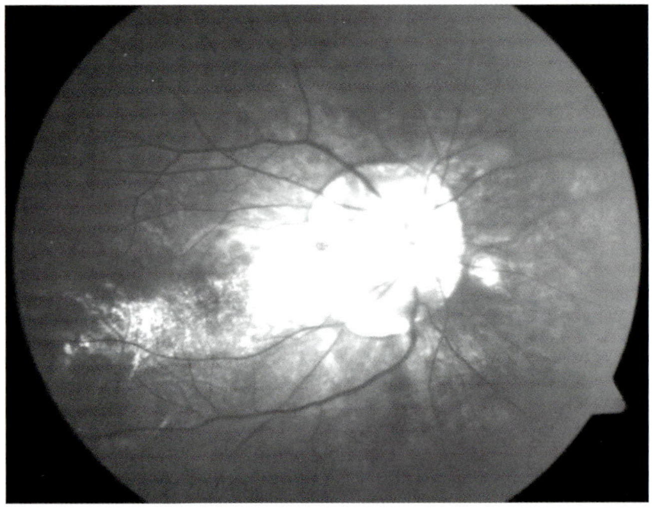

Red free photograph showing the myopic changes at the posterior pole

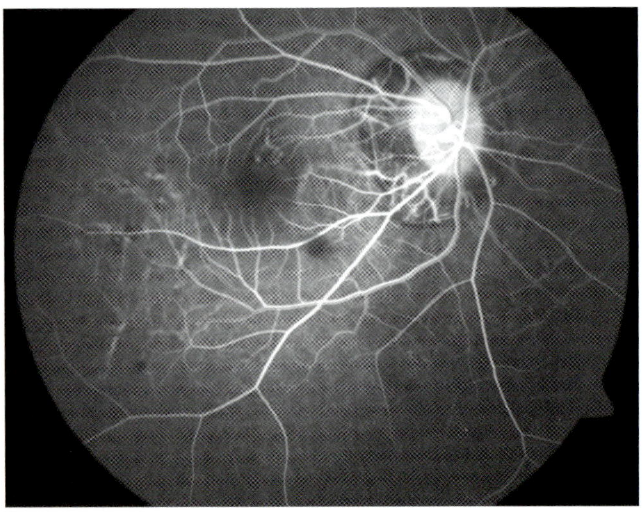

Early part of the arteriovenous phase showing faint hyperfluorescence in the region of the CNVM, just superior to the fovea. Temporally linear hyperfluorescent lines are seen suggestive of lacquer cracks

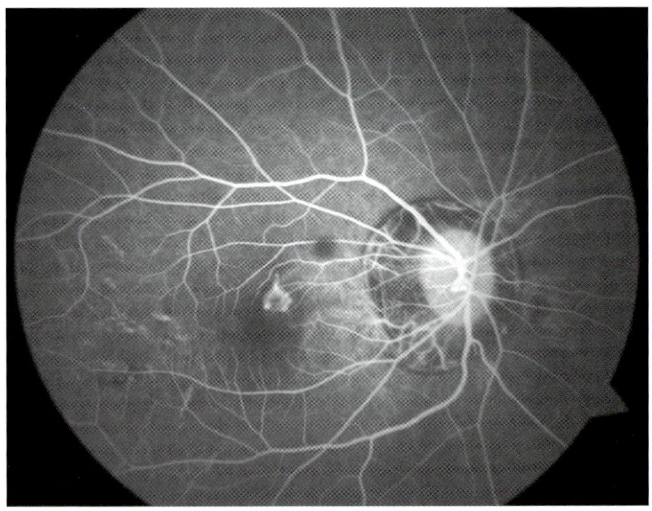

Increased hyperfluorescence of the CNVM is noted in the arteriovenous phase

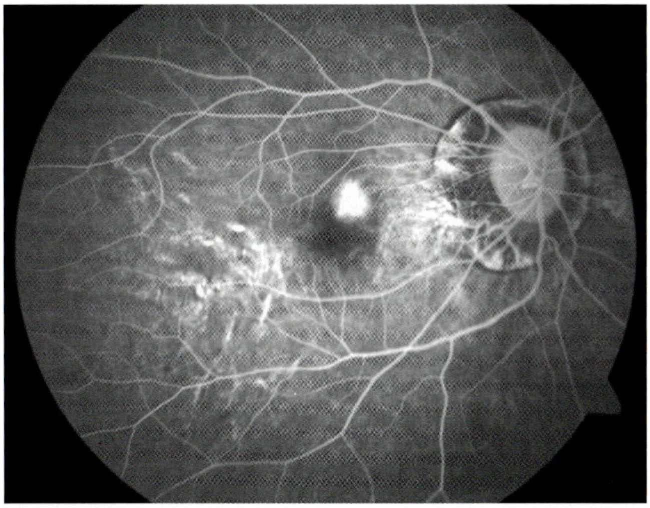

Late phase of the angiogram showing the hyperfluorescent CNVM with fuzzy margins

COMMENT

Myopic CNVM tend to be pigmented, small and close to the foveal center. They leak minimally in the late phase.

CASE 2

A 38-year-old high myope, presented with reduced vision in the right eye of one month duration. Visual acuity was 3/60 in the right eye.

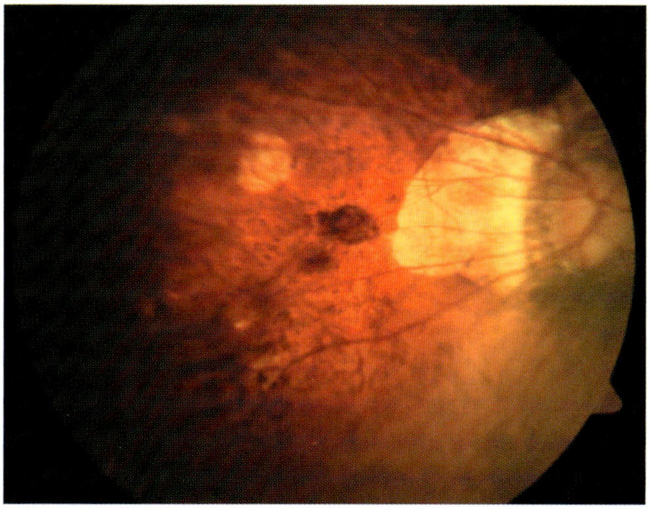

Fundus photograph of the right eye showing high myopic changes at the posterior pole. A small, pigmented CNVM is seen very close to the foveal center

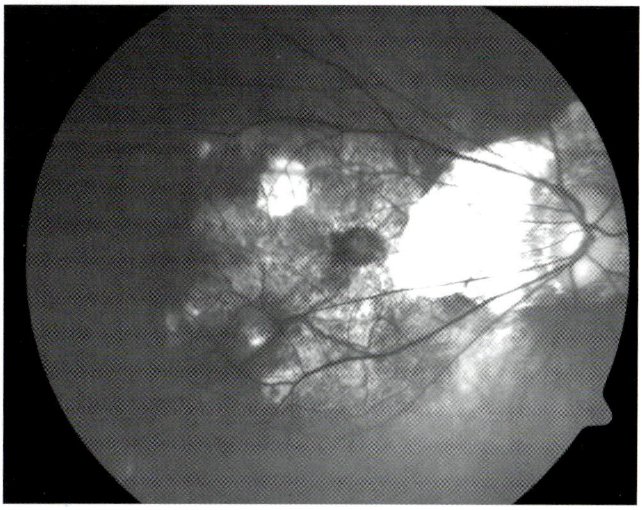

Red free photograph of the right eye

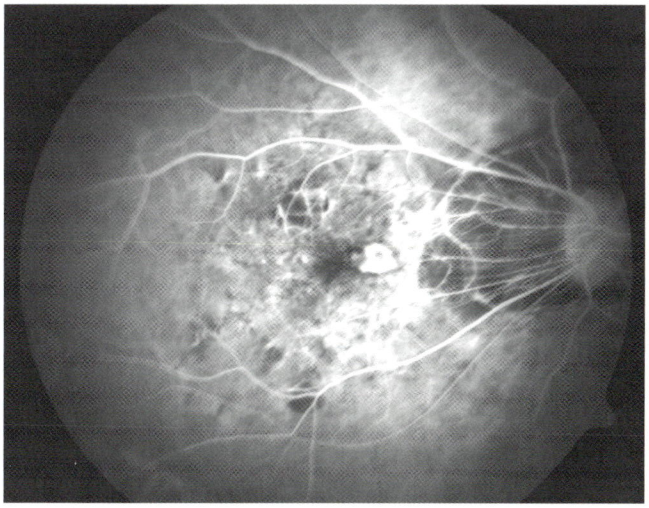

Arteriovenous phase showing hyperfluorescence of the CNVM

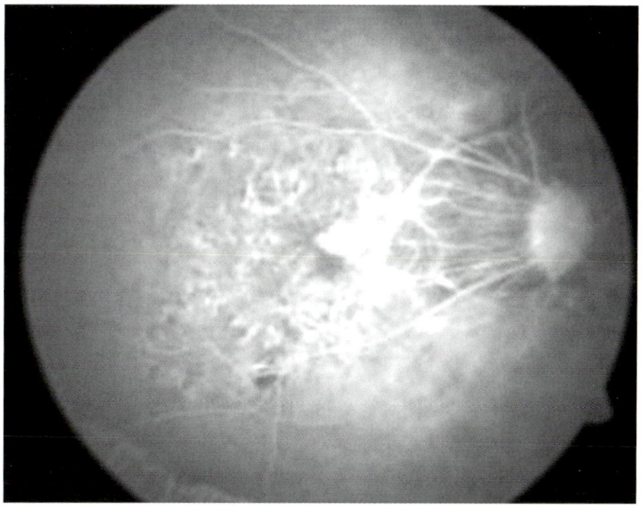

Increased hyperfluorescence is seen in the later part of the angiogram

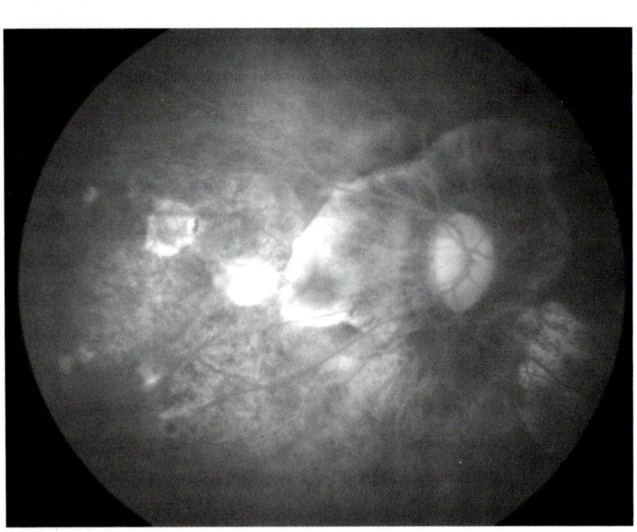

Staining of the CNVM with fuzzy margins is seen in the late film

COMMENT

A small subfoveal myopic CNVM is seen in this case.

IDIOPATHIC CNVM

CASE 3

A 32-year-old female presented with blurring of vision in the left eye for the past one week. Visual acuity was 6/9; N8.

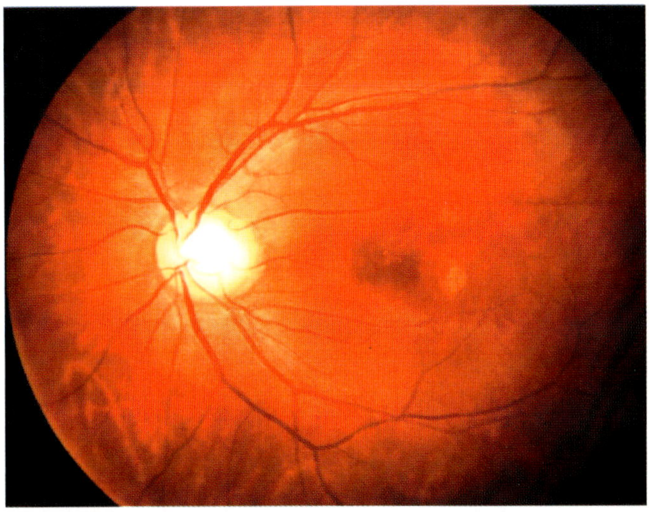

Fundus photograph of the left eye showing a small subretinal membrane temporal to the fovea

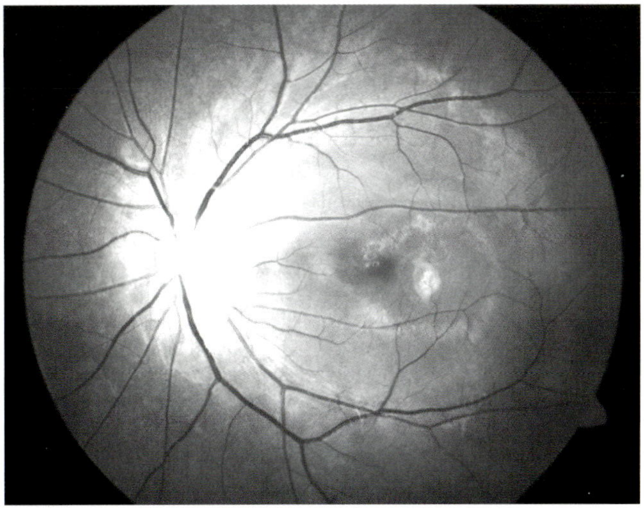

Red free photograph showing the CNVM

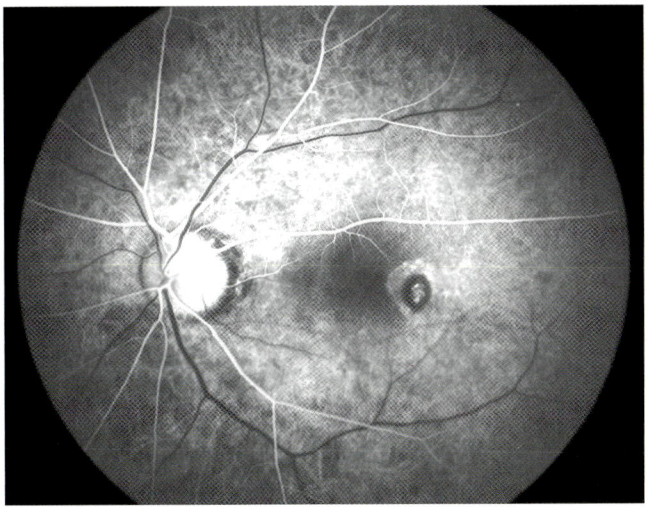

The CNVM is seen to fill in the arterial phase of the angiogram. A rim of hypofluorescence is seen surrounding the CNVM. This is further surrounded by a zone of hyperfluorescence

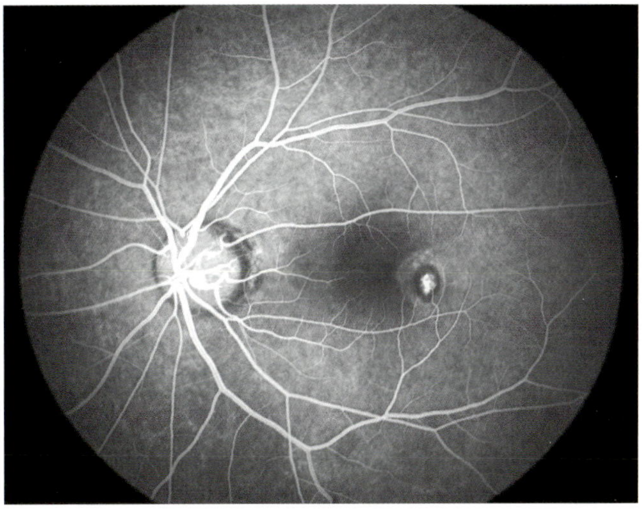

Arteriovenous phase showing increased hyperfluorescence of the CNVM

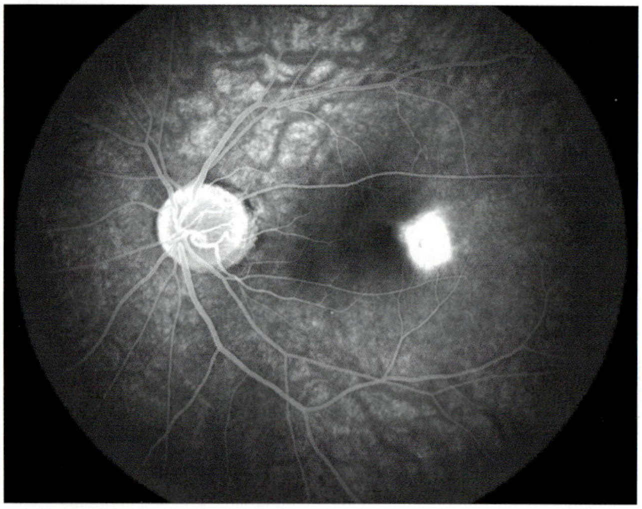

Late phase showing increased hyperfluorescence of the CNVM. The margins are fuzzy

COMMENT

An extrafoveal idiopathic CNVM is seen in this case.

CASE 4

A 29-year-old male presented with reduced vision in the right eye, accidentally noted on closing the fellow eye. Visual acuity was 6/24; N18. Left eye was normal.

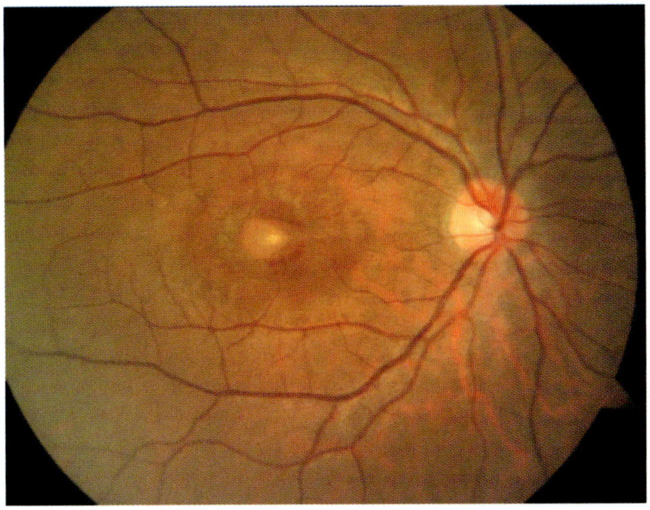

Fundus photograph of the right eye showing a subfoveal scarred CNVM

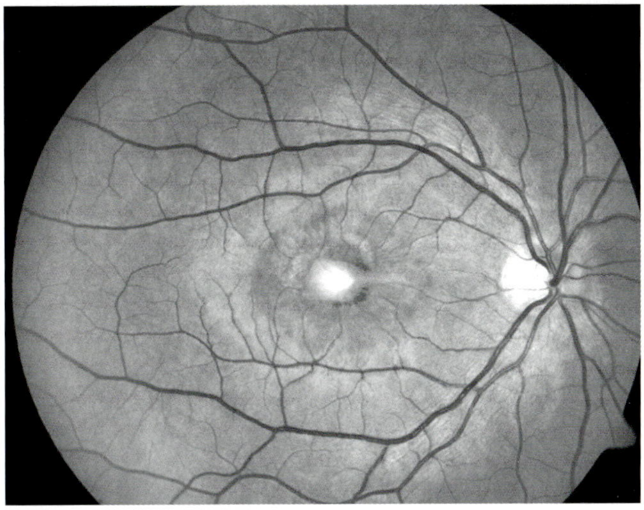

Red free photograph showing the subfoveal scar

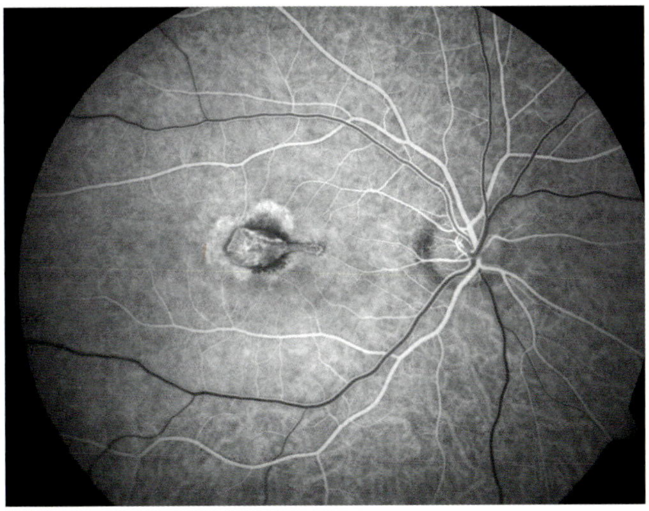

Arteriovenous phase of the angiogram showing filling up of the CNVM, the vessels within which are well made out

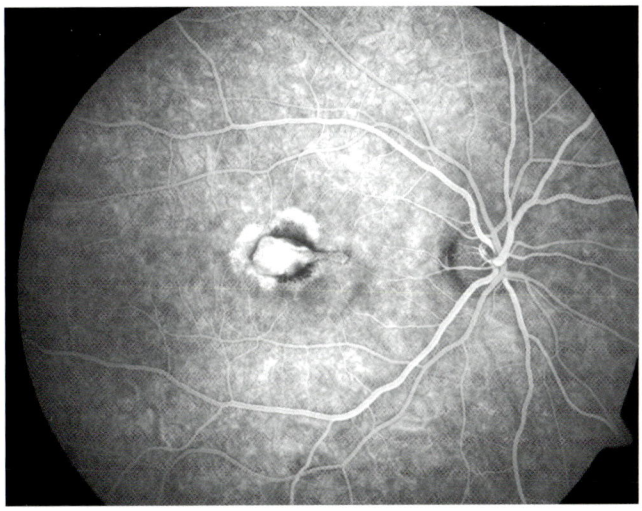

Increased hyperfluorescence of the CNVM is seen. A zone of hypofluorescence surrounded by another zone of hyperfluorescence is seen around the CNVM

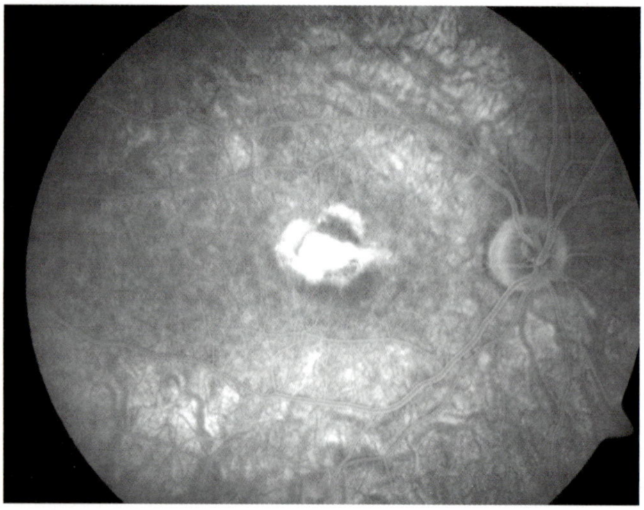

Staining of the CNVM is seen. The margins are still well defined. Some fading is seen in the surrounding zone of hyperfluorescence indicating transmission defect

COMMENT

This case shows a cicatrized idiopathic CNVM.

JUXTAPAPILLARY CNVM

CASE 5

A 25-year-old male presented with metamorphopsia in the left eye of two weeks duration. Visual acuity was 6/12; N8. He had previously been diagnosed to have a juxtapapillary CNVM in the right eye which was treated with laser photocoagulation.

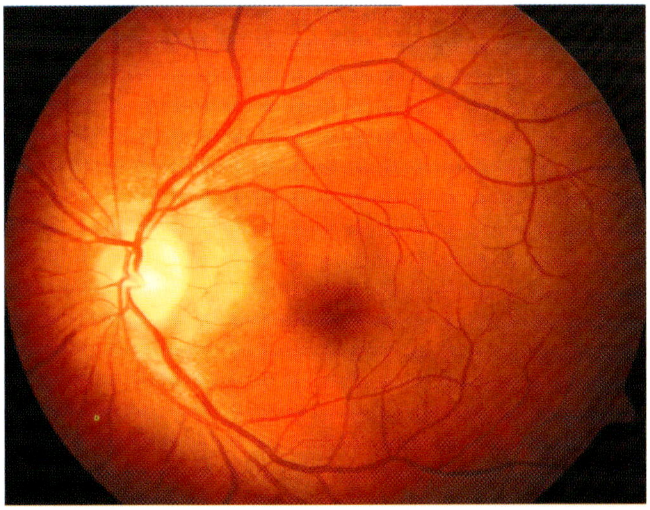

Fundus photograph of the left eye showing a juxtapapillary CNVM. Associated subretinal fluid and hemorrhage are present

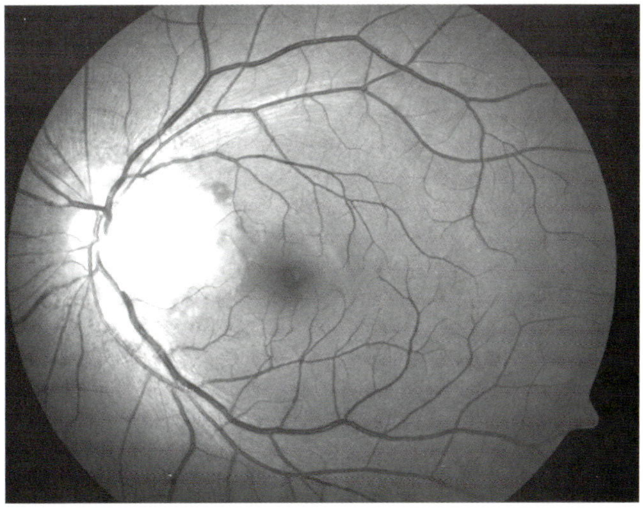

Red free photograph showing a spot of subretinal hemorrhage at the superotemporal edge of the membrane

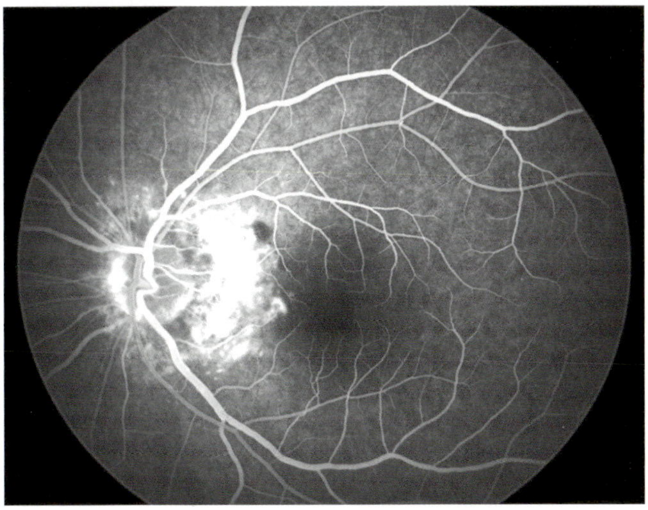

Arteriovenous phase showing filling up of the vessels of the juxtapapillary membrane

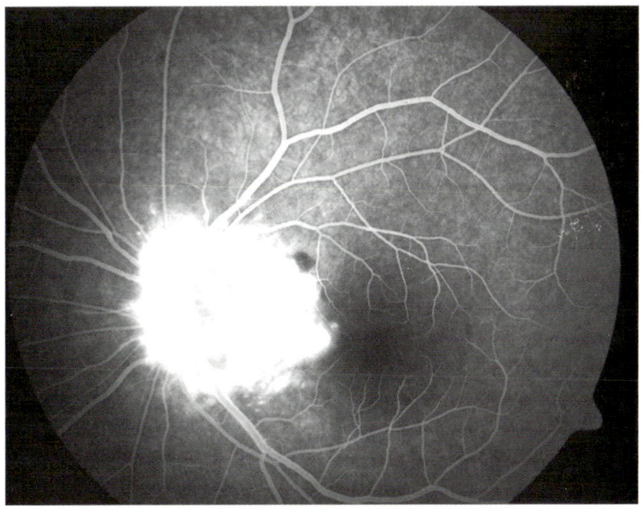

Increased leakage of the dye from the CNVM is seen, blurring the underlying details

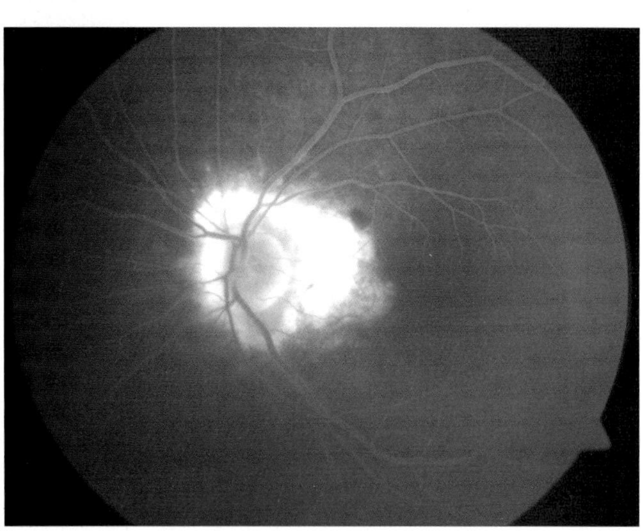

Staining of the CNVM and pooling of the dye in the subretinal space is seen in the late phase

COMMENT

A large juxtapapillary CNVM is seen extending towards but not yet reaching the foveal center.

CASE 5 (*Continued*)

Argon laser photocoagulation was done to the juxtapapillary CNVM. One month later the visual acuity was 6/6; N6.

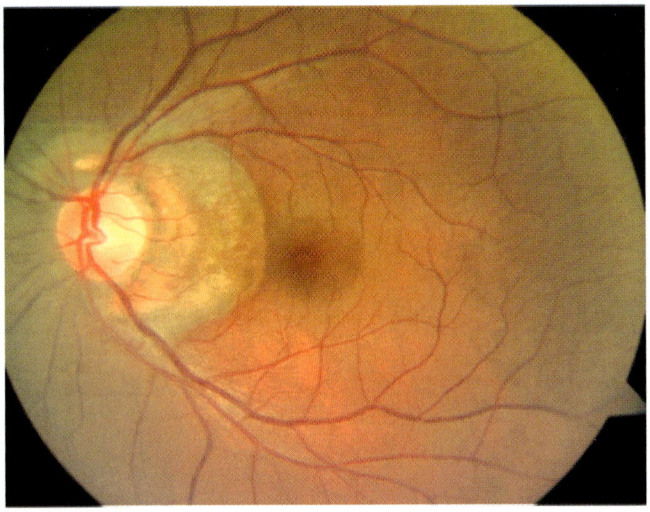

Fundus photograph of the left eye showing a flat chorioretinal atrophy in the juxtapapillary region

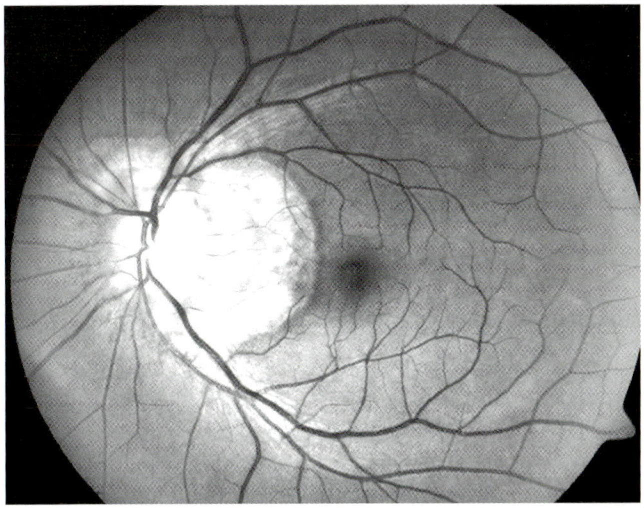

Red free photograph of the left eye

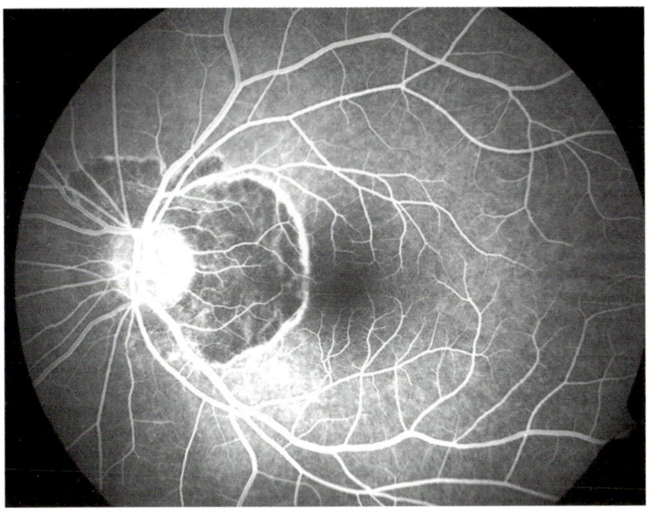

Early part of the arteriovenous phase of the angiogram showing hypofluorescense in the juxtapapillary region. A rim of hyperfluorescence is seen at the edge

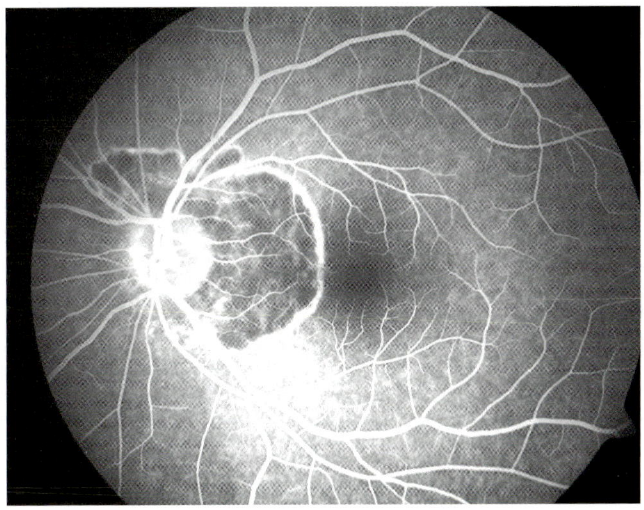

Arteriovenous phase showing persistence of the hypofluorescence

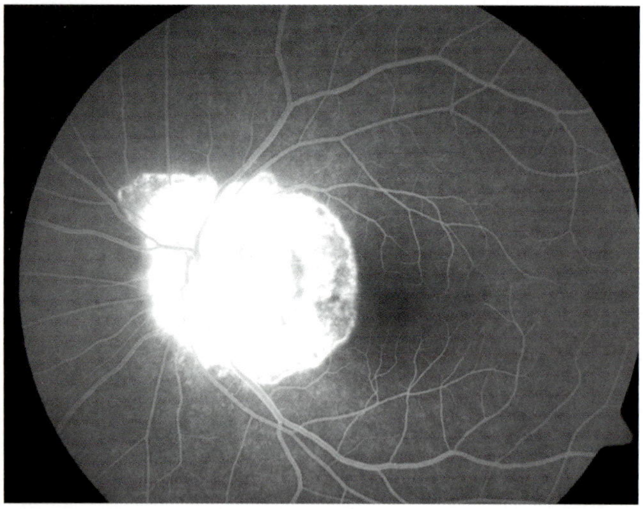

Late hyperfluorescence due to staining of the sclera and the tissue in the juxtapapillary region is seen. Note that the margins are still well defined

COMMENT

A well ablated CNVM is seen. There is no evidence of persistence of the CNVM.

POSTINFLAMMATORY CNVM—GHPC

CASE 6

A 36-year-old male with GHPC in both eyes, presented with distortion of vision in the right eye of four days duration. Visual acuity was 6/9; N6 in the right eye.

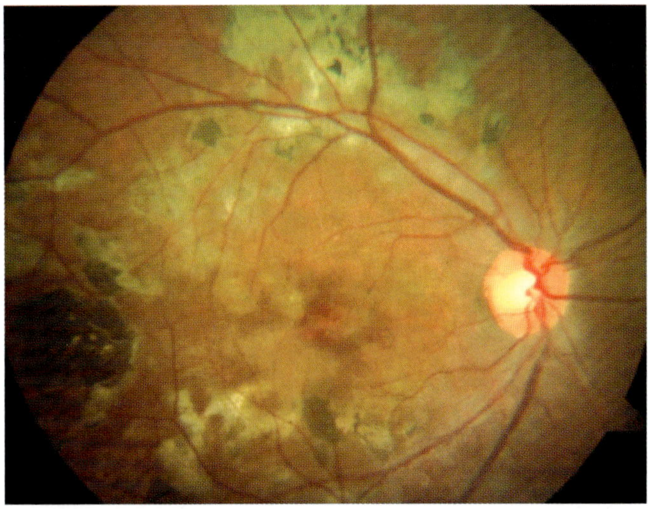

Fundus photograph of the right eye showing healed GHPC. A CNVM and associated subretinal fluid was noted inferior to the foveal center

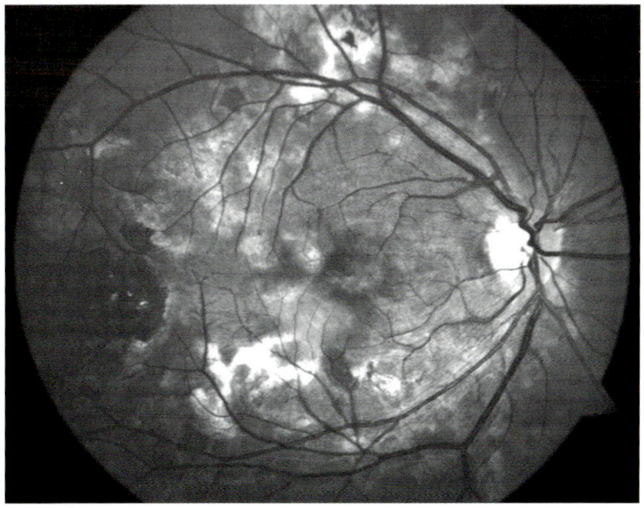

Red free photograph of the right eye showing the CNVM inferior to the fovea

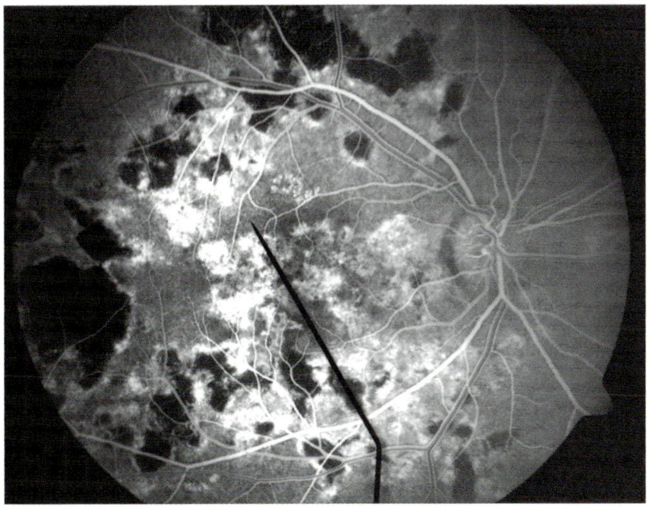

The fine lacy network of vessels are seen in the CNVM located inferotemporal to the foveal center

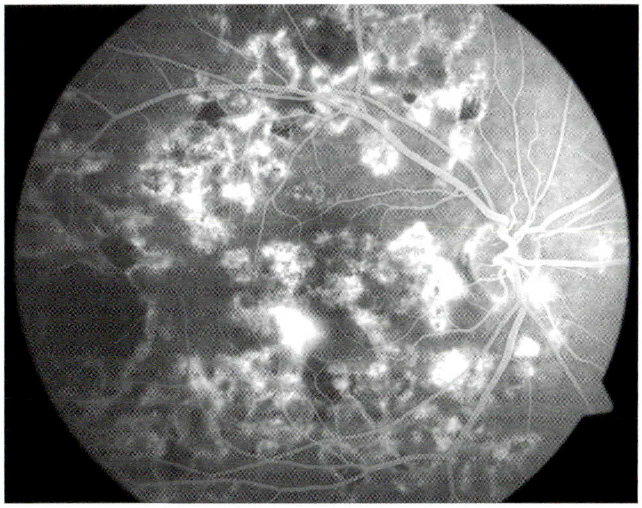

Leakage of the dye is seen from the CNVM in the arteriovenous phase of the angiogram. The healed choroiditis patches are seen as an area of hypofluorescence surrounded by a rim of hyperfluorescence. Hyperfluorescence due to transmission defect is seen at the fovea

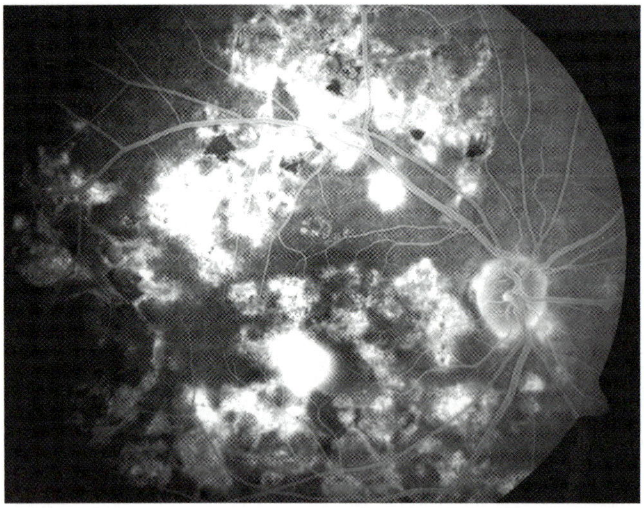

Intense hyperfluorescence is seen at the CNVM in the late phase

COMMENT

The lacy pattern of the vessels of the CNVM is well seen in the angiogram. Late intense hyperfluorescence with fuzzy margins is seen. Active GHPC lesion also shows late hyperfluorescence. However, they are hypofluorescent in the early phase.

POSTINFLAMMATORY CNVM—TOXOPLASMOSIS

CASE 7

A 27-year-old male presented with drop in vision in the right eye of two weeks duration. Visual acuity was 6/36; N36. He had been previously diagnosed to have a healed toxoplasmic retinochoroiditis scar close to the fovea in the right eye.

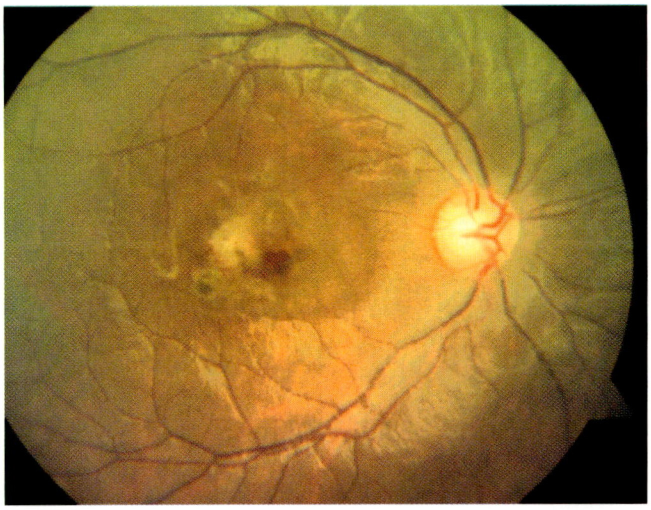

Fundus photograph of the right eye showing a CNVM at the fovea. A healed retinochoroiditis patch is seen inferior to the CNVM. Adjacent retinal hemorrhage is seen

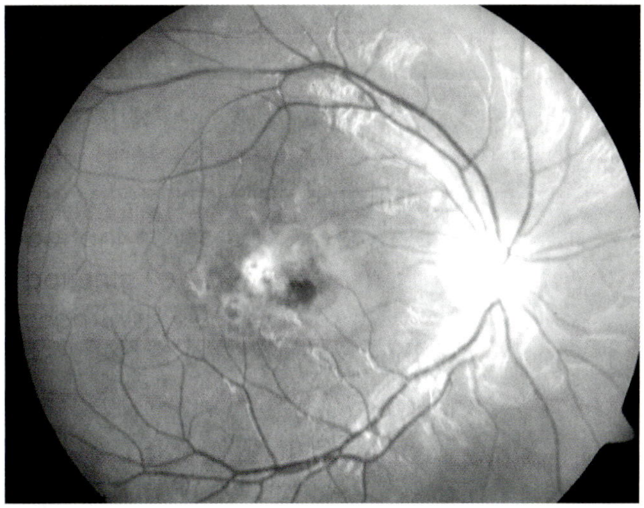

Red free photograph of the right eye

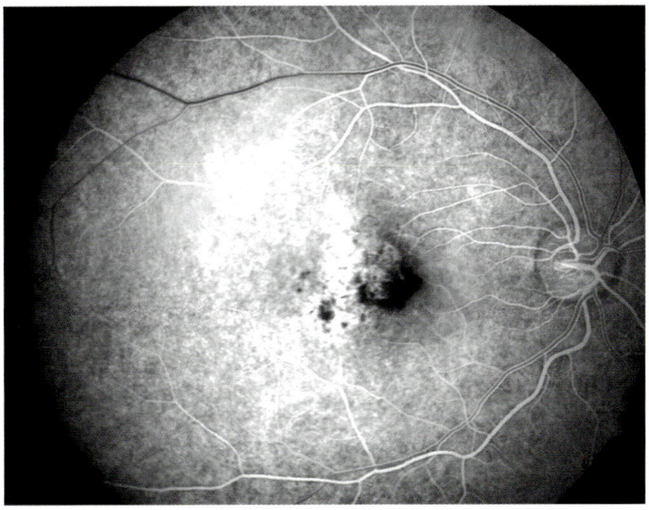

Early arteriovenous phase of the angiogram shows a lacy network of vessels in the subfoveal region

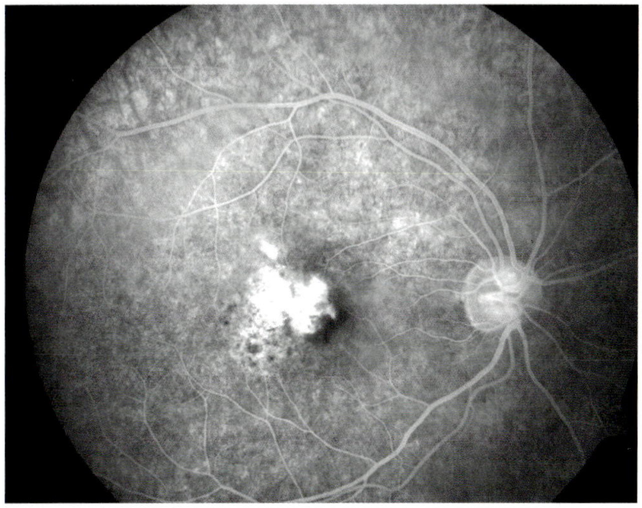

Increased leakage of the dye from the CNVM is seen in the arteriovenous phase of the angiogram. Blocked fluorescence due to hemorrhage and pigment is seen nasal and inferotemporal to the CNVM, respectively

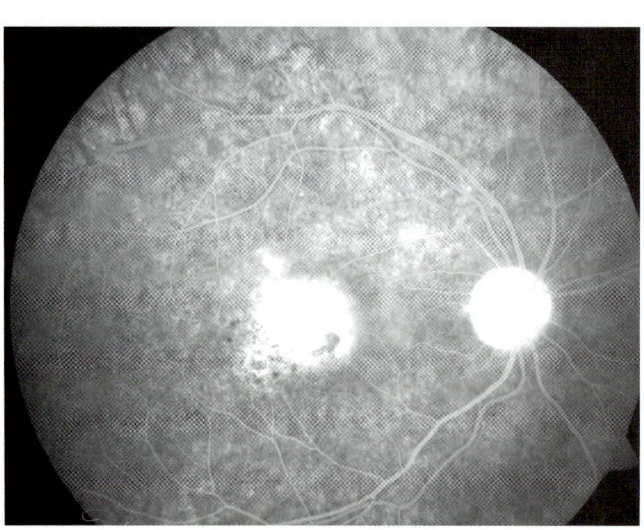

Intense hyperfluorescence with fuzzy margin is noted in the late phase

COMMENT

CNVM in toxoplasmic retinochoroiditis usually occurs at the edge of the healed scar.

CASE 8

A 14-year-old girl presented with defective vision in both eyes, noticed since 1 year. At presentation, BCVA in right eye was CF, <N36 and that in the left was 6/18; N18. She was diagnosed of having chorioretinal atrophy secondary to toxoplasmosis in both eyes with CNV in the left eye. The patient underwent combination photodynamic therapy (PDT) and intravitreal bevacizumab for treatment of the CNV in the left eye.

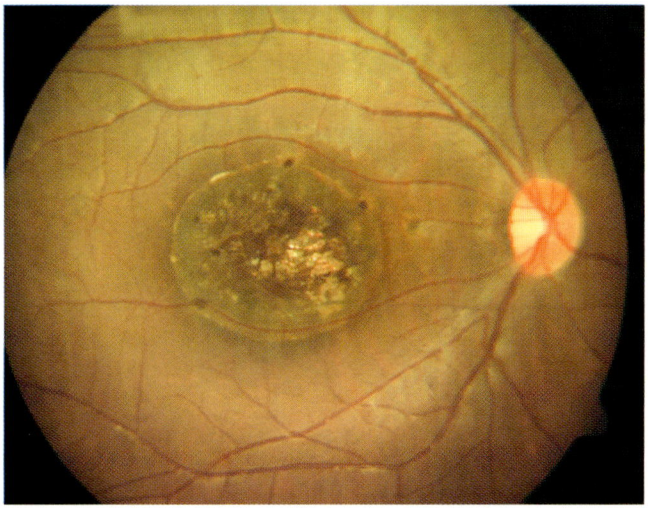

Color fundus of the right eye reveals a punched-out, pigmented, chorioretinal atrophic scar suggestive of toxoplasma chorioretinitis sequelae

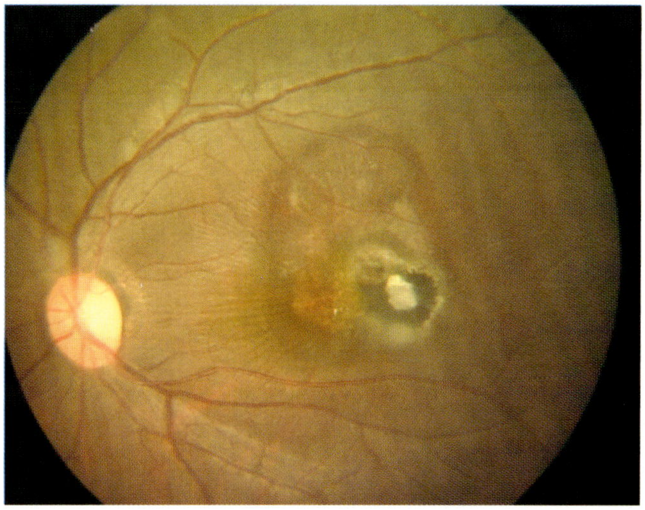

Color fundus photograph of the left eye reveals a pigmented macular scar with a yellow-gray CNVM and contiguous submacular hemorrhage

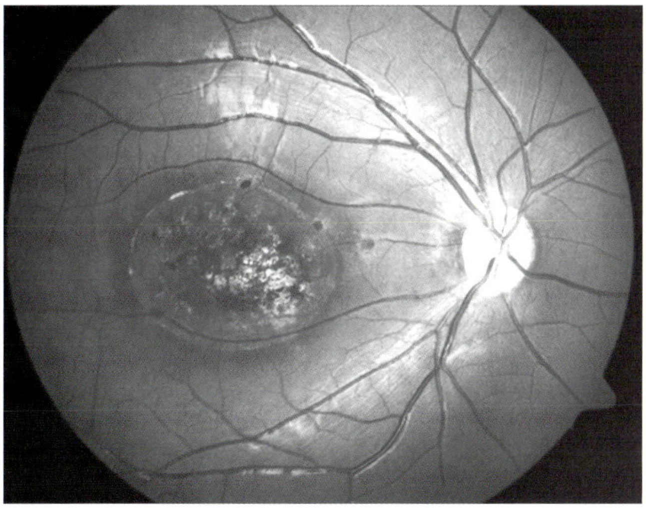

Red free photograph of the right eye highlights the extent of the macular scar

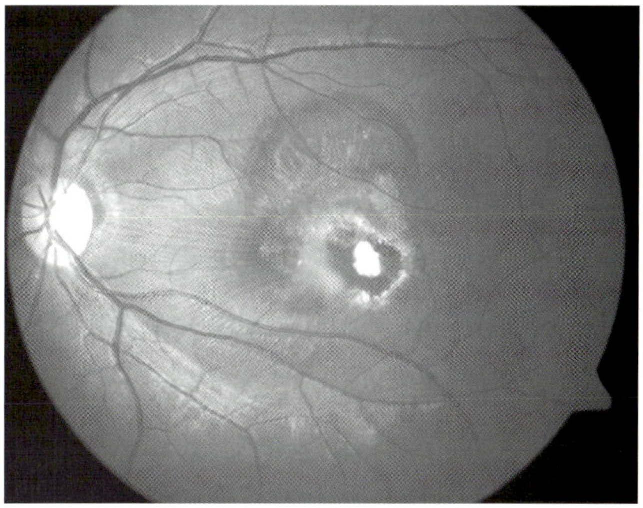

Red free photograph of the left eye highlights the extent of the macular scar

Two months later, visual acuity improved to 6/36; N8 in the left eye. CNVM had regressed. Clinical findings were confirmed on OCT. At the last follow-up, 2 years later, visual acuity had improved to 6/9; N6 in the left eye.

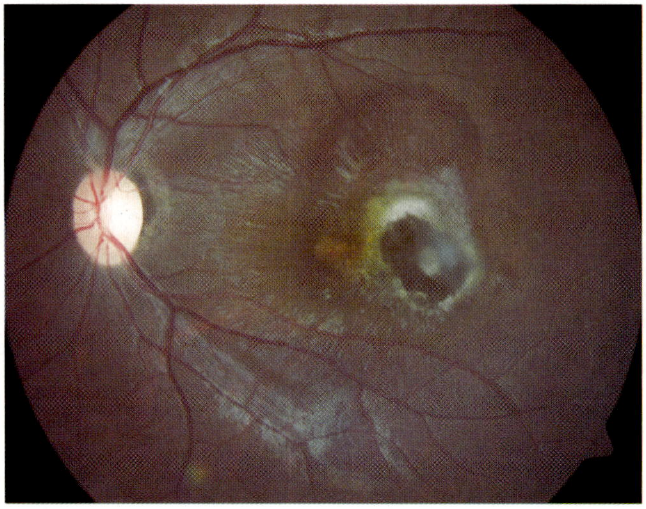

Color fundus photograph of the left eye reveals the regressed CNV with the pigmented macular scar

CNVM AT DEMARCATION LINE

CASE 9

A 46-year-old female who had undergone a scleral buckling surgery in the left eye, presented with sudden drop in vision of one month duration. Visual acuity was 6/60; N36. The retina was attached.

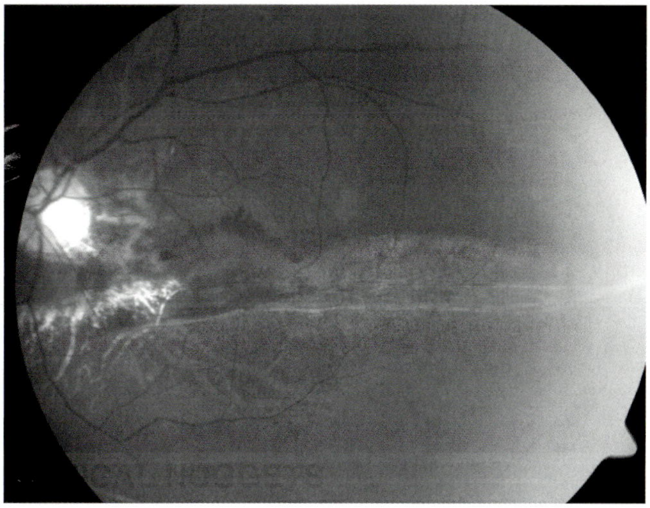

Red free photograph of the left eye showing a demarcation line running across the fundus inferior to the disc. A subfoveal CNVM with adjacent subretinal hemorrhage is noted. Lower half of the fundus shows RPE alteration

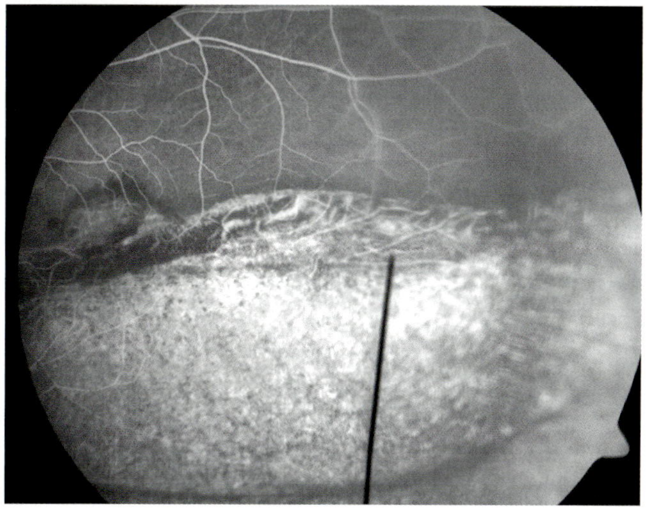

Early arteriovenous phase showing the lacy network of the subfoveal CNVM

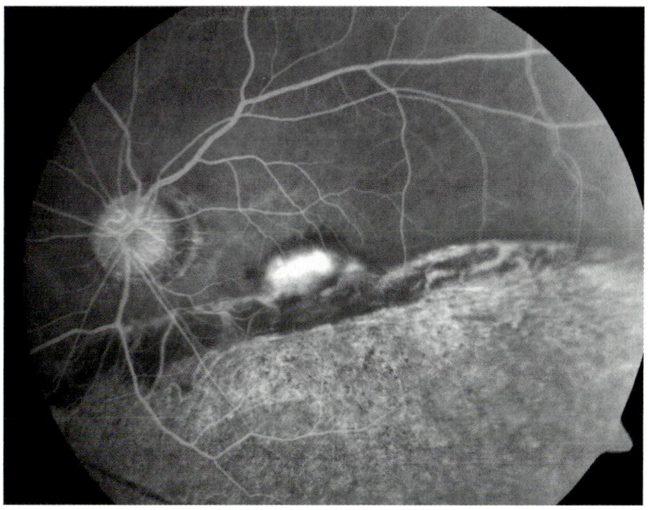

Increased leakage of the dye is noted at the CNVM

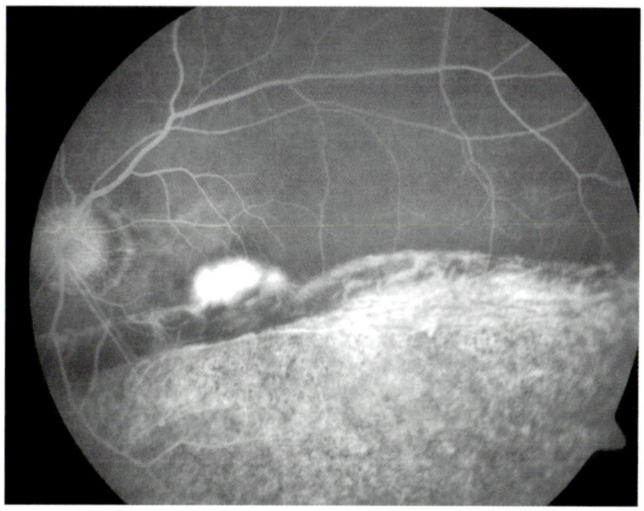

Increased hyperfluorescence due to leakage of the dye is noted at the CNVM in the later part of the arteriovenous phase

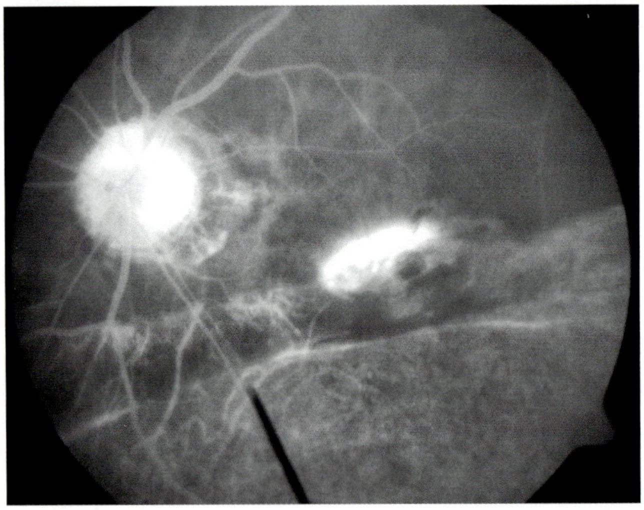

Late phase shows staining of the CNVM with fuzzy margins

COMMENT

This case shows rare occurrence of a CNVM at the demarcation line that develops at the junction of attached and detached retina in cases of long-standing rhegmatogenous retinal detachment.

CNVM AT MARGIN OF RETINOCHOROIDAL COLOBOMA

CASE 10

An 18-year-old boy presented with BCVA of CF in right eye and 6/9; N6 in the left. Examination revealed iris coloboma with retinochoroidal coloboma in both eyes with total retinal detachment in the right eye. He underwent vitreous surgery with silicone oil injection in that eye. BCVA at 1 month postoperative period was 6/45; N18.

1 year later, he underwent uneventful cataract surgery with IOL implantation and silicone oil removal. BCVA 1 month post surgery was 6/12; N6. 5 years later, he experienced decreased vision again in the right eye (BCVA 6/35; N18) and was found to have CNVM at the edge of the coloboma margin.

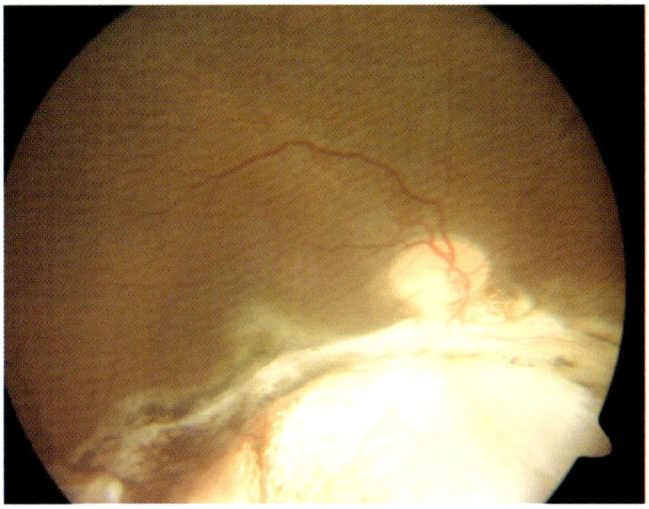

Color fundus of the right eye reveals a retinochoroidal coloboma with a yellow-gray subfoveal CNVM

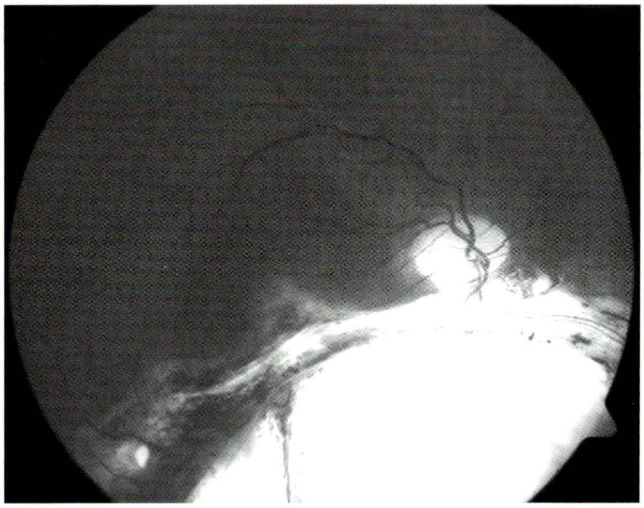

Red free photograph of the right eye

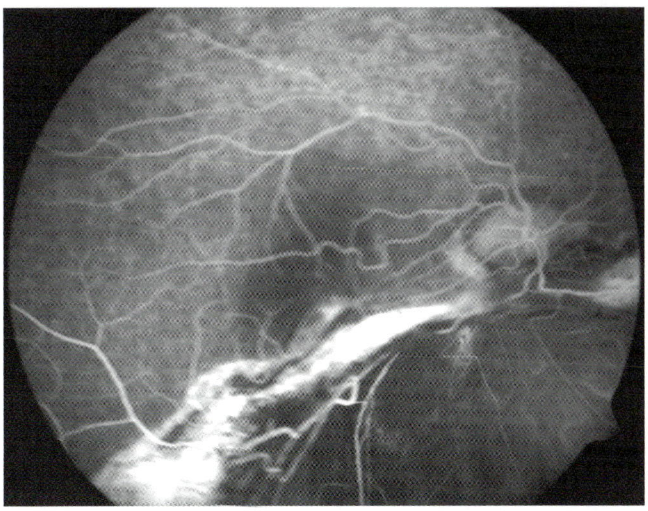

Late A-V phase angiogram reveals lacy pattern of hyperfluorescence at the fovea suggestive of classic CNVM

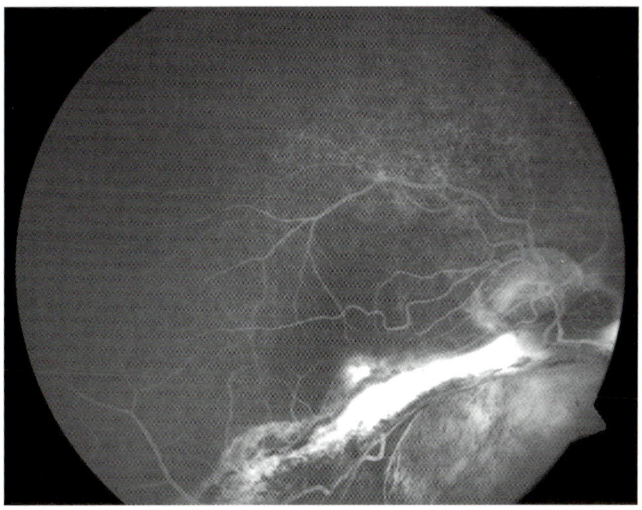

Late phase angiogram reveals intense hyperfluorescence at the fovea due to leakage from the CNVM

COMMENT

The patient underwent intravitreal injection bevacizumab following which the CNVM scarred and visual acuity was maintained till last follow-up, 18 months later.

CNVM AFTER VITREORETINAL SURGERY

CASE 11

A 69-year-old gentleman presented with diminution of vision in the left eye since six weeks. He had undergone surgery for retinal detachment elsewhere. On evaluation, fundus showed total retinal detachment with severe PVR. Visual acuity was HM. The patient underwent IOL removal, re-vitrectomy, membrane peeling, LPFC injection, 360 degrees relaxing retinotomy, endolaser and silicone oil infusion. At a follow-up 6 months postoperatively, he was found to have large subfoveal CNVM in the operated eye (Silicone oil filled eye).

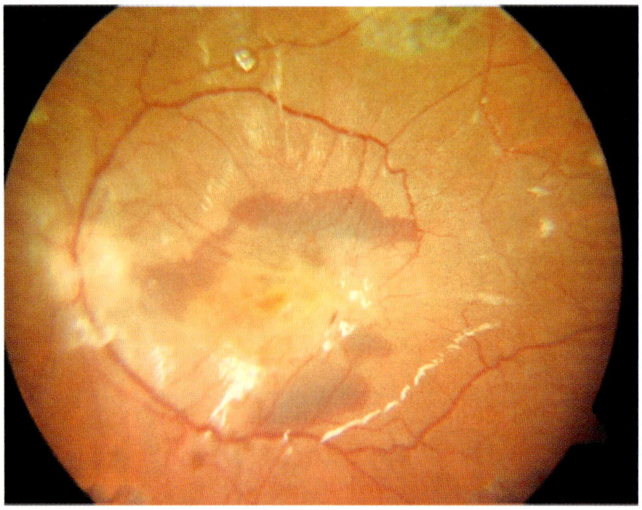

Color fundus photograph reveals silicone oil reflexes, epimacular membrane, attached retina, submacular hemorrhages and large CNVM

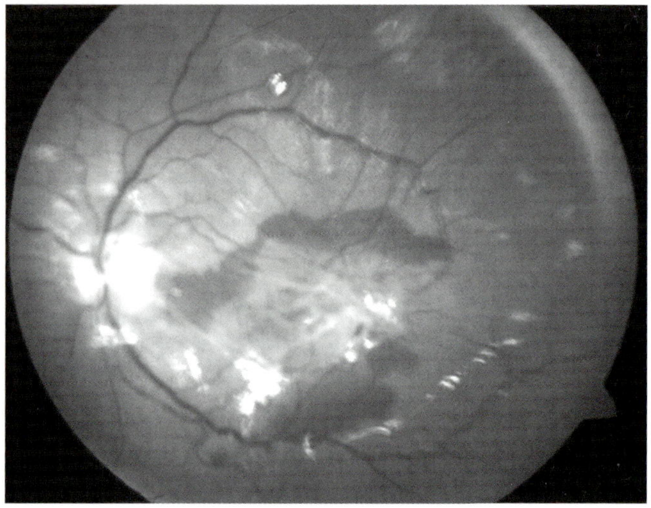

Red free photograph of the left eye highlights the extent of submacular hemorrhage. Silicone oil reflexes can be made out

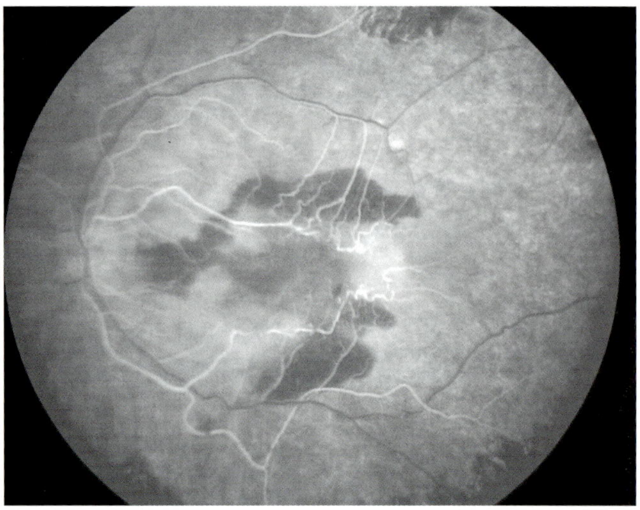

Early A-V phase angiogram reveals retinal vascular tortuosity due to ERM, blocked fluorescence due to submacular hemorrhage and lacy pattern filling of CNVM

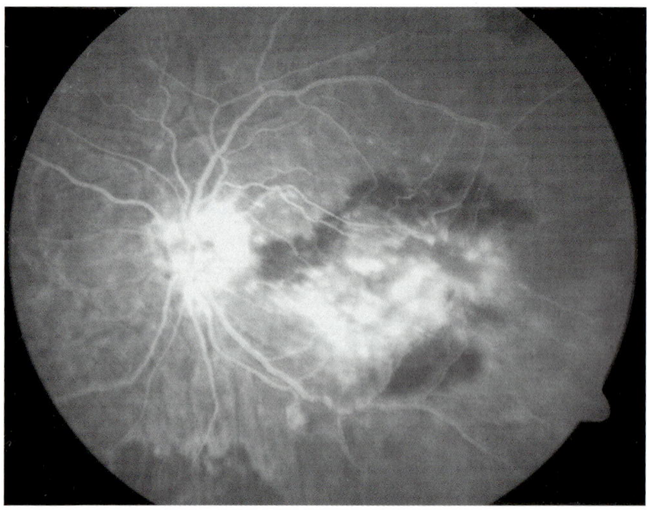

Late A-V phase angiogram reveals cystoid pooling of dye in the macula with intense hyperfluorescence due to leakage from CNVM. Blocked fluorescence persists

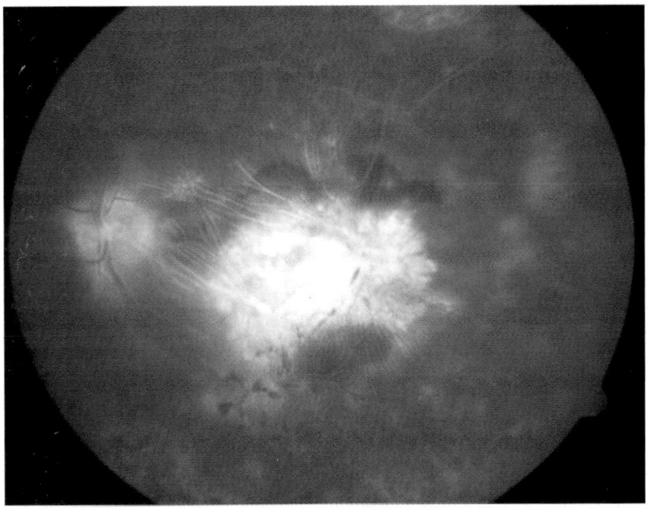

Late phase angiogram reveals intense hyperfluorescence due to leakage from CNVM. Blocked fluorescence persists

CNVM SECONDARY TO HEALED CHORIORETINAL SCAR

CASE 12

A 34-year-old lady complained of sudden diminution of vision in the left eye. She had macular scars in both the eyes secondary to healed fungal endogenous endophthalmitis, treated 2 years back. She was diagnosed of CNV in the left eye.

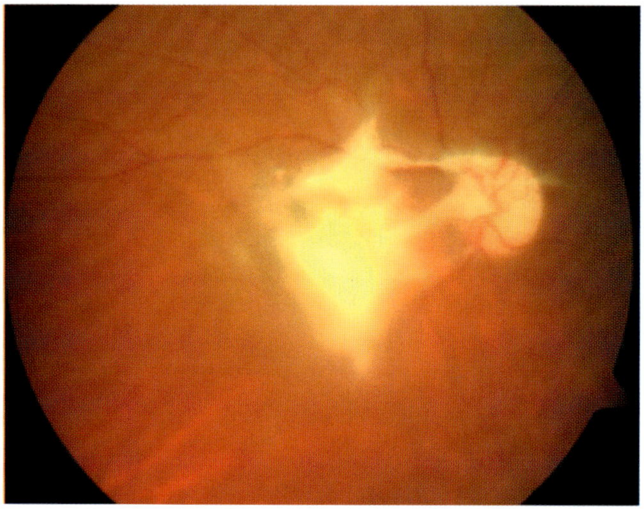

Color fundus photograph of the right eye showing healed granuloma over the posterior pole

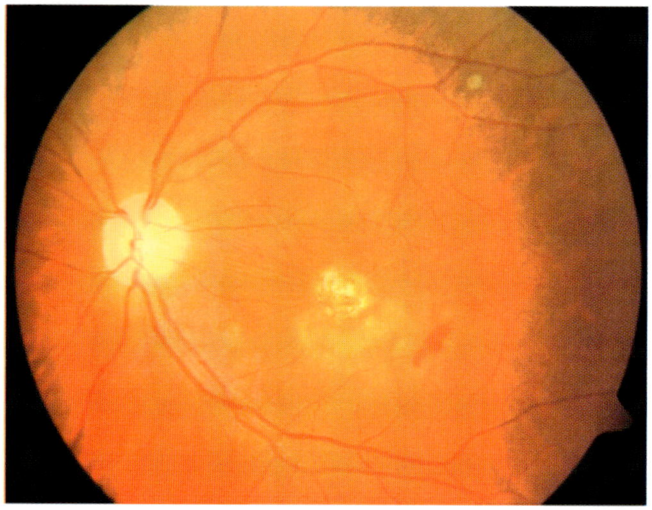

Color fundus of left eye showing a subfoveal scar and a yellowish-gray subretinal neovascular membrane with adjacent subretinal hemorrhage

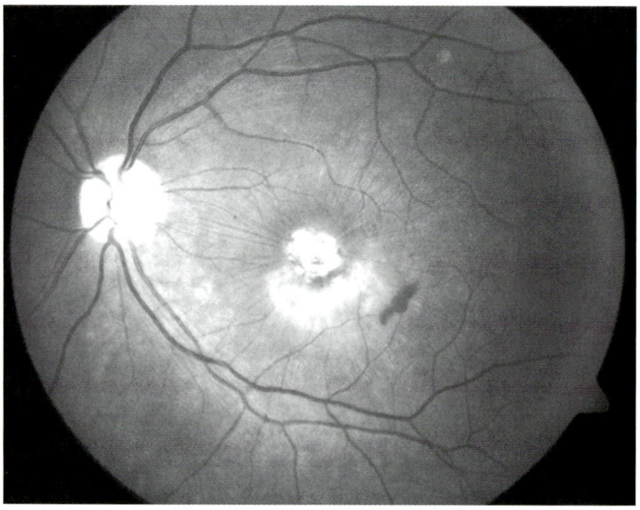

Red free picture of left eye showing the lesions clearly

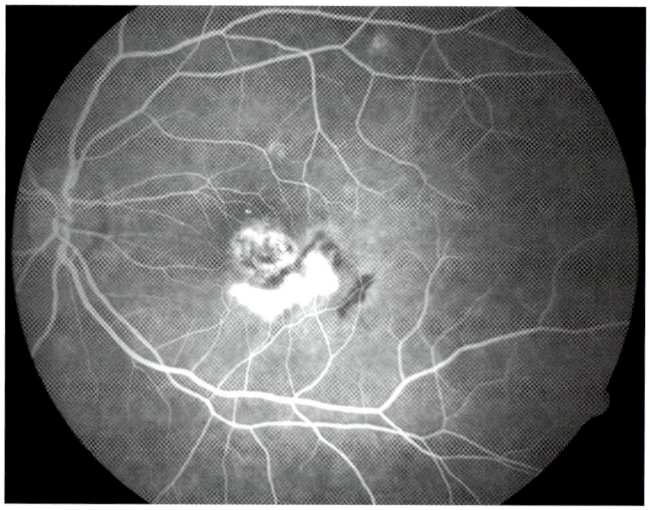

A-V phase showing intense hyperfluorescence inferotemporal to scar with adjacent blocked fluorescence due to hemorrhage

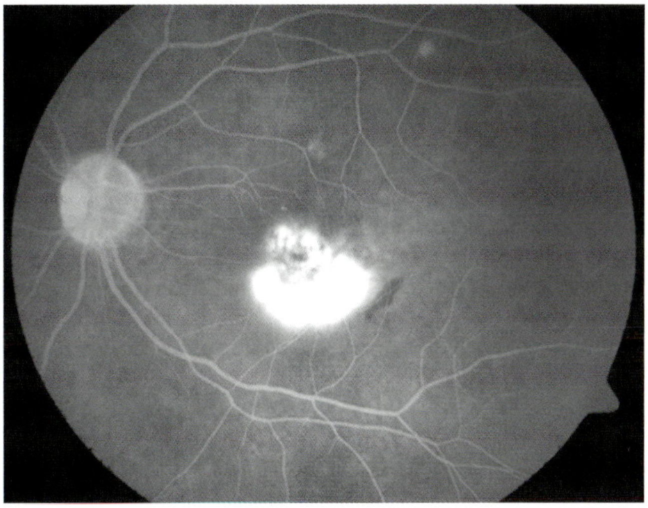

Late phase showing central staining, increasing leakage inferotemporally suggestive of active lesion

The patient underwent treatment with intravitreal bevacizumab. Six weeks later, examination revealed regressed CNVM.

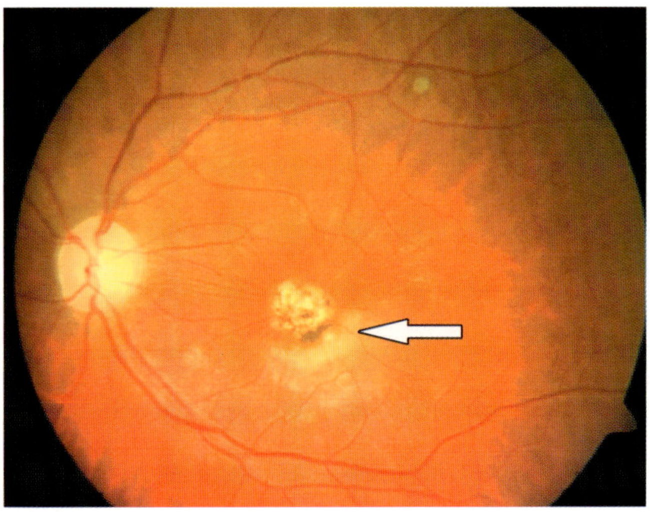

Color fundus photograph of the left eye showing scarred CNVM (arrow)

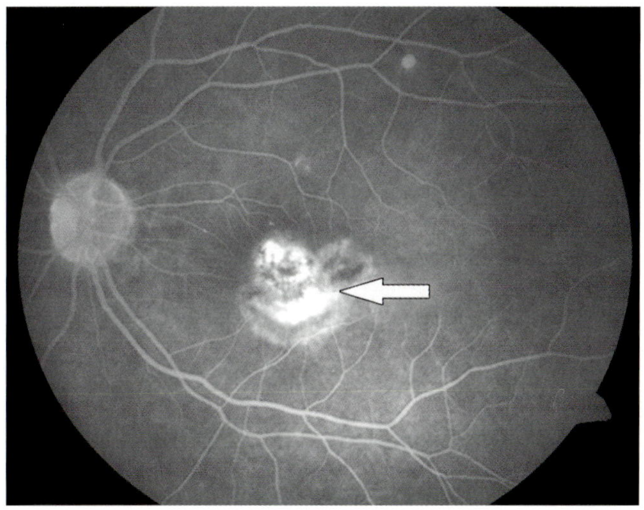

Late phase FFA showing staining of the lesion with no leakage (arrow)

CLINICAL NUGGETS

1. Visual prognosis in idiopathic CNVM is significantly better than that in age related macular degeneration.
2. CNVM associated with myopia appears as a grayish circumscribed lesion occurring close to fovea.
3. Natural history of CNVM in myopia is variable.
4. Photodynamic therapy can be considered as a treatment modality for the treatment of subfoveal myopic CNVM.

BIBLIOGRAPHY

1. Bhende M, Suganeswari G, Gopal L, Bhende PS, Gopal L, Rao C. Choroidal neovascularization associated with coloboma of the choroid: A series of three cases. Indian J Ophthalmol 2011; 59(2):148-51.
2. Gass JDM. Stereoscopic atlas of macular diseases. Diagnosis and treatment, 4th edn, CV Mosby, Chapter 3, 1997;2:1045.
3. Ho AC, Yannuzzi LA, Pisicano K, DeRosa J. The natural history of idiopathic subfoveal choroidal neovascularisation. Ophthalmology 1995;102:782-9.
4. Hotchkiss ML, Fine SL. Pathologic myopia and choroidal neovascularisation. Am J Ophthalmol 1981;91:177-83.
5. Jampol LM, Orth L, Daily MT, Rabb MF. Subretinal neovascularisation with geographic (serpiginous) choroiditis. Am J Ophthalmol 1979;88:683-9.
6. Nachiappan K, Kadekar A, Gopal L, Sharma T. Intravitreal Ranibizumab in the Treatment of Fungal Endophthalmitis Scar-Related Choroidal Neovascular Membrane. RETINAL Cases & Brief Reports. 03 September 2010. doi: 10.1097/ICB.0b013e3181d8e814
7. Rishi P, Venkataraman A, Rishi E. Combination photodynamic therapy and bevacizumab for choroidal neovascularization associated with toxoplasmosis. Indian J Ophthalmol 2011; 59(1):62-4.
8. Wojno T, Meredith TA. Unusual findings in serpiginous choroiditis. Am J Ophthalmol 1982;94:650-5.

17

Chapter

Retinal Pigment Epithelial Rip

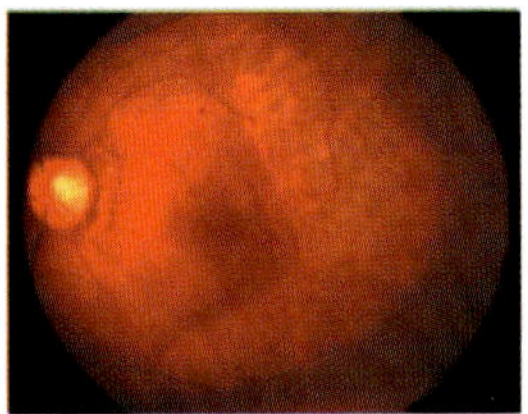

- Retinal pigment epithelial (RPE) rip or tears can occur in patients with a pigment epithelial detachment associated with central serous chorioretinopathy or with a choroidal neovascular membrane. It may follow laser photocoagulation as well.
- RPE layer is torn from one edge of the pigment epithelial detachment and scrolls under the opposite edge.

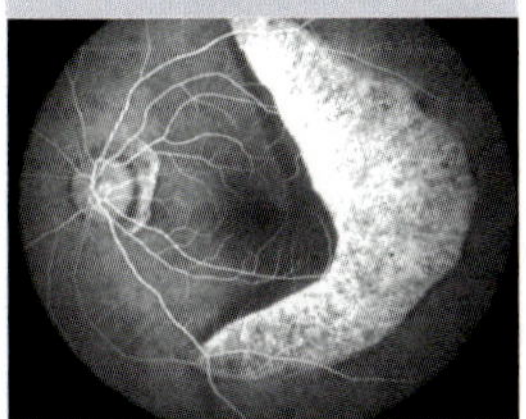

- The area devoid of RPE appears hyperfluorescent due to transmission of the underlying choroidal fluorescence that is easily seen through.
- Staining of the choroidal tissue and the underlying sclera causes the rip to appear hyperfluorescent in the late phase.
- The area of scrolled RPE appears hypofluorescent throughout the angiogram. However, if this scrolled edge harbors a choroidal neovascular membrane, some irregular hyperfluorescence may be seen.

CASE 1

A 45-year-old male presented with history of metamorphopsia in the left eye for the past two months; visual acuity was 6/6; N6.

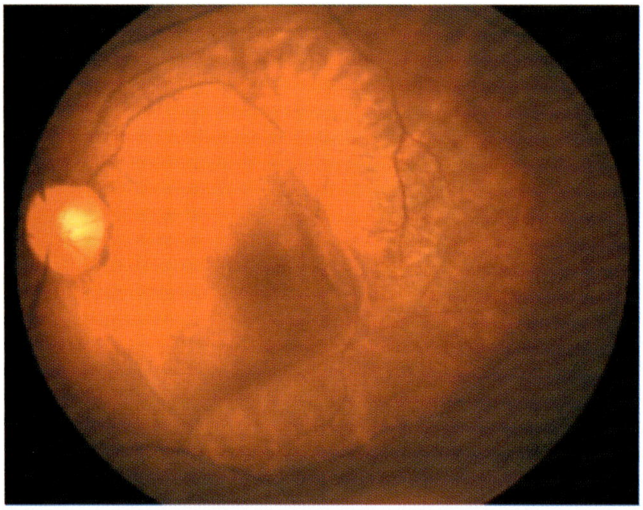

Fundus photograph of the left eye shows a broad crescentic depigmented zone in the temporal macula

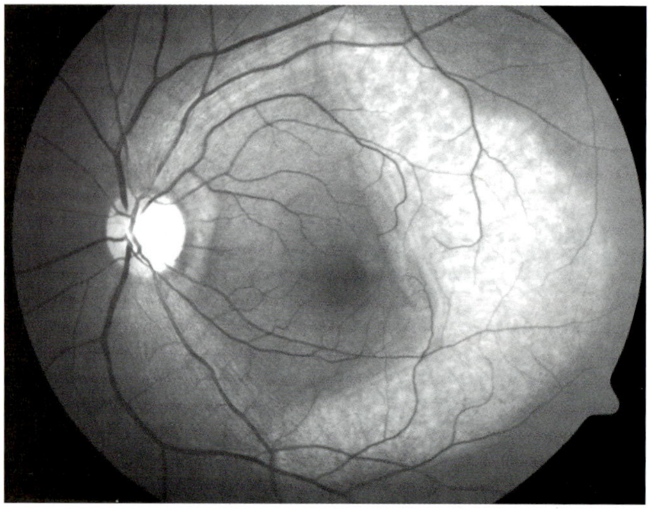

Red free photograph shows the large RPE tear. The scrolled up RPE layer is seen along the inner margin of the tear

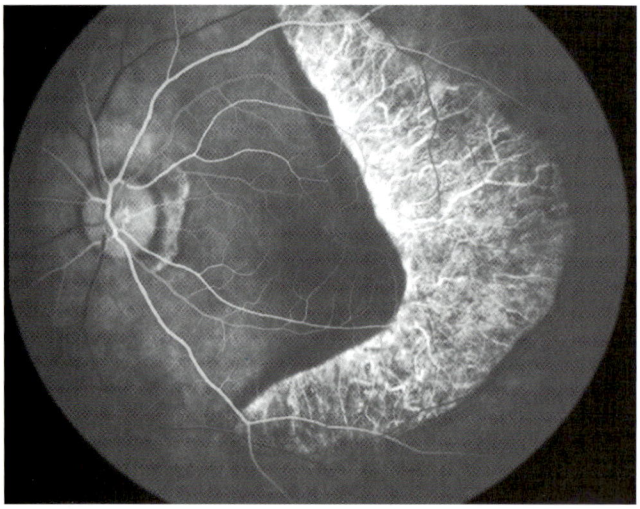

The background choroidal fluorescence and choroidal vasculature is clearly seen through the area of RPE rip. The scrolled up RPE blocks the background fluorescence and is visible as a band of hypofluorescence on the inner margin

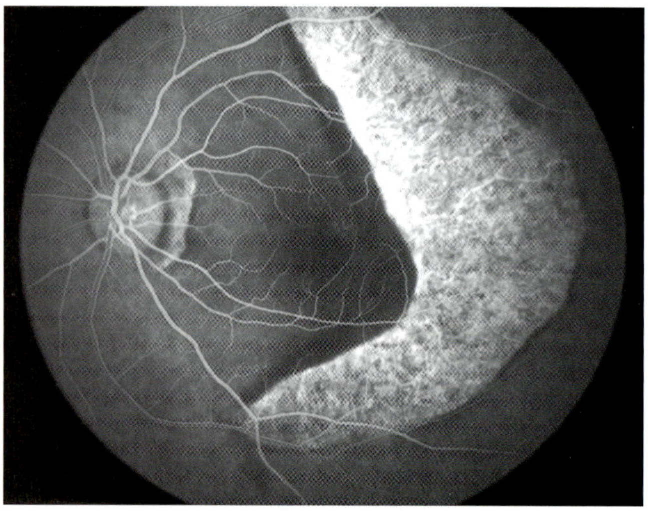

Increased hyperfluorescence is seen in the area of RPE rip. The hypofluorescence along the inner margins is better appreciated

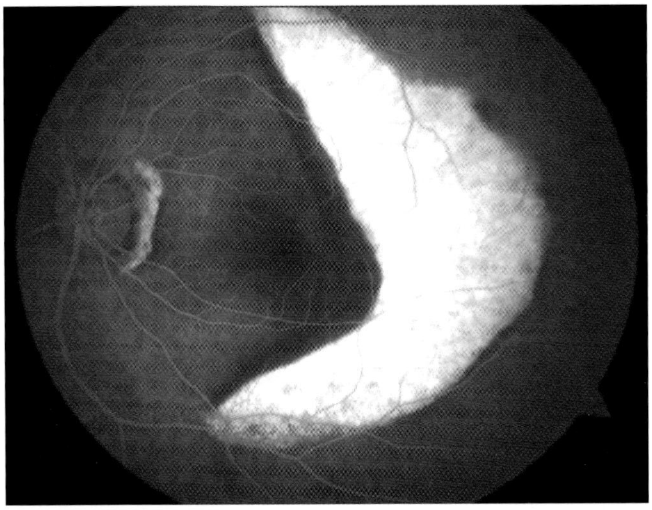

Late staining of the choroidal tissue and the sclera is seen through the area of absent RPE. Note that the scrolled RPE remains hypofluorescent throughout the angiogram

COMMENT

Absence of the overlying RPE in the region of the tear allows increased visibility of the choroidal fluorescence.

The scrolled edge of the RPE blocks the back-ground choroidal fluorescence throughout the angiogram.

CASE 2

A 64-year-old presented with reduced vision in the right eye for the past three months; visual acuity was 3/60.

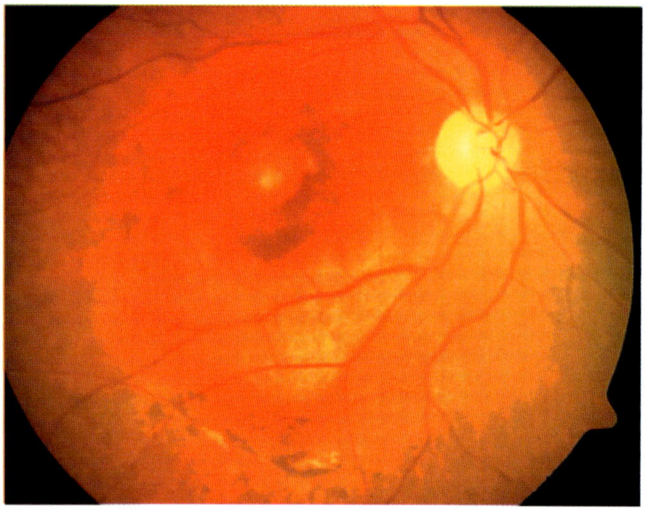

Fundus photograph of the right eye shows a CNVM in the foveal region. A broad crescent shaped depigmented zone is seen in the inferior macula

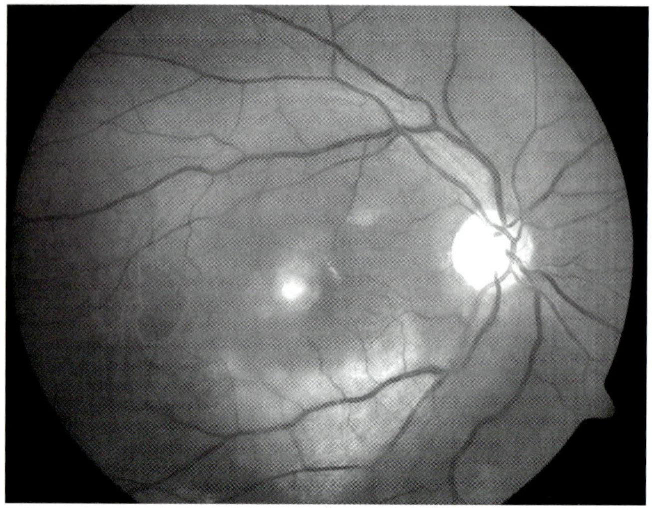

Red free photograph shows the area of RPE rip in the inferior macula

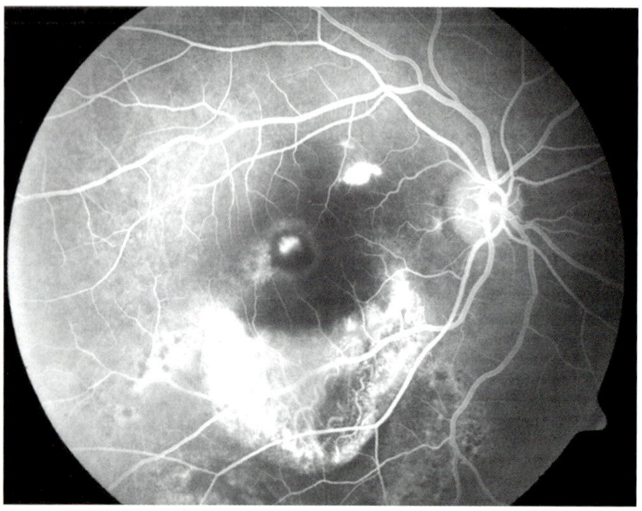

Hyperfluorescence is seen in the area of RPE rip. The scrolled RPE appears as a zone of hypofluorescence on the foveal side of the rip. Hyperfluorescence from a CNVM is seen at the fovea

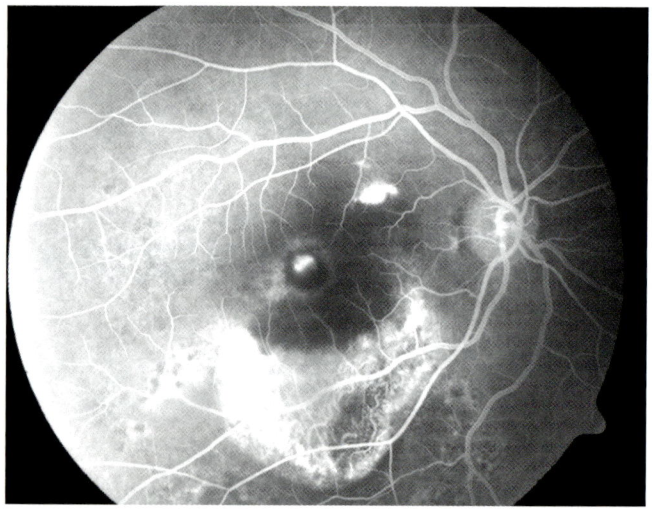

Increased hyperfluorescence is seen in the area of RPE rip in the later part of the arteriovenous phase

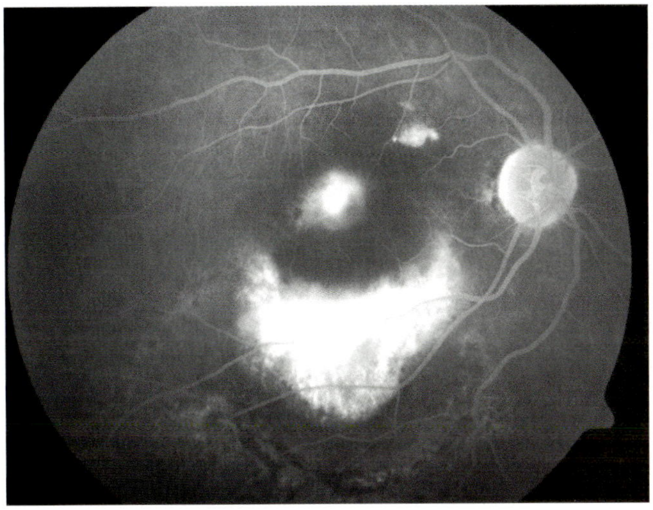

Retinal pigment epithelial (RPE) rip appears hyperfluorescent in the late phase due to staining of the choroidal tissue and the underlying sclera. Fuzzy hyperfluorescence is seen at the CNVM. The scrolled RPE remains hypofluorescent

COMMENT

In cases of RPE rip associated with CNVM, the torn RPE usually scrolls towards the CNVM.

CLINICAL NUGGETS

1. RPE rip involving the fovea can cause a sudden drop in vision.
2. There is no effective treatment for RPE rip.

BIBLIOGRAPHY

1. Bressler NM, Finkelstein D, Sunness JS, et al. RPE Tears through the fovea with preservation of good visual acuity. Arch Ophthalmol 1990;108:1694-97.
2. Gass JDM. Retinal pigment epithelium rip during krypton red photocoagulation. Am J Ophthalmol 1984;98:700-6.
3. Gass JDM. Stereoscopic atlas of macular diseases. Diagnosis and treatment. CV Mosby 4th edn. Chapter 3, 1997;2:81-91.
4. Machemer R, Heriot W. RPE Tears through fovea with preservation of good visual acuity. Arch Ophthalmol 1991;109:1492-93.

18 Chapter Choroidal Rupture

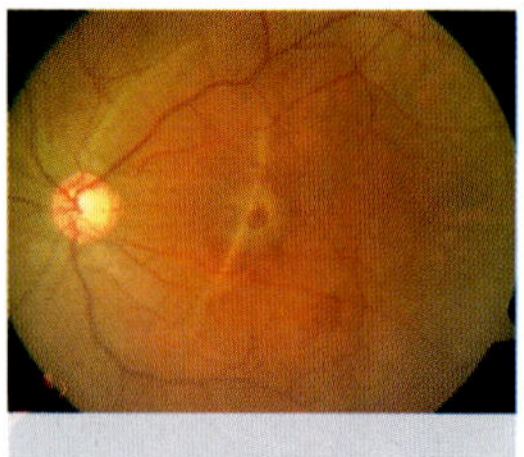

- It follows blunt injury to the eye.
- Due to distortion of the globe, the relatively inelastic Bruch's membrane ruptures along with the closely apposed RPE and choriocapillaries.
- They are usually crescent shaped and occur concentric to the optic disc.
- Associated with intrachoroidal, subretinal or intraretinal hemorrhage.
- It can be associated with fibrous proliferation, RPE hyperplasia and development of choroidal neovascular membrane.

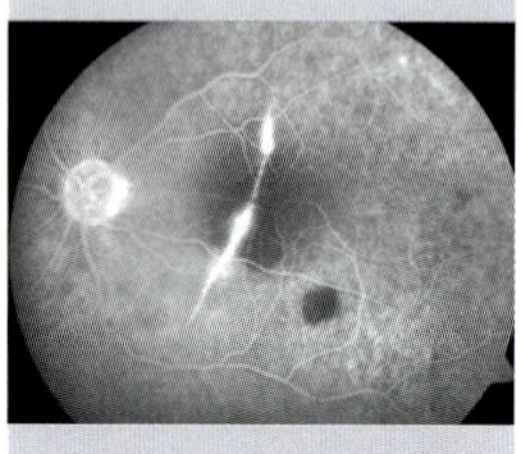

- Early phase may show relative hypofluorescence due to absence of the choriocapillaries. The underlying larger choroidal vessels may be seen through.
- Late hyperfluorescence is seen due to staining of the tissue at the choroidal rupture and the sclera.
- Areas of RPE hyperplasia are associated with blocked fluorescence.
- Fibrous tissue within the rupture stains in the late film.
- CNVM appears as an hyperfluorescent area which increases and has fuzzy margins in the late phase.

CASE 1

A 42-year-old male was seen with history of blunt injury to the eye two months back; visual acuity was 1/60.

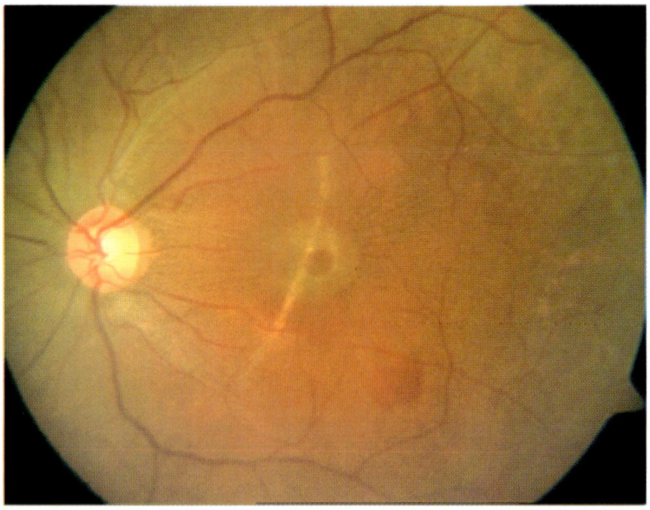

Fundus photograph of the left eye shows a choroidal rupture running through the fovea. A macular hole with a shallow cuff of subretinal fluid is seen

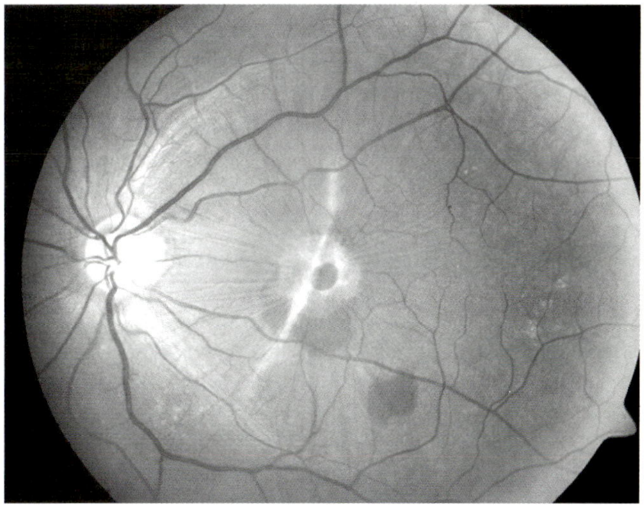

Red free photograph of the left eye. A small patch of subretinal hemorrhage is seen inferotemporal to the fovea

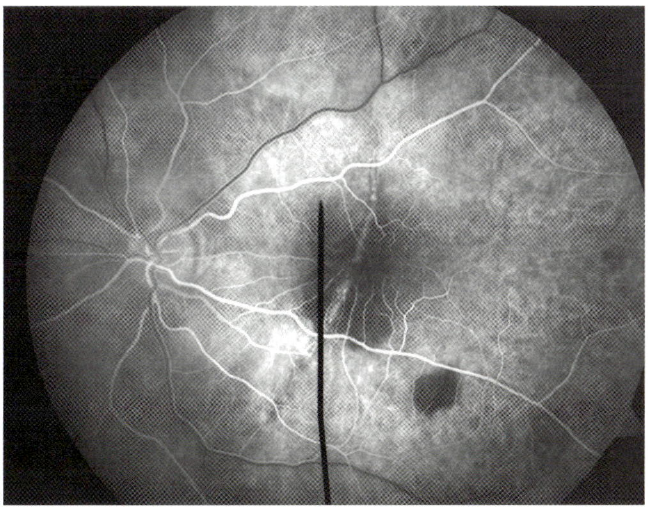

Early arteriovenous phase showing hyperfluorescence along the choroidal rupture due to transmission defect

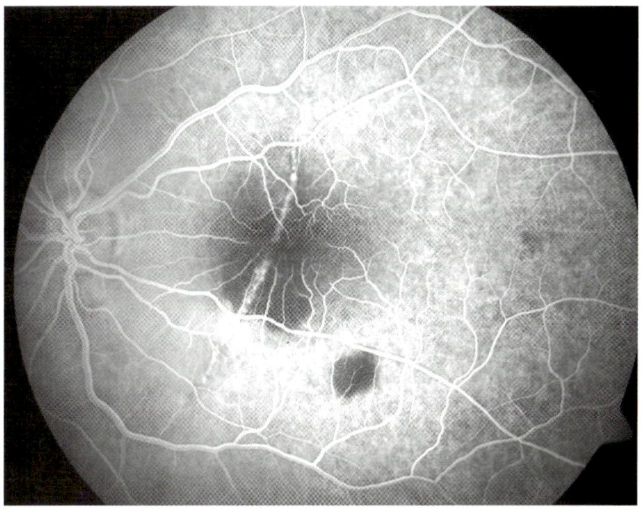

The hyperfluorescence along the choroidal ruptures has increased in the midarteriovenous phase. Blocked choroidal fluorescence is noted inferotemporal to the fovea caused by the subretinal hemorrhage

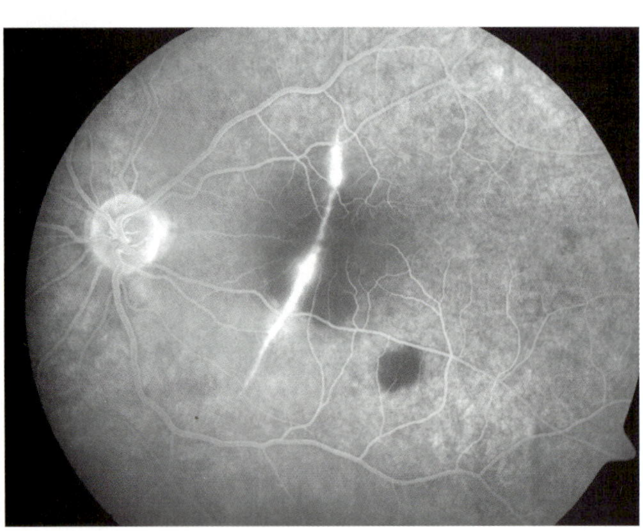

Late phase shows staining of the tissue along the choroidal rupture

COMMENT

This case shows the choroidal rupture traversing close to the foveal center. It shows minimal hyperfluorescence in the early phase which increases in the late phase of the angiogram.

CASE 2

A 25-year-old female presented with history of injury to the right eye with a tennis ball, one year back; visual acuity was 6/18; N18.

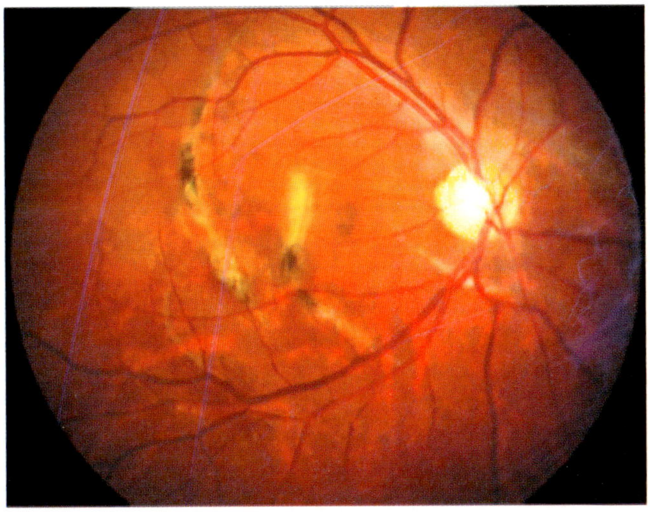

Fundus photograph of the right eye showing multiple choroidal ruptures at the macula. Areas of scarring and pigmentation are seen along the ruptures

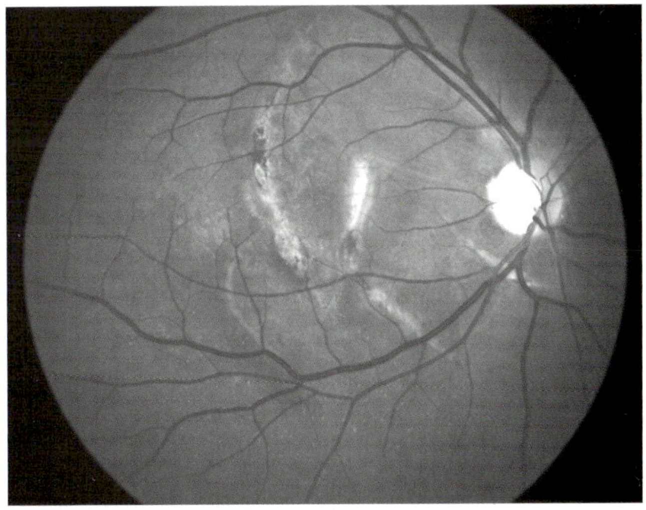

Red free photograph of the right eye

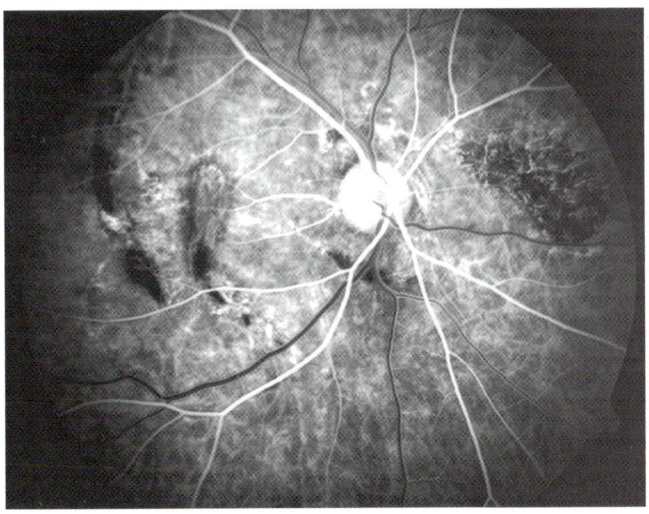

Early arteriovenous phase showing variable fluorescence along the choroidal rupture. Vascular network can be made out in the scar at the fovea. Blocked fluorescence is seen in areas of pigmentation

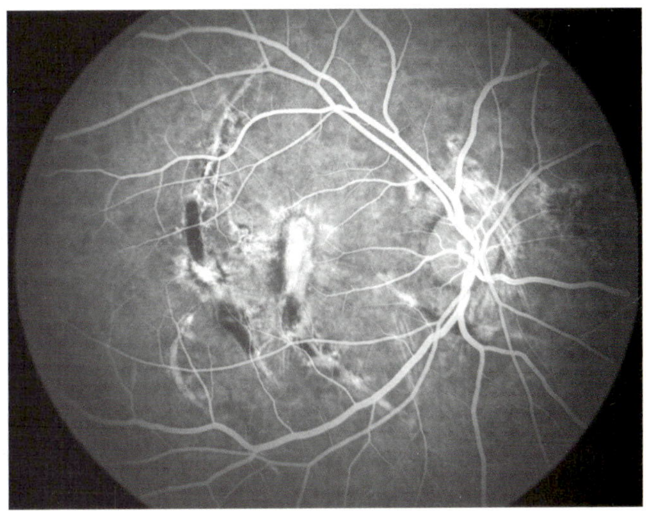

The hyperfluorescence at the scar has increased in the midarteriovenous phase. Areas of blocked fluorescence and transmission hyperfluorescence are seen in the other areas of choroidal rupture

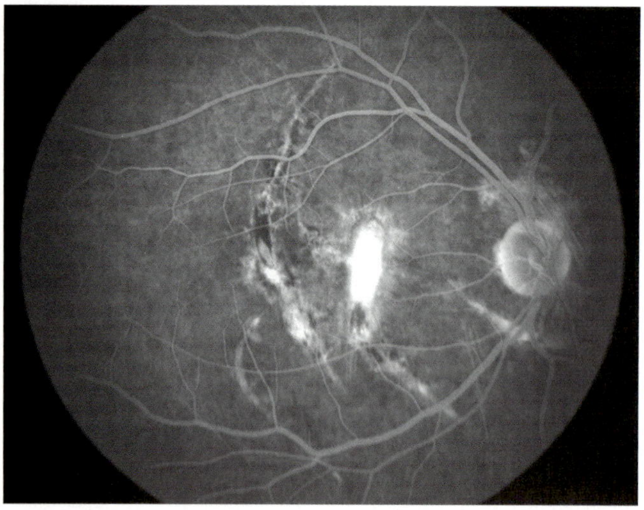

Intense staining is seen in the scar at the fovea. Hyperfluorescence elsewhere along the choroidal rupture has faded

COMMENT

Growth of CNVM through the choroidal tear is common. The CNVM shows intense hyperfluorescence with leakage and fuzzy margins in the late phase.

CASE 3

An 18-year-old healthy lady presented with blurred vision in OD following trauma with a tennis ball, 1 month back. At presentation, her BCVA was 6/9; N6 in OD and 6/6; N6 in OS. Examination showed choroidal rupture temporal to fovea with CNVM which was confirmed on FFA/OCT.

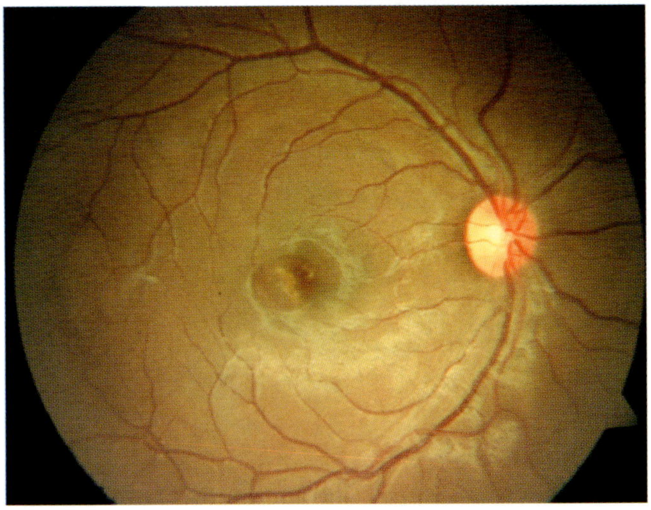

Color fundus photo of the right eye reveals a pale, curvilinear subretinal lesion inferotemporal to the fovea (choroidal rupture) with associated subretinal hemorrhage

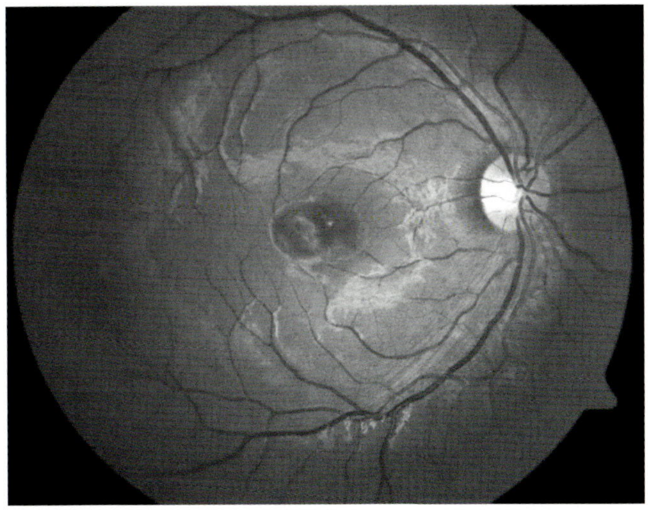

Red free photograph enhances the visualization of the extent of submacular hemorrhage

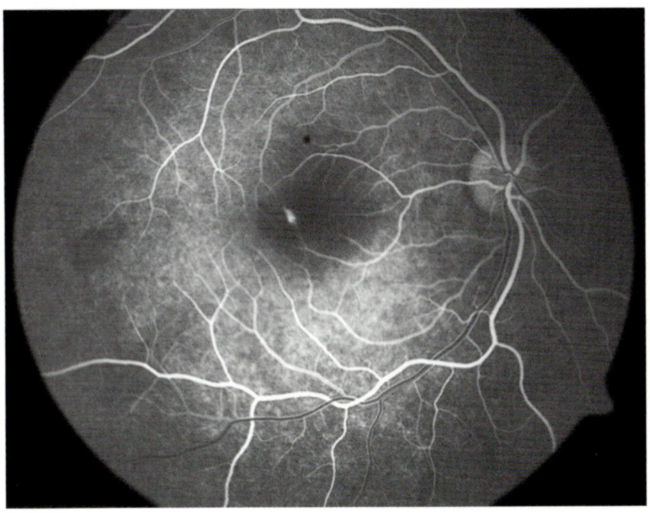

Early arteriovenous phase reveals hyperfluorescence related to the choroidal rupture

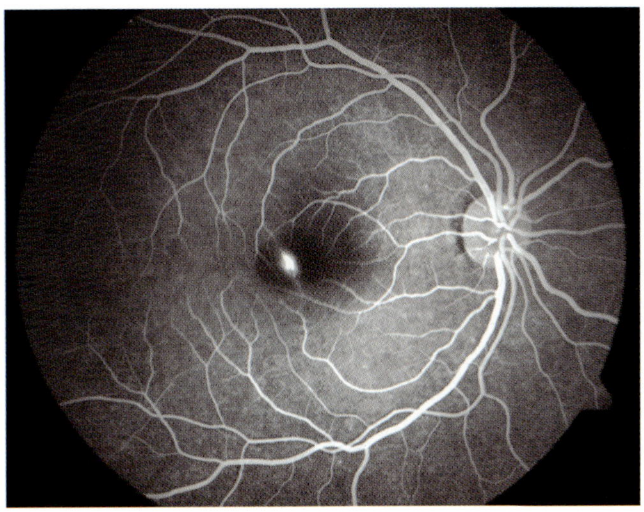

Late arteriovenous phase reveals hyperfluorescence increase in extent and intensity suggestive of underlying CNVM

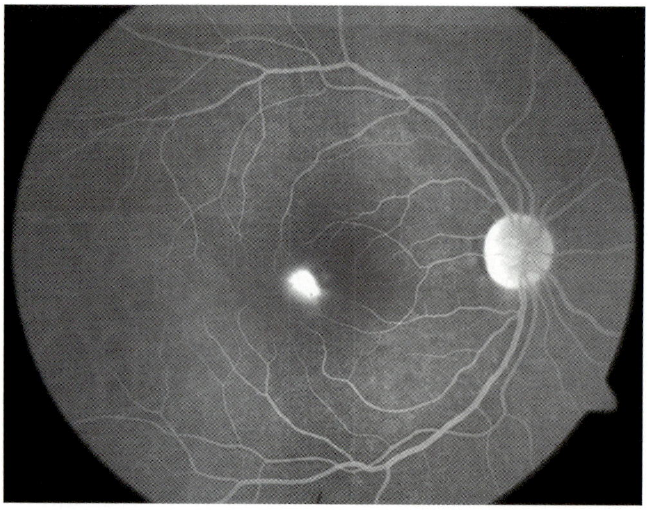

Late phase angiogram reveals intense hyperfluoresence confirmatory of CNV

The patient underwent intravitreal injection bevacizumab and was followed up after a month. CNVM regressed and fundus remained stable till the last follow-up of six months post-treatment.

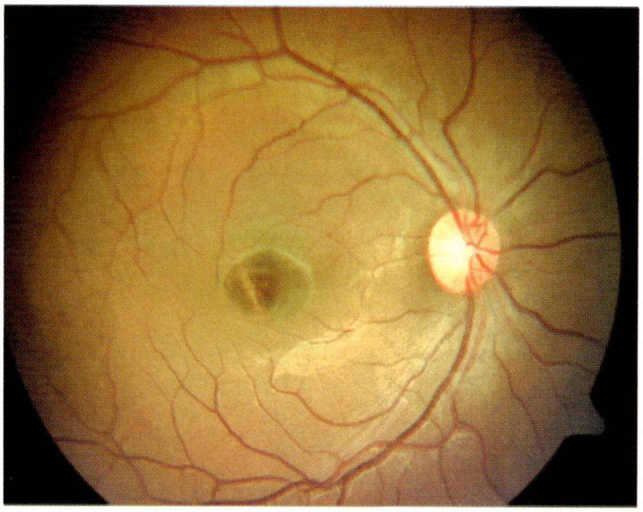

Color fundus photograph reveals resolution of submacular hemorrhage with regression of CNVM

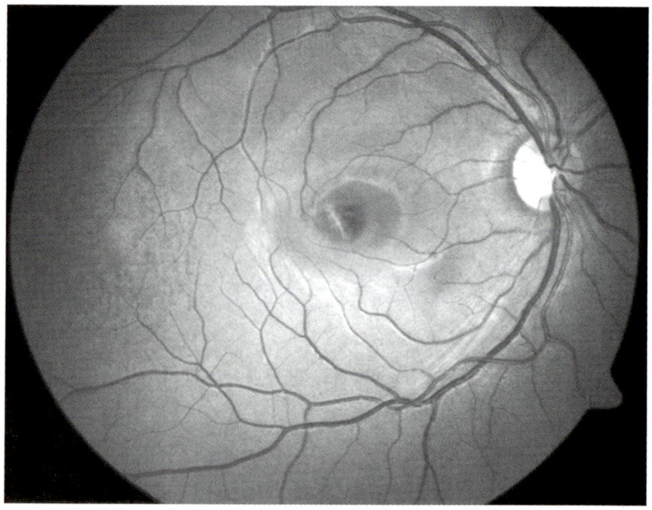

Red free photograph reveals just the choroidal rupture

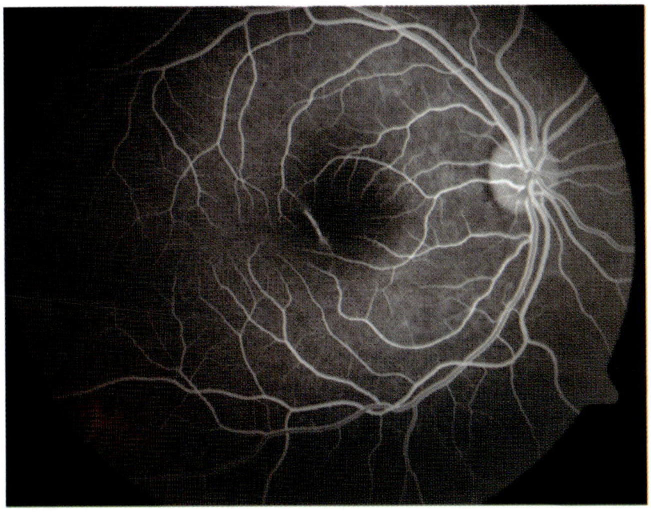

Early arteriovenous phase reveals hyperfluorescence due to the transmission effect of the choroidal rupture

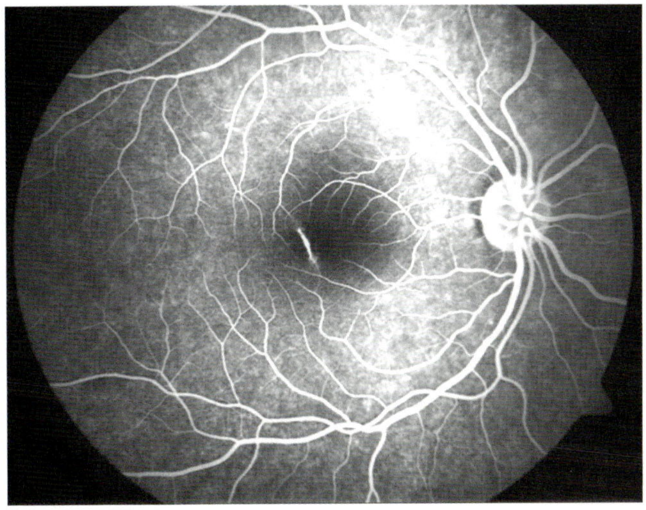

Late arteriovenous phase reveals hyperfluorescence due to the transmission effect of the choroidal rupture with no leakage

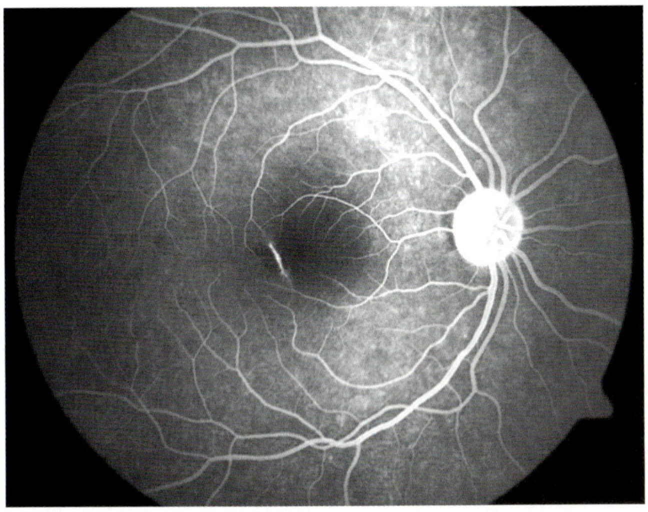

Late phase angiogram reveals hyperfluorescence due to scleral staining in the area of the choroidal rupture with no leakage

CLINICAL NUGGET

Eyes with choroidal ruptures should be followed-up for the development of choroidal neovascular membrane.

BIBLIOGRAPHY

1. Aguilar JP, Green WR. Choroidal rupture: a histopathological study of 47 cases. Retina 1984;4:269-75.
2. Duke-Elder WS. Textbook of Ophthalmology, Vol 6. St Louis: CV Mosby Co 1954;5829-37.
3. Gass JD. Stereoscopic Atlas of Macular Disease. Diagnosis and Treatment, 3rd edn. St Louis: CV Mosby Co 1987;170.
4. Rishi P, Shroff D, Rishi E. Intravitreal bevacizumab in the management of post-traumatic choroidal neovascular membrane. RETINAL Cases and Brief Reports. 2008;2(3):236-8.
5. Wyszynski RE, Grossniklaus HE, Frank KE. Indirect choroidal rupture secondary to blunt ocular trauma: a review of eight eyes. Retina 1988;8:237-43.

19 Chapter

Angioid Streaks

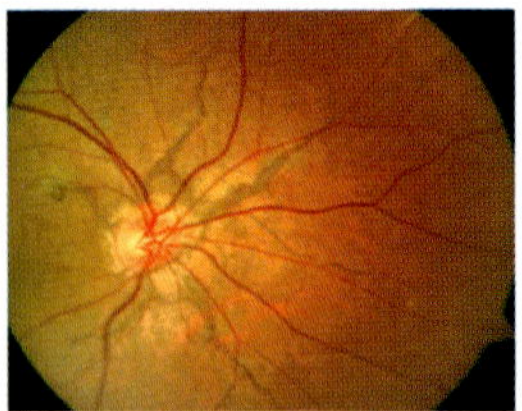

- Angioid streaks are usually bilateral and represent visible breaks in the Bruch's membrane.
- They appear as irregular radiating, reddish brown, ribbon like bands extending from the peripapillary area towards the periphery. Near the optic disc they are interconnected by circular ring. The retina, especially temporal to the macula has a mottled 'orange peel' or 'peau d'orange' appearance.
- Excessive deposition of calcium in the Bruch's membrane has been found in patients with angioid streaks. This deposition makes the layer brittle and susceptible to breaks.
- The systemic association of angioid streaks includes pseudoxanthoma elasticum, Ehlers-Danlos syndrome, Paget's disease, sickle cell disease, etc.

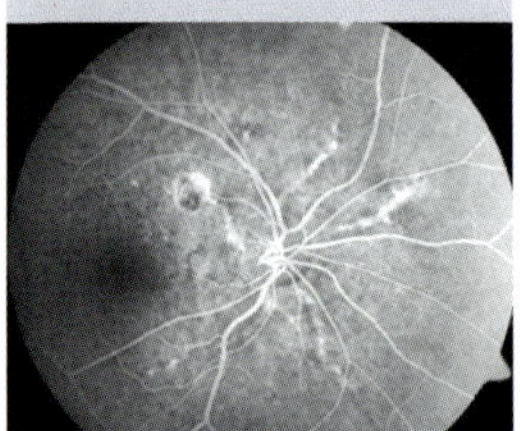

- Angiographic pattern of angioid streaks depends on the status of the overlying RPE, the degree of pigmentation in the region of the streaks and the status of the underlying choriocapillaris.
- Typically, angioid streaks become hyperfluorescent in the arterial phase due to transmitted choroidal fluorescence, which increases slightly in the later phases. No leakage of dye is seen.
- Choroidal neovascular membranes are common in patients with angioid streaks.

CASE 1

A 48-year-old female presented with history of floaters in both eyes. Visual acuity was 6/9; N6 in the right eye and 6/12; N6 in the left eye. She was found to have angioid streaks with CNVM in both eyes.

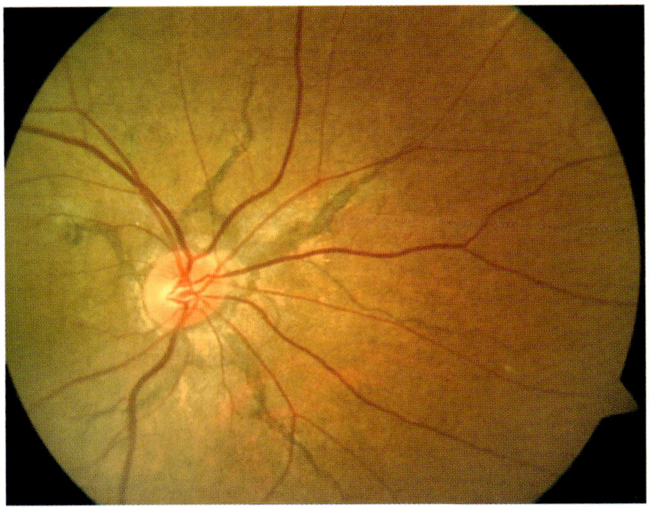

Fundus photograph of the right eye showing prominent angioid streaks radiating from an annular ring around the disc. Note the pigment clump seen along the angioid streak superotemporal to the disc. A CNVM is noted just superior to this pigment clump

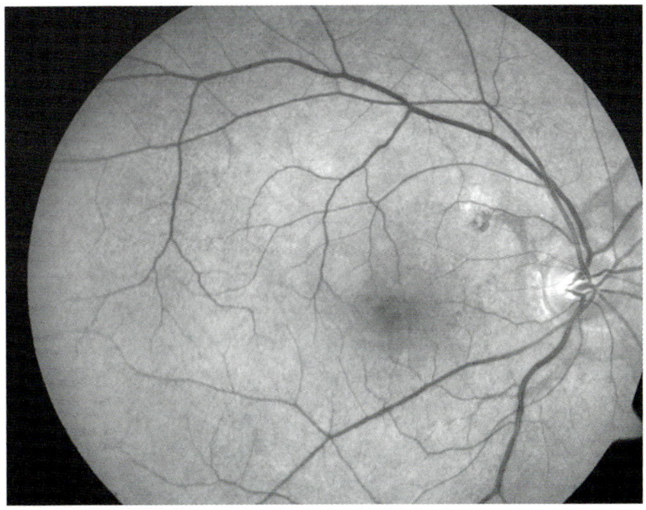

Red free photograph highlights the changes seen in the fundus photograph

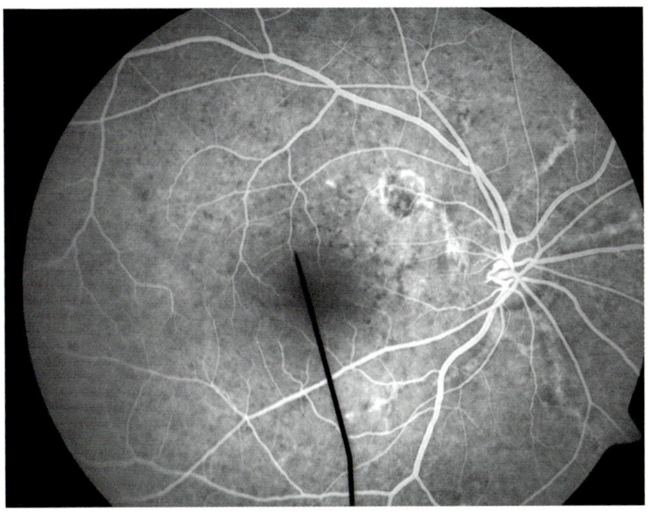

The angioid streaks are well seen in the arteriovenous phase as hyperfluorescent radiating lines. Faint mottled hyperfluorescence is seen temporally. Note the speckled hyperfluorescence seen just superior to the blocked hypofluorescence caused by the pigment clump

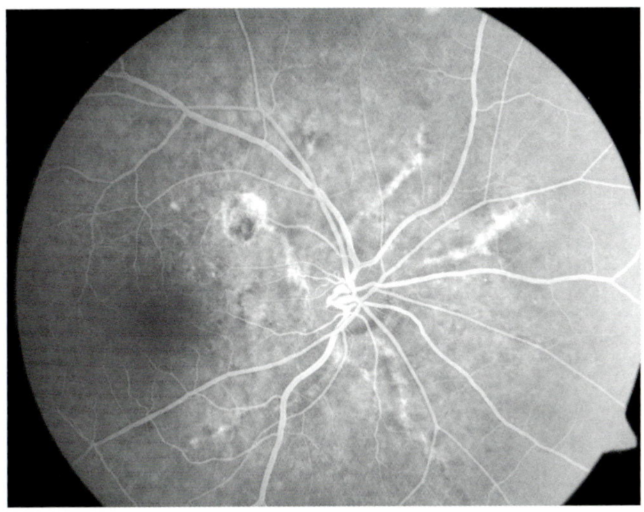

Increased hyperfluorescence is seen along the angioid streaks in the late arteriovenous phase. There is marked increase in the hyperfluorescence in the lesion superotemporal to the disc suggesting the presence of a CNVM

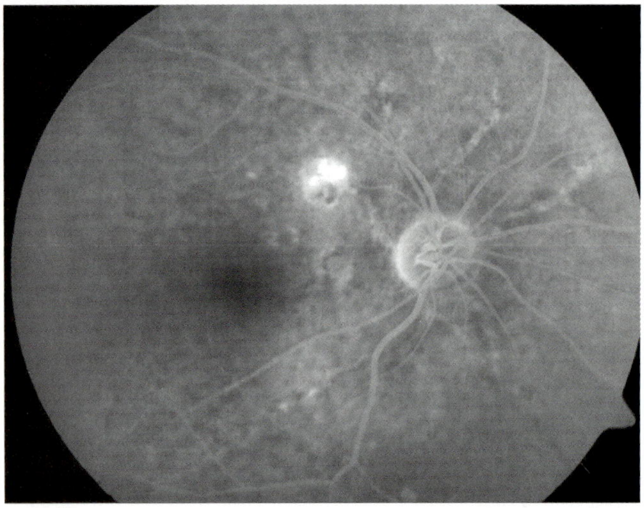

Late phase shows fading of the hyperfluorescence along the angioid streaks. Leakage of dye is noted in the area of the suspected CNVM

COMMENT

In this patient, the angioid streaks are much better seen clinically than on the angiogram. This is probably due to pigment and fibrous tissue within the angioid streak blocking the transmitted fluorescence to some extent.

CNVM occurs very commonly in eyes with angioid streaks and should be particularly looked for in the angiogram.

CASE 1 (*Continued*)

Left Eye of the Patient

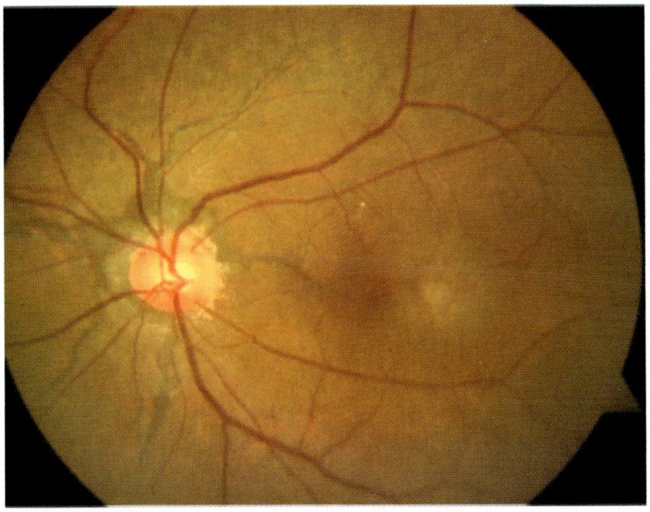

Fundus photograph of the left eye showing the prominent angioid streaks radiating from an annular ring around the disc. A CNVM is noted temporal to the fovea

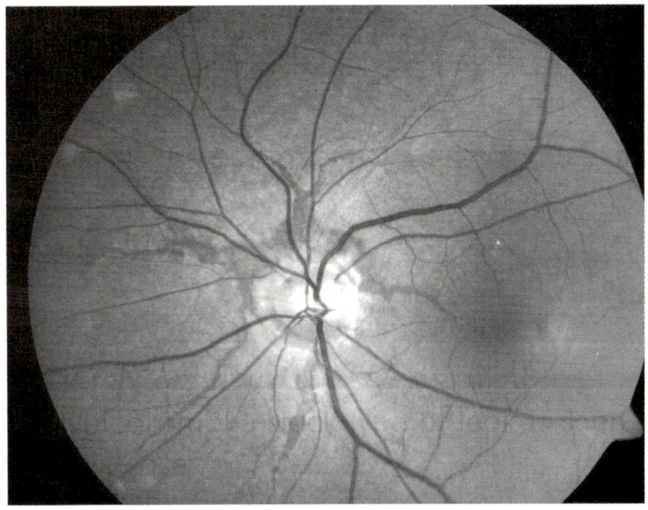

Red free photograph highlights the changes seen in the fundus photograph

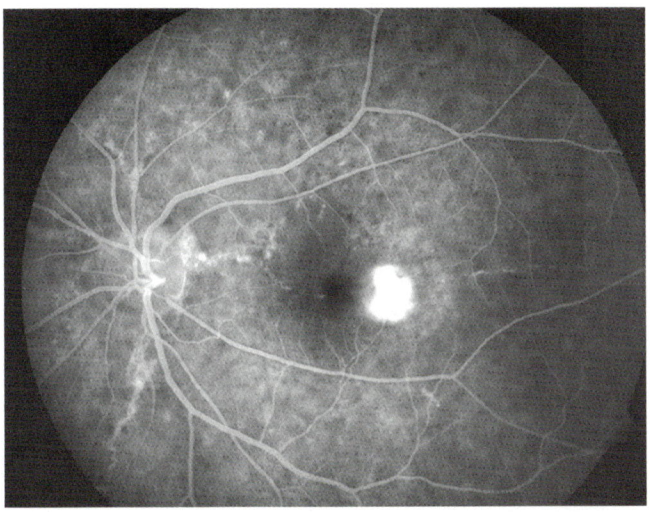

The late arteriovenous phase shows hyperfluorescence along the angioid streaks. Marked hyperfluorescence is noted in the region of the CNVM

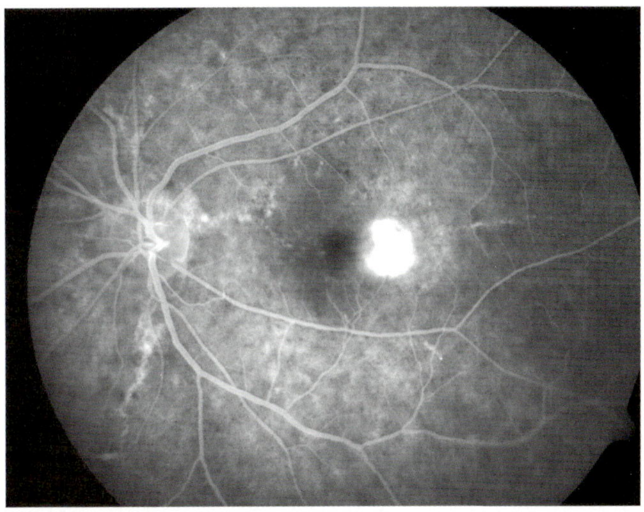

Late phase angiogram showing fading of the hyperfluorescence along the angioid streaks. Leakage of dye from the CNVM is seen

COMMENT

Growth of the CNVM through the breaks in the Bruch's membrane is common in patients with angioid streaks.

CASE 2

A 55-year-old patient with a visual acuity of 6/9; N6 in the left eye. He was noted to have angioid streaks in both eyes.

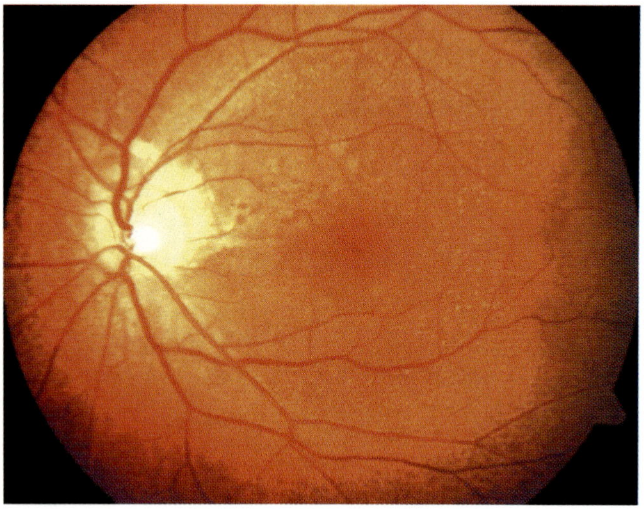

Fundus photograph of the left eye showing RPE alterations over and superior to the papillomacular bundle. Peripapillary atrophy is seen temporal and superior to the disc

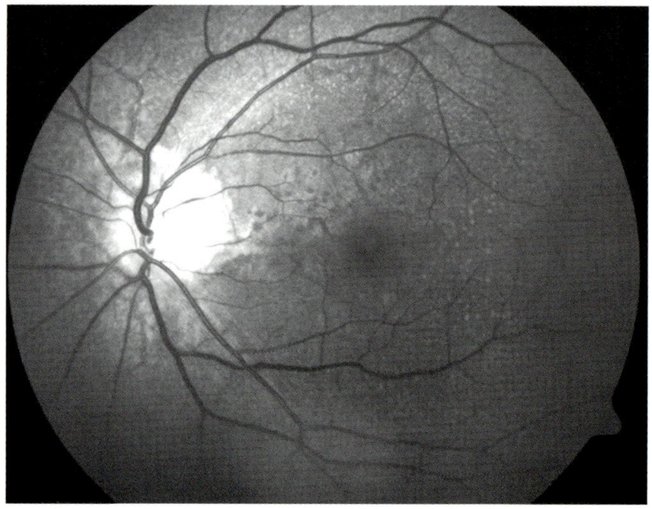

Red free photograph shows the angioid streaks as dark bands radiating away from the disc — both superior and inferior to the disc

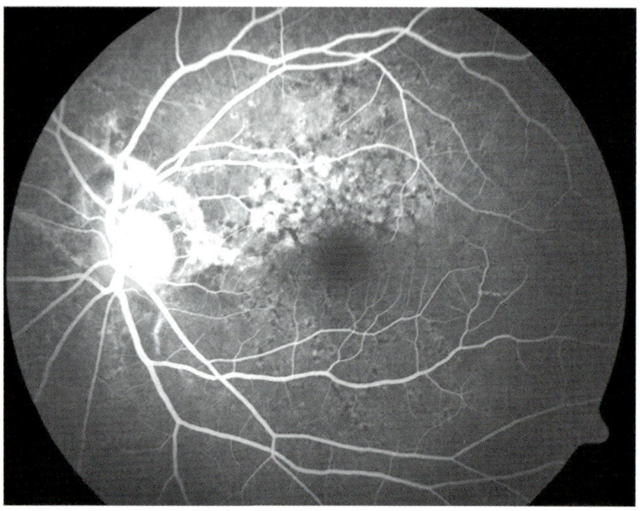

Mid arteriovenous phase shows transmission defect in the form of radiating bands seen superior, nasal and inferior to the disc. A mottled hyperfluorescence is seen in the macular region more prominent superiorly

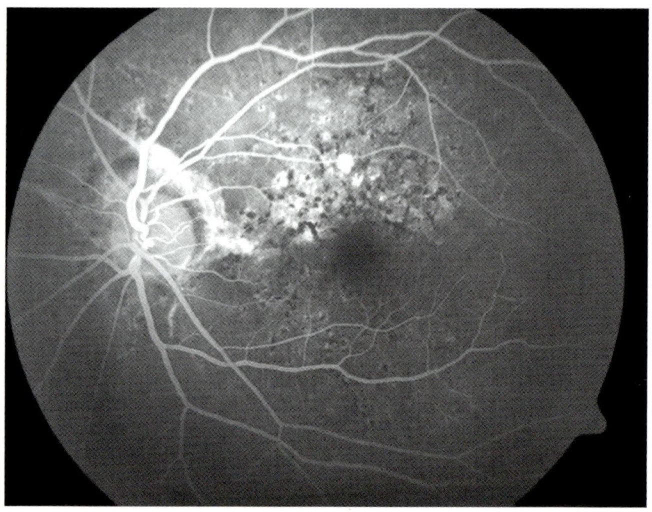

Recirculation phase shows increased mottled hyperfluorescence in the macular region

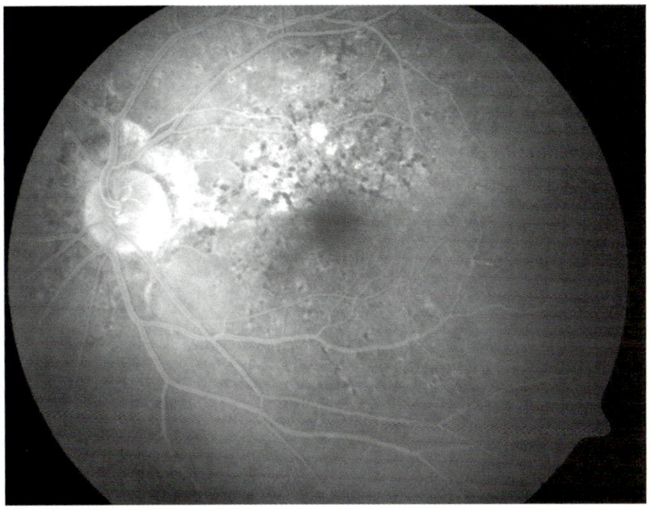

Late phase of the angiogram shows some fading of the hyperfluorescence. Staining of the scleral tissue is seen in the temporal and superior peripapillary region

COMMENT

Angioid streaks are seen as hyperfluorescent bands, more prominent in the mid arterio-venous phase. The mottled or stippled pattern of hyperfluorescence is a common finding in patients with angioid streaks and is usually seen at the posterior pole-especially the temporal macular region. It is caused by small clumps of pigment epithelium which block the choroidal fluorescence.

CASE 3

A 55-year-old male patient presented with decreased vision in the right eye. Visual acuity was 6/36; N36. He was noted to have angioid streaks in both eyes with a choroidal neovascular membrane in the right eye.

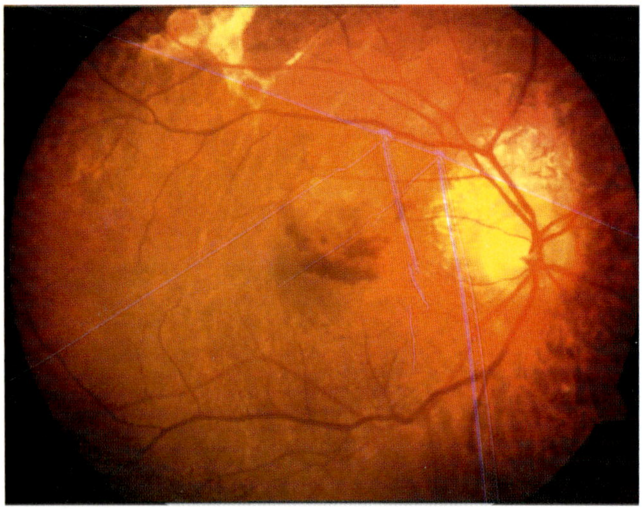

Fundus photograph of the right eye shows a CNVM surrounded by subretinal hemorrhage, just superior to the foveal center. Concentric white lines (choroidal rupture) are seen along the superior arcade with a large subretinal scar seen superotemporally

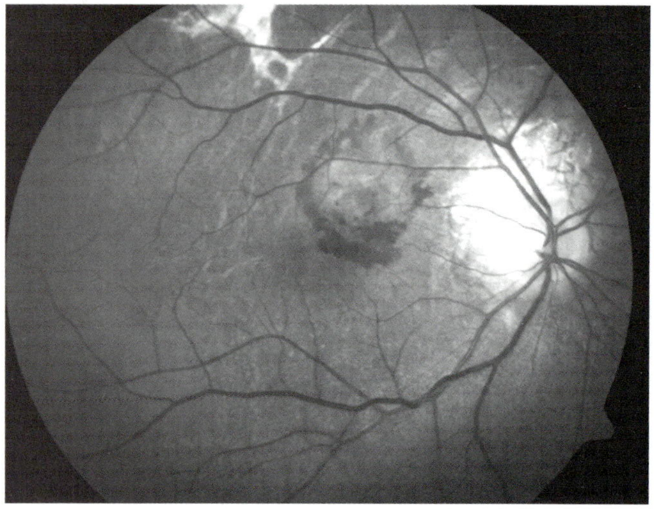

Red free photographs highlights these changes. The peripapillary atrophy is well-made out temporal and superior to the optic nerve head

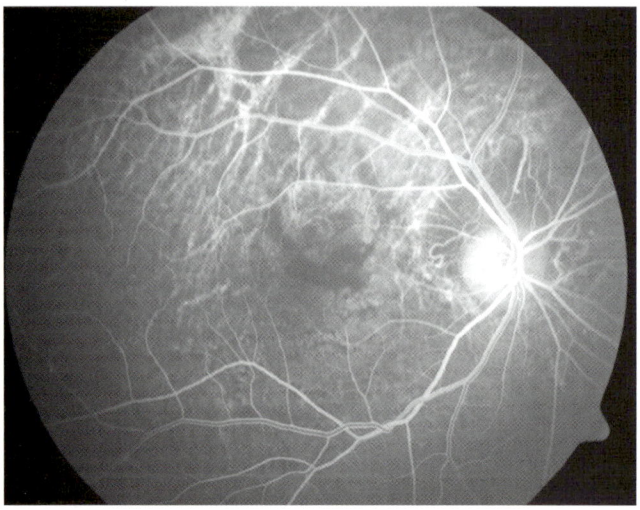

Mid arteriovenous phase shows the filling of the CNVM. Hyperfluorescent lines (due to transmission defect) concentric to the disc margin are noted superotemporal to the disc

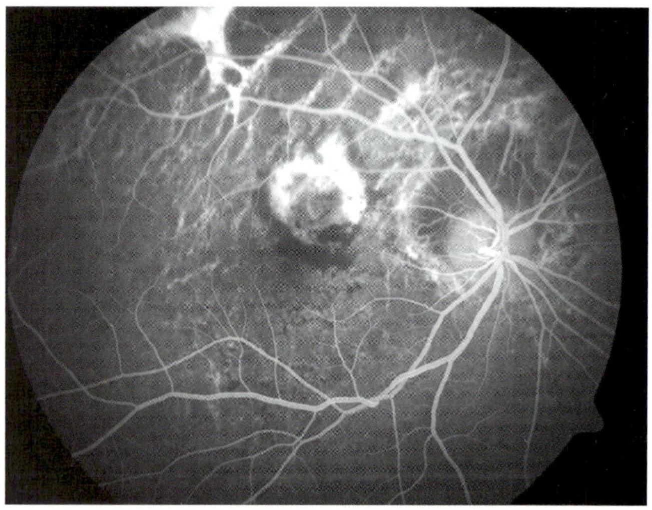

Arteriovenous phase shows increased filling of the CNVM. Faint linear hyperfluorescent bands are noted radiating away from the disc—nasally and inferiorly

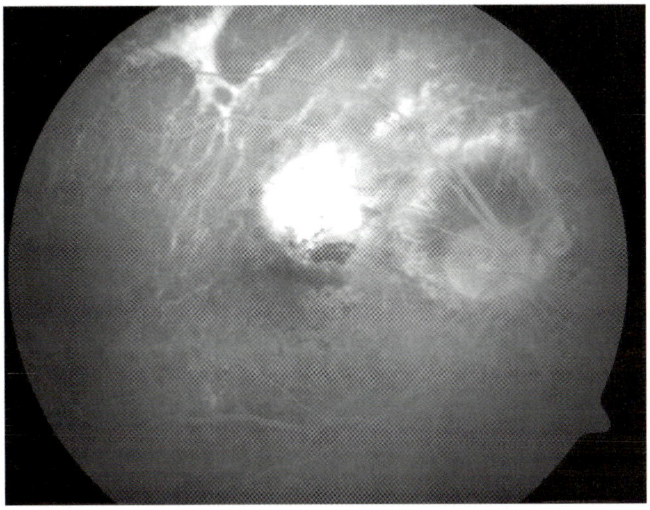

Late phase of the angiogram shows leakage of the dye from the CNVM. Some fading of the hyperfluorescence is seen in the region of the choroidal rupture. Staining of the scar in the superotemporal region is also seen

COMMENT

Eyes with angioid streaks are very susceptible to trauma. The concentric lines seen along the superotemporal arcade do not follow the general pattern of the angioid streaks and probably represents choroidal rupture due to some trivial eye injury in the past. The fellow eye of this patient had typical pattern of angioid streaks.

CASE 4

A 36-year-old male patient diagnosed to have pseudoxanthoma elasticum presented with decreased vision in the right eye. Visual acuity was 6/24; N36.

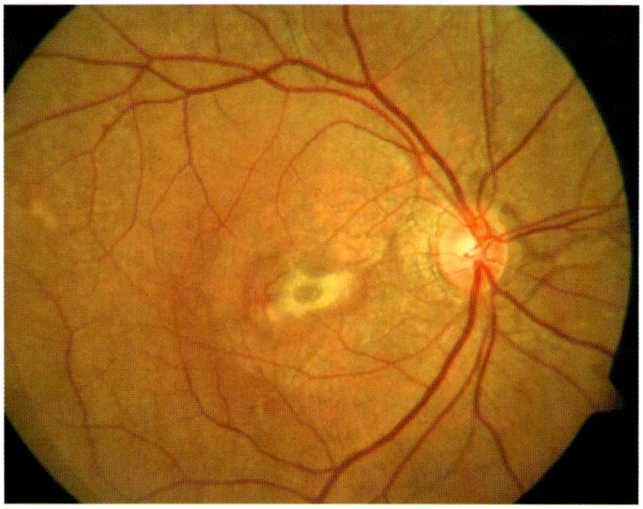

Fundus photograph of the right eye of a patient with angioid streaks with a partly cicatrized CNVM. The angioid streaks are seen as dark brown bands radiating away from the disc

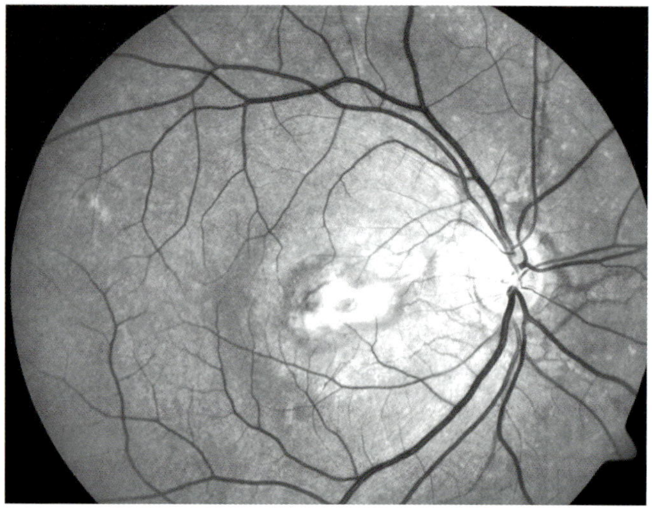

The angioid streaks are well-made out in the red free photograph

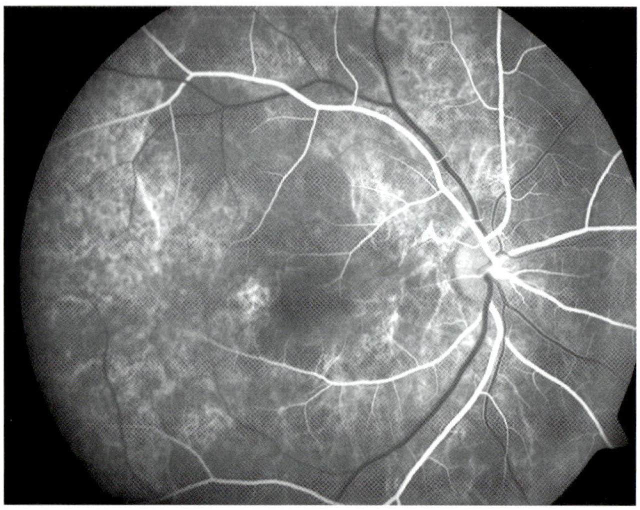

In this case the angioid streaks are not evident in the arterial phase of the angiogram. The normal patchy choroidal filling is well-seen in this phase

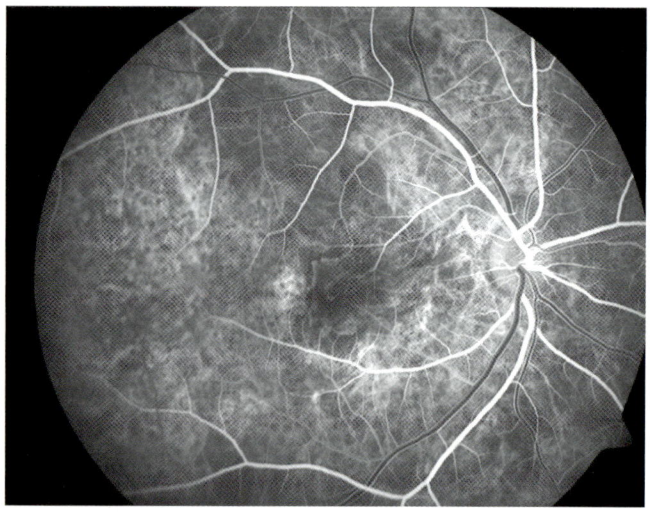

The early arteriovenous phase shows filling of the CNVM. The normal choroidal patchy filling is persisting. The angioid streaks are not yet clearly seen. There is mottled hyperfluorescence in the temporal macular region

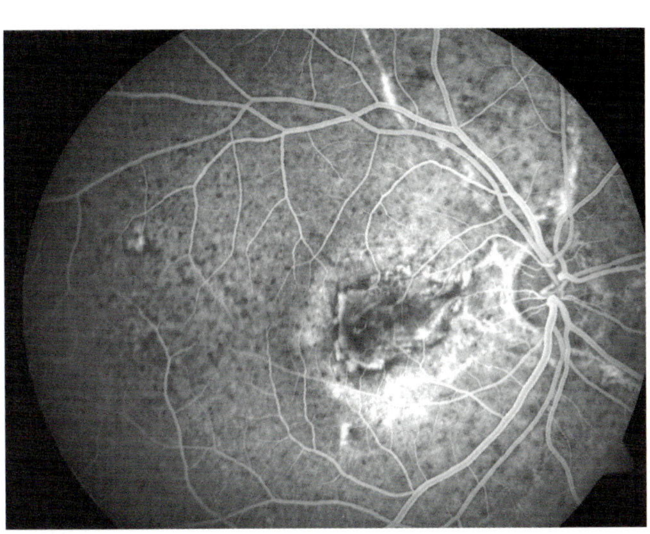

Angioid streaks became evident in the late arteriovenous phase of the angiogram as hyperfluorescent bands. The mottled hyperfluorescence in the temporal macular region is better seen

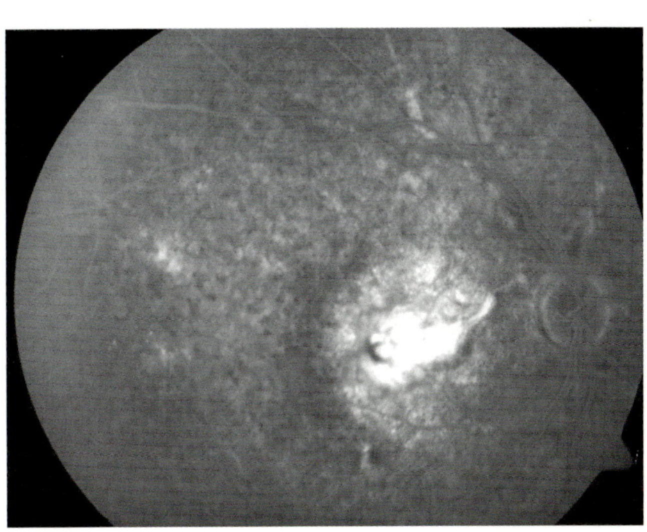

Late phase angiogram shows increased staining of the scarred CNVM. The hyperfluorescence along the angioid streaks has faded to some extent. The temporal mottled hyperfluorescence is persisting

CASE 5

A 47-year-old male patient presented with a history of decreased vision in the right eye for the past two years. Visual acuity was 3/60 in the right eye.

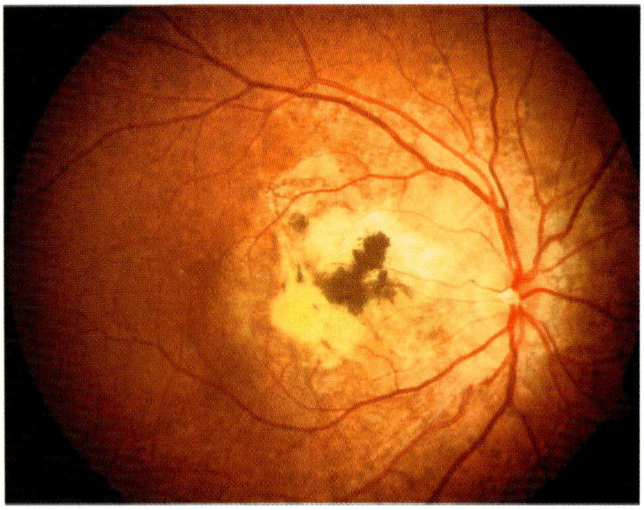

Fundus photograph of the right eye showing a large disciform scar in the macular region. Prominent pigment hypertrophy is seen within the scar. Angioid streaks were noted (not evident in this photo)

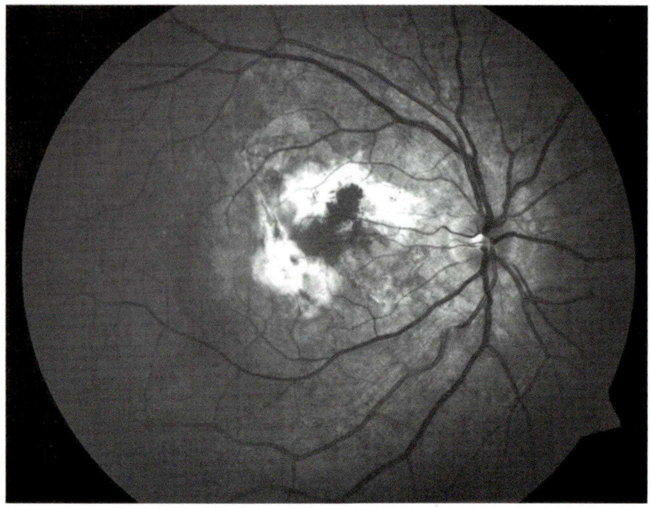

Red free photograph highlights the changes seen in the fundus photograph

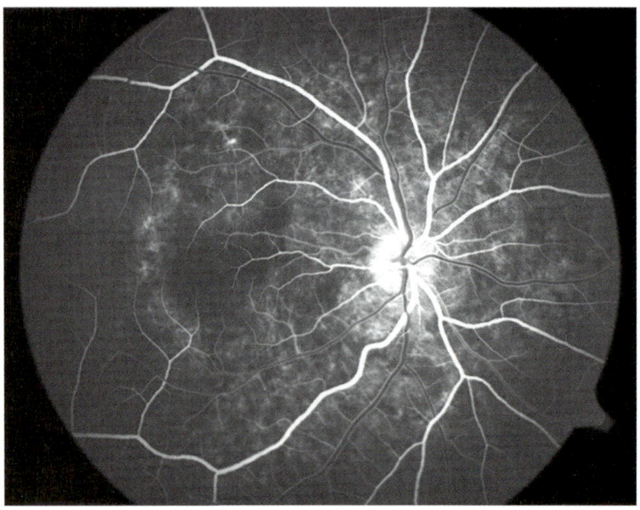

Early arteriovenous phase shows some hypofluorescence in the region of the scar. Faint hyperfluorescence is seen along the angioid streaks

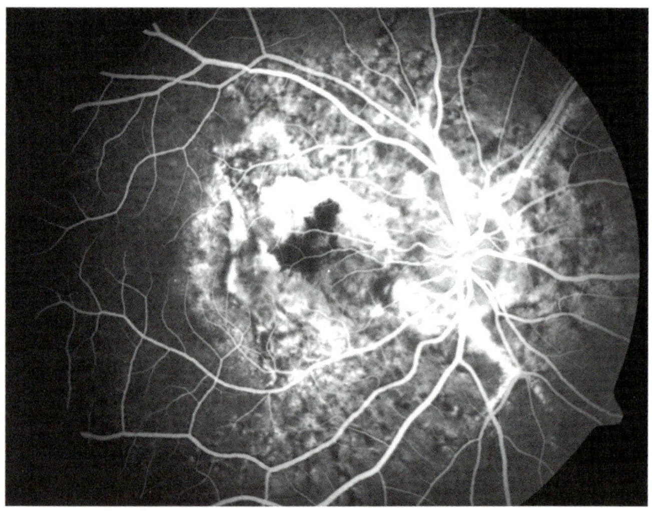

The mid arteriovenous phase showing the hyperfluorescence along the angioid streaks. Some hyperfluorescence is noted in the disciform scar due to the filling of its vasculature. Mottled hyperfluorescence is seen in the adjacent retina

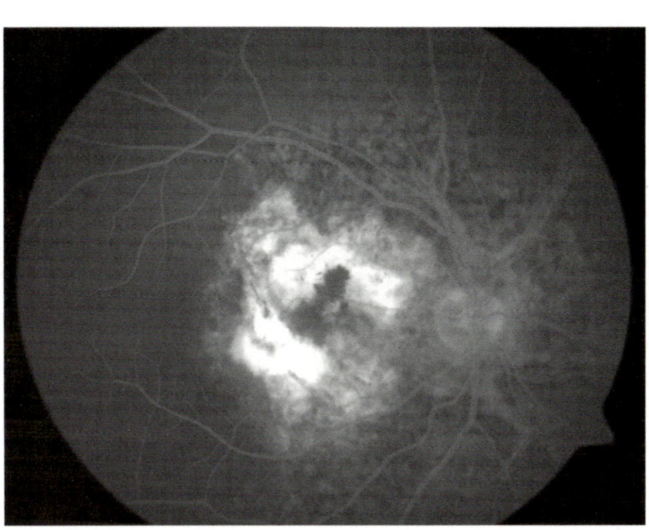

Late phase shows fading of the hyperfluorescence along the angioid streaks. Staining of the disciform scar is seen

COMMENT

Untreated or recurrent CNVM in patients with angioid streaks, usually results in the formation of a disciform scar. This is an important cause of severe visual loss in these patients.

CASE 6

A 48-year-old lady presented with distortion of vision in the right eye since one week. Vision in the right eye was 6/6p; N6 and CF 1 mt in the left eye.

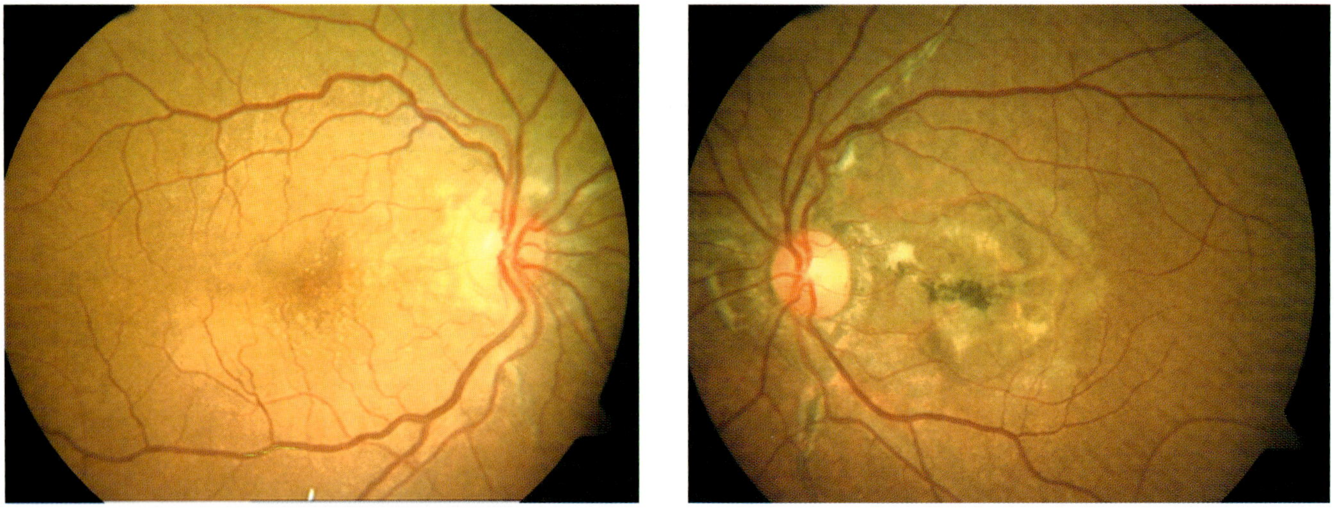

Fundus examination revealed the presence of peripapillary angioid streaks in both eyes, associated with a large, partially active CNVM in the left eye and a small, extrafoveal CNVM under the papillomacular bundle in the right. Intravitreal bevacizumab (1.25 mg in 0.05 ml) was injected in the right eye, thrice at monthly intervals.

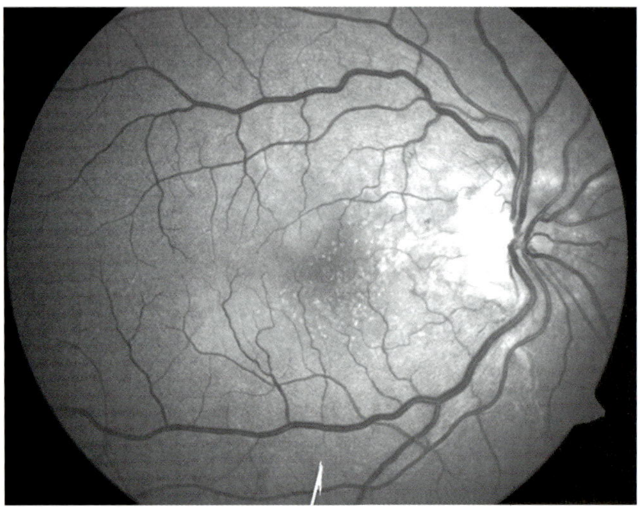

Red free photograph highlights the angioid streaks in both eyes

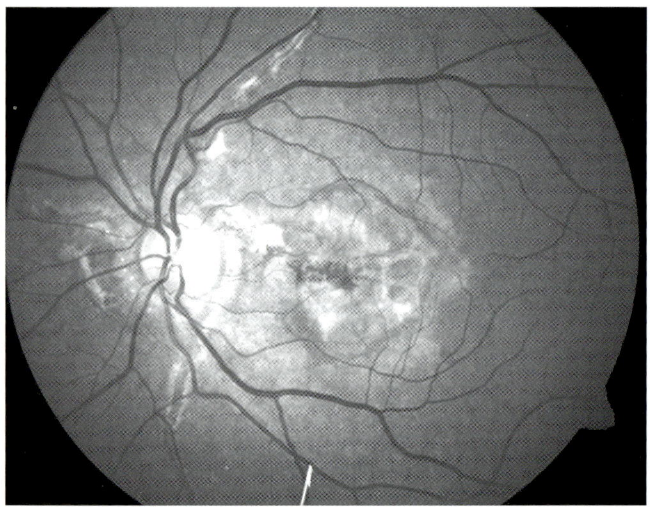

A scarred CNV with pigmentation is noted at the macula

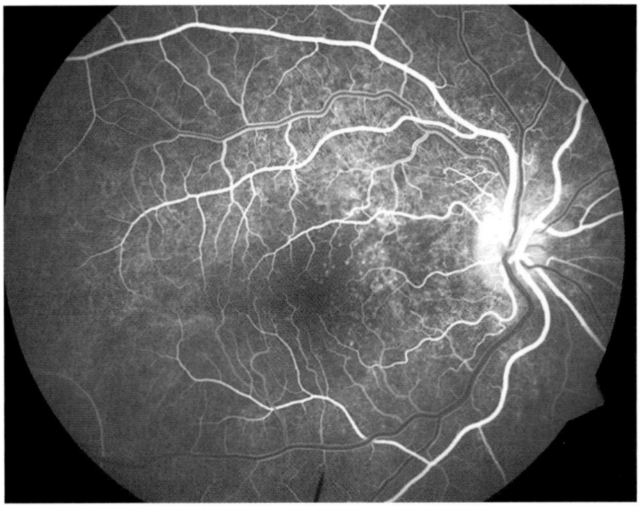

Stippled hyperfluorescence is noted in the early arterio-venous phase

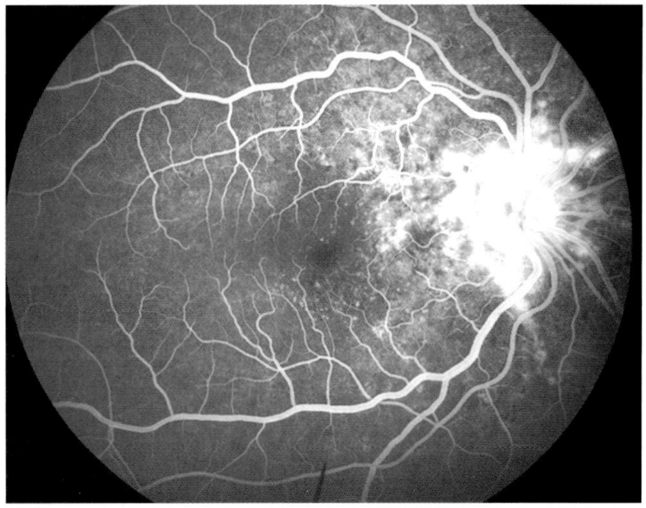

Lacy pattern of the CNVM underlying the papillomacular bundle is highlighted in the late arteriovenous phase

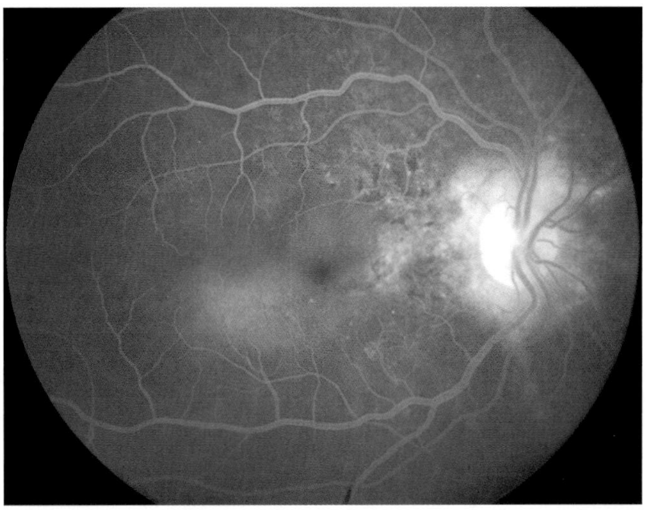

Diffuse leakage of fluorescein is noted in the late phase

Visit 2

Six weeks after the last injection, the patient complained of severe visual loss.

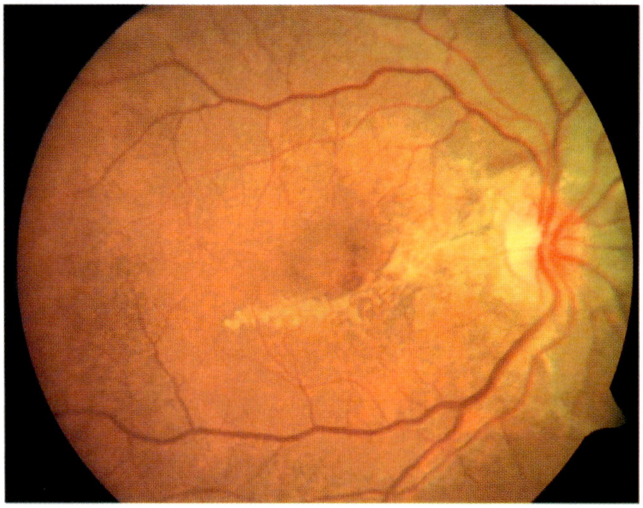

Clinical examination revealed a fresh, curvilinear, subretinal lesion, akin to angioid streaks and in continuity with it, involving the fovea in the right eye

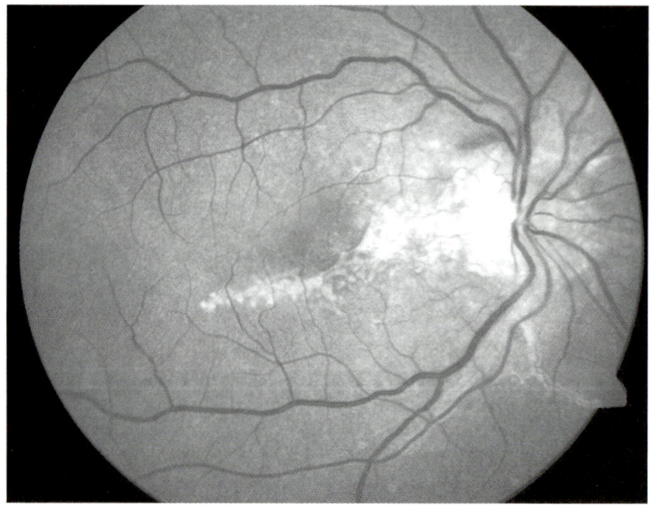

Red free photograph highlights the newly developed angioid streak running just below the fovea

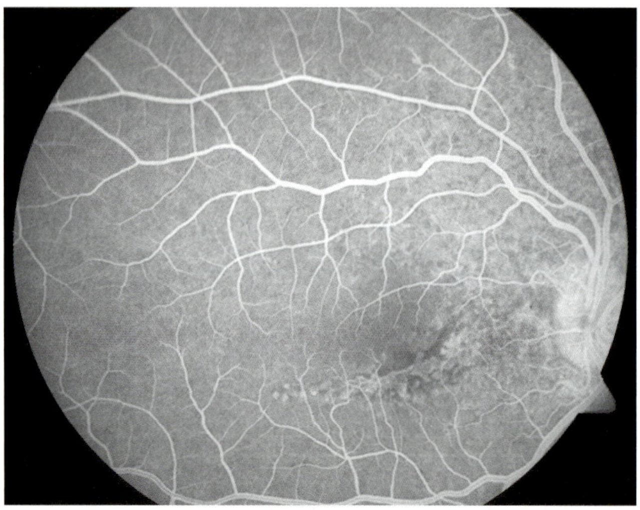

Hyperfluorescence due to the transmission effect corresponding to the angioid streaks is made out in the early arteriovenous phase

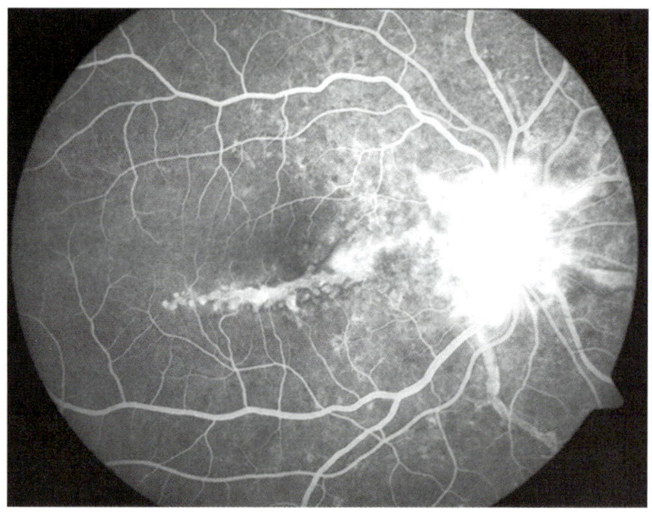

Increased hyperfluorescence is seen in the late arteriovenous phase

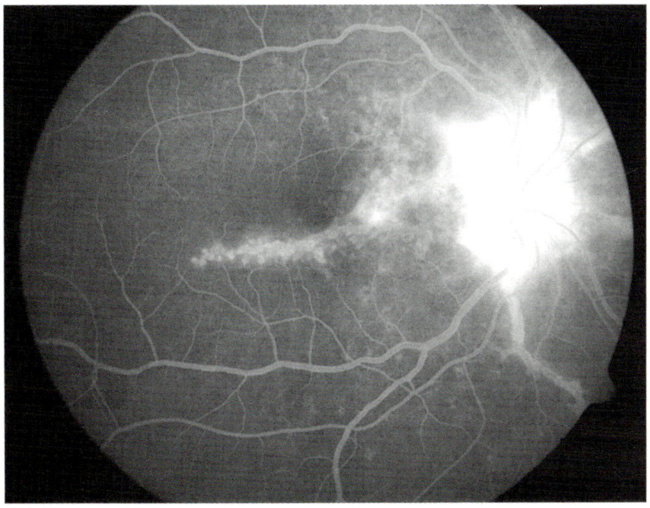

Scleral staining and leakage of the dye is made out in the late phase

CLINICAL NUGGETS

1. Eyes with angioid streaks are susceptible to trivial trauma and the patient should be advised accordingly.
2. Causes for poor vision in eyes with angioid streaks is either due to involvement of the fovea by the breaks in the Bruch's membrane or development of choroidal neovascular membrane.

BIBLIOGRAPHY

1. Clarkson JG, Altman RD. Angioid streaks. Surv Ophthalmol 1983;26:235-46.
2. Federman JL, Shields JA, Tomer TL. Angioid streaks II. Fluorescein angiographic features. Arch Ophthalmol 1976;93:921-6.
3. Gass JD, Clarkson JG. Angioid streaks and disciform macular detachment in Paget's disease. Am J Ophthalmol 1974;30:955-68.
4. Gass JD. Stereoscopic Atlas of Macular Diseases, 3rd edn, St Louis, CV Mosby Co 1987;102-9.
5. Hagedoorn A. Angioid streaks and traumatic rupture of Bruch's membrane. Br J Ophthalmol 1975;59:267.
6. Sen PR, Rishi P, Sen P, Rishi E, Shroff D. Rapid progression of angioid streaks following intravitreal bevacizumab. Can J Ophthalmol. 2009; 44(5):e39-40.

2nd Section

20 Chapter
Choroidal Folds

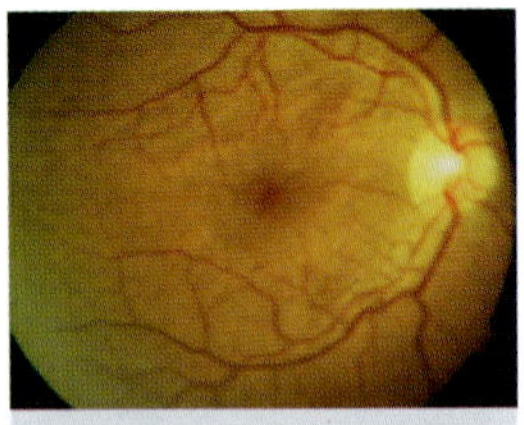

- Choroidal folds or chorioretinal folds can be either idiopathic or secondary to hypotony, posterior scleritis, retrobulbar mass lesion, choroidal neovascular membrane, focal chorioretinal scarring, etc.
- They involve the inner layers of the choroid, Bruch's membrane and the retinal pigment epithelium.
- The folds may be horizontal, vertical or oblique and are parallel to each other.
- They are usually present at the posterior pole and appear as alternate yellow and dark streaks–yellow corresponding to the crest of the folds.

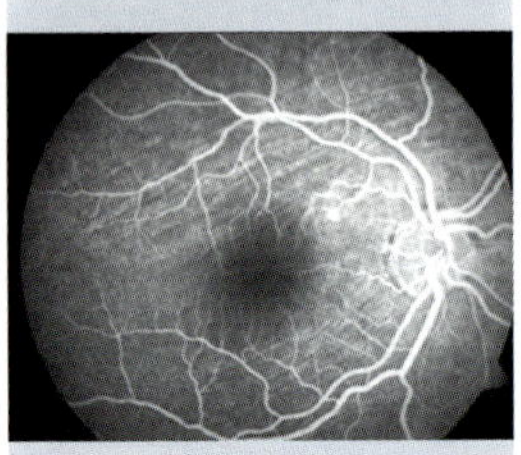

- Alternate dark and light bands are seen corresponding to the choroidal folds.
- The crest of the fold appears hyperfluorescent. This could be due to thinning of the retinal pigment epithelium at the crest of the folds.
- The trough appears as hypofluorescent streaks probably due to crowding of the retinal pigment epithelium causing blockage of the choroidal fluorescence.

CASE 1

A 43-year-old female was noted to have choroidal folds in both eyes on a routine eye examination. Visual acuity was 6/6; N6 in both eyes.

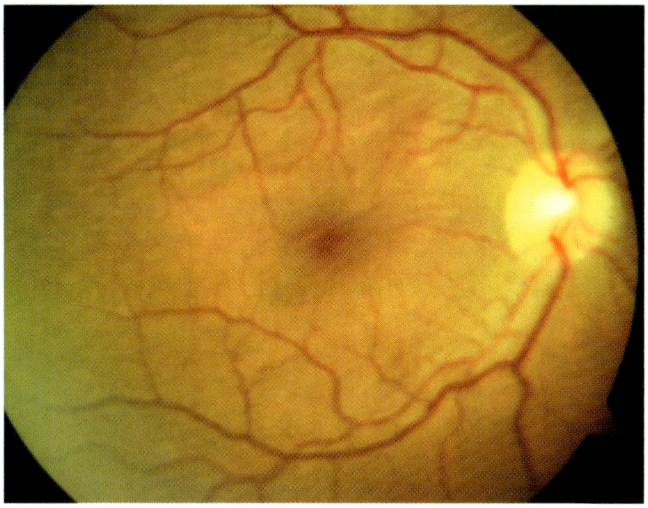

Fundus photograph of the right eye showing parallel choroidal folds

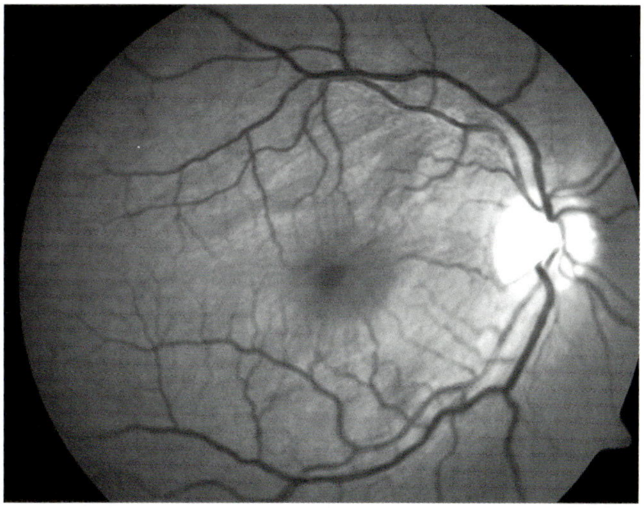

Red free photograph highlighting the choroidal folds

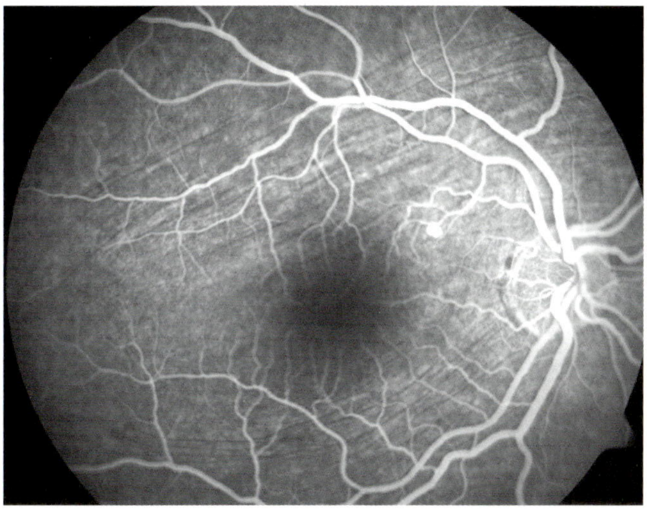

Arteriovenous phase showing obliquely running choroidal folds. A hyperfluorescent spot is noted superonasal to the fovea

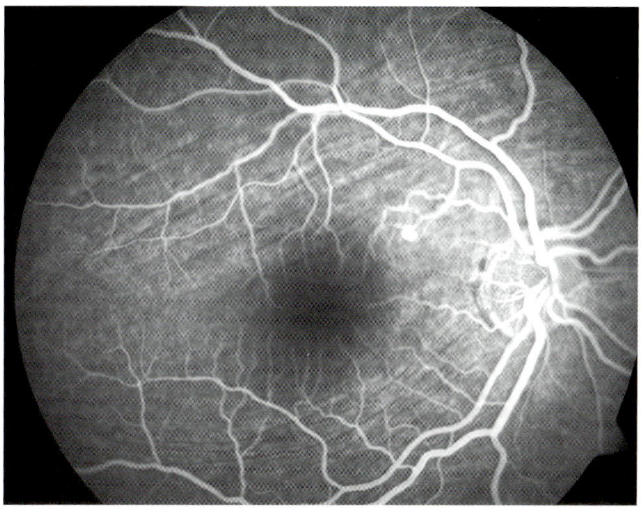

The alternating hypo and hyperfluorescent streaks due to choroidal folds are well seen in the later part of the arteriovenous phase

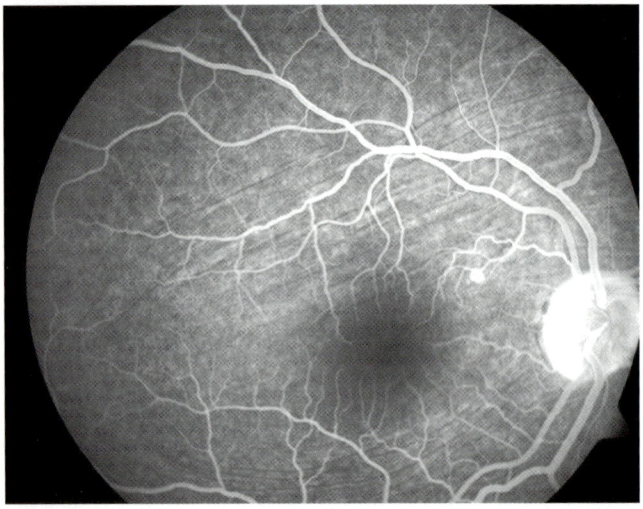

Some fading of the hyperfluorescent lines is noted in the late film. The hyperfluorescent spot persists. However, it remains discrete with minimal fading probably representing a RPE defect

COMMENT

The crest of the choroidal folds appears hyperfluorescent whereas the through appears hypofluorescent

CASE 2

A 51-year-old male came for a routine eye examination. Visual acuity was 6/6; N6 in both eyes. Both eyes had choroidal folds at the posterior pole. Myelinated nerve fibers were noted at the right optic nerve head.

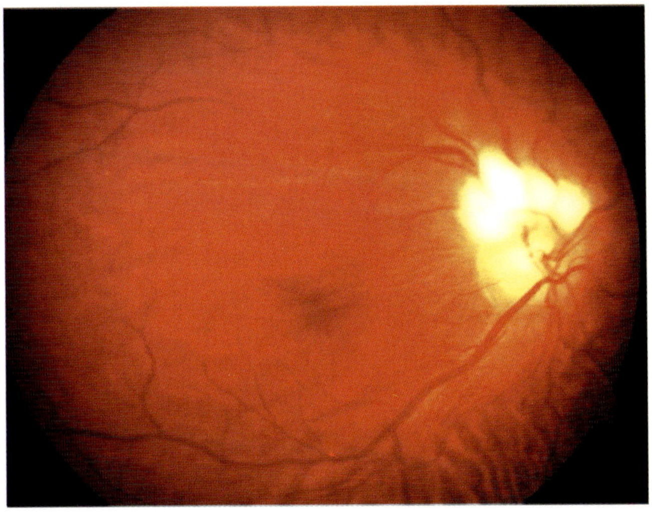

Fundus photograph showing the parallel horizontal choroidal folds at the posterior pole. Myelinated nerve fibers are noted at the optic nerve head

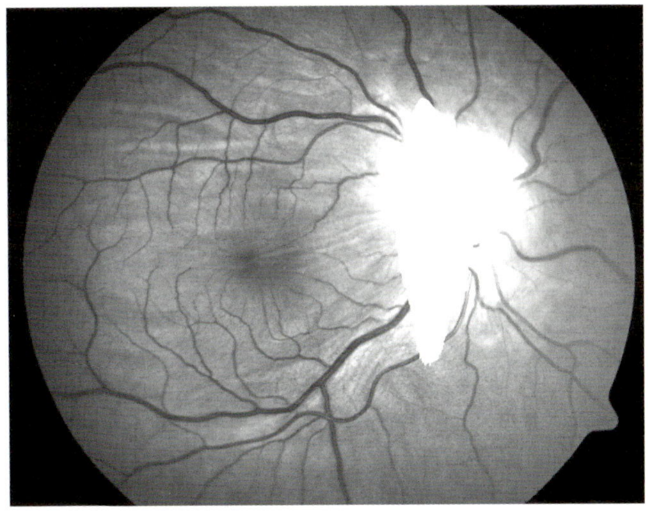

The red free photograph shows the choroidal folds. A bloomimg artifact is noted at the optic nerve head

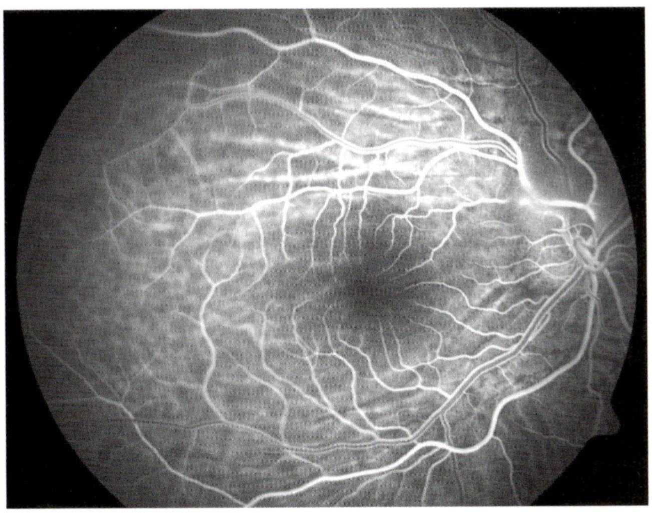

Early arteriovenous phase showing the parallel dark and light streaks, which are more prominent along the arcades

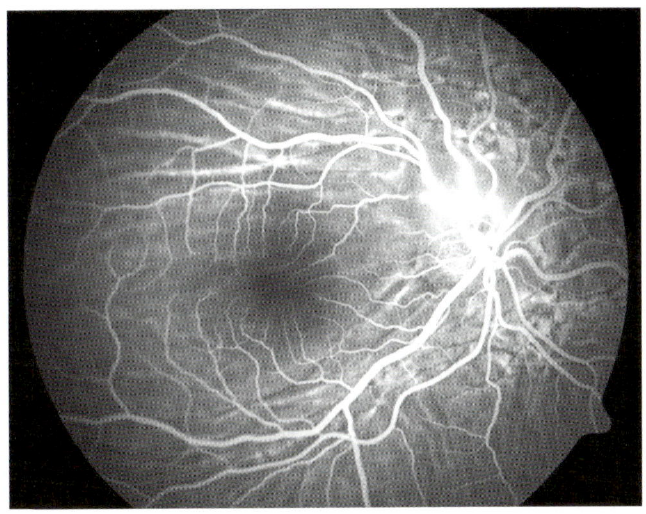

The choroidal folds appear more prominent in the late arteriovenous phase. Note the irregular appearing folds nasal to the disc. Minimal blurring of details is noted in the superior part of the disc due to myelinated nerve fiber

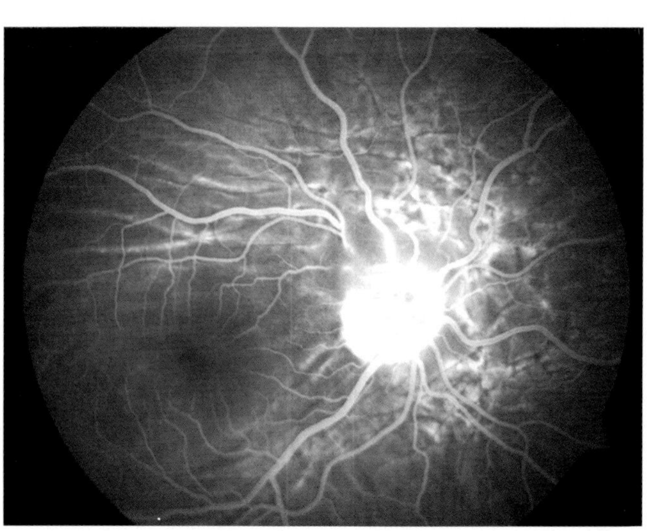

Late phase shows some fading of the hyperfluorescence along the crests of the choroidal folds. The irregular folds nasally are well-made out

CASE 3

A 45-year-old male presented with blurring of vision in the both eyes. The visual acuity was 6/9; N10 in the right eye and 6/9; N6 in the left eye. Both eyes had similar fundus findings.

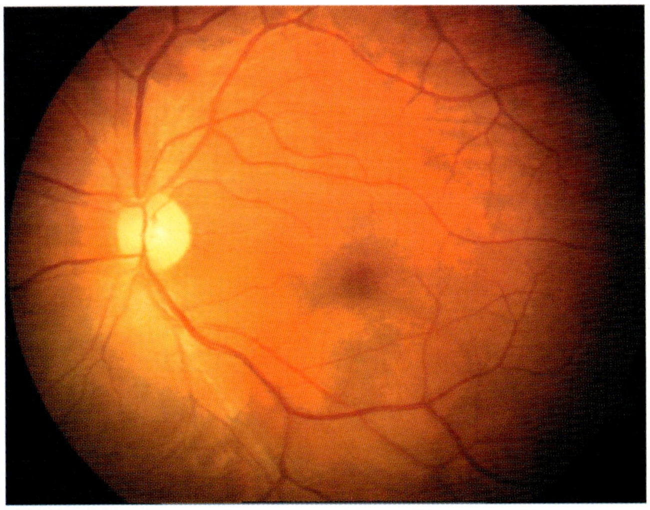

Fundus photograph showing very subtle choroidal folds in the upper part of the macula. There is an elevation of the sensory retina inferiorly

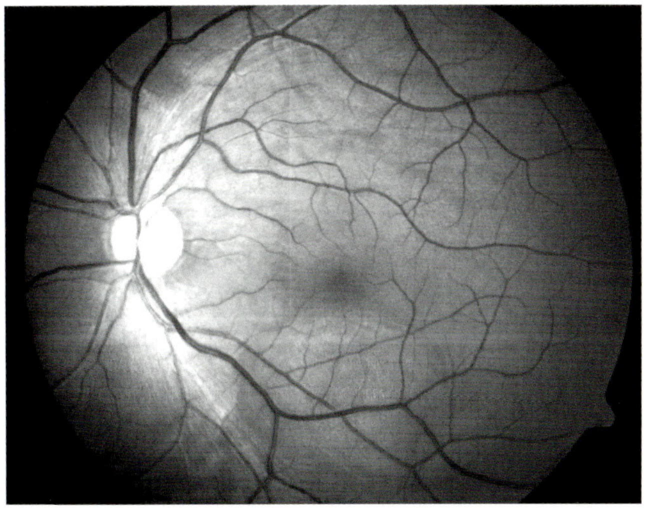

Red free photograph highlights the sensory retinal elevation in the inferior part of the macula

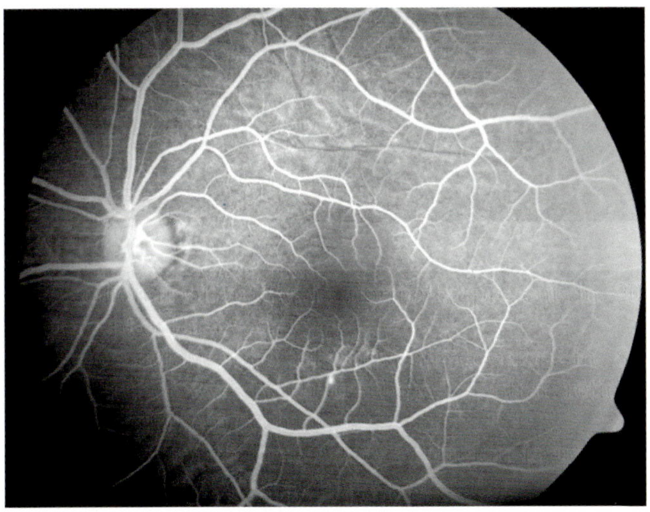

Arteriovenous phase shows a hyperfluorescent dot in the inferior macula. Note subtle choroidal folds in the superior part of the macula

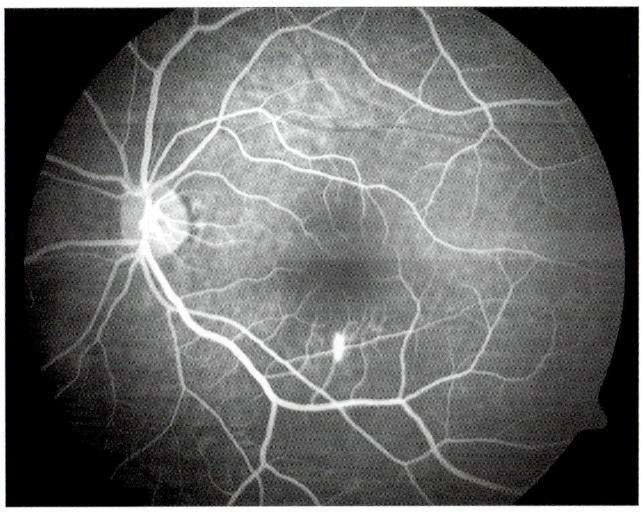

The dye is seen to leak from the hyperfluorescent point and ascend upwards

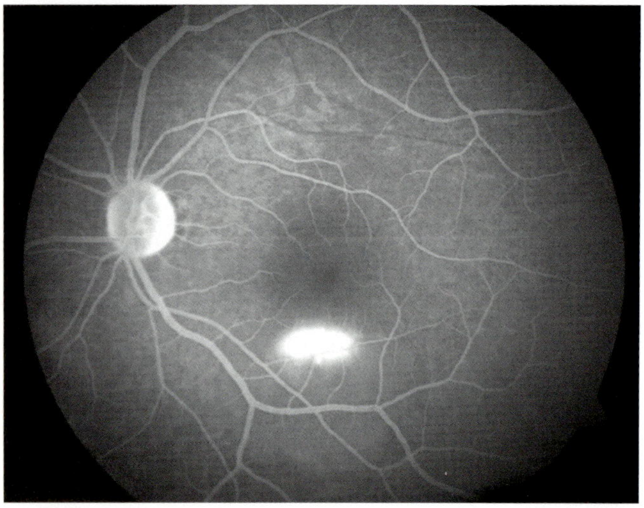

Late phase shows pooling of dye in the upper part of the sensory retinal detachment. The hyperfluorescence along the choroidal folds has diminished

COMMENT

Central serous chorioretinopathy can occur with idiopathic choroidal folds.

CASE 4

A 43-year-old female was referred for pain and decreased vision in the right eye of 6 months duration. Visual acuity was 6/18; N36 at presentation. Left eye was normal. Based on clinical and ultrasound findings she was diagnosed to have posterior scleritis in the right eye. Vision improved to 6/6; N6 following treatment with systemic steroids.

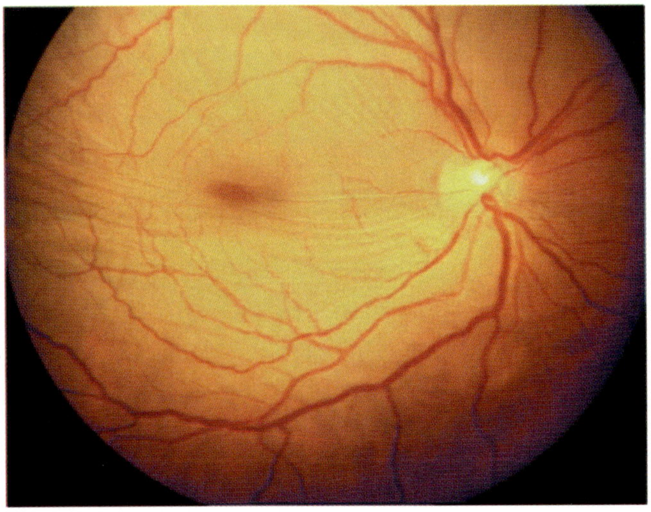

Fundus photograph of a patient who presented with very prominent chorioretinal folds at the posterior pole

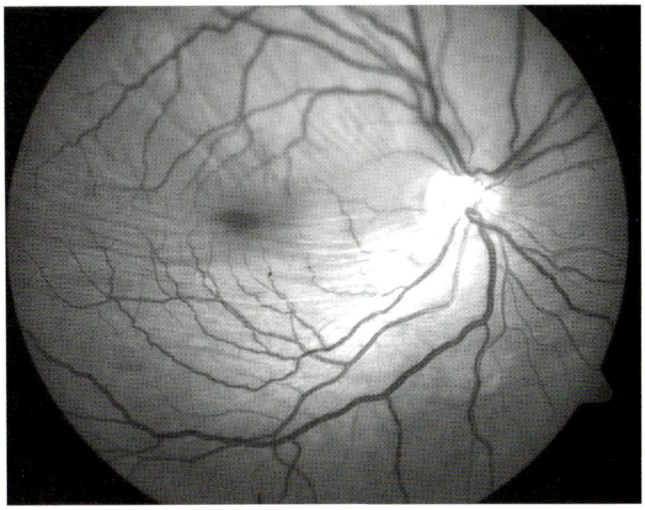

Red free photograph showing the parallel choroidal folds at the posterior pole

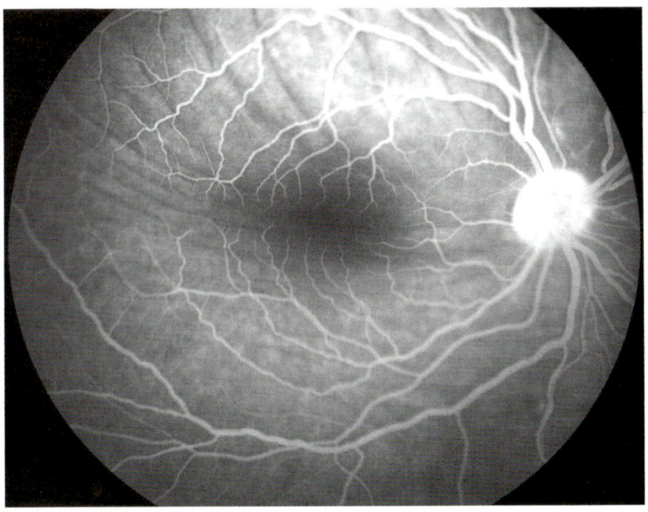

The hyperfluorescent crest is more broader than the hypofluorescent trough which appears as narrow streaks. These represent broad choroidal folds

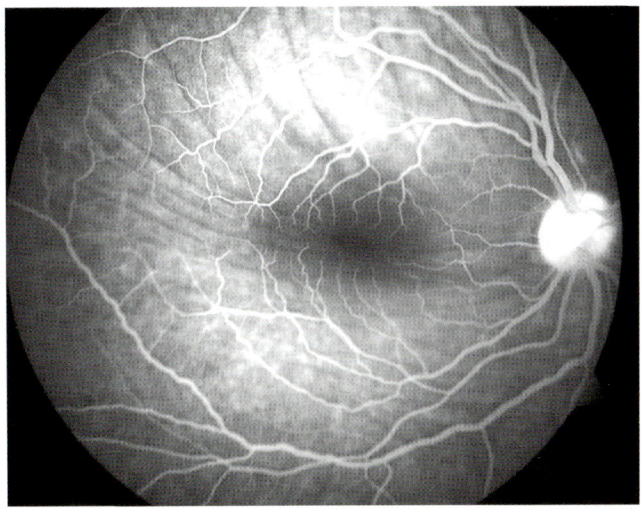

Late broad choroidal folds are well made out in the late arteriovenous phase

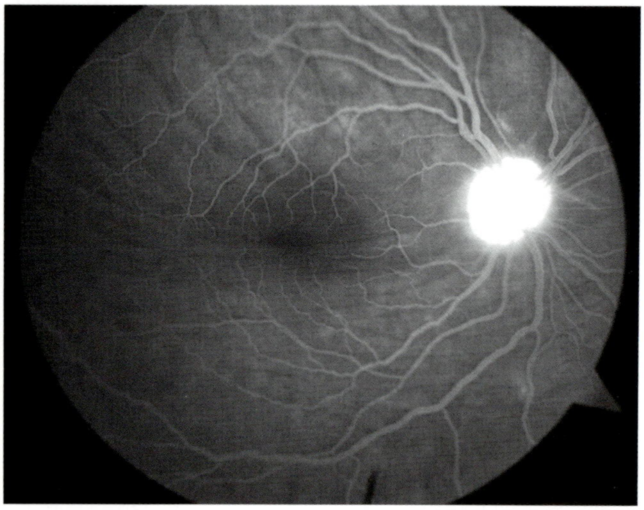

There is fading of the hyperfluorescence seen along the choroidal folds. Increased staining of the disc is seen

COMMENT

In scleritis, increased thickening of the sclera and the choroid results in the inner choroidal layers, Bruch's membrane and the RPE to be thrown into folds.

CLINICAL NUGGETS

1. Idiopathic choroidal folds, *per se do* not affect the visual acuity and do not require any treatment.
2. Acquired choroidal folds have been seen to cause acquired hyperopia, flattening of the posterior pole and widening of optic nerve sheath.
3. Autofluorescence images show reversal of the banding pattern seen on FA, with the crests appearing hypoautofluorescent and the throughs hyperautofluorescent.

BIBLIOGRAPHY

1. Fine HF, Cunningham ET, Kim E, Theodore Smith R, Chang S. Autofluorescence imaging findings in long-standing chorioretinal folds. Retin Cases Brief Rep 2009;3(2):137-9.
2. Francois De Laey JJ. Fluorescein angiographic aspects of acquired chorioretinal folds-Mod. Probl Ophthalmol 1970;9:29-135.
3. Gass JDM. Stereoscopic atlas of macular diseases: Diagnosis and treatment. 3rd edn St. Louis Mosby Year Book, 1987.
4. Norton EWD. A characteristic fluorescein angiographic pattern in choroidal folds. Proc R Soc Med 1969;62: 119-28.
5. Paz-Moreno J, Jiménez-Parras R. Choroidal folds: a presentation of two cases. Arch Soc Esp ophthalmol 2010;85(1):38-40.

21

Chapter

Acute Macular Neuroretinopathy

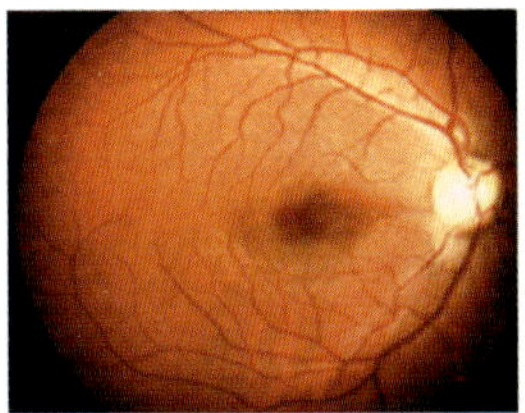

- It is one of the conditions grouped under the AZOOR (Acute Zonal Occult Outer Retinopathy) complex.
- Women are more commonly affected.
- Presentation is with sudden onset of unilateral or bilateral paracentral scotomas
- Rare type of maculopathy associated with wedge-shaped red-brown lesions located at the center of the macula.
- Lesions may vary in size from barely detectable to one disc diameter or more in size.
- Lesion is most likely located at the outer neurosensory retina.
- Optical coherence tomography shows defect in the inner and outer segment junction of photoreceptors and thinning of the outer nuclear layer.
- Pathogenesis is speculated to be vasculogenic with increased association with hypertension, oral contraceptive pills and heavy caffeine intake.
- Autoimmune origin with a viral prodrome is also thought to be responsible for the condition.

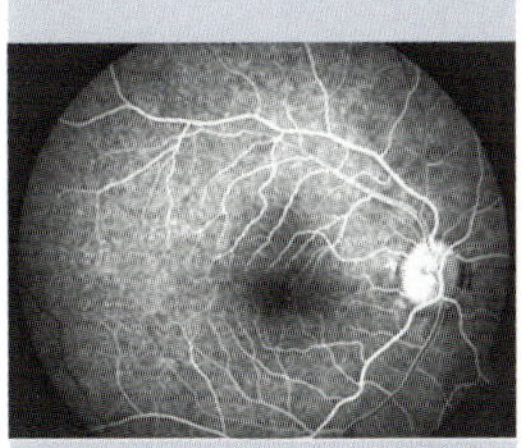

- Fluorescein angiogram shows relative hypofluorescence corresponding to the lesion.

CASE 1

A 16-year-old male patient presented with complaints of reduced vision in the left eye of two months duration. Visual acuity was 6/6; N6 in the right eye and 6/36; N36 in the left eye. The right eye fundus was normal.

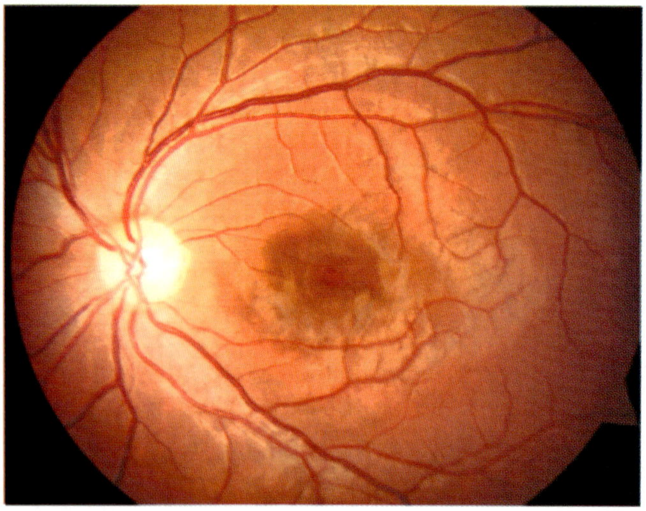

Fundus photograph of the left eye showing a red-brown irregular lesion located at the fovea

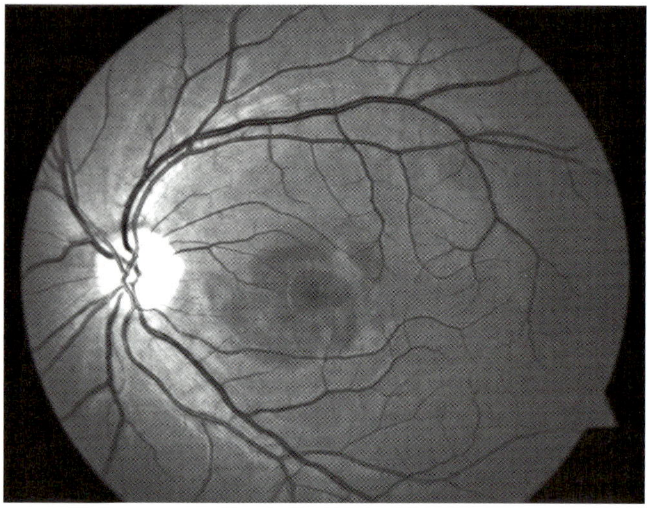

The lesion at the fovea is well seen in the red free photograph

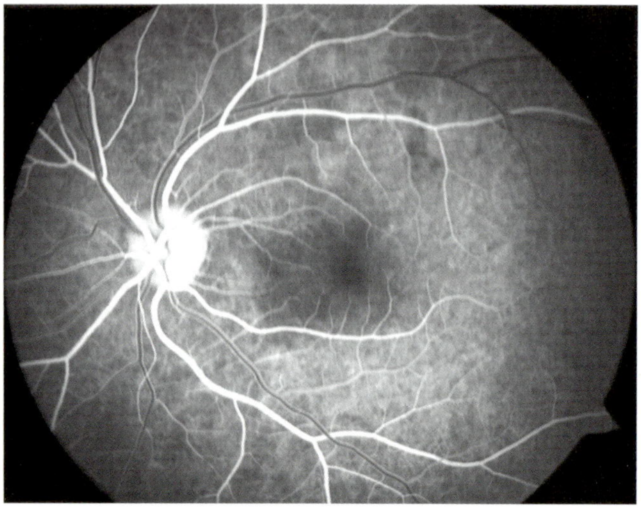

Early arteriovenous phase shows a relative hypofluorescence in the region of the foveal lesion

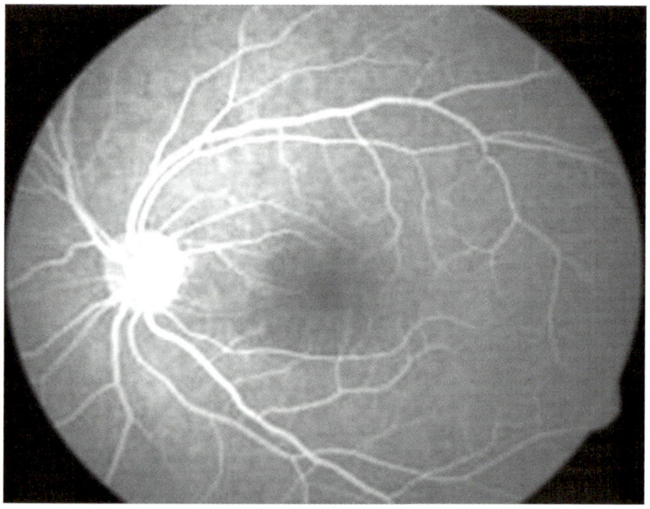

Some hypofluorescence persists at the fovea in the arteriovenous phase

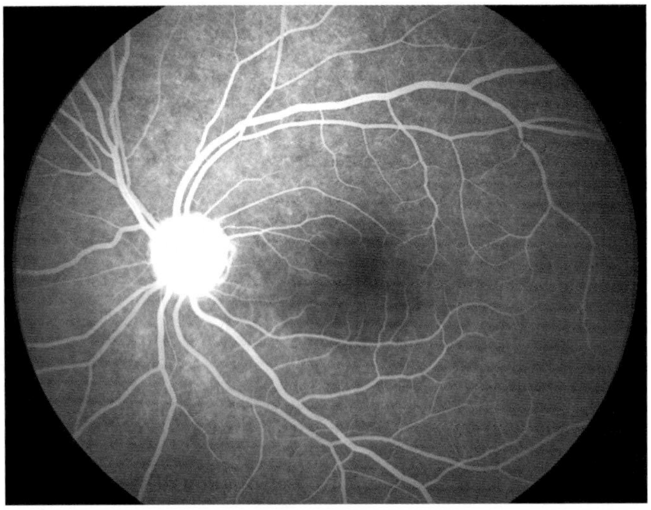

Late phase shows persistence of the hypofluorescence corresponding to the lesion seen clinically

COMMENT

Minimal hypofluorescence is seen at the site of the lesion in the macula.

This lesion usually persists for a long time.

CASE 2

A 39-year-old male patient presented with a history of being involved in a road accident one month back. He sustained injuries to the mandible without any injury to the eye. Four days after the injury he noticed decreased vision in the left eye. Visual acuity was 6/6; N6 in the right eye and 1/60 in the left eye.

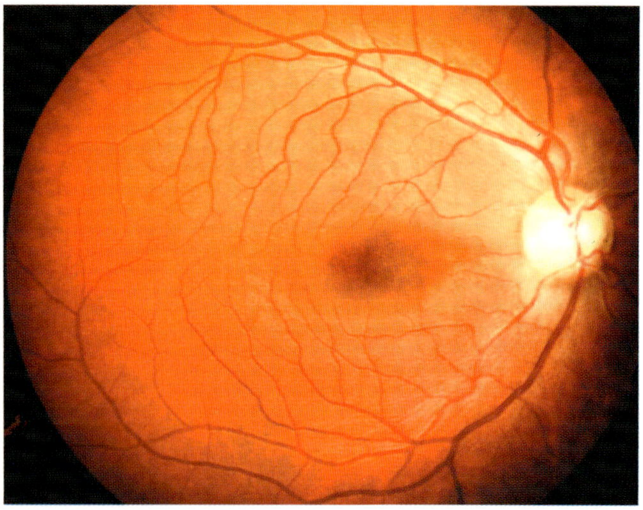

Fundus photograph of the right eye showing a red-brown wedge shaped defect at the fovea

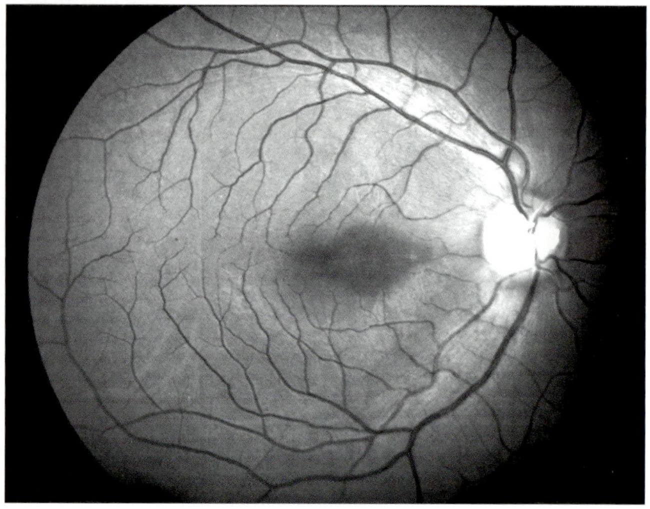

Red free photograph demarcates the lesion

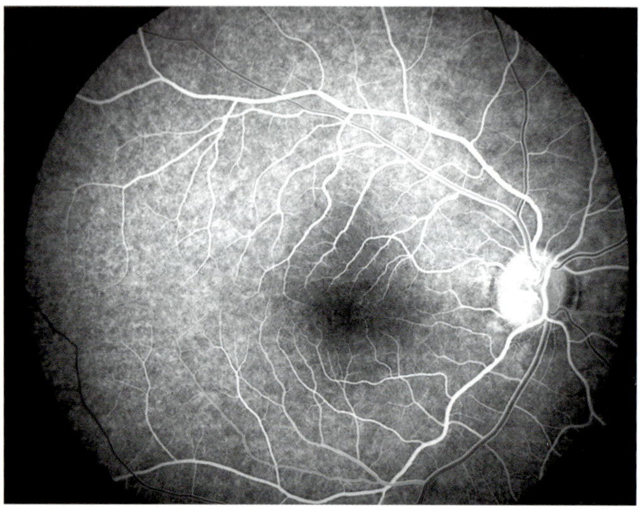

Early arteriovenous phase of the angiogram showing hypofluorescence at the site of the lesion

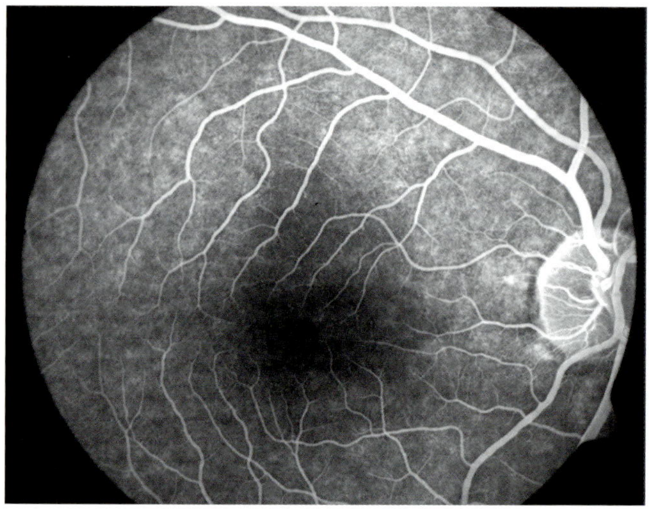

Hypofluorescence persists in the arteriovenous phase

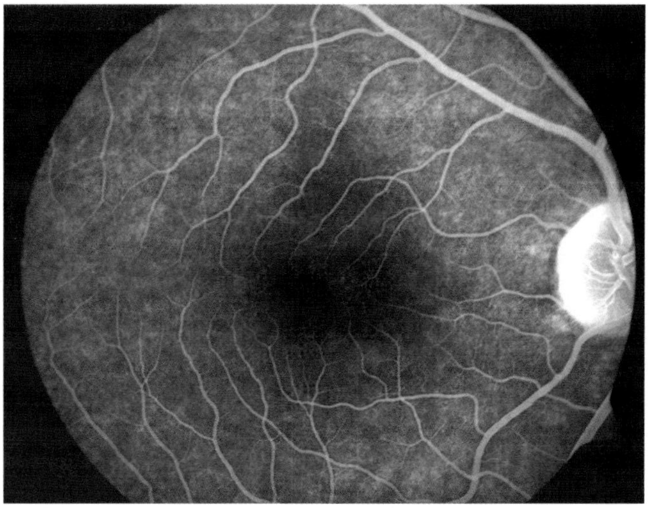

Late phase showing hypofluorescence at the lesion site

CASE 2 (*Continued*)

Left Eye of the Patient

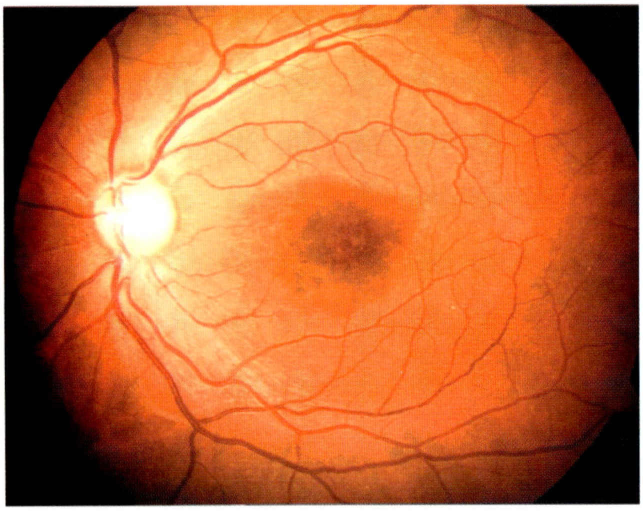

Fundus photograph of the left eye showing a red-brown irregular lesion located at the fovea

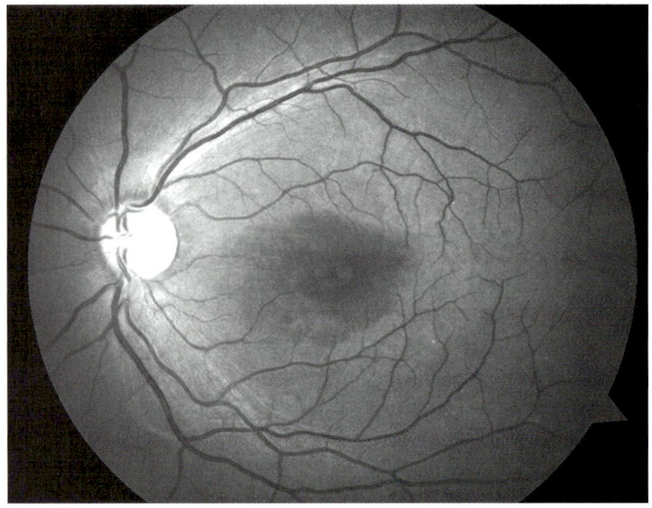

Red free photograph highlights the lesion

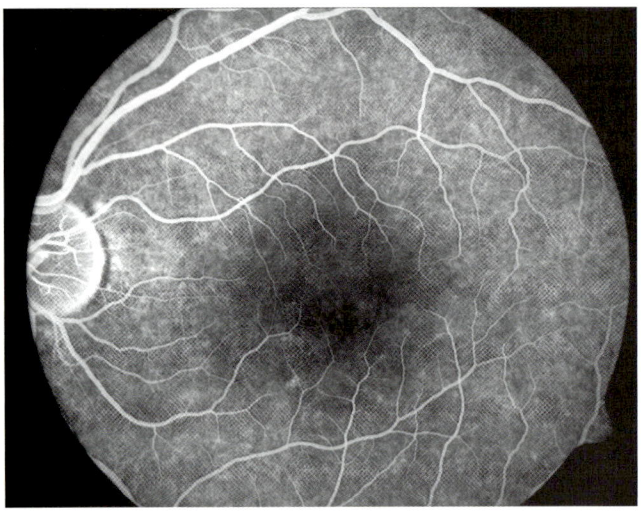

Arteriovenous phase showing hypofluorescence at the site of the lesion

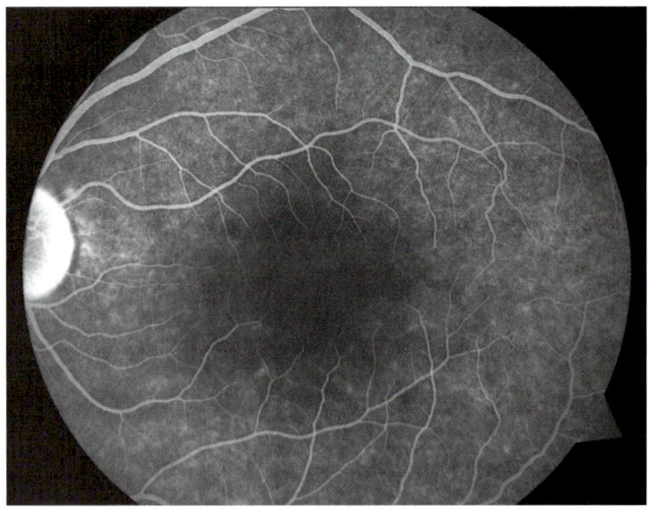

Late phase showing persistence of the hypofluorescence

CLINICAL NUGGETS

1. In patients with acute macular neuroretinopathy, the scotoma seen on the Amsler grid corresponds exactly to the lesion seen at the macula and may persist for a long time.
2. There is no effective treatment for acute macular neuroretinopathy. It is self-limiting, however multiple recurrences are known.
3. The macular lesion in acute macular neuroretinopathy may persist for a very long time.

BIBLIOGRAPHY

1. Bos PJ, Deutman AF. Acute macular neuroretinopathy. Am J Ophthalmol 1975;80:573-84.
2. Maschi C, Schneider-Lise B, Paoli V, Gastaud P. Acute macular neuroretinopathy: contribution of spectral-domain optical coherence tomography and multifocal ERG. Graefes Arch Clin Exp Ophthalmol 2010; Nov 20. [Epub ahead of print]
3. Miller MH, Spalton DJ, Fitzke FW, Bird AC. Acute macular neuroretinopathy. Ophthalmology 1989;96: 265-9.
4. O'Brfen DM, Farmer SG, Kalina RE, Leon JA. Acute macular neuroretinopathy following intravenous sympathomimetics. Retina 1989;9:281-6.
5. Salom D, Díaz-Llopis M, Cervera E, García-Delpech S, Hernández-Garfella M, García-Pous. Acute macular neuroretinopathy. Arch Soc Esp Oftalmol. 2007;82(5): 307-9.
6. Turbeville SD, Cowan LD, Gass JDM. Acute macular neuroretinopathy. A review of the literature. Surv Ophthalmol 2003;48:(1):1-11.
7. Vance SK, Spaide RF, Freund KB, Wiznia R, Cooney MJ. Outer retinal abnormalities in acute macular neuroretinopathy. Retina 2011;31(3):441-5.

22 Chapter

Central Serous Chorioretinopathy

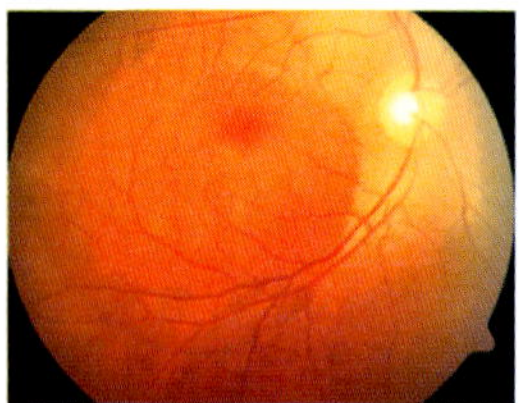

- Central serous chorioretinopathy (CSC) is characterized by accumulation of clear fluid at the posterior pole, causing a well circumscribed area of retinal detachment.
- Leakage of fluid occurs through a discrete defect in the retinal pigment epithelial (RPE) layer and accumulates in the subretinal space.

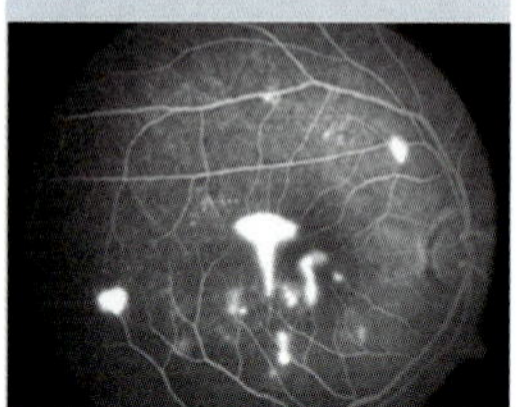

Leakage

The different leakage patterns seen in CSC include:

Ink blot type of leakage

- Starts as a point leak at the RPE level and spreads symmetrically in all directions in the subretinal space.
- Initial diffusion of the dye occurs quickly, however, the dye usually does not fill the entire area of neurosensory detachment even in the late films taken at 30 minutes.

Smoke-stack phenomenon

- Dye enters as a point leak, but instead of spreading in all directions, it ascends to reach the highest point of the neurosensory detachment and then expands laterally in a umbrella or a mushroom like pattern.
- This is said to be due to the osmotic gradient resulting from the different protein concentrations in the content of the fluid within the neurosensory detachment and the fluid entering through the point of leakage.

Inverse smoke-stack appearance

- Starts as a point leakage, but instead of ascending the dye tends to track down towards the lower limit of the neurosensory detachment.

Multiple leaks

- Sometimes more than one leak may be seen. They may behave either as an ink blot leak or a smoke-stack leak or a combination of both.

Diffuse leakage

- No definite leakage pattern is seen, instead a diffuse area of leakage may be seen.

No leakage seen even though neurosensory detachment is present

- This probably indicates a resolving stage of CSC where the leakage has resolved; however, the fluid has not yet absorbed; in such cases optic pit associated sensory retinal elevation should also be looked for.
- Important to look at the retina superior to the neurosensory elevation, or outside the arcade to look for causative leaks.

Pigment epithelial detachment

- May be located within the neurosensory detachment or outside it.
- Entire area of the PED shows hyperfluorescence in the early film. This increases in intensity towards the later films; however the extent remains the same.
- Area of hypofluorescence may be noted within the PED; this occurs due to pigment clumping and can produce a cruciate or a triradiate pattern of hypofluorescence within the PED.

Retinal pigment epithelial transmission defects

- Seen in resolved CSC cases.
- Usually quite extensive, extent depending on the area of previous neurosensory detachment.

Retinal pigment epithelial tracts

- Transmission defects seen in the form of a tract extending downwards from the posterior pole and expanding inferiorly to have a 'flask', 'teardrop', 'dumb-bell', or 'hourglass' shaped appearance.

CASE 1

A 32-year-old male presented with history of noticing a scotoma in front of the right eye for the past one month. Visual acuity was 6/9; N6 in the right eye and 6/6; N6 in the left eye. The right eye shows a shallow sensory elevation of the retina at the macula. A small PED was seen in the temporal part of the macula in the left eye.

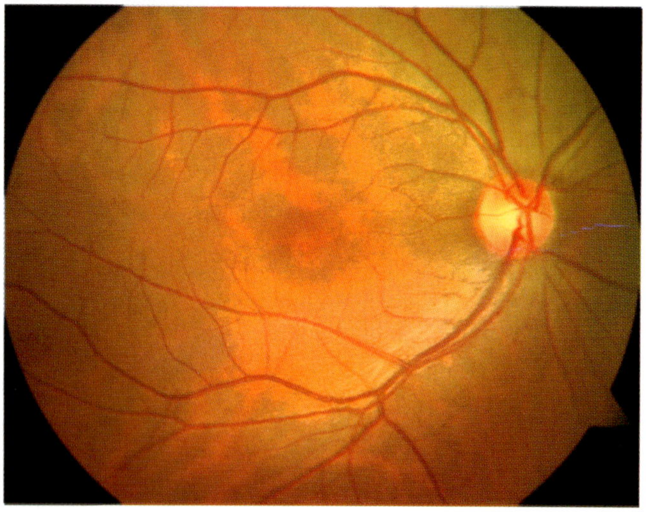

Fundus photograph of the right eye showing a sensory elevation of the retina at the macula

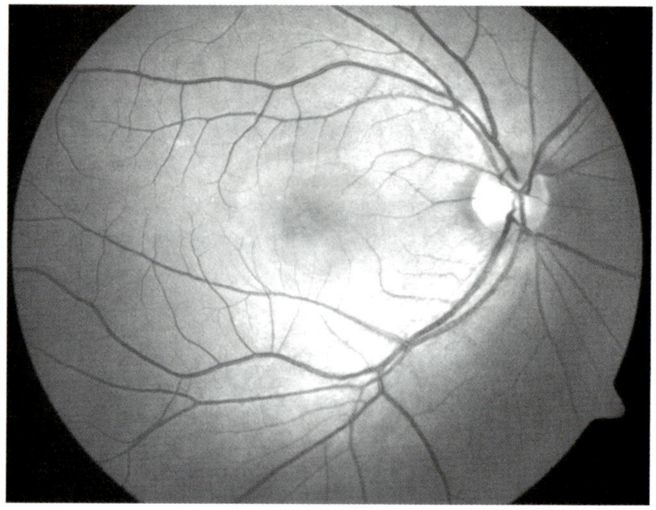

The sensory retinal detachment is well seen in the red free photograph

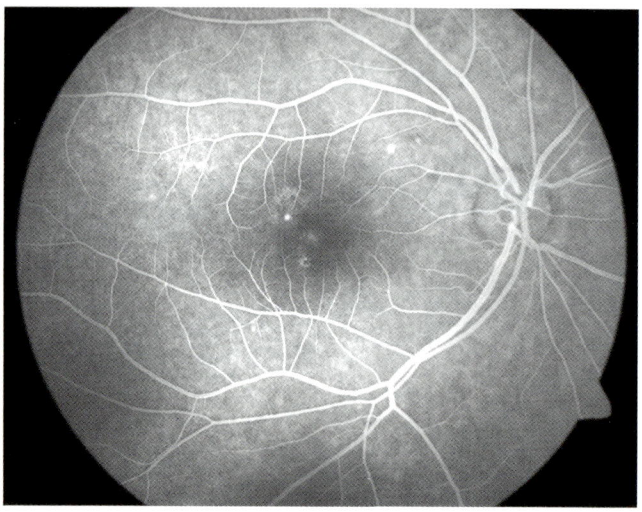

An intense dot hyperfluorescence is noted superotemporal to the foveal center. Few faint hyperfluorescent areas are noted within the FAZ and also superotemporal to the disc

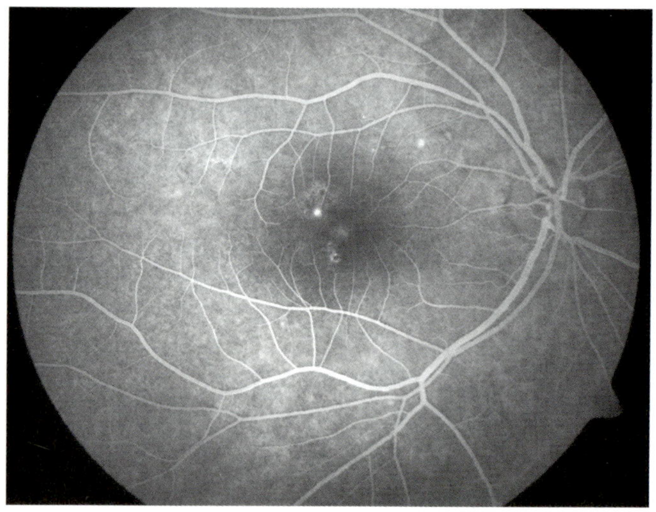

The intensity of the hyperfluorescent dot superotemporal to the fovea has marginally increased in the late arteriovenous phase

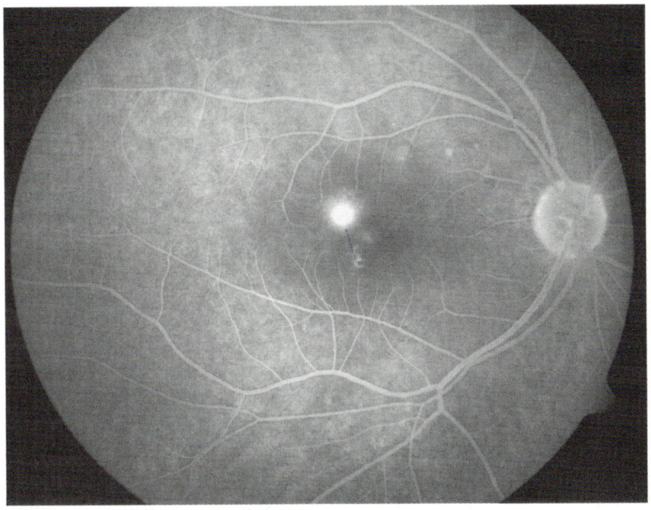

The dot hyperfluorescence has increased in intensity and extent in the late films, showing the typical ink blot appearance of CSC. The other areas of hyperfluorescense have faded suggestive of a window transmission defect

COMMENT

A typical ink blot type of leak in seen in this case.

CASE 2

A 30-year-old male presented with history of blurring of vision in the right eye of one month duration; visual acuity was 6/12; N6.

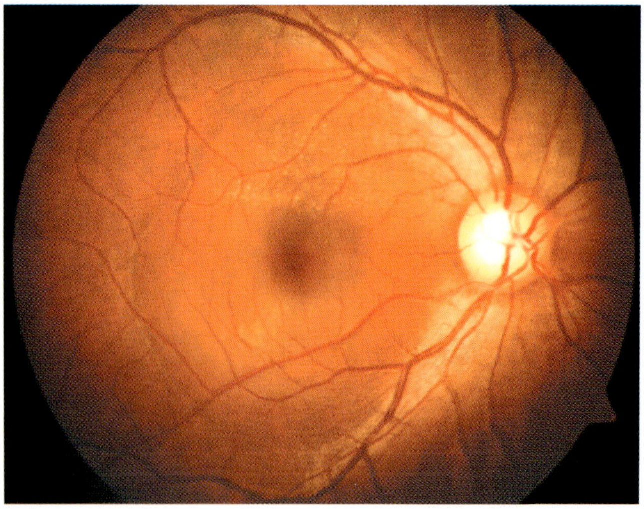

Fundus photograph of the right eye showing a serous elevation of the retina at the macula

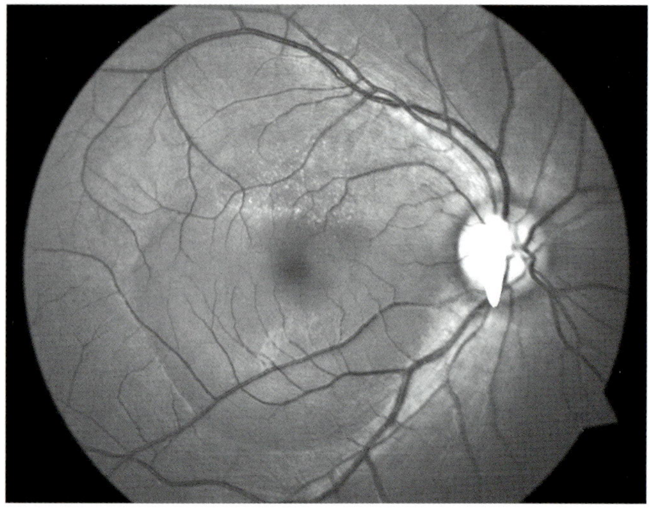

Subretinal precipitates superior to the fovea and RPE alterations inferior to the fovea are well made out in the red free photograph

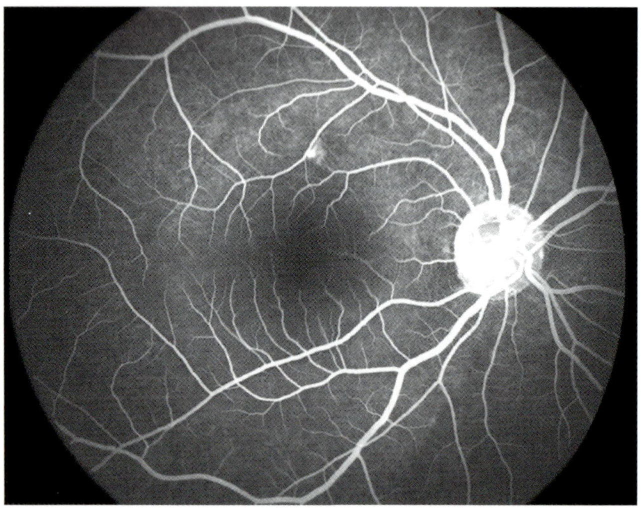

The arteriovenous phase shows a point hyperfluorescence superior to the fovea

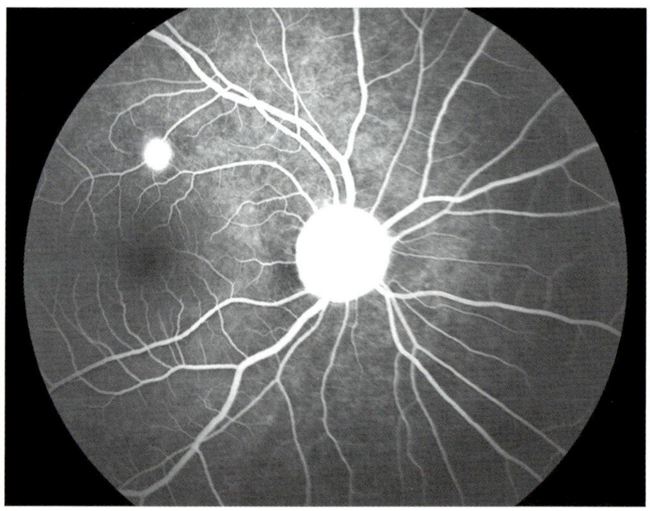

The hyperfluorescence has increased in intensity and extent due to leakage in fovea

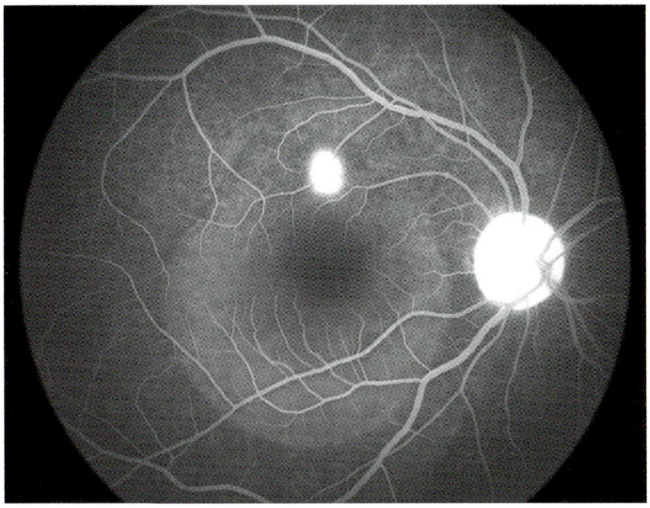

Typical ink blot appearance of the leak is seen in the late film. The extent of the detachment is well made out

COMMENT

Leakage of dye never fills up the entire extent of the sensory detachment even in very late films.

CASE 3

A 30-year-old male presented with history of sudden onset of blurring of vision in the left eye of 15 days duration. Visual acuity was 6/12; N18. He gave history of being treated with periocular steroid injection. The right eye was normal.

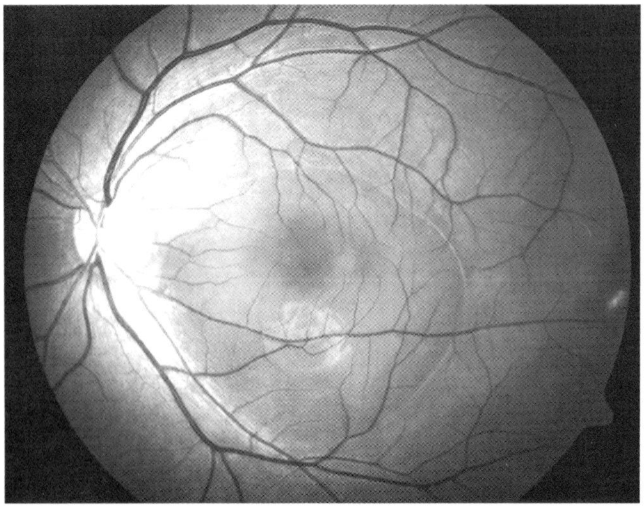

Red free photograph of the left eye showing a serous RD at the macula

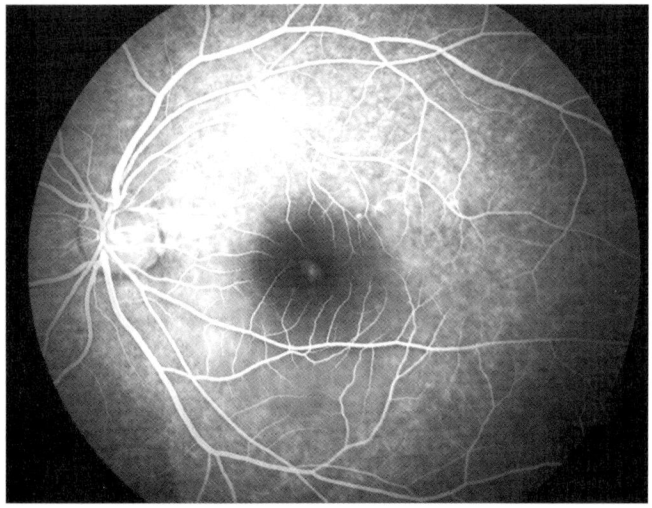

Faint hyperfluorescence is seen at the fovea in the mid-arteriovenous phase

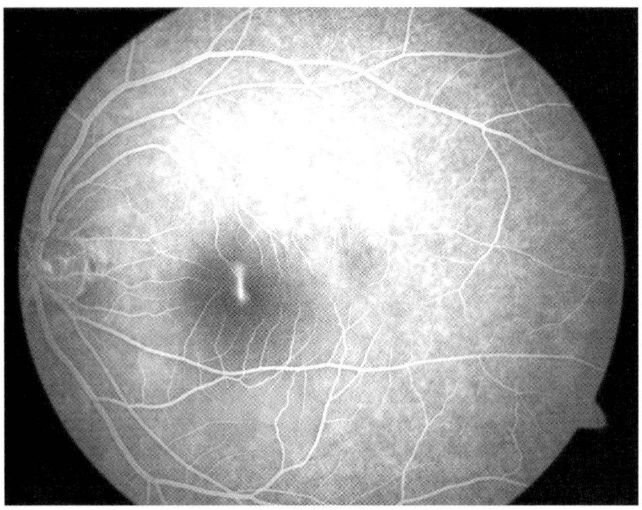

Dye is seen to leak out from the central hyperfluorescence and ascend vertically

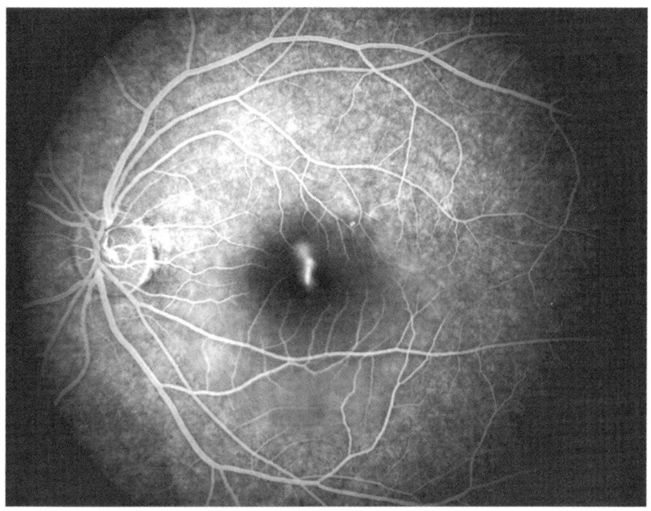

Further leakage of the dye is seen

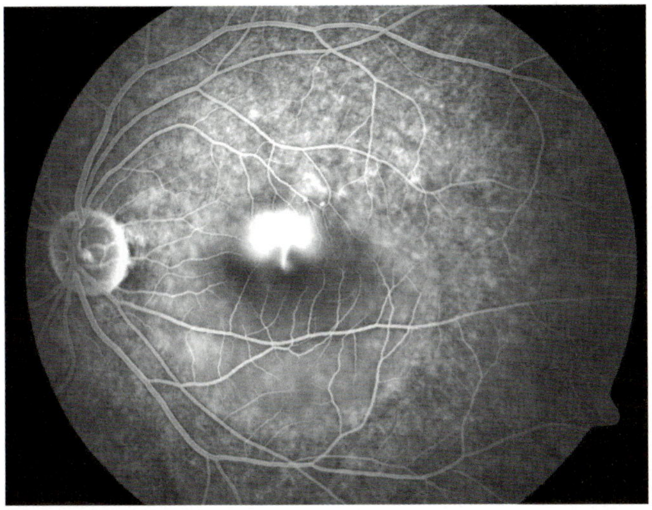

A typical smoke stack leak is seen. The dye has reached the upper border of the detachment and is seen to spread sideways

COMMENT

A typical smoke stack type of leak is seen in this case.

CASE 4

A 46-year-old male presented with history of decrease in vision in the left eye of 2 weeks duration. He was being treated for allergic rhinitis—details of the medication were not known. The visual acuity was 6/9; N6 in the left eye. Right eye was normal.

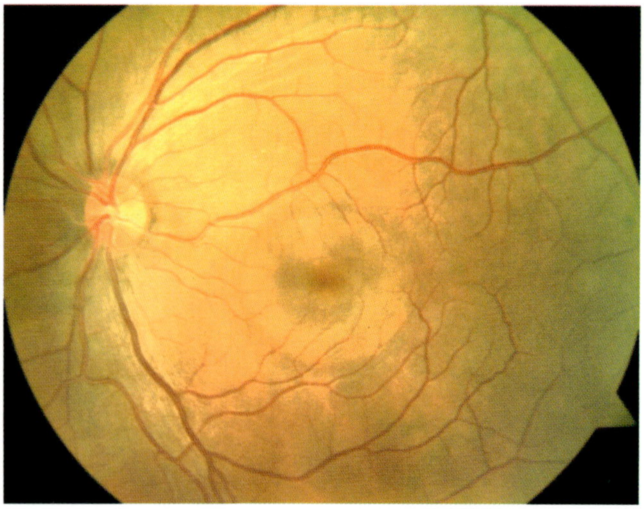

A serous elevation of the retina is seen involving the fovea

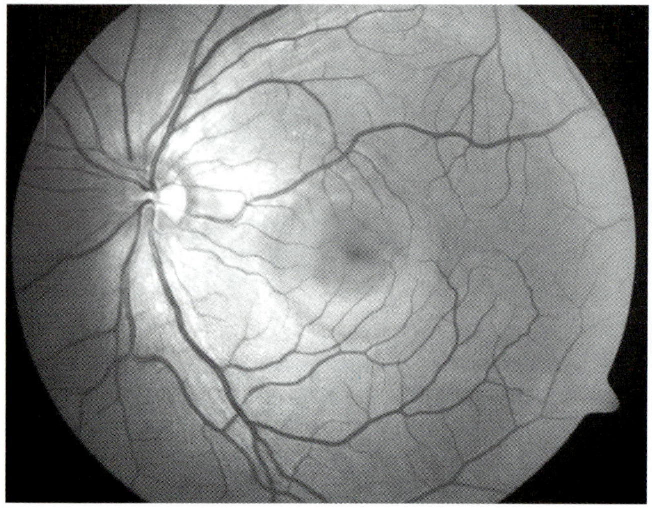

Red free photograph clearly showing the extent of the detachment

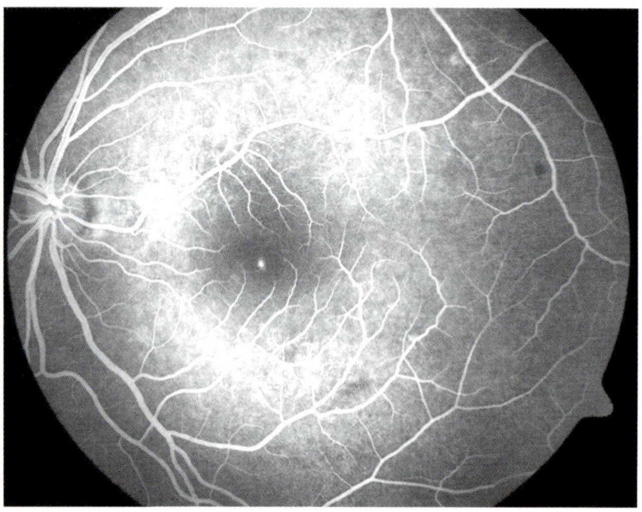

A point hyperfluorescence is seen within the foveal avascular zone

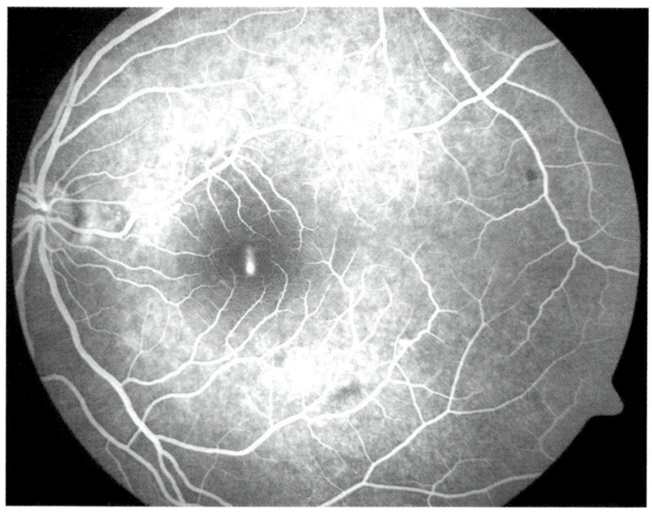

Dye is seen to leak out and ascend vertically upwards

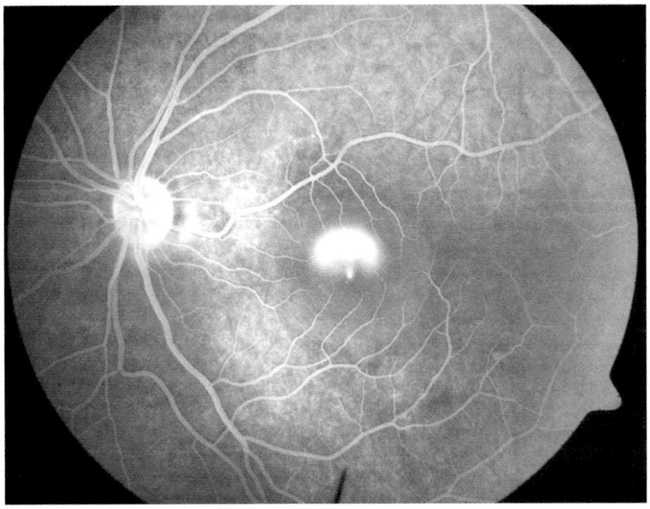

A smoke stack appearance is seen in the late phase. Even though the dye has not filled the entire detachment, its extent is well highlighted

COMMENT

CSC leaks can occur within the FAZ. The resultant RPE alterations that follow resolution of CSC, may compromise the final visual outcome.

CASE 5

A 37-year-old male presented with history of noticing distorted image in his right eye of 4 days duration. He gave history of using steroid inhalers which was prescribed for treatment of his asthma. His visual acuity was 6/6; N6 in both eyes.

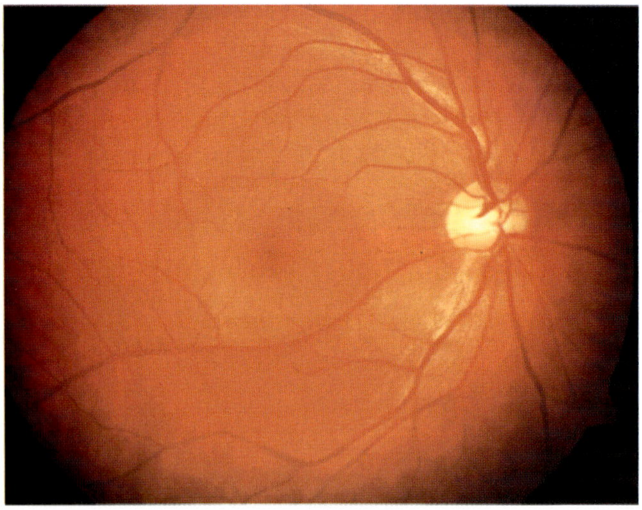

A serous elevation of the retina is seen at the macula

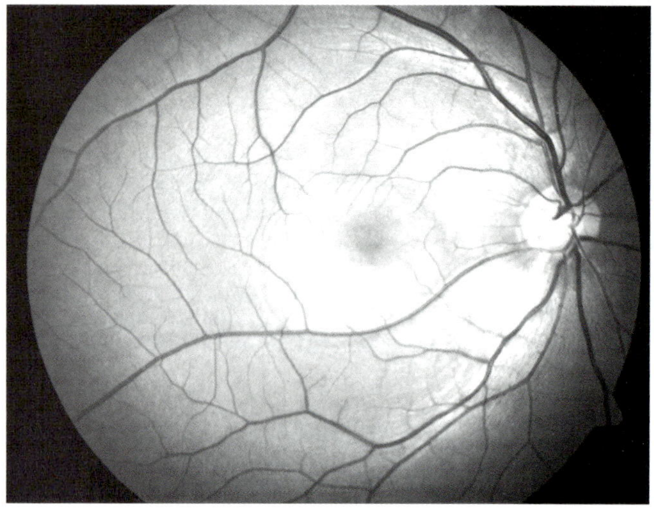

The extent of the detachment is well made out in the red free photograph

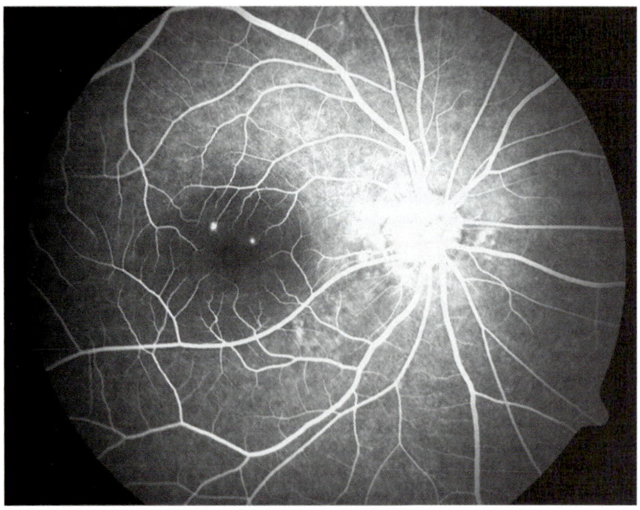

Multiple hyperfluorescent spots are seen in the mid-arteriovenous phase

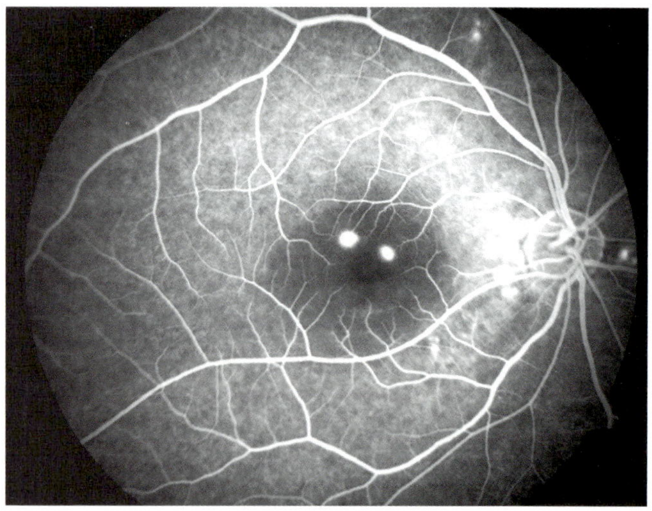

The hyperfluorescent spots have increased in intensity and size indicating leakage of the dye

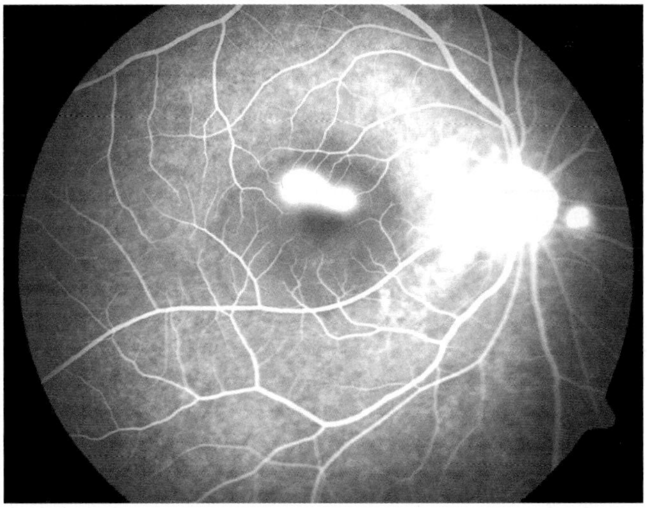

Multiple ink blot leaks are seen in the late phase of the angiogram indicating a multiple leak CSC

COMMENT

Multiple leak CSC is more commonly associated with the use of steroids.

CASE 6

A 41-year-old male presented with history of blurred vision in the right eye of three months duration. He gave history of being treated with systemic steroids. His visual acuity was 6/9; N6.

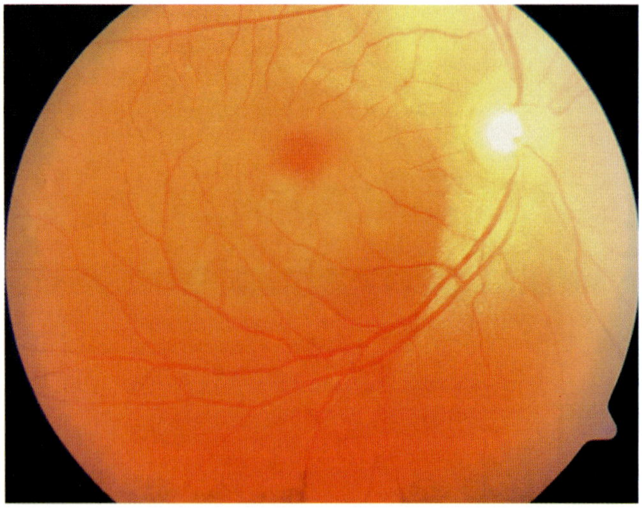

Fundus photograph of the right eye showing the large sensory retinal elevation at the macula. An additional pocket of fluid is noted superotemporal to the disc

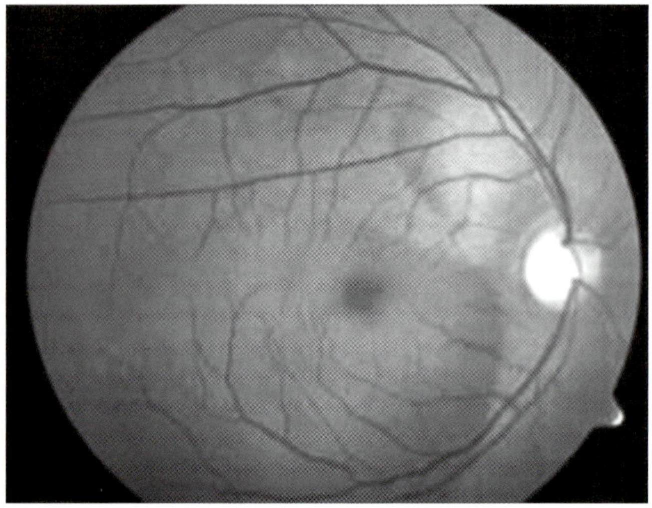

Red free photograph shows the two areas of sensory retinal detachment

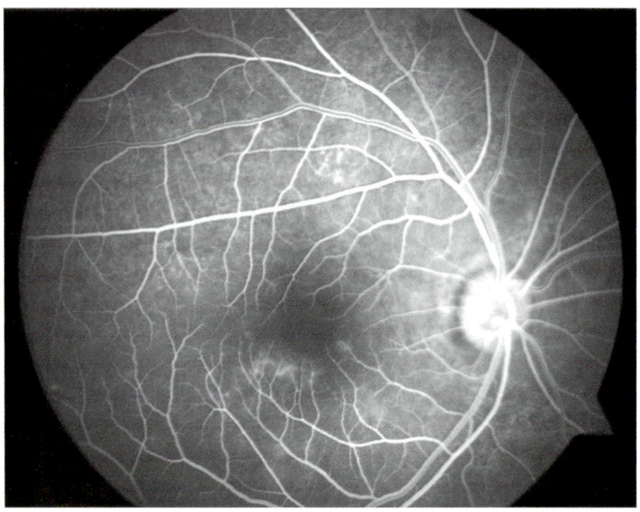

In the early arteriovenous phase, faint hyperfluorescence is seen inferior to the fovea and in the superior macula

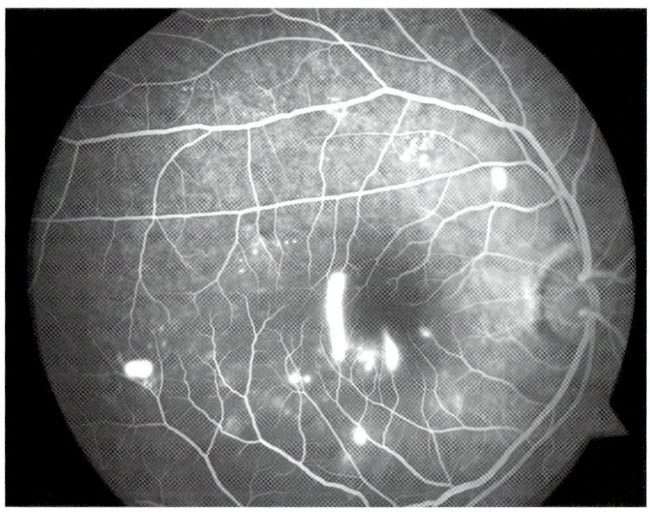

The arteriovenous phase shows multiple points of leakage of dye. At two points inferior to the fovea, the dye is seen to ascend vertically

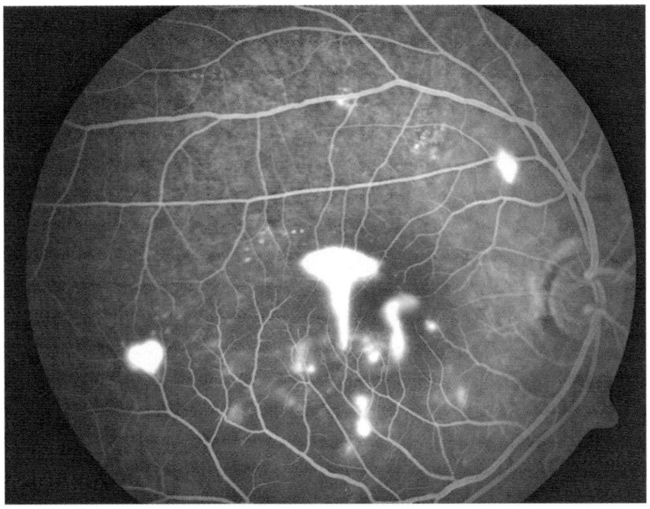

Multiple smoke stack and ink blot leaks are seen in the late arteriovenous phase

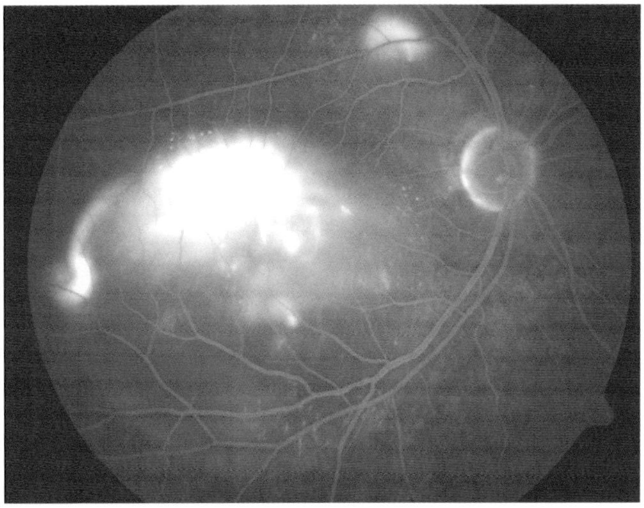

The dye has leaked from multiple points and pooled in the upper part of the detachment in the late phase of the angiogram

CASE 7

A 40-year-old male patient presented with history of blurred vision in the left eye for the past three months. Visual acuity was 6/12; N8. Right eye was normal.

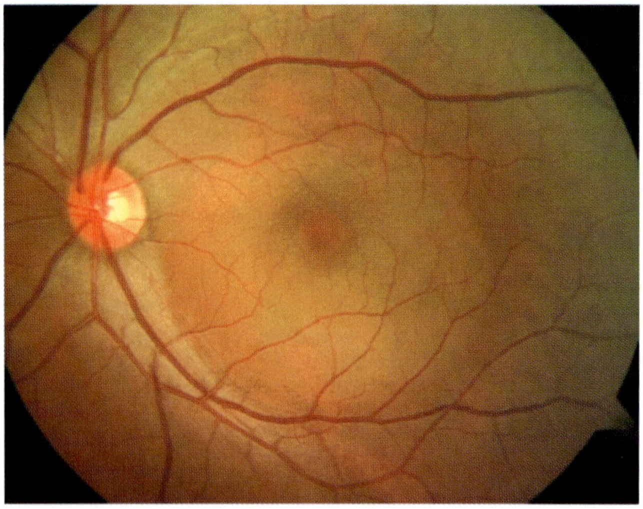

A serous elevation of the retina is seen at the macula. A pigment epithelial detachment is in the center

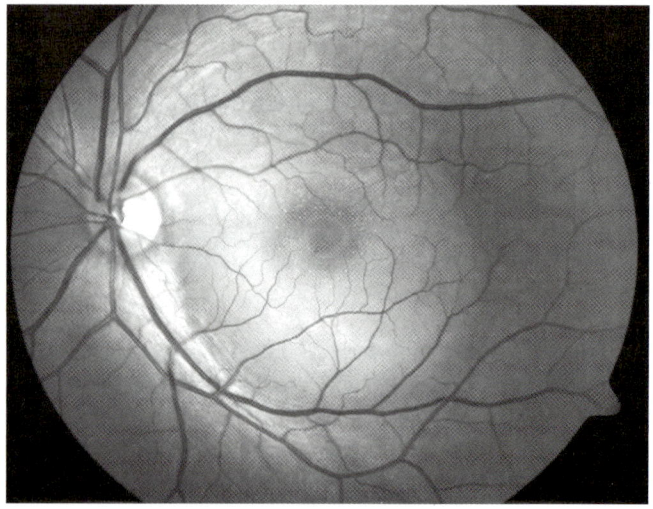

Red free photograph of the left eye showing the extent of the detachment. The pigment epithelial detachment is seen at the fovea

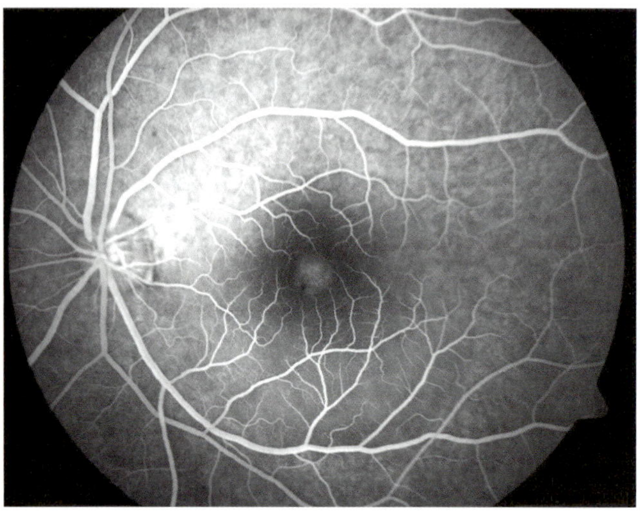

Midarteriovenous phase of the angiogram showing hyperfluorescence due to leakage of the dye into the pigment epithelium detachment

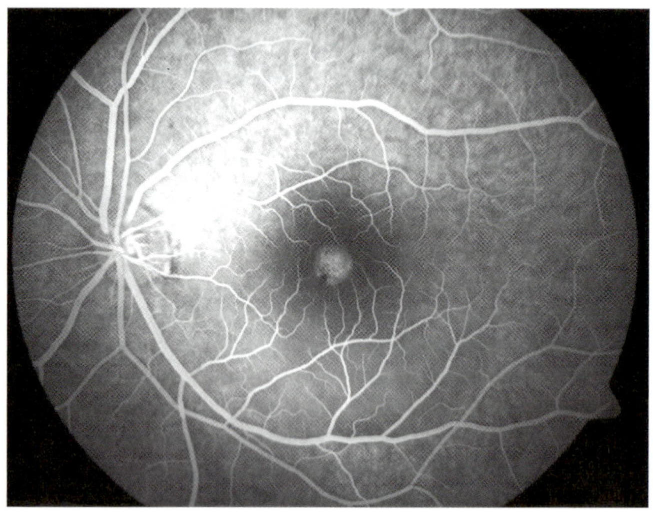

Increase in hyperfluorescence is seen at the pigment epithelium detachment

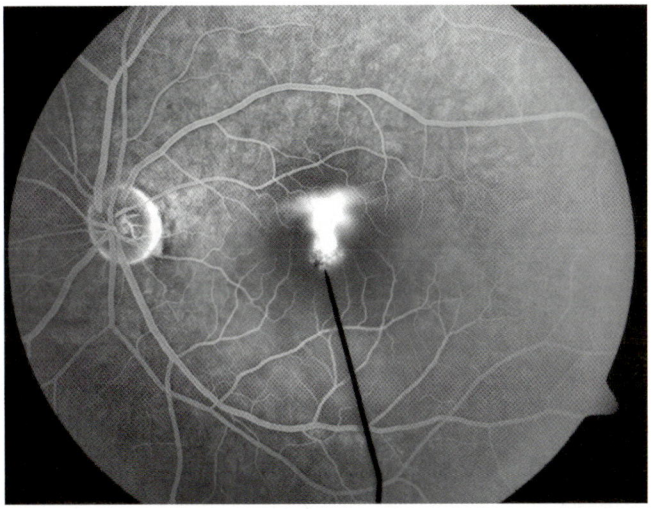

Dye leakage from the pigment epithelial detachment into the subretinal space is seen. The dye is seen to ascend and reach the upper border of the detachment

COMMENT

Leakage of the dye from the PED itself is seen in this case.

CASE 8

A 32-year-old female patient gave history of reduced vision in the left eye of three months duration. She had been diagnosed elsewhere as having choroiditis and was started on systemic steroids. At presentation her vision in the left eye was 6/18; N36. She was found to have central serous chorioretinopathy in the left eye.

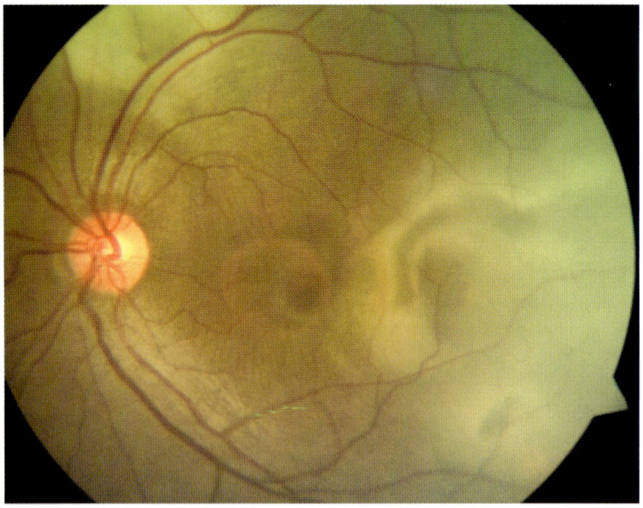

Fundus photograph of the left eye showing multiple PEDs at the macula. Extensive subretinal whitening (fibrin) is seen temporally and superiorly

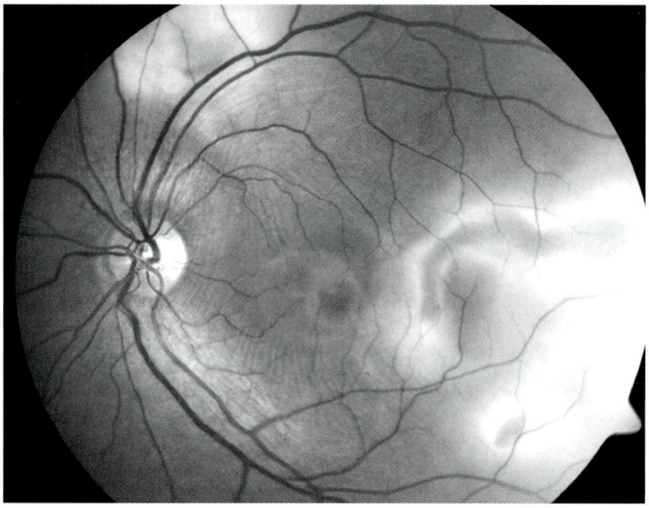

Red free photograph highlighting the features seen in the fundus photograph

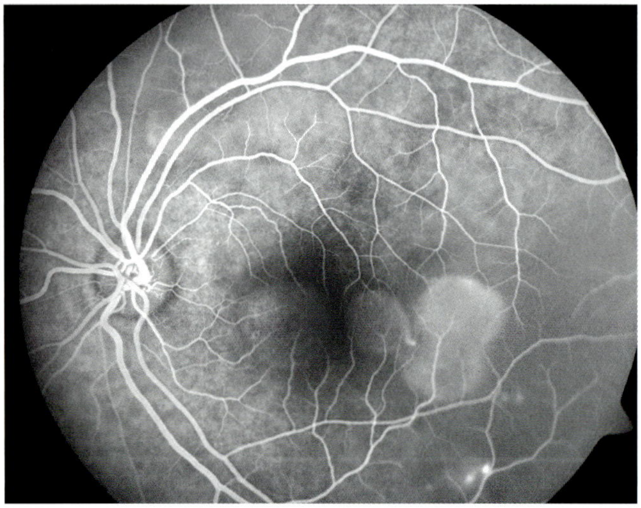

Hyperfluorescence due to early filling of the PED is seen. Point hyperfluorescence are also seen: one point leak temporal to the fovea and two point leaks inferotemporally

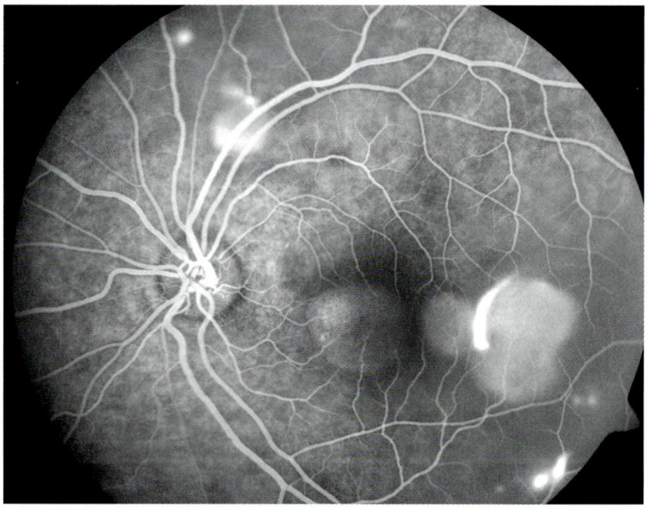

Leakage of the dye is seen from the hyperfluorescent points. Increased filling of the PEDs is seen

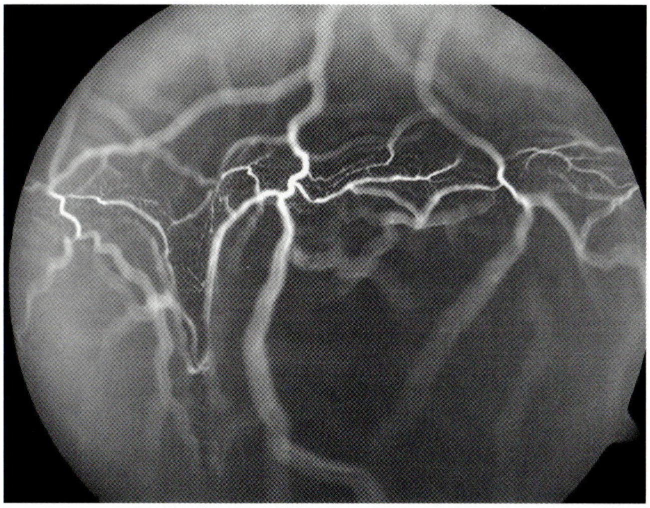

The bullous inferior retinal detachment is seen. Blurring of vascular details due to retinal elevation; choroidal pattern is not seen

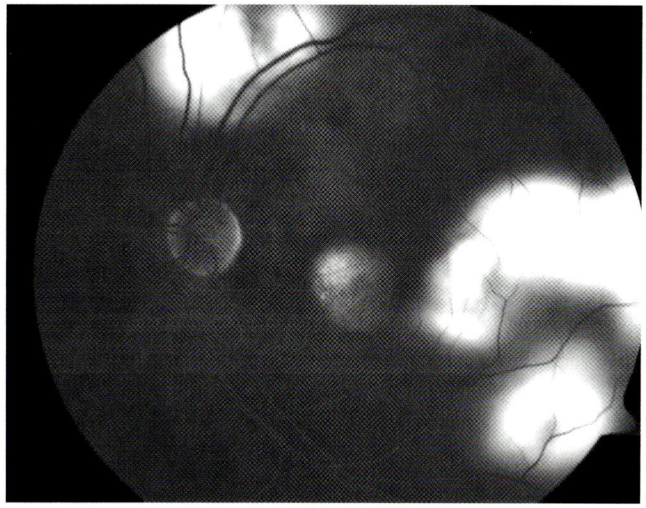

Extensive pooling of the dye in the subretinal space is seen in the late phase

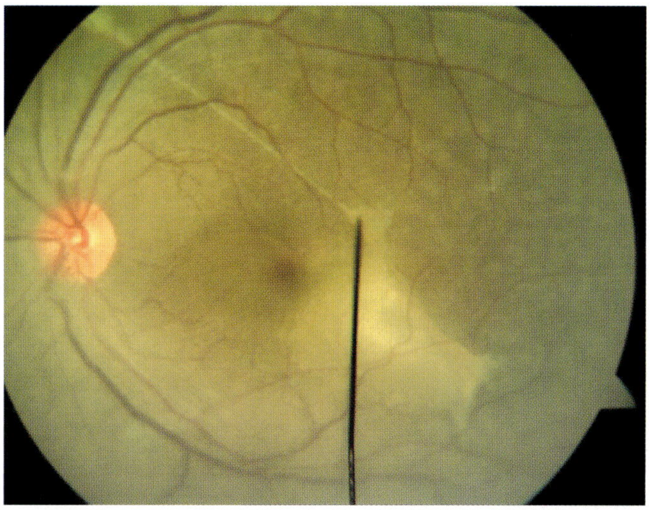

One month later vision was 6/24;N18. The subretinal fibrin is seen to be organizing. The fluid has reduced considerably

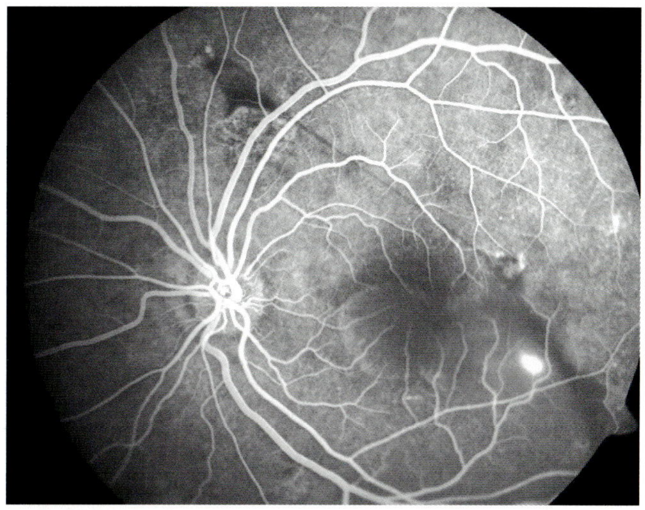

Arteriovenous phase showing a point leak temporally. Blocked choroidal fluorescence (temporal to fovea) is seen caused by the subretinal fibrin

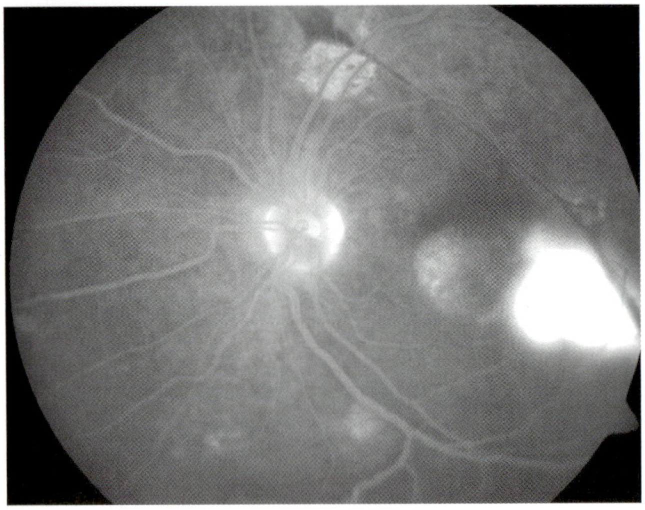

Leakage and pooling of the dye is seen temporally

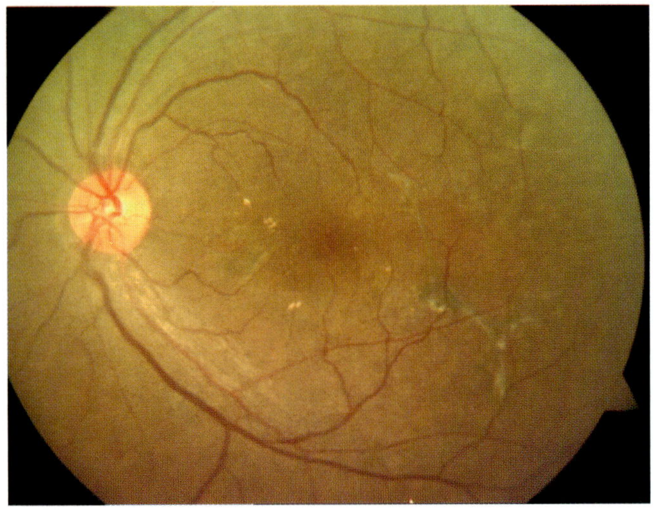

Three months later, visual acuity was 6/24; N6. RPE alteration is seen at the macula.The subretinal fibrin has resorbed. Subretinal gliotic band is seen inferotemporally

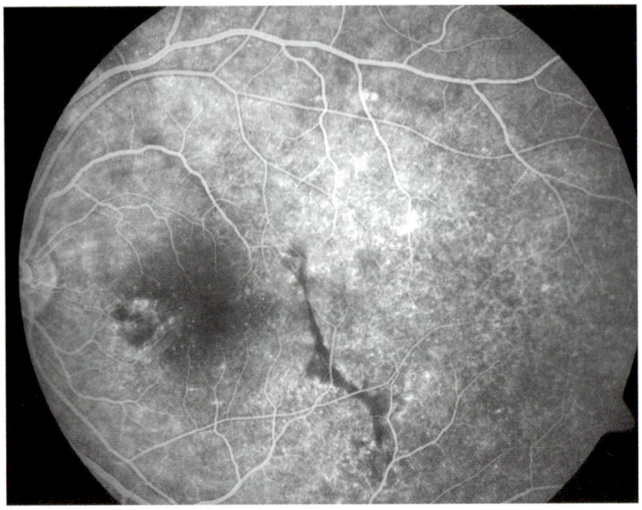

Transmission window defects are seen thoughout the macula. Blocked choroidal fluorescence is seen caused by subretinal gliosis

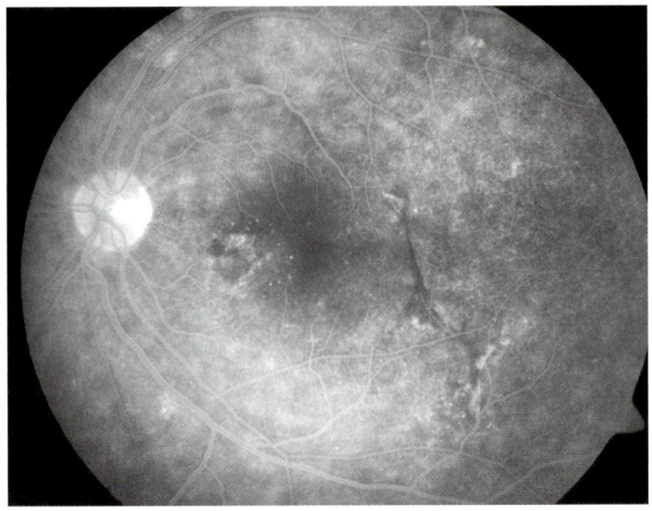

Late phase picture shows minimal fading of the hyperfluorescence temporally suggestive of window defects

CASE 9

A 39-year-old male presented with history of decreased vision in the left eye one month back. Visual acuity was 6/9; N6 in the left eye. The right eye was normal.

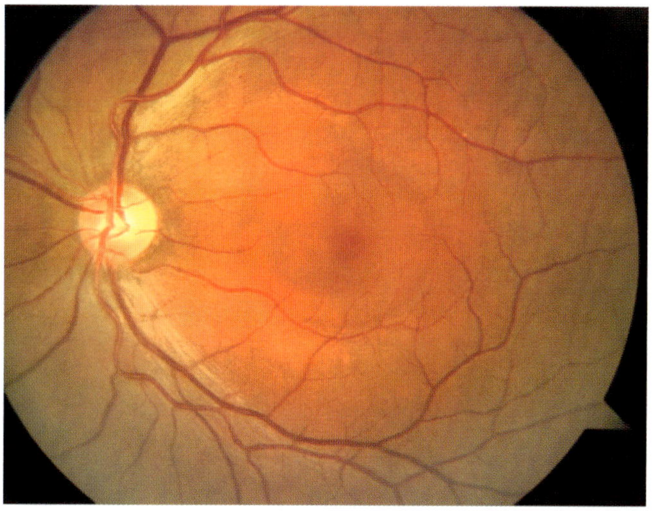

Fundus photograph of the left eye showing the sensory retinal detachment at the center of macula

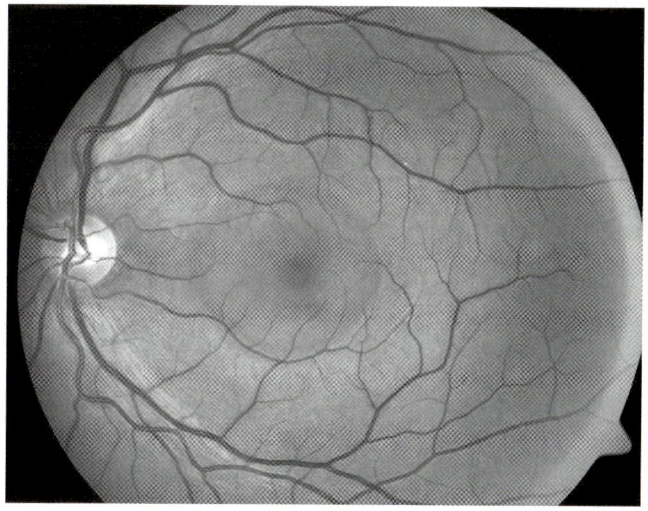

Red free photograph clearly shows the extent of the detachment

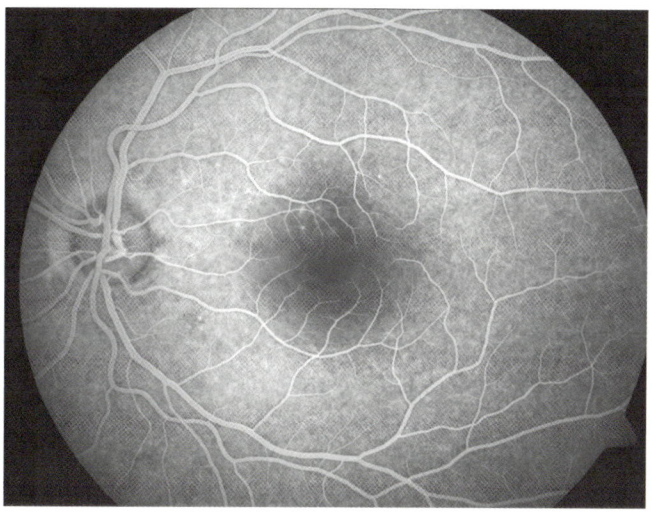

Arteriovenous phase showing faint point hyperfluorescent spots superonasal to the fovea

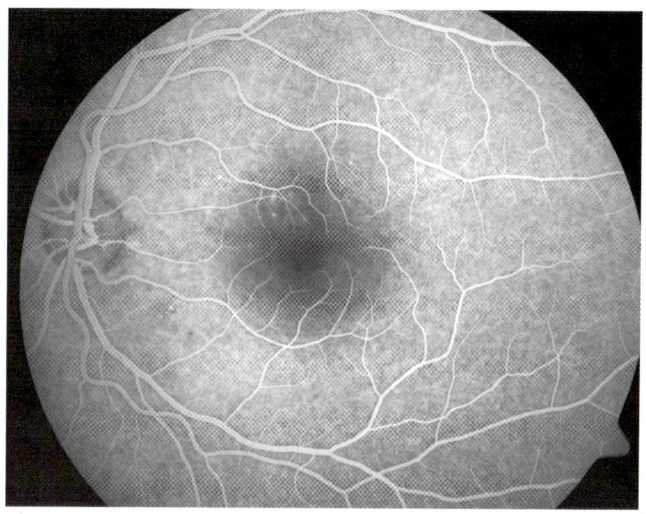

The hyperfluorescent spots have remained the same without leakage of dye

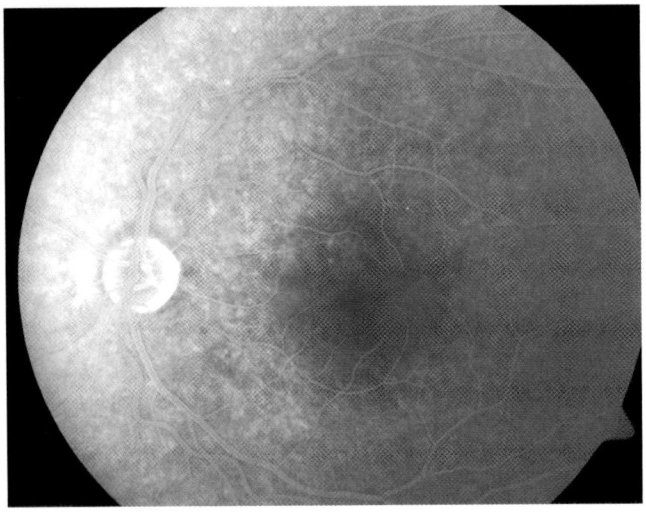

No leakage of dye is seen even in the late films

COMMENT

Absence of leakage on the angiogram, despite clinical evidence of subretinal fluid probably indicates a resolving stage of central serous chorioretinopathy.

It is important to rule out the presence of a leak outside the area of sensory detachment or the presence of an optic pit.

CASE 10

A 48-year-old male presented with decreased vision in the right eye for the past five months. He gave history of an episode of decreased vision in the left eye eleven years back. Visual acuity was 6/36; N18 in the right eye and 6/6; N6 in the left eye. Both eyes had features of resolved central serous chorioretinopathy.

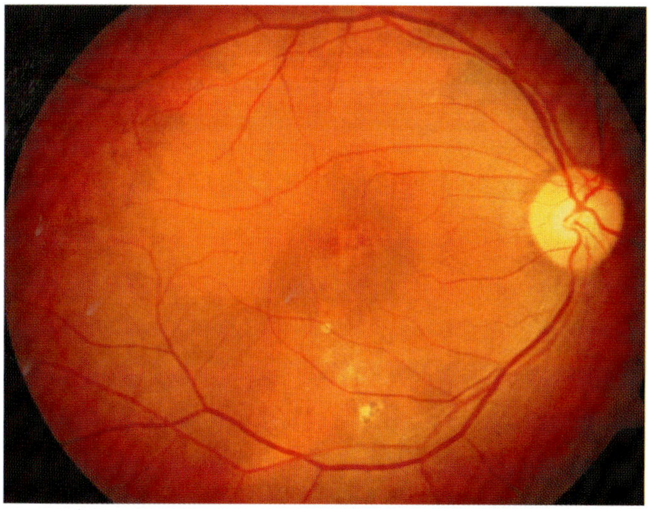

Fundus photograph of the right eye showing RPE alterations in the inferior macular region

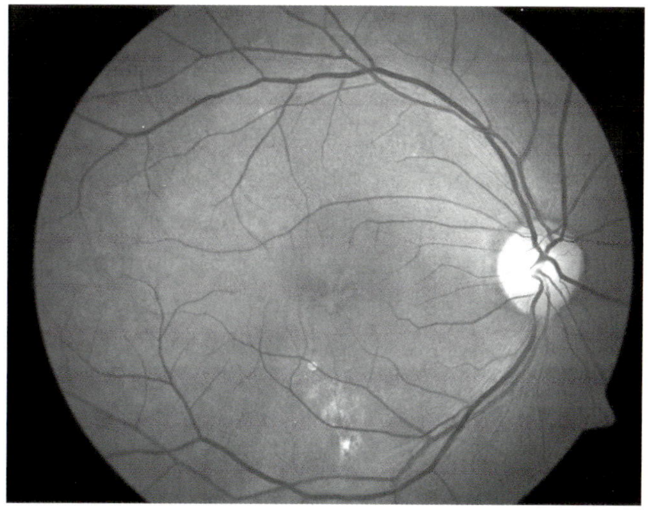

Red free photograph shows RPE alterations in the inferior part of the macula

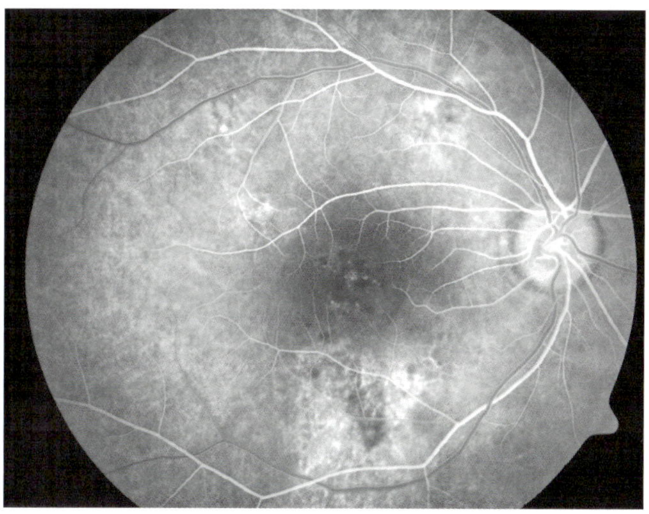

Stippled hyperfluorescence is noted corresponding to the region of RPE alteration. Hyperfluorescence is also noted superotemporal to the disc and to the fovea

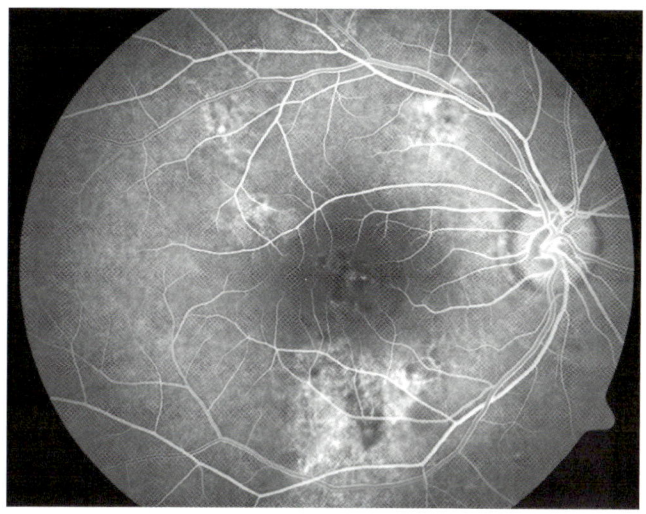

Increase in hyperfluorescence in these areas is seen. Hyperfluorescence is also noted at the foveal center

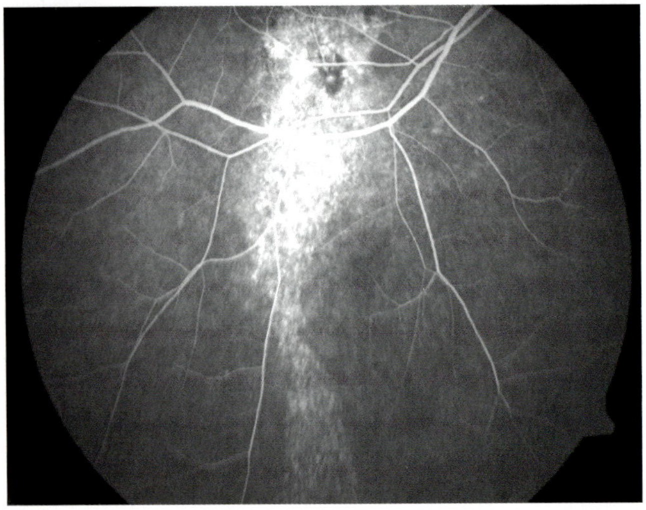

An RPE track is seen extending from the macula inferiorly

COMMENT

Presence of widespread RPE alterations at the posterior pole and the characteristic RPE track are hallmarks of old resolved central serous chorioretinopathy.

CLINICAL NUGGETS

1. Use of corticosteroids in any form should be avoided in patients with central serous chorioretinopathy.
2. Argon laser photocoagulation to the leaks can be considered in cases of nonresolving central serous chorioretinopathy that hampers daily activities; majority of leaks gets obliterated spontaneously.
3. Discontinuation of corticosteroids may be the only treatment required in most of the cases where use of steroid is responsible for CSC.
4. Reduced fluence photodynamic therapy, antivascular endothelial growth factor agents and transpupillary thermotherapy have shown to be useful in chronic CSC where the leak is close to the fovea.

BIBLIOGRAPHY

1. Bennett G. Central serous chorioretinopathy. Br J Ophthamol 1955;39:605-18.
2. Castro-Correia J, Coutinho MF, Rosas V, Maia J. Long-term follow-up of central serous retinopathy in 150 patients. DOC Ophthalmol 1992;81(4):379-86.
3. Friberg TR, Campagna J. Central serous chorioretinopathy: An analysis of the clinical morphology using image processing techniques. Graefes Arch Clin Exp Ophthalmol 1989;227:201-5.
4. Fujisawa Y. Clinical studies on central serous chorioretinitis by fluorescein fundus photography. Jpn J Ophthalmol 1966;10:19-26.
5. Gass JDM. Idiopathic central serous chorioretinopathy. Stereoscopic atlas of macular diseases. Diagnosis and Treatment. 4th edn, St Louis; Mosby 1997;52-70.
6. Schaal KB, Hoeh AE, Scheuerle A, Schuett F, Dithmar S. Intravitreal bevacizumab for treatment of chronic central serous chorioretinopathy. Eur J Ophthalmol. 2009;19(4):613-7.
7. Sharma T, Parikh SD. Transpupillary thermotherapy for juxtafoveal leak in central serous chorioretinopathy. Ophthalmic Surg Lasers Imaging 2010;9:1-3.
8. Sharma T, Shah N, Rao M, Gopal L, Shanmugam MP, Gopalakrishnan M, Bhende P, Bhende M, Shetty NS, Baluswamy S. Visual outcome after discontinuation of corticosteroids in atypical severe central serous chorioretinopathy. Ophthalmology 2004;111(9):1708-14.
9. Shin JY, Woo SJ, Yu HG, Park KH. Comparison of efficacy and safety between half-fluence and full-fluence photodynamic therapy for chronic central serous chorioretinopathy. Retina 2011;31(1):119-26.
10. Spitznas M, Huke J. Number, shape and topography of leakage points in acute type I central serous retinopathy. Graefes Arch Clin Exp Ophthalmol 1987;225: 437-40.
11. Yamada K, Hayasaka S, Setogawa T. Fluorescein angiographic patterns in patients with central serous chorioretinopathy at initial visit. Ophthalmologica 1992;205: 69-76.

Chapter 23

Drug Toxicity

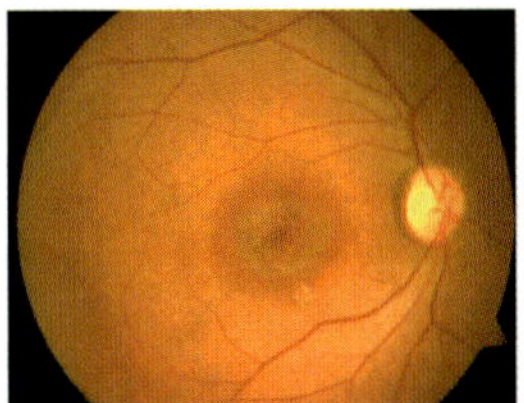

CHLOROQUINE TOXICITY

Antimalarials are used for long-term treatment of patients with arthritis. Hydroxychloroquine (HQ) is less toxic as compared to chloroquine and other disease-modifying drugs. Because of its retinotoxicity, chloroquine is no longer the preferred drug. Clinical presentation in early stages is limited to the macula, typically showing hypopigmented patch at the macula, a typical Bull's eye maculopathy.

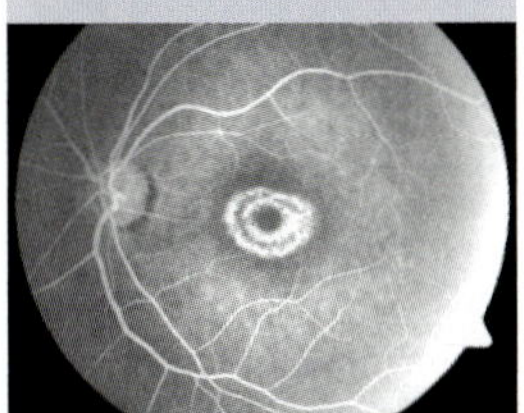

FFA reveals window defects with blocked fluorescence.

CASE 1

A 64-year-old female presented with history of gradual progressive decrease in vision in both the eyes for past 6 months. Her BCVA was 6/36; N36 in right eye and 6/6; N6 in left eyes. She had been on chloroquine 150 mg/day for treatment of rheumatoid arthritis for past 5 years.

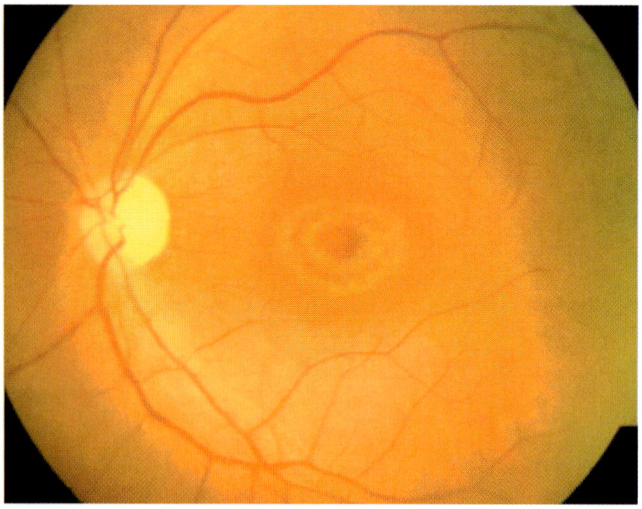

Fundus photograph of the left eye showing hypo-pigmented patch at the macula (noted in symmetrical distribution in both the eyes)

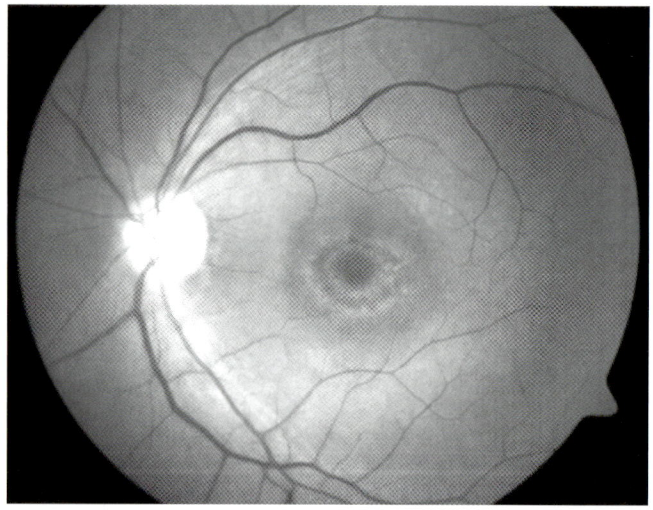

Red free photograph of the left eye highlights the pigmentary changes

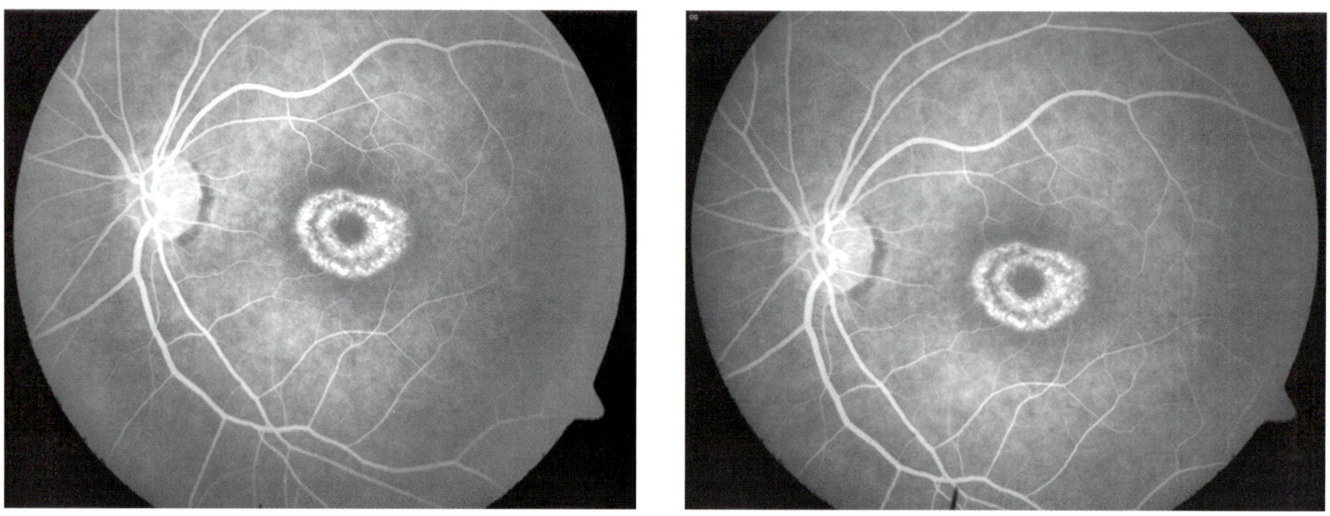

FFA revealed window defects with blocked fluorescence corresponding to the clinically seen areas in the macular region

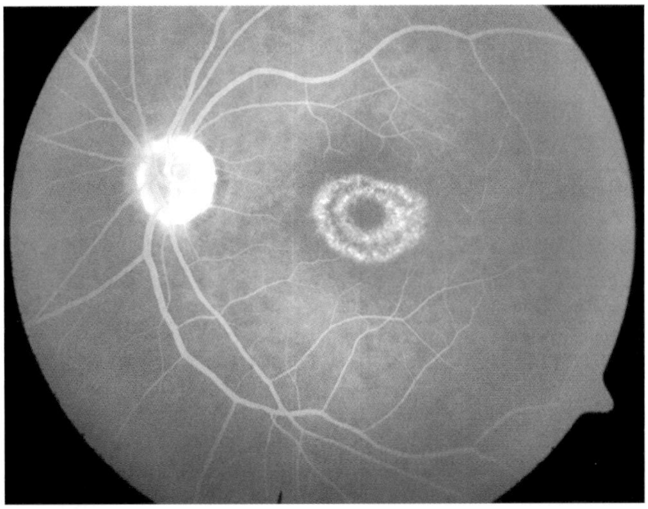

Late phase FFA does not reveal any leakage

HYDROXYCHLOROQUINE TOXICITY

Clinical presentation may vary from a near normal looking macula to a Bull's eye maculopathy.

Though, hydroxychloroquine (HQ) is safer than chloroquine, long-term hydroxychloroquine use may also be associated with retinal toxicity. Sight threatening retinopathy in these patients is less at the recommended dose of 400 mg daily.

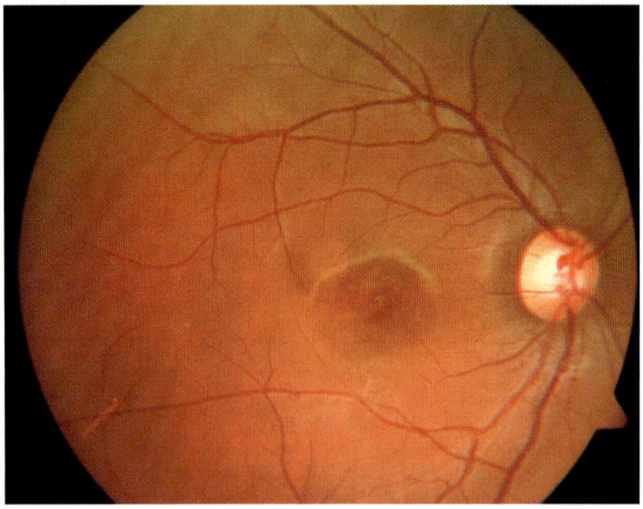
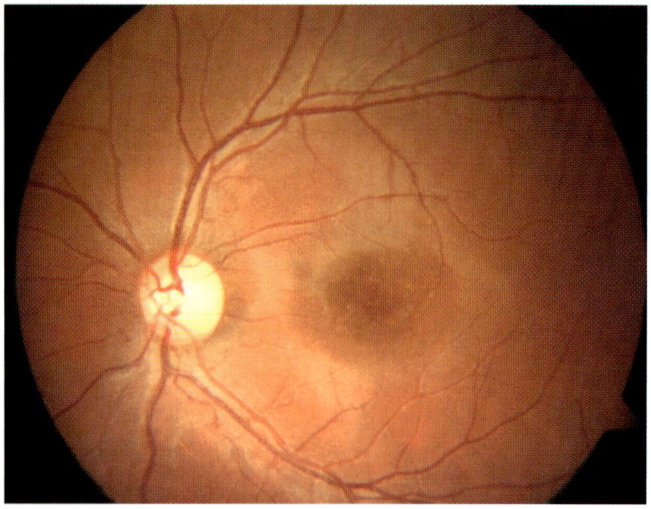

Color fundus photographs of the right and left eye reveal pigment alterations at the fovea

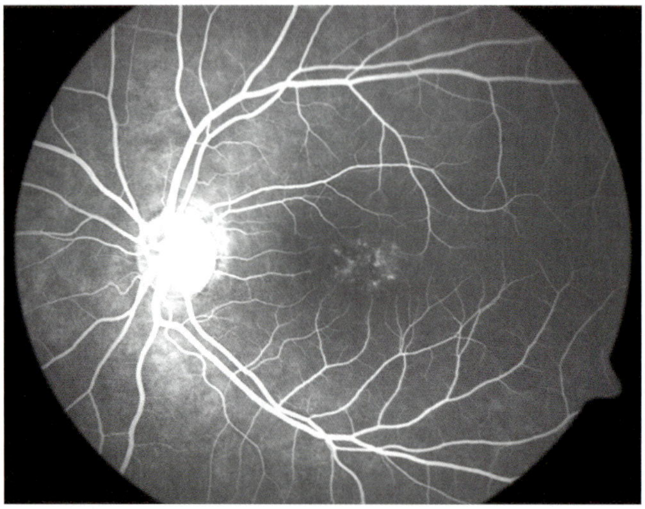

Fundus fluorescein angiography (FFA) reveals presence of retinal pigment epithelium (RPE) alteration with hyperfluorescence due to window defects

Damage caused by it is reversible in the early stages of the disease.

Retinal toxicity due to HQ is also monitored using other investigations like visual acuity, Amsler charting, color vision, automated perimetry, mfERG, OCT and EOG. Multifocal ERG can point towards macular toxicity due to HQ even when other investigations are normal.

CASE 1

A 20-year-old girl presented with a history of gradual decrease in vision since 2 years. She gave a history of Hydroxychloroquine intake for the last 3 years for rheumatoid arthritis. The dosage of the drug was 500 mg/day for 1 year followed by 200 mg/day for the last 2 years. Her best corrected visual acuity (BCVA) was 6/18 in both eyes.

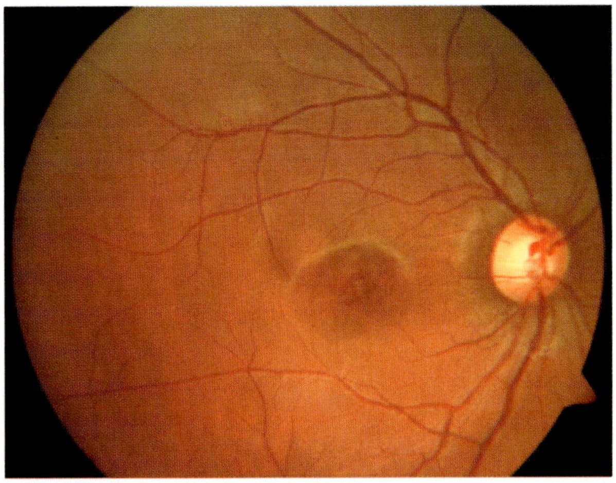

Fundus photograph of right eye showing few faint yellowish lesions at RPE at the macula in both eyes with normal disc and the vessels

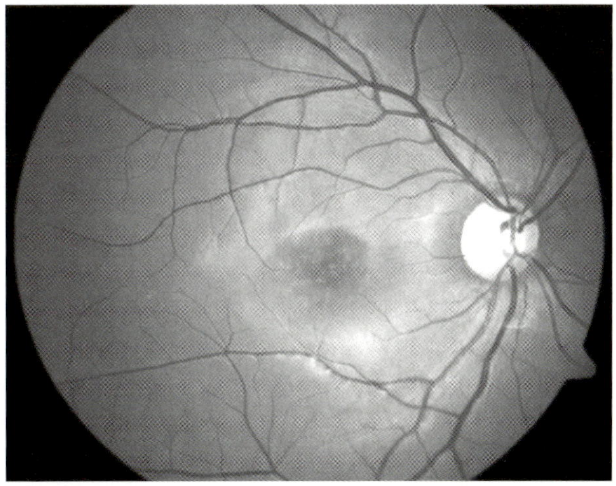

Red free photograph of the right eye highlights the pigmentary changes

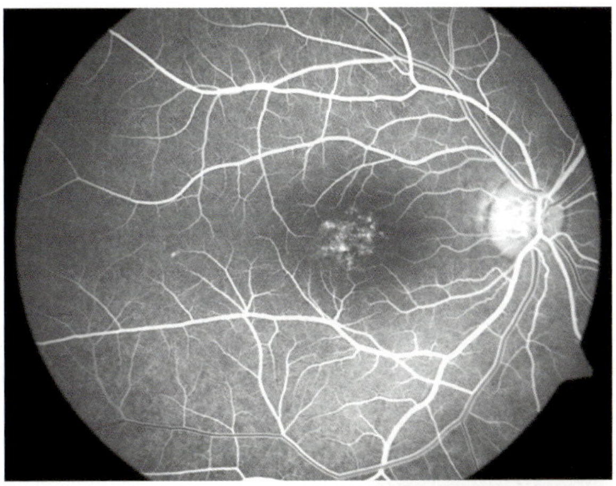

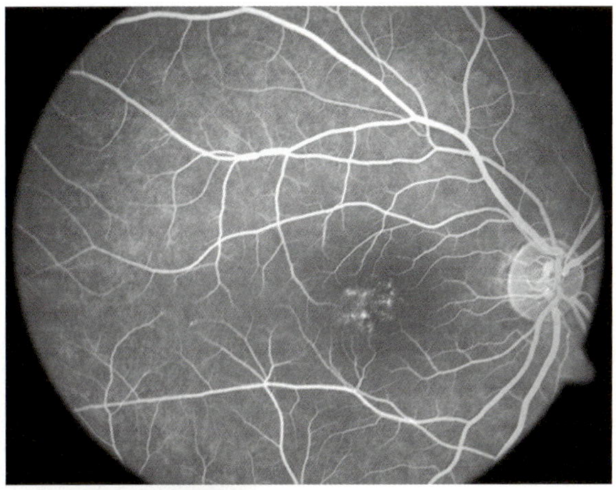

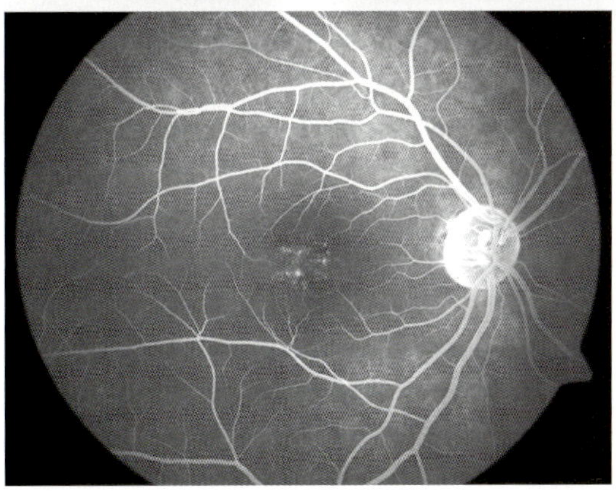

Arteriovenous and late phase of right eye shows window defects corresponding to the RPE lesions

DESFERRIOXAMINE TOXICITY

Desferrioxamine is used for the treatment of chronic iron overload and acute iron poisoning.

Ocular toxicity secondary to prolonged treatment with desferrioxamine is known to cause night blindness, visual field defects, cataract, pigmentary retinopathy, maculopathy and optic neuropathy.

To avoid such complications a routine ophthalmic screening is recommended for patients taking desferrioxamine.

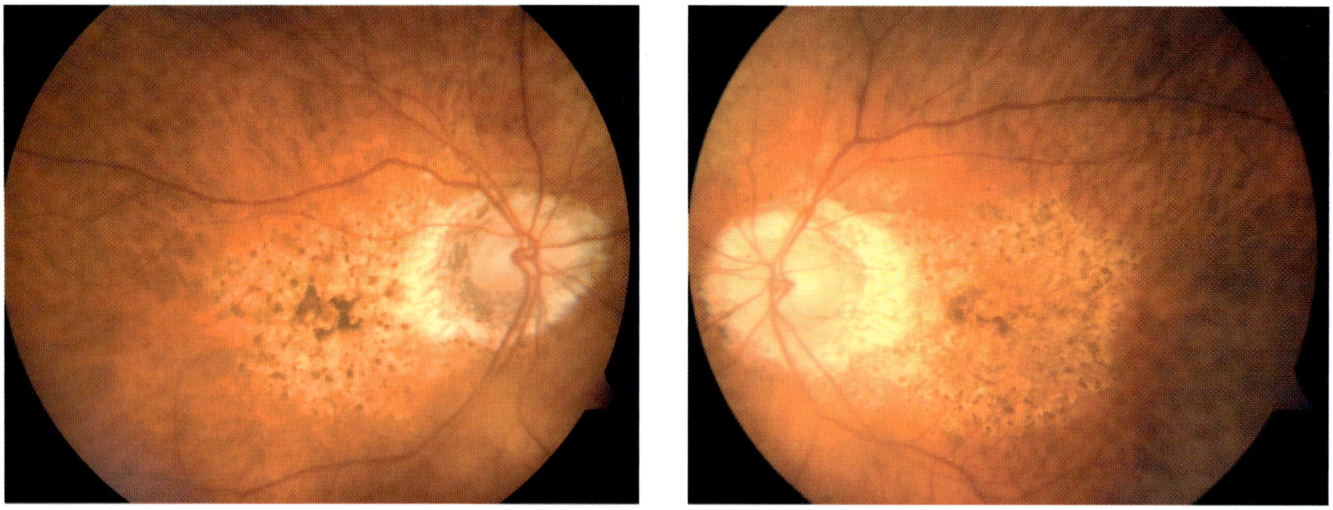

Color fundus photographs of the right and left eye show marked pigmentary changes at the macula

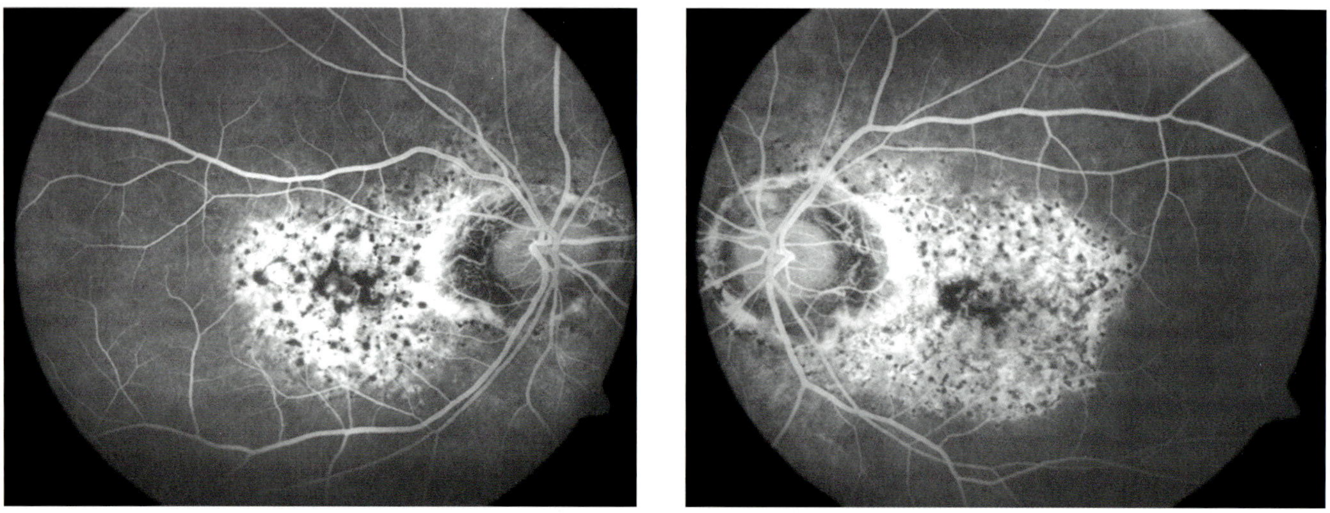

FFA reveals areas of hyperfluorescence (window defects due to RPE atrophy) and blocked fluorescence (due to pigmentary changes) corresponding to the clinical picture

CASE 1

A 77-year-old gentleman presented with history of refractory anemia for which he was taking regular blood transfusions every 7-10 days. Patient was on desferrioxamine since the last 5 years. His visual acuity in both eyes was 6/36; N12.

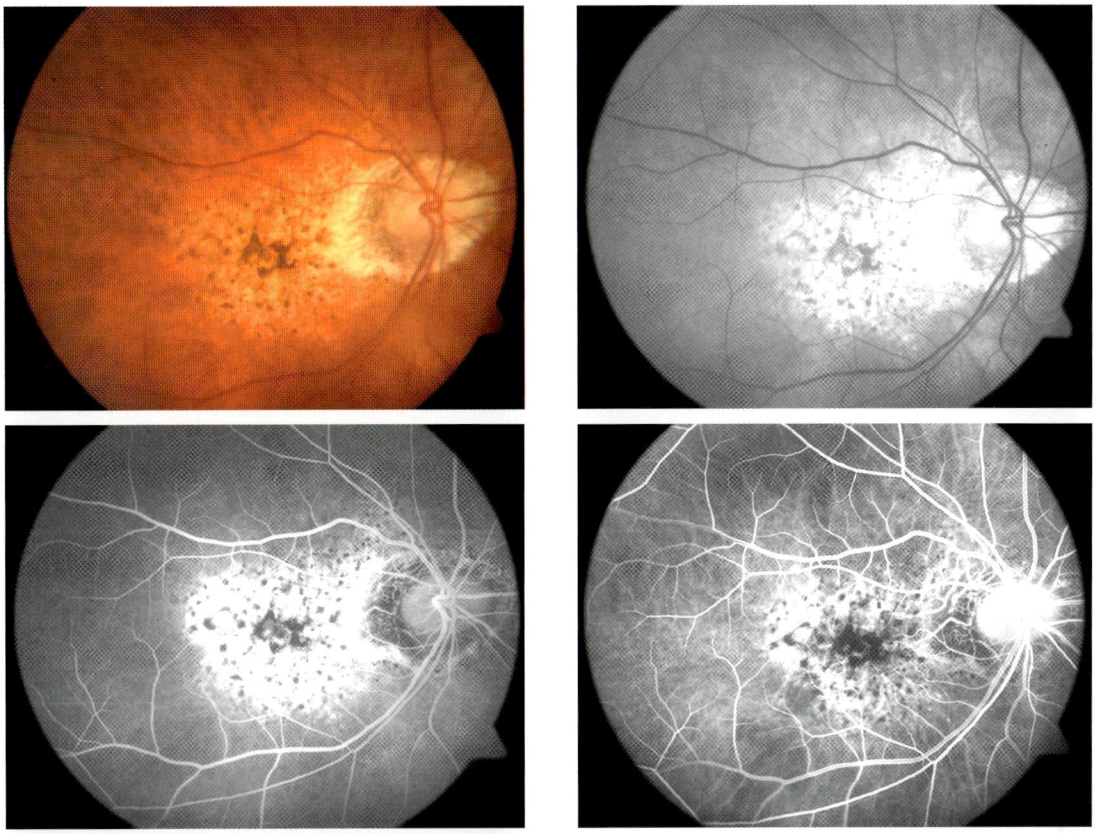

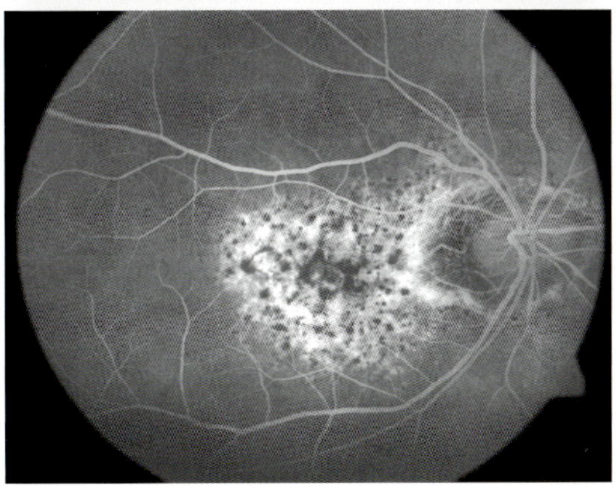

Fundus photograph of the right eye (upper left) shows pigment mottling of the macula which is highlighted in the red free photograph (upper right). FFA frames show hyperfluorescence at the macula due to underlying RPE atrophy and mottled hypofluorescence due to blockage from pigment clumps (middle and lower frames)

BIBLIOGRAPHY

1. Genead MA, Fishman GA, Anastasakis A, Lindeman M. Macular vitelliform lesion in desferrioxamine-related retinopathy. Doc Ophthalmol. 2010;121:161-6.
2. Gonzales CR, Lin AP, Engstrom RE, Kreiger AE. Bilateral vitelliform maculopathy and deferoxamine toxicity. Retina. 2004;24:464-77.
3. Sen P, Bhende M, Ravi P, Roy R. Multifocal Electroretinogram in Desferrioxamine-Related Macular Toxicity. Retinal Cases & Brief Reports. 2010;4: 224-8.
4. Xiaoyun Ma, Liang Yan, Linping He, Dongyi He, Hao Lu. Ocular fundus manifestation of two patients following long-term chloroquine therapy: a case report. Diagn Pathol. 2010;5:20.
5. Yam JC, Kwok AK. Ocular toxicity of hydroxychloroquine. Hong Kong Med J. 2006;12:294-304.

24

Chapter

Photic Maculopathy

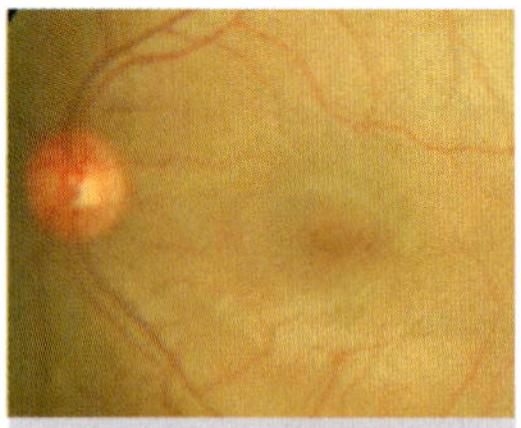

- Most cases of solar maculopathy are due to retinal phototoxicity rather than retinal photocoagulation.
- However, solar observation with a dilated 7 mm pupil produces a 22°C retinal temperature increase, well above the 10°C threshold for retinal photocoagulation.
- Telescope-assisted solar observation can cause higher retinal temperature increases.
- Solar eclipse observation is particularly hazardous because of possible pupil dilation.
- Injuries have been reported after sungazing during severe hypoglycemia and drug abuse.
- There are many indirect methods for safely viewing solar eclipses
- Other causes of photic damage include postsurgical, welding-arc and accidental laser exposure:
  - Early changes can be yellow dot at the fovea and RPE alterations. Late changes can be lamellar macular hole, CNVM.
  - Visual acuity depends on the extent of retinal damage. Usually between 20/40–20/100 range.
  - Fundus fluorescein angiogram reveals RPE window defects in the early stages
  - Spectral domain OCT and multifocal ERG help in diagnosis
  - mfERG reveals localized attenuated first order kernel responses.

CASE 1

A 63-year-old male presented with defective vision in both eyes since 16 years following unprotected viewing of solar eclipse. VA was 6/24 in right eye and 6/9 in left eye.

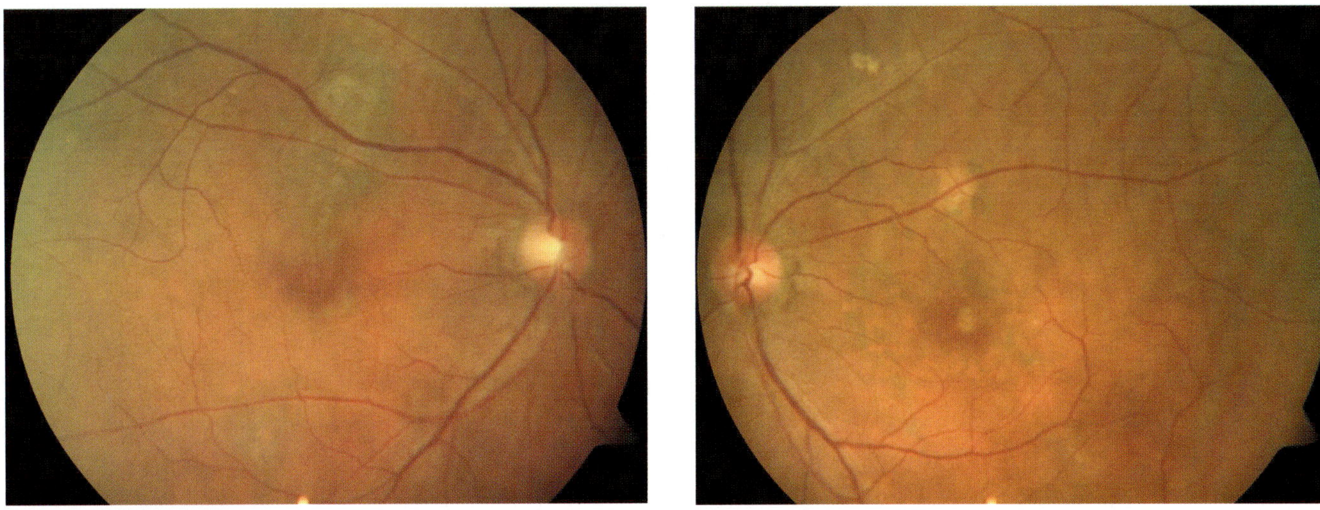

OU fundus shows RPE alterations at the posterior pole

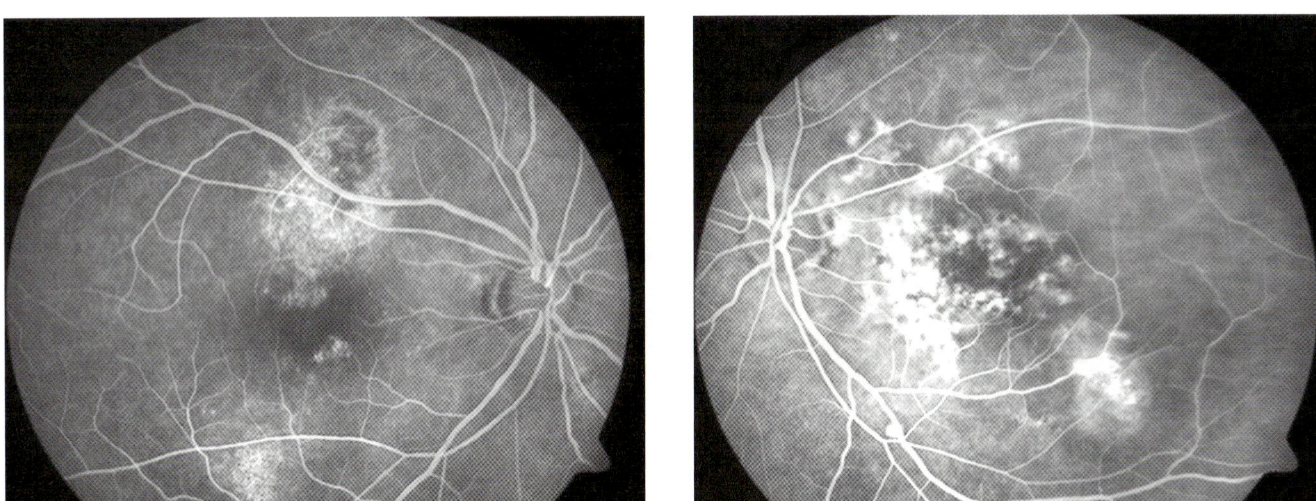

OU FA shows hyperfluorescent areas suggestive of transmission defects due to RPE alterations

CASE 2

A 30-year-old man presented with a history of painless decreased vision in both the eyes following unprotected viewing of the solar eclipse 10 years ago. Ocular or medical history was otherwise unrevealing. Best corrected visual acuity was 6/36; N12 in both the eyes.

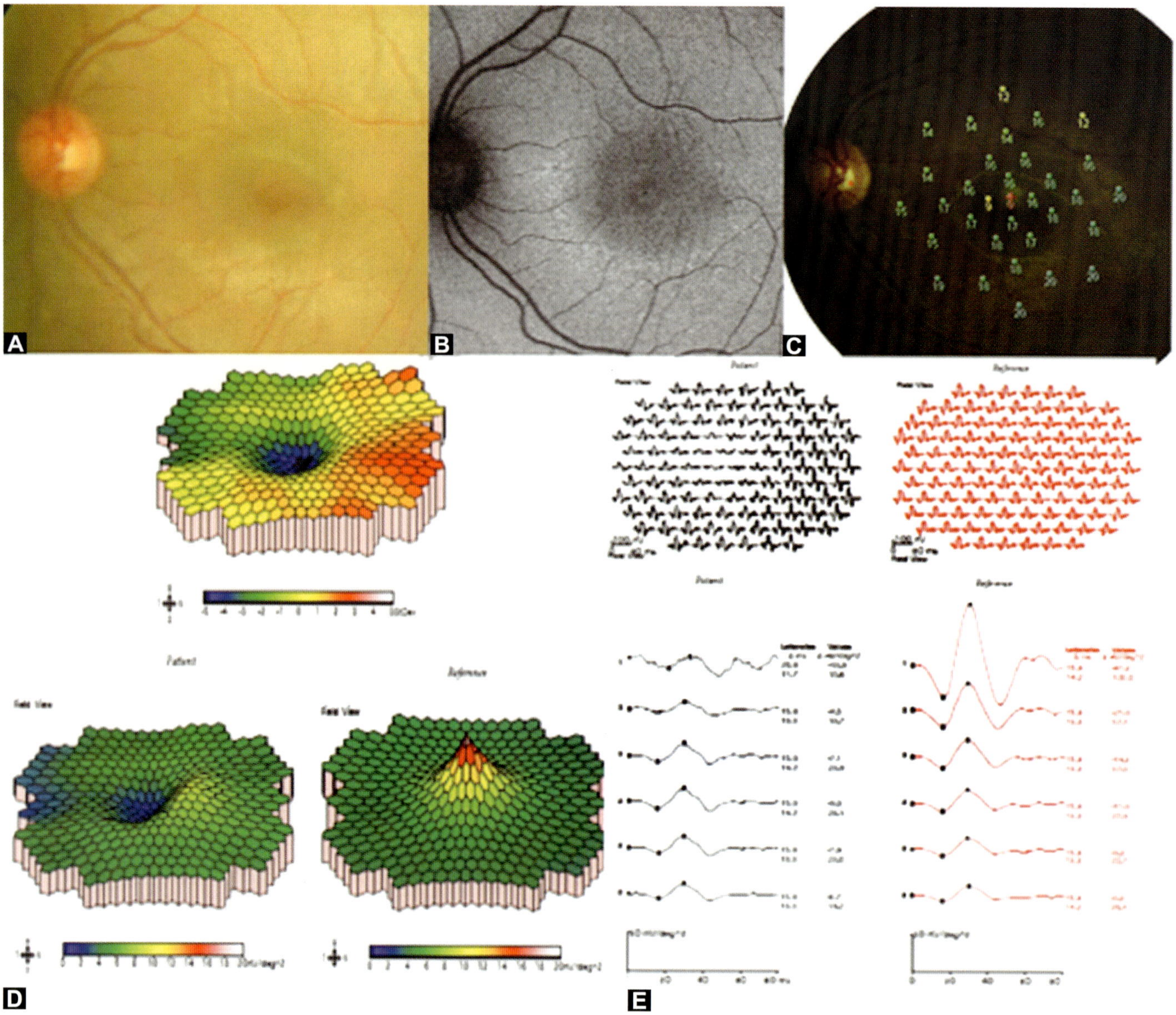

A: Fundus photograph of the left eye showing retinal pigment epithelium alterations
B: Fundus Autofluorescence of left eye showing mottled increased signal in the foveal and parafoveal area
C: Microperimetry in the left eye showing dense central scotoma with reduced mean sensitivity
D and E: Multifocal electroretinogram trace array and plot showing reduced P1 and N1 ring amplitude in the foveal and the parafoveal area without any change in latency

BIBLIOGRAPHY

1. Huang SJ, Gross NE, Costa DL, Yannuzzi LA. Optical coherence tomography findings in photic maculopathy. Retina 2003;23(6):863-6.
2. Kallmark FP, Ygge J. Photo-induced foveal injury after viewing a solar eclipse. Acta Ophthalmol Sc and 2005;83(5):586-9.
3. Long VW, Woodruff GH. Bilateral retinal phototoxic injury during cataract surgery in a child. AAPOS. 2004; 8(3):278-9.
4. Lund DJ, Stuck BE, Edsall P. Retinal injury thresholds for blue wavelength lasers. Health Phys. 2006; 90(5):477-84.
5. Wu J, Seregard S, Algvere PV. Photochemical damage of the retina. Surv Ophthalmol. 2006;51(5):461-81. Review.

25

Chapter

Cystoid Macular Edema

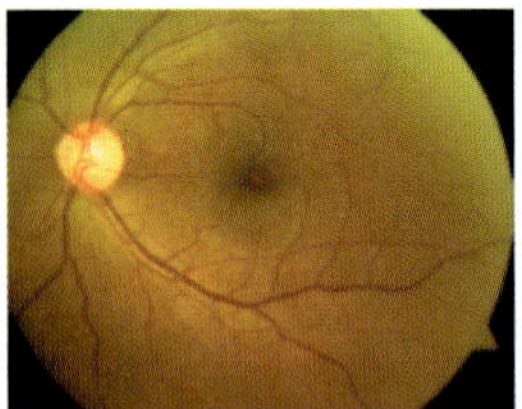

- Fluid accumulation in cystic spaces localized to the outer plexiform and inner nuclear layers of the retina is called cystoid macular edema.
- The common causes of cystoid macular edema include.

1. Postsurgical cystoid macular edema
    - Angiographic macular edema: The macular edema is not obvious on clinical examination, however, the fluorescein angiography shows leakage of the dye. The visual acuity is usually unaffected.
    - Clinically significant macular edema: Here the macular edema is associated with a drop in visual acuity.
    - The area of dye leakage on fluorescein angiography correlates poorly with the visual acuity. A better predictor in such cases would be the estimation of the retinal thickness.
2. Diabetic macular edema
    - In addition to cystoid macular edema, the other changes occurring in diabetic maculopathy are well-seen on the angiogram. This includes capillary leakage, microaneurysms, capillary dropout areas and intraretinal microvascular abnormalities. In patients with diabetic retinopathy undergoing cataract surgery it may be difficult to determine whether the postoperative macular edema is due to the surgical intervention or occurring as part of the diabetic process. In diabetic macular edema the leakage may be more diffuse and not localized to the perifoveal region. In addition the late disc staining, which is commonly seen in postsurgical cystoid macular edema, is absent in diabetic macular edema.
3. Intermediate uveitis
4. Vascular occlusions
5. Epiretinal membrane
6. Retinitis pigmentosa
7. Drug toxicity, e.g. epinephrine, nicotinic acid and rarely after infliximab therapy for Behçet's disease
8. Dominantly inherited cystoid macular edema
9. After bone marrow transplantation

In addition to fluorescein angiography, optical coherence tomography (OCT) is an important investigation, which clearly delineates the cystoid spaces. OCT is useful in the comparative evaluation and detection of subtle edema. Fundus autofluorescence (FAF) has also been used to evaluate cystoid macular edema. Petalloid pattern seen on angiography is known to be identical to what is seen on fundus autofluorescence. Interestingly, there is a difference in the pattern seen on FAF done with 488 nm excitation Vs that done with 580 nm. Macular pigments normally block 488 nm light more than 580 nm. Hence, when macular edema pushes the pigment away from center, there is enhanced FAF when autofluorescence is elicited with 488 nm light (Heidelberg SLO) compared to that elicited with 580 nm light (Topcon Camera).

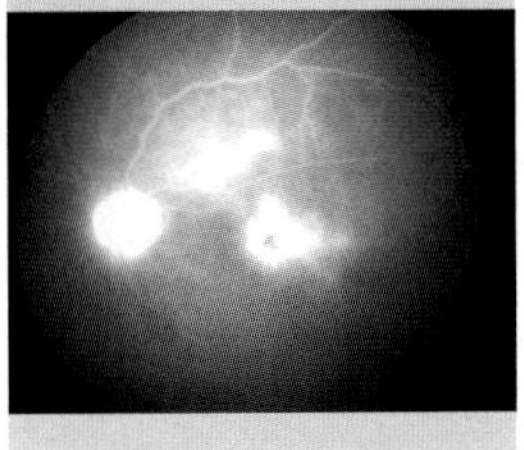

- In the early phase of the angiogram, capillary dilation is seen in the perifoveal region.
- Late pooling of the dye is seen, occurring in a petaloid pattern in the perifoveal region. The fusiform cystoid spaces are arranged in a radial pattern.
- Often patchy hyperfluorescence is seen extending beyond the region of the cystic spaces indicating more widespread capillary leakage.
- Leakage of the dye from the disc capillaries gives rise to late staining of the optic nerve head.
- When cystoid spaces occur outside the perifoveal area, fluorescein angiography shows a 'honeycomb' appearance rather than a petalloid pattern.

CASE 1

A 62-year-old female gave history of reduced vision in the right eye. She had undergone a cataract surgery with intraocular lens implantation in the past, with no visual improvement seen in the postoperative period. Vision was 2/60 in the right eye.

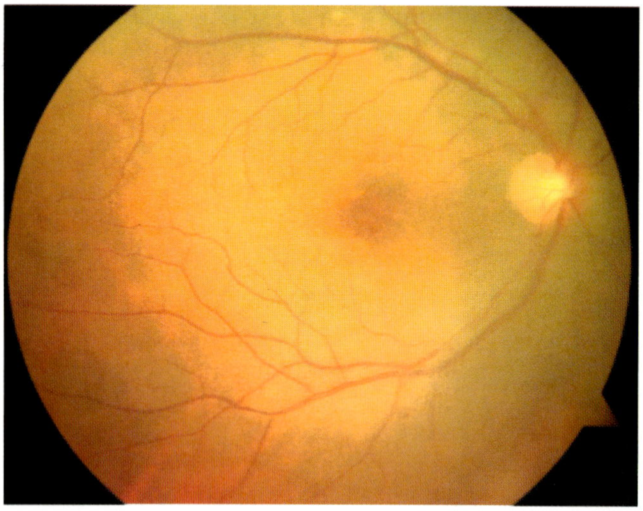

Fundus photograph of the right eye. A large lamellar macular hole with surrounding cystoid changes are seen

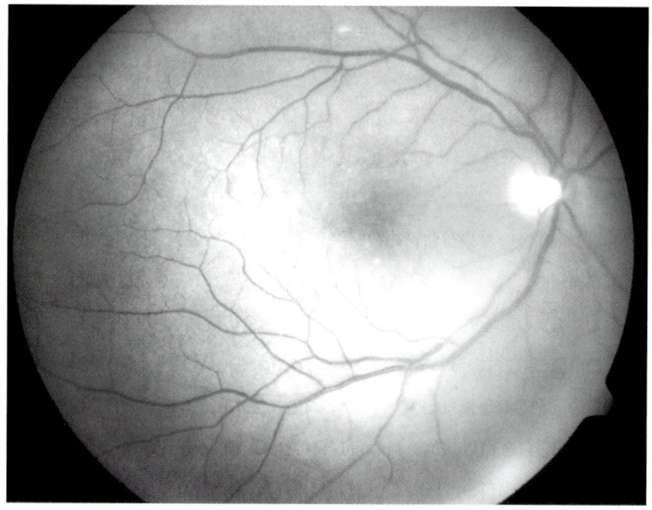

Red free photograph of the right eye. Large cystoid changes are seen in the foveal region with a large central lamellar macular hole

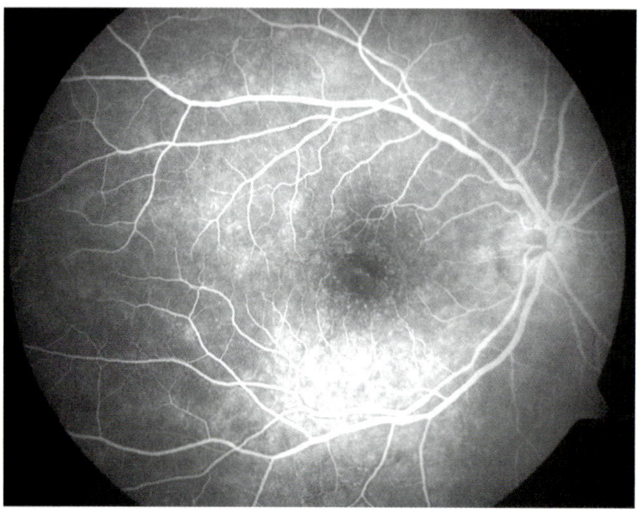

Dilation of the perifoveal capillaries is seen. Early leakage of the dye is seen from the capillaries in the inferior macular region

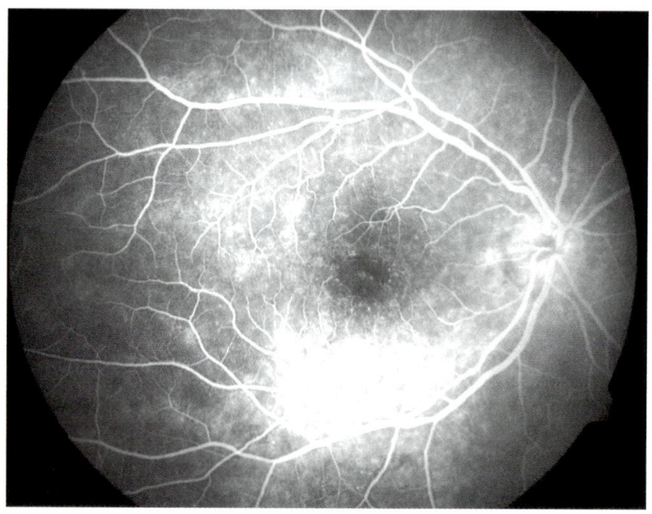

Increased leakage from the capillaries in the macula is evident

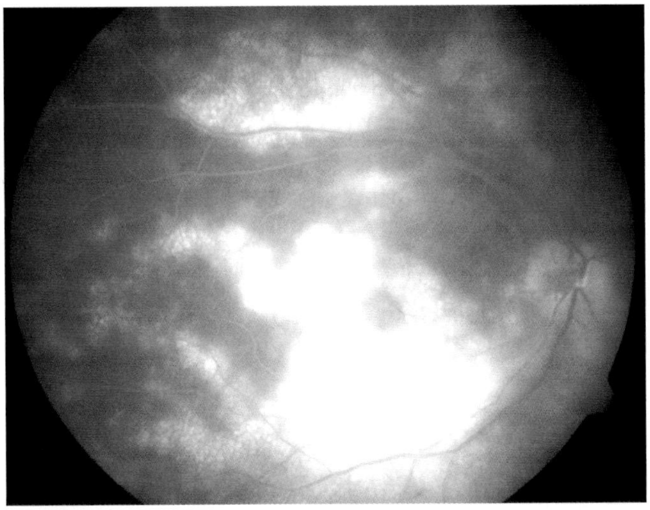

Significant accumulation of the dye is noted throughout the macula. Honeycomb pattern of cystoid macular edema is noted in the areas outside the fovea. Note the hypofluorescent appearing lamellar macular hole

COMMENT

No dye accumulation occurs in the lamellar macular hole as the dye which leaks into its cavity easily escapes into the vitreous. Hence, it appears hypofluorescent.

Cystoid changes occurring outside the fovea assumes a honeycomb pattern.

CASE 2

A 36-year-old female presented with history of blurring of vision in both eyes for the past one month. Visual acuity was 6/9; N6 in the right eye and 6/24; N8 in the left eye. Examination revealed exudates over the pars plana in both eyes suggestive of intermediate uveitis.

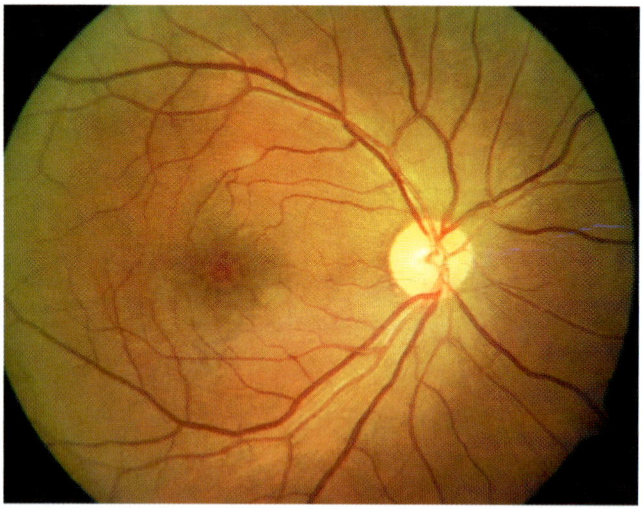

Cystoid changes are seen in the foveal region of the right eye

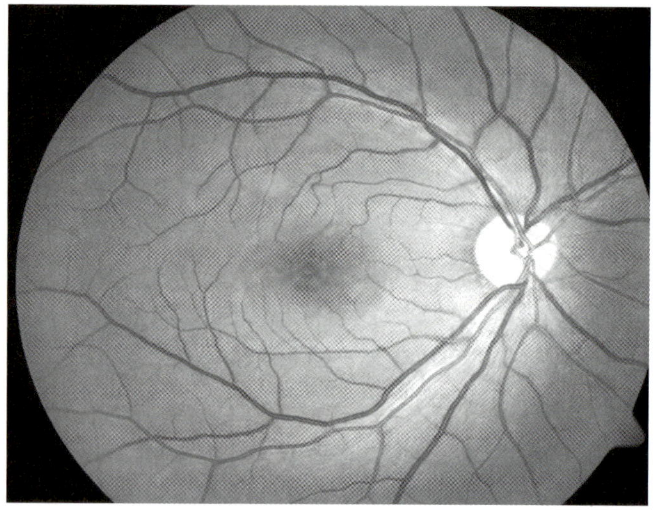

Red free photograph clearly demarcates the cystoid changes

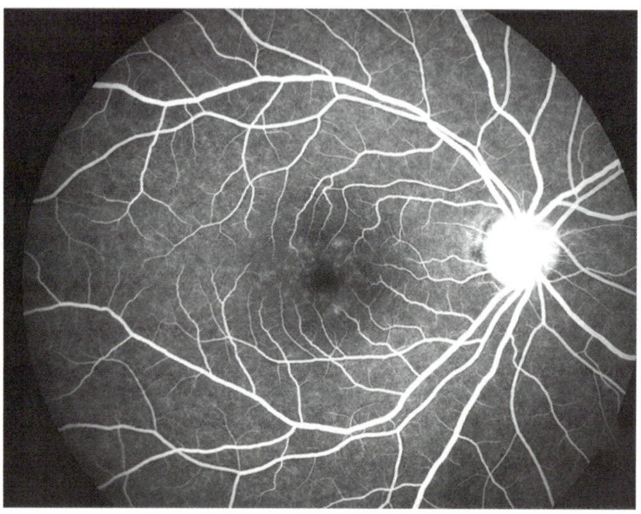

The arteriovenous phase shows dilation and early leakage of the dye from the perifoveal capillaries

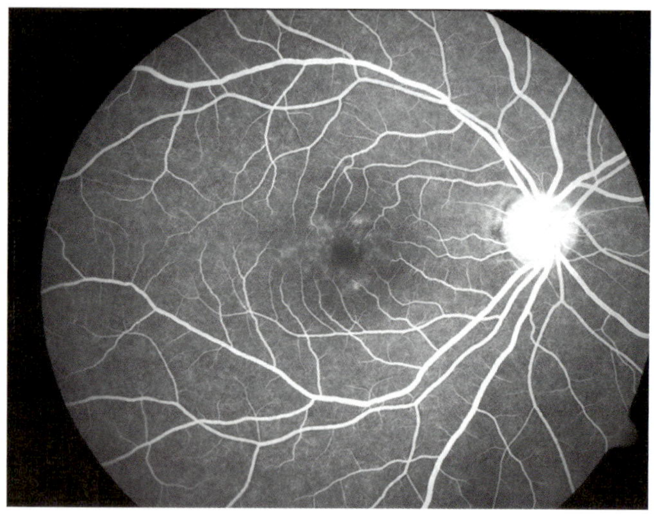

Increased leakage of the dye is noted in the perifoveal region

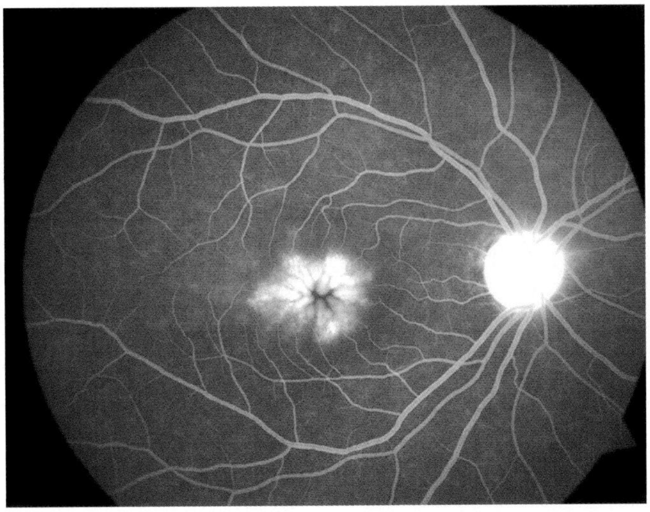

Late leakage and accumulation of the dye in cystoid spaces in seen. Increased staining of the disc is seen

CASE 2 (*Continued*)

Left Eye of the Patient

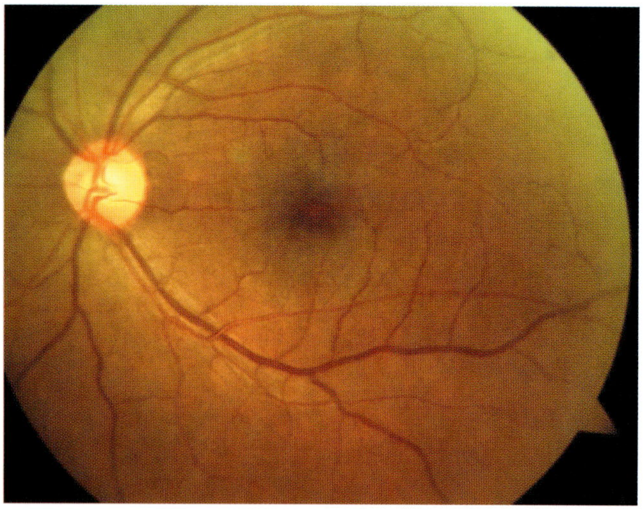

Fundus photograph of the left eye of the same patient showing cystoid changes at the fovea

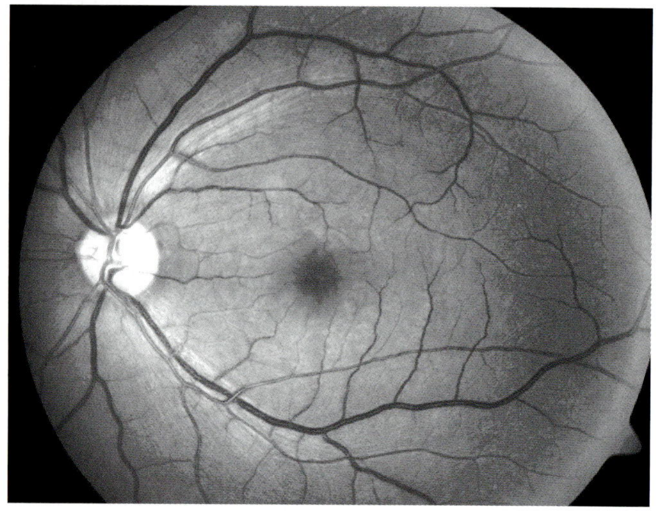

Red free photograph of the left eye

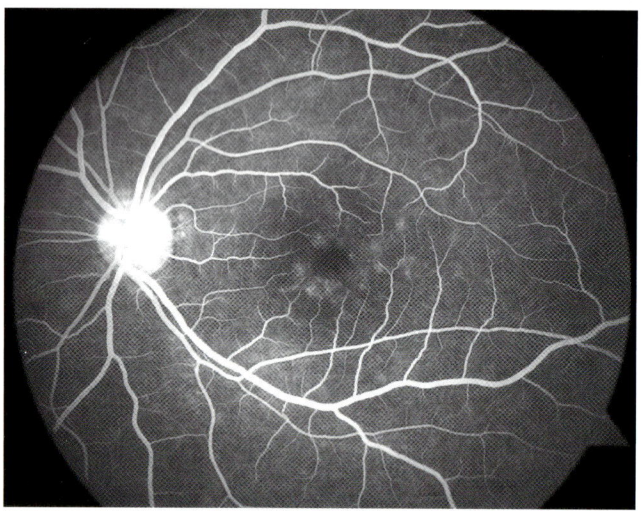

Dilation of the perifoveal capillaries is well seen. Minimal leakage of the dye from these dilated capillaries is seen

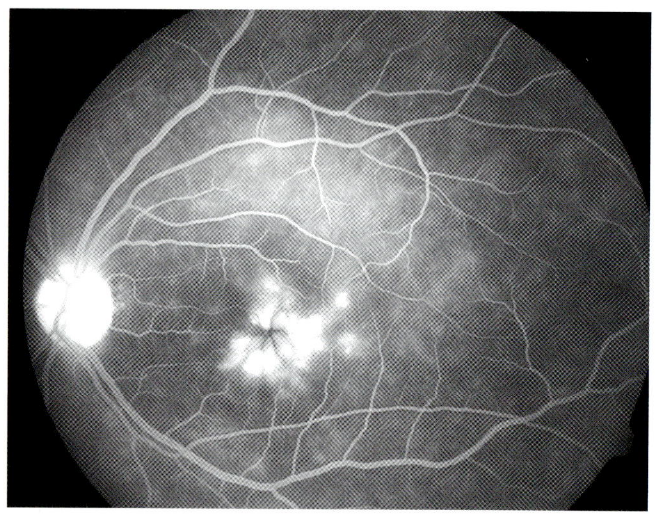

Petalloid pattern of cystoid macular edema is well seen. Noncystoid accumulation of the dye is noted in the superior macular region

COMMENT

Intraocular inflammation caused by intermediate uveitis results in the dilation of the perifoveal capillaries and leakage of fluid; this leads to cystoid macular edema.

CASE 3

A 56-year-old presented with diminution of vision in the left eye, one month following an uneventful phacoemulsification with intraocular lens implantation surgery. The visual acuity was 6/60; N18.

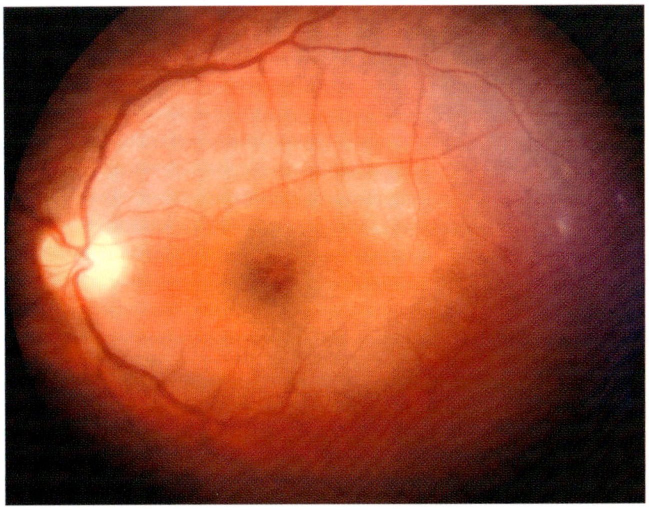

Fundus photograph of the left eye showing cystoid changes at the fovea

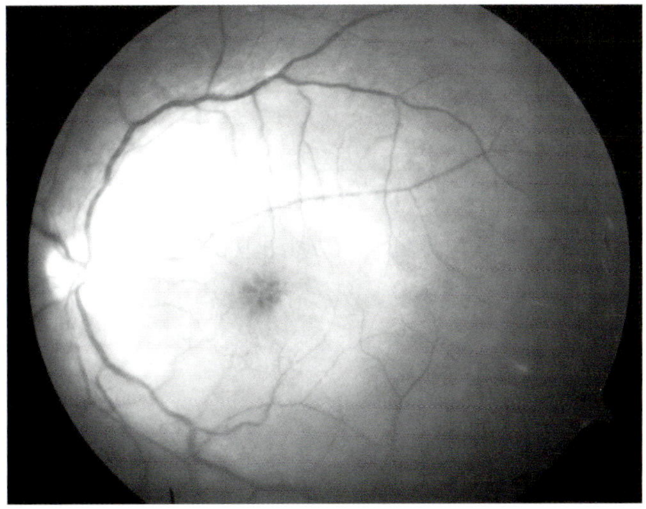

Red free photograph shows the large cystoid spaces at the fovea

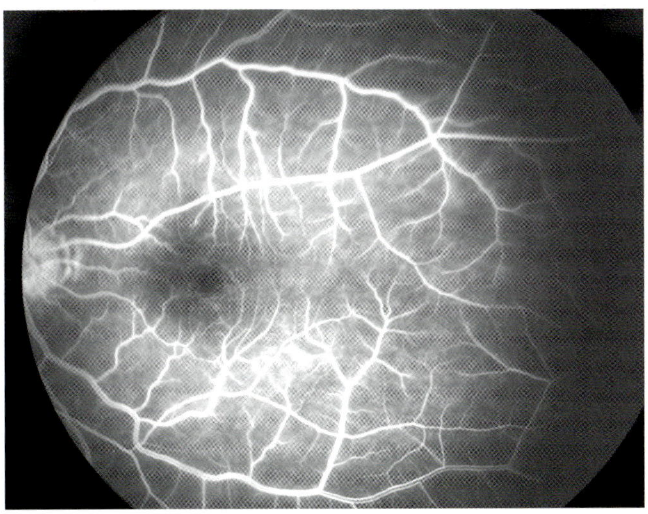

Arteriovenous phase showing the dilated perifoveal capillaries

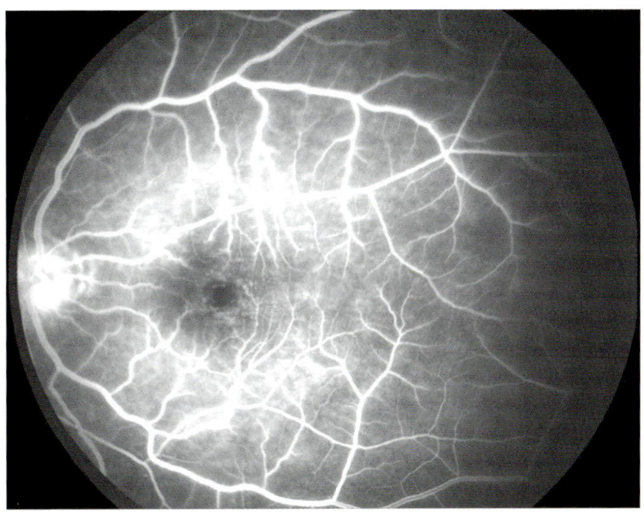

Early leakage from the dilated perifoveal capillaries is seen

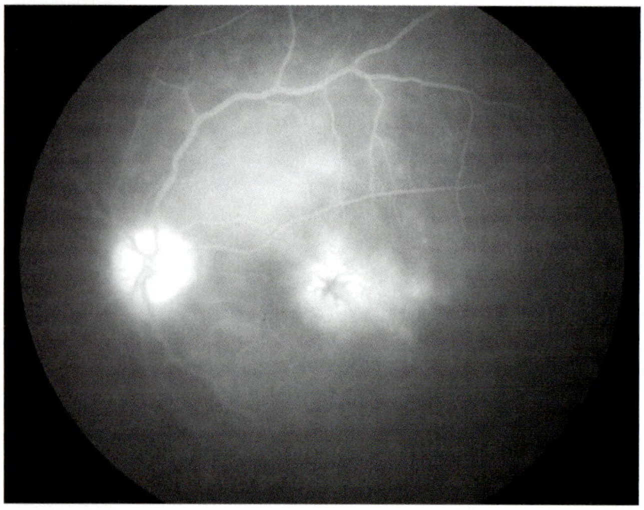

Late leakage of the dye and its collection in cystoid spaces is seen. The cystoid spaces are arranged in a petalloid pattern. Noncystoid accumulation of the dye is noted in the superior macular region. Increased staining of the disc is seen

COMMENT

Leakage of the dye from the perifoveal capillaries causes the cystoid pattern.

CLINICAL NUGGETS

1. The petalloid pattern of cystoid macular edema is best seen in the late phase of the angiogram.
2. Fluorescein angiography and OCT are useful investigative tools to document and follow-up eyes with cystoid macular edema.

BIBLIOGRAPHY

1. Allen AW, Jaffe NS. Cystoid macular edema: a preliminary study. Trans Ame Acad Ophthalmol and Otolaryngology 1976;81:133-4.
2. Bessho K, Gomi F, Harino S, Sawa M, Sayanagi K, Tsujikawa M, Tano Y. Macular autofluorescence in eyes with cystoid macular edema, detected with 488 nm excitation, but not with 580 nm excitation. Clin Exp Ophthalmol 2009;247:729.
3. Fine BS, Bruker AJ. Macular edema and cystoid macular edema. Am J Ophthalmol 1981;92:466-81.
4. Gass JDM, Anderson DR, Davis EB. A clinical fluorescein angiographic and electron microscopic correlation of cystoid macular edema. American Journal of Ophthalmol 1985;100:82-6.
5. Gass JDM, Mortan EWD. Cystoid macular edema and papilledema following cataract extraction, a fluorescein fundoscopic and angiographic study. Arch Ophthalmol 1966;76:646-66.
6. Ikewaki J, Nono H, Shinoda K, Kubota T, Nakatsuka K. Cystoid macular edema: Possible complication of Infliximab therapy in Behcet's disease. Case report ophthalmol. 2010;11:14-9.
7. Jaffe NS, Luscombe SM, Clayman HM, Gass JDM. A fluorescein angiographic study of cystoid macular edema. Am J Ophthalmol 1981;92:775-80.
8. Khetan V, Chaudhary SP, Gopal L. Cystoid macular edema after bone marrow transplantation. Indian J Ophthalmol 2009;57(1):55-7.
9. Peng XJ, Su LP. Characteristics on fundus autofluorescence of cystoid macular edema. Chin Med J (Engl). 2011;124:253-7.
10. Wright PL, Wilkinson CP, Balyeat HB, et al. Fluorescein angiographic study of cystoid macular edema after PCI-OL. Arch Ophthalmol 1988;106:740-44.

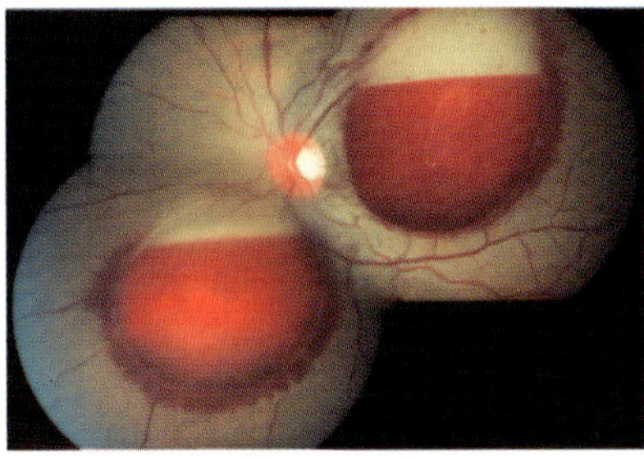

Section 3
Vascular Disorders

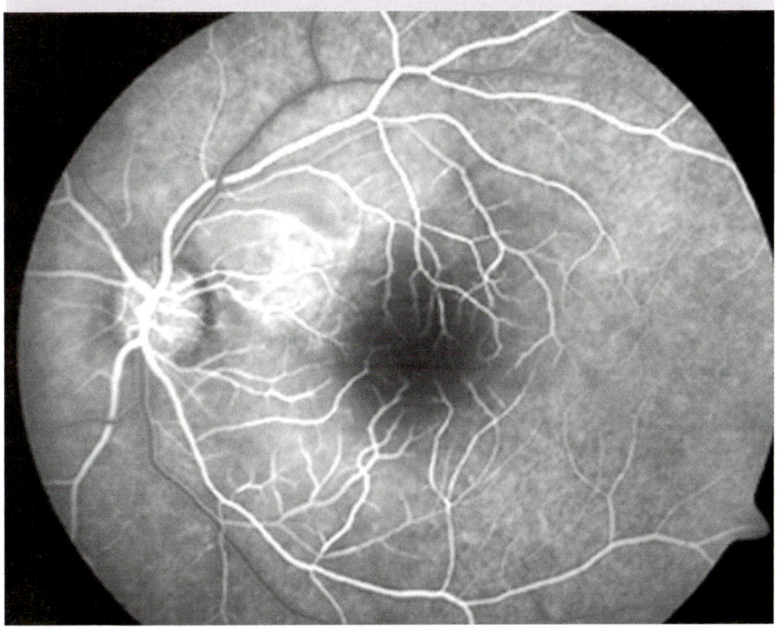

26

Chapter

Arterial Occlusion

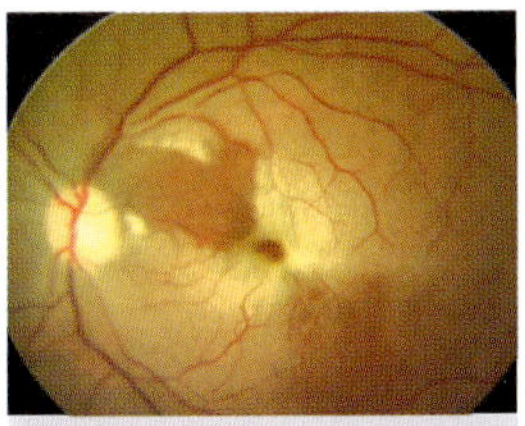

- Acute central retinal artery occlusion causes a sudden painless visual loss occurring over several seconds.
- The fundus is characterized by opacification of retina especially at the posterior pole; the opacification may take hours to become apparent.
- A cherry red spot is present in most of the cases.
- The retinal arterioles are thinned and may show 'boxcarring' of the blood column.
- Approximately 25 percent of eyes with central retinal artery occlusion have a patent cilioretinal artery, in which case the retinal area supplied by this is spared.
- Sometimes, the occlusion may involve only the branch arteriole, in which case the changes are restricted to the affected segment.
- Isolated occlusion of the cilioretinal artery can also occur by itself or in association with a central retinal vein occlusion.

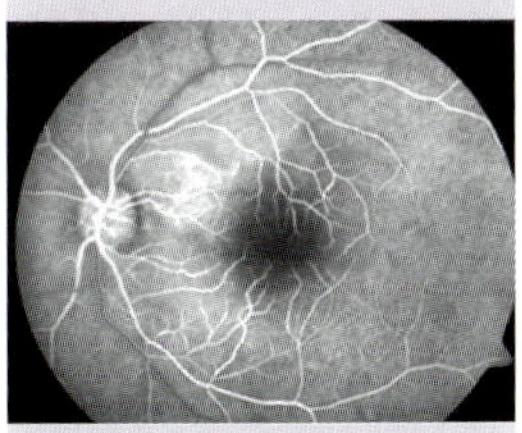

- In the acute stage there may be considerable amount of masking of choroidal fluorescence due to the cloudy swelling of the overlying retina.
- The arterial phase is extremely delayed; it is often possible to see the slow progress of the dye front in the arteriole. There is marked delay in the arteriovenous transit time. The column of blood is seen to be broken into segments and hardly any dye reaches the capillaries. Venous return is also delayed and incomplete.
- By about the 2nd week following the occlusion, dye begins to flow into the vessels but shows a high degree of irregularity of caliber. Venous return improves, however the capillary details do not recover. Optic disc shows staining during the late phase of the angiogram.

CASE 1

A 42-year-old male presented with sudden loss of vision in the right eye of one week duration. Visual acuity was perception of light with inaccurate projection of rays in the right eye. Left eye was normal.

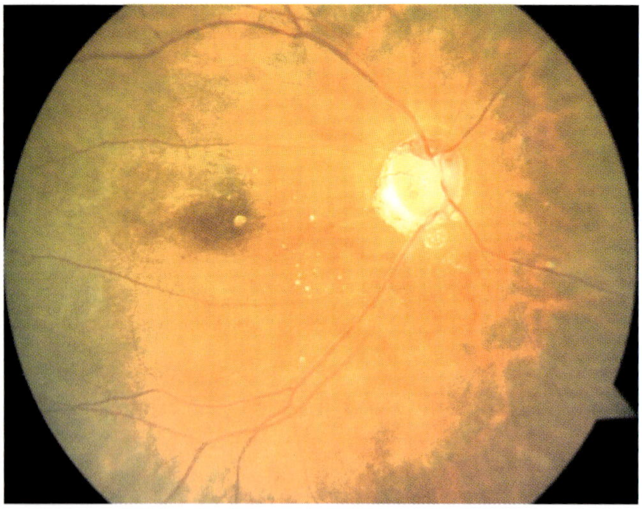

Fundus photograph of the right eye showing a pale optic disc with markedly narrowed arterioles. Few white deposits are seen in the inferior macular region

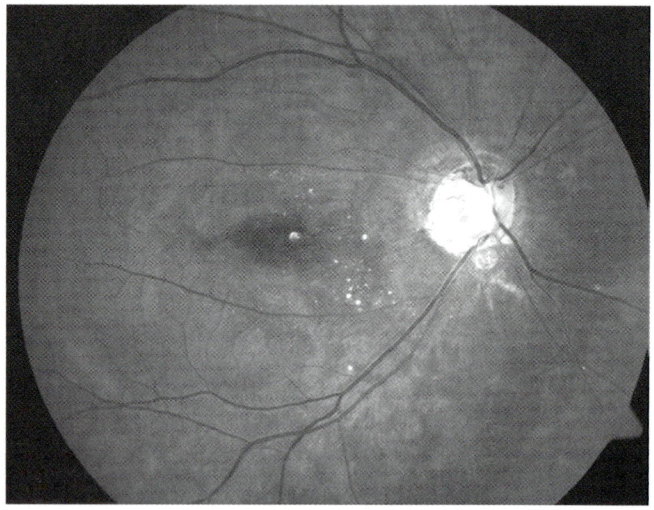

Red free photograph of the right eye shows an optic pit in the inferotemporal part of the disc

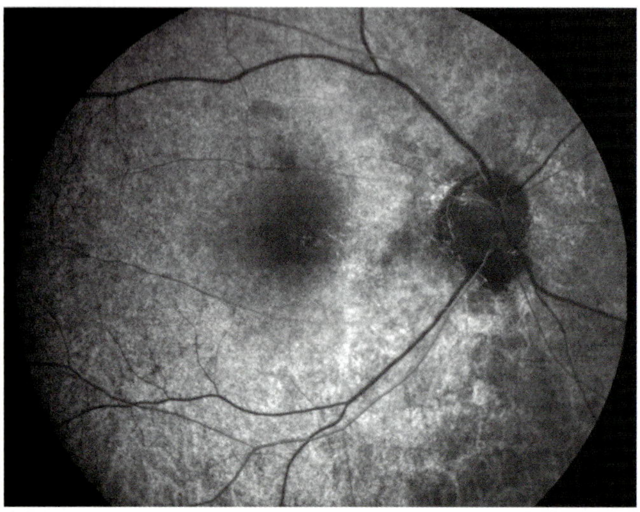

Delayed filling of the arteries is evident from the fact that the arteries show only minimal hyperfluorescence whereas the choroidal filling is more or less complete

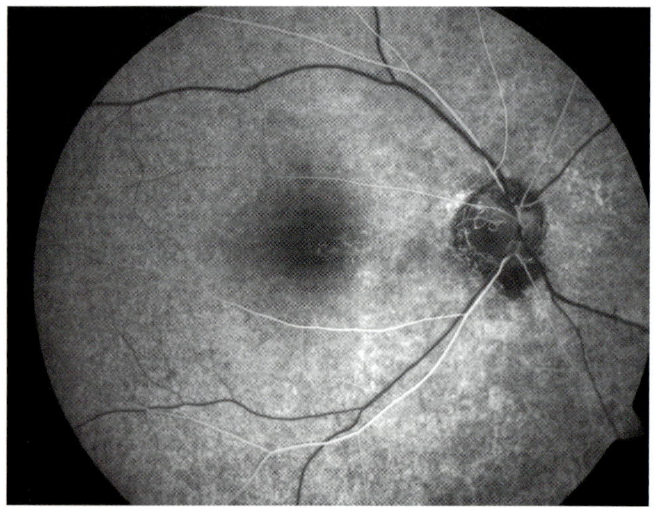

The concentration of the dye in the arteries has increased. Hypofluorescence due to optic pit is seen in the inferotemporal part of the optic nerve head

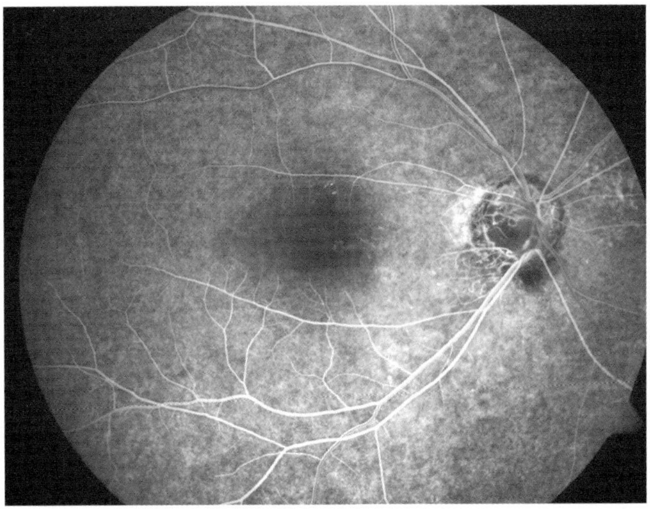

Markedly delayed filling of the veins is seen. All the vessels appear narrowed. The optic pit is still hypofluorescent

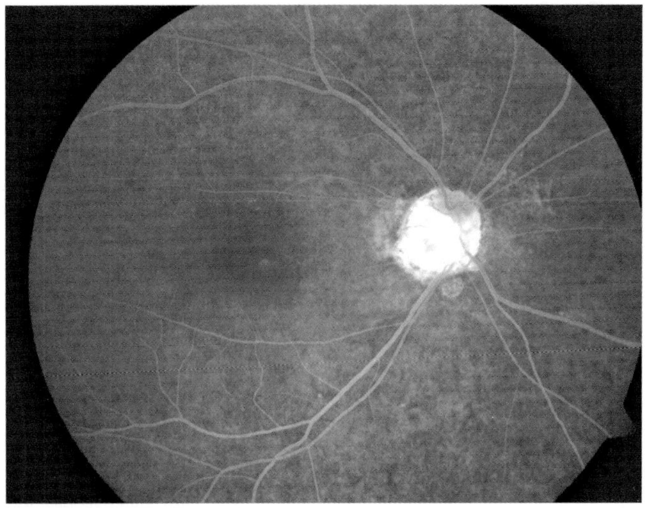

Late phase shows the washout of the dye. Hyperfluorescence of the optic pit is seen

CASE 2

A 29-year-old female with systemic lupus erythematosus presented with sudden loss of vision in the right eye of one day duration. Visual acuity was perception of light.

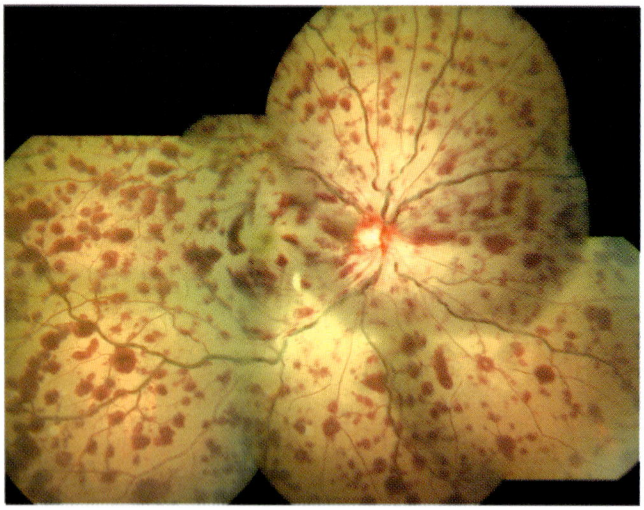

Fundus photograph showing multiple scattered retinal hemorrhages and retinal whitening at the posterior pole. Note the dilated retinal veins

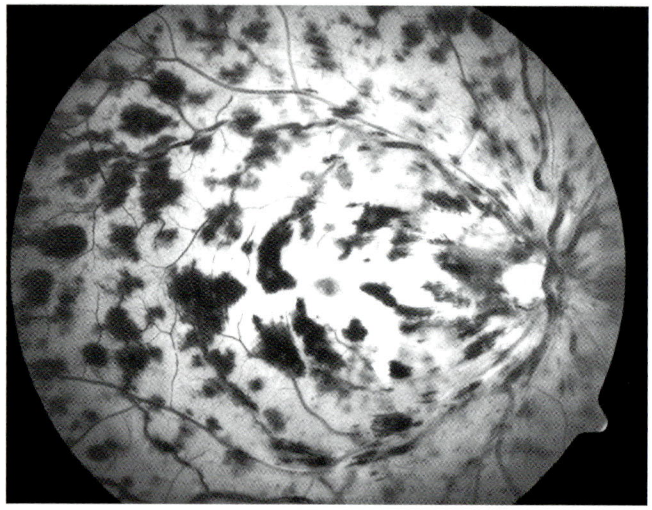

Red free photograph shows retinal hemorrhages

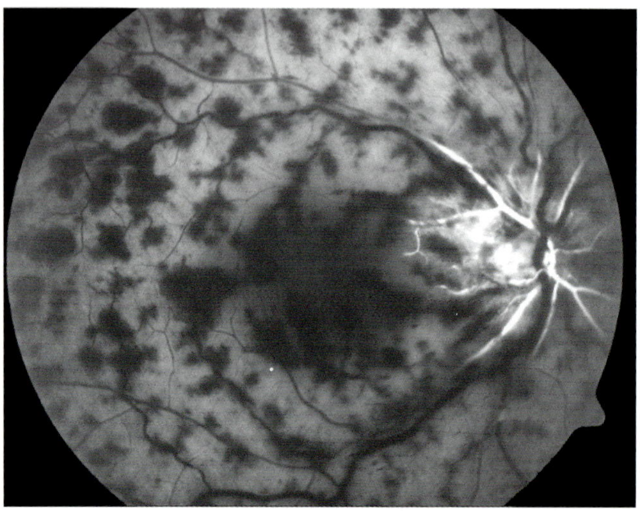

Filling of the arteries is markedly delayed with dye appearing in the arteries only after 40 seconds. The leading edge of the dye column is seen within the arteries

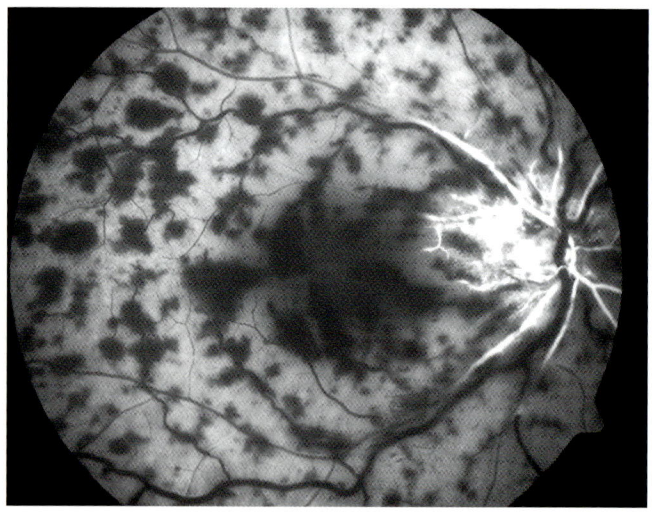

The dye has not progressed much in the arteries even at 2 minutes

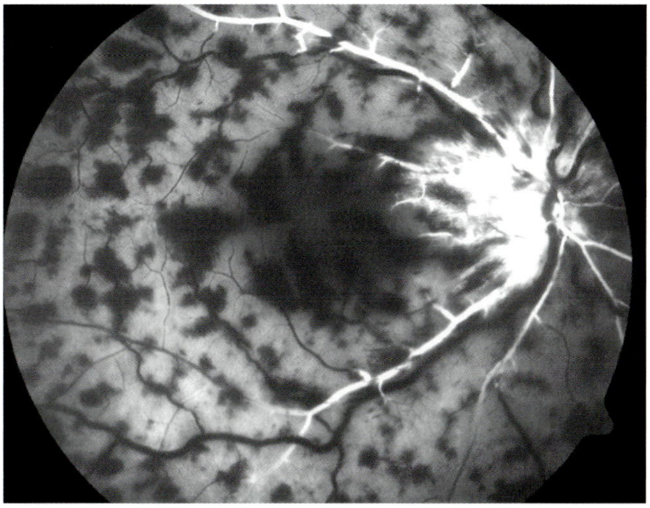

Further filling of the arteries is seen at 5 minutes. However, the dye has not yet entered the veins

COMMENT

This type of fundus appearance is suggestive of a combined central retinal artery and a central retinal vein occlusion.

CASE 3

A 51-year-old patient with history of hypertension for the past fifteen years presented with loss of vision in the right eye of one month duration; visual acuity was perception of light.

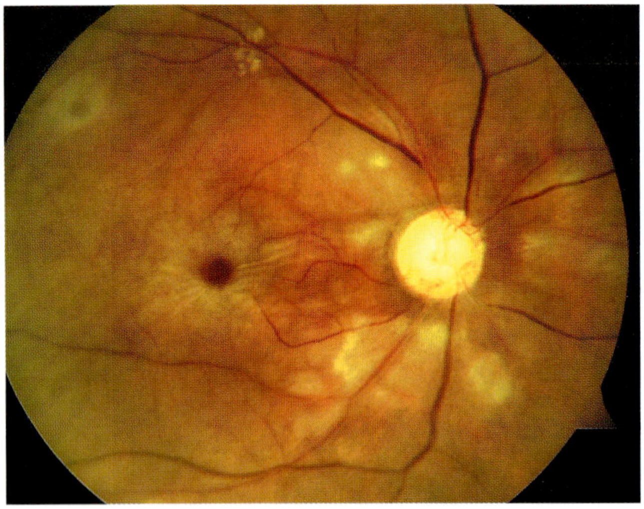

Fundus photograph of the right eye showing areas of retinal whitening at the posterior pole; cherry red spot is seen. An area of subretinal whitening with associated subretinal fluid is seen superotemporally

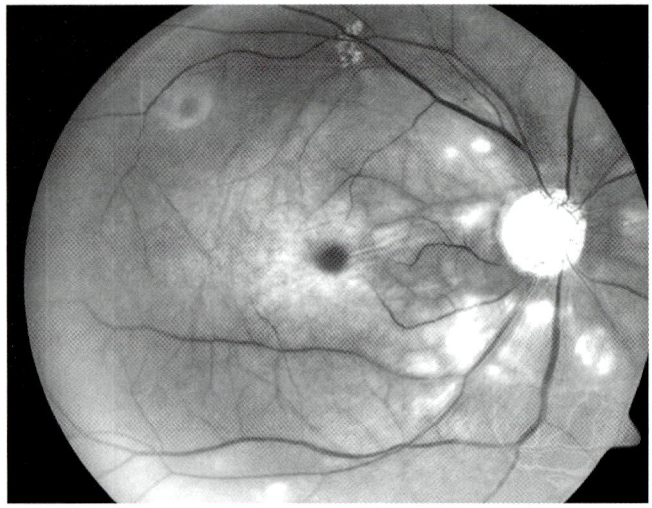

Red free photograph highlights the features seen in the color photograph

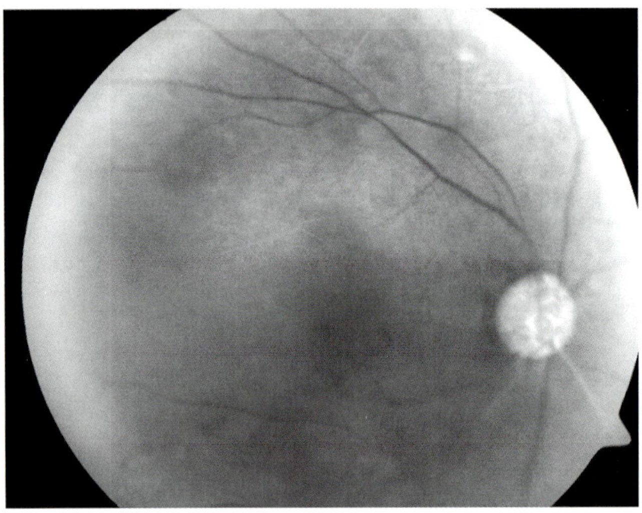

Early disc hyperfluorescence is seen. However, the dye has not entered the arteries even at 28 seconds

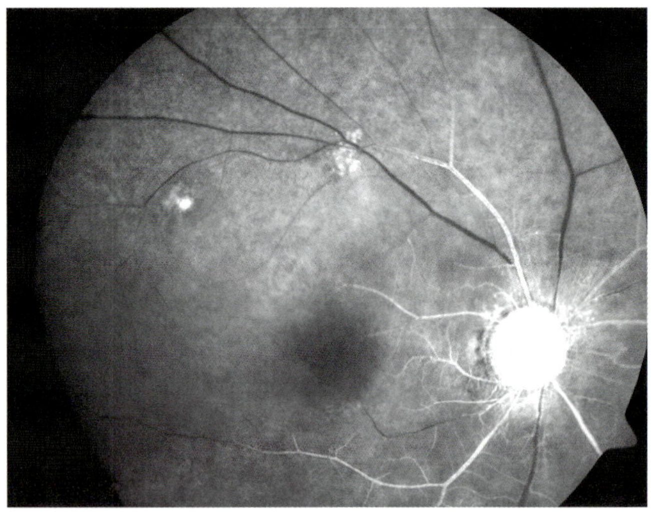

Delayed entry of the dye is noted in the arteries. The disc capillaries have filled. A point leak is noted superotemporally

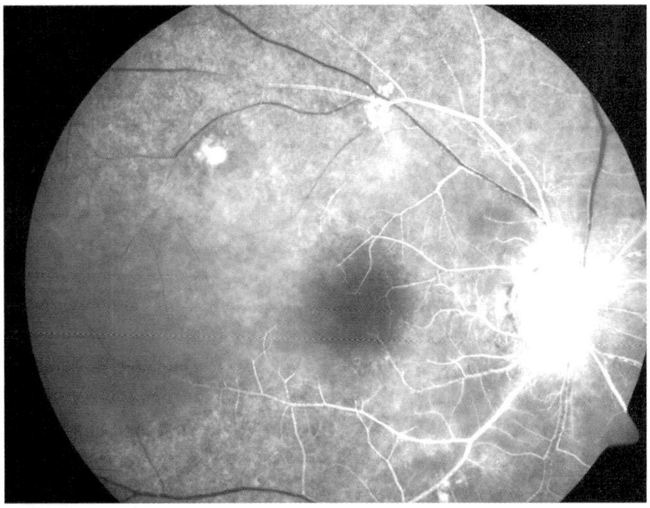

The dye has progressed in the arteries and some venous return is noted in the veins close to the disc. The point leak superotemporally has increased in intensity and extent

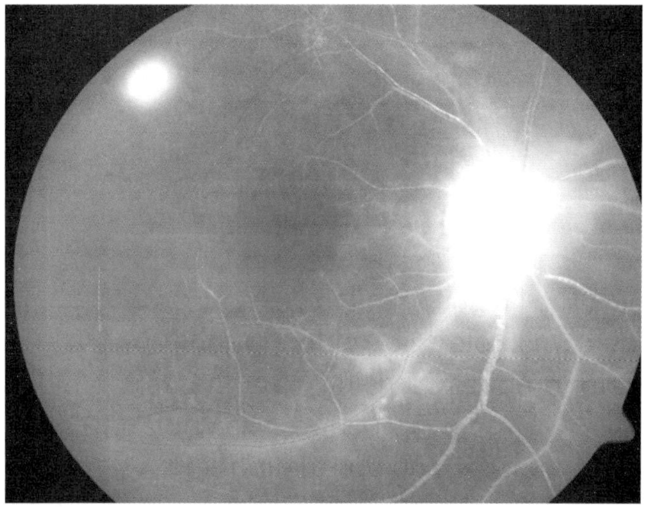

Increased staining of the disc and the arteries is seen in the late film. A smoke stack like leak is seen superotemporally

CASE 4

A 52-year-old male presented with sudden loss of vision in the left eye of 2 days duration. He was a diabetic for the past fifteen years and had undergone pars plana vitrectomy in the left eye eight months back with a postoperative visual acuity of 6/24; N36. His visual acuity was recorded as perception of light in the left eye.

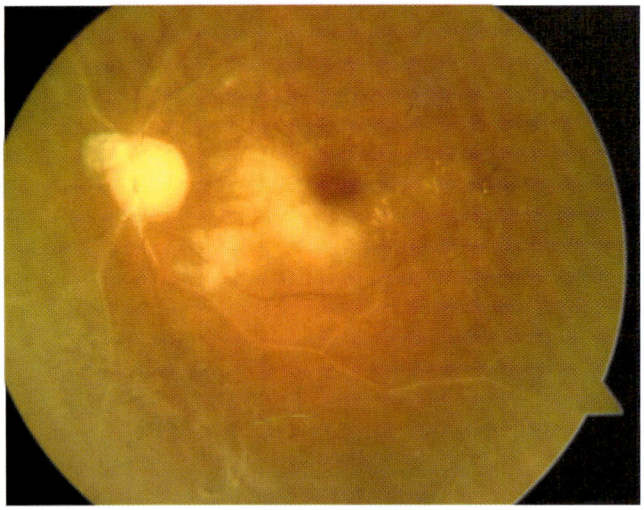

Fundus photograph of the left eye showing retinal whitening and cherry red spot in the macula

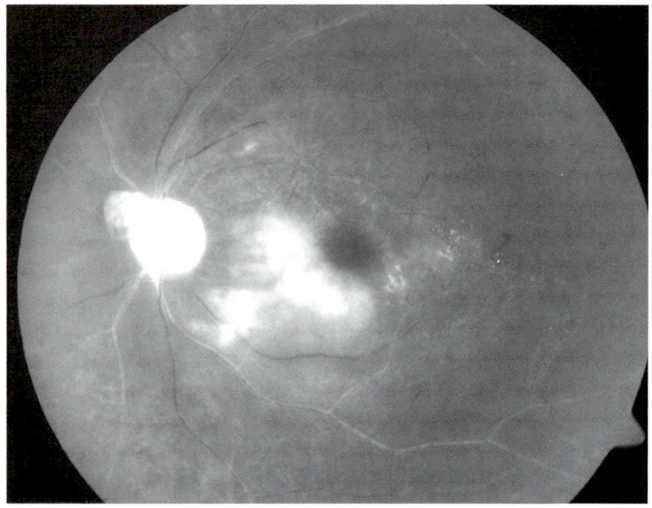

The red free photograph shows very clearly the areas of retinal whitening

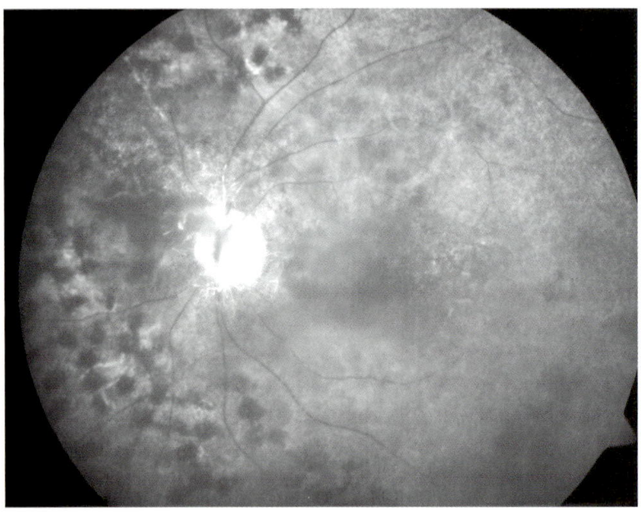

At 25 seconds, filling of few disc capillaris is seen. However, the dye has not yet entered the arteries

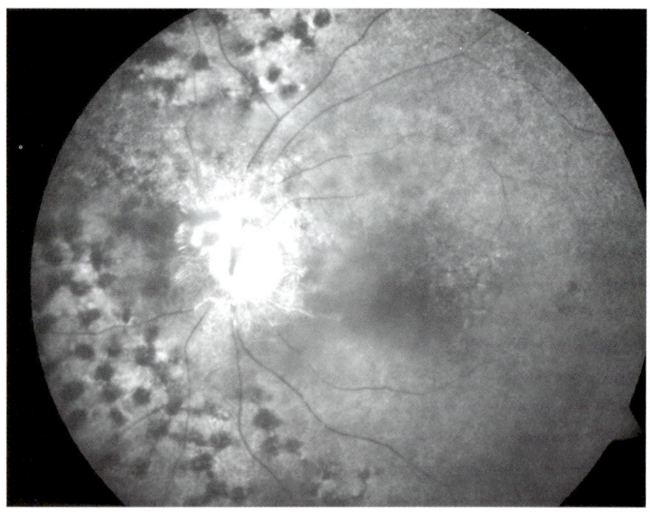

At 45 seconds, dye is seen entering the arteries near the disc. The leading edge of the dye column within the arterioles is seen

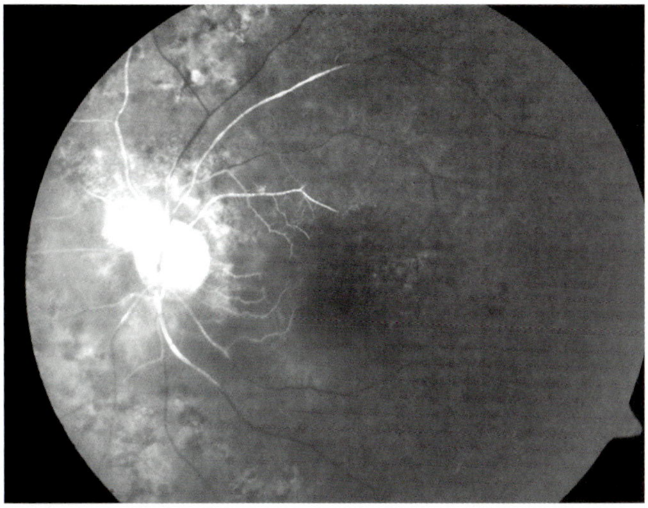

At 5 minutes the dye has progressed to some extent in the arterioles, however it has not yet completely filled. Some filling of the veins close to the disc is seen

COMMENT

There is marked delay in the filling of the arterioles and filling is incomplete even in the late phase. The leading edge of the dye column in the arterioles is clearly seen.

CASE 5

A 25-year-old male presented with sudden decrease in vision of the left eye of fifteen days duration. Visual acuity was 6/36; N18 in the left eye.

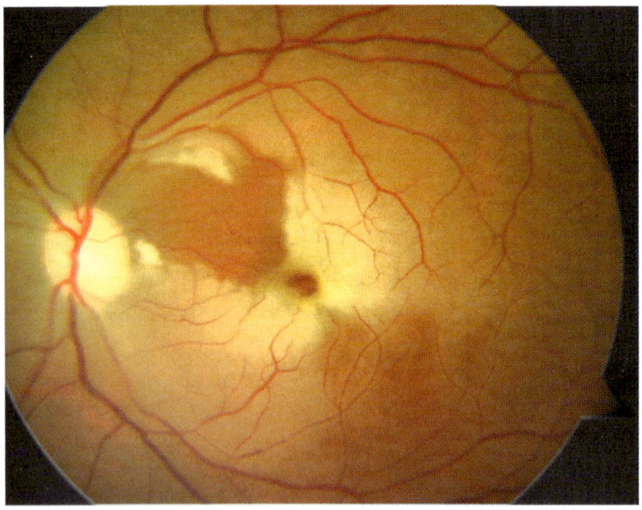

Fundus photograph of the left eye showing areas of retinal whitening. A small island of retina adjacent to the disc is spared due to the presence of a cilioretinal artery

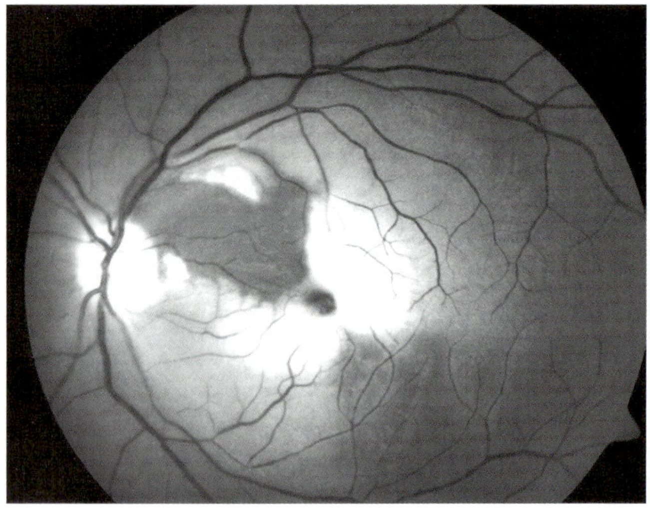

Red free photograph shows the cilioretinal artery in the superotemporal part of the disc

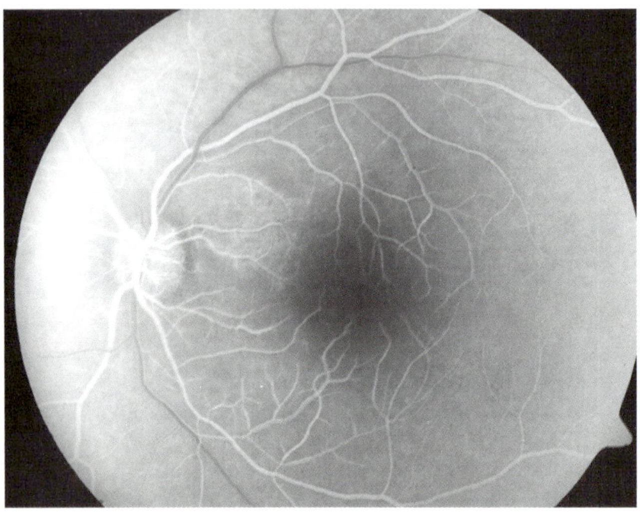

Arterial filling is delayed and low concentration of the dye is seen initially in the arteries due to its sluggish filling

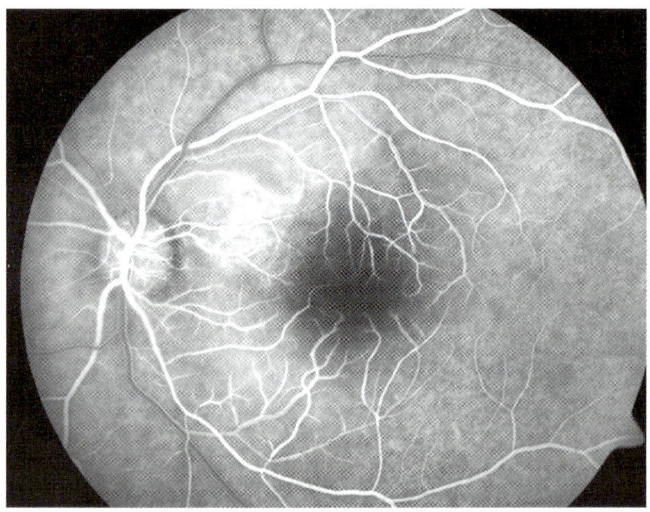

Early arteriovenous phase showing the laminar flow in the veins. Capillary filling is not well seen except superotemporal to the disc in the region of the cilioretinal artery

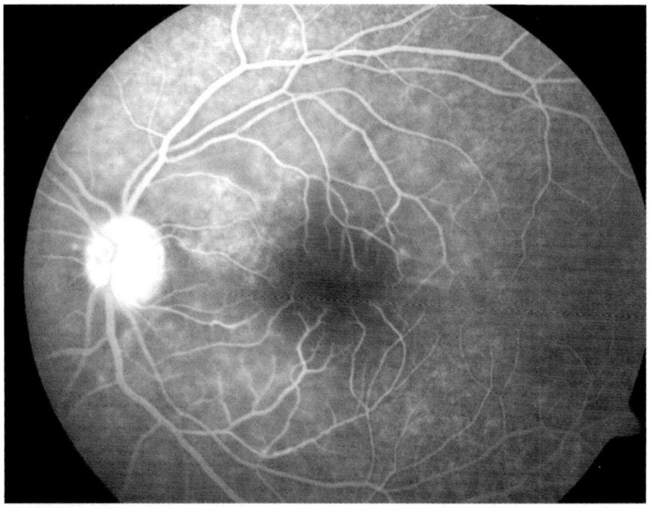

Arteriovenous phase showing capillary filling only in the region of the cilioretinal artery

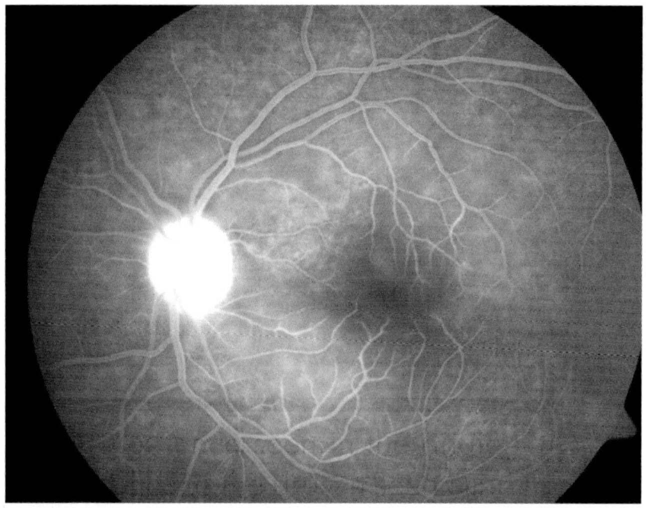

Late phase showing increased staining of the disc

CASE 6

A 49-year-old male presented with history of a scotoma in front of the left eye for the past four days. He gave history of having undergone some dental procedure one month back. Visual acuity in the left eye was 6/9; N6.

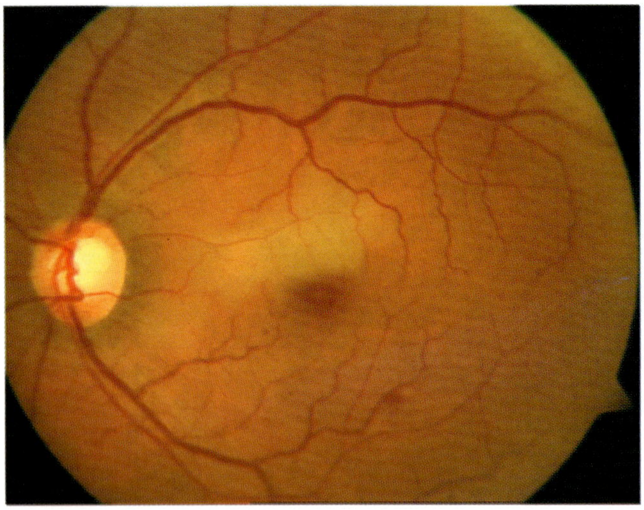

Fundus photograph of the left eye showing a band of retinal whitening extending temporally from the disc. A cilioretinal arteriole is seen coming out from the superotemporal part of the disc

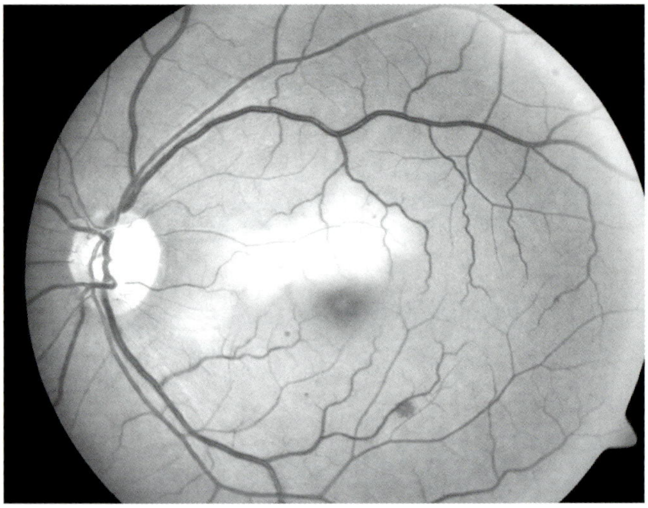

Red free photograph shows the area of retinal whitening and the cilioretinal vessel. Few specks of retinal hemorrhage are seen in the inferior macular region

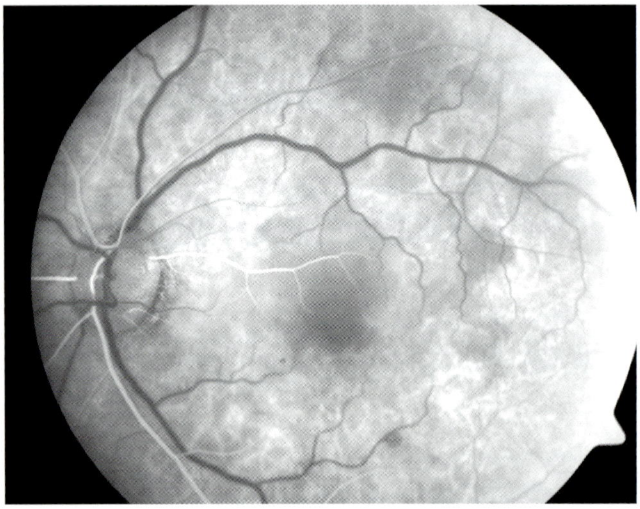

Arterial phase of the angiogram shows the normal filling of the cilioretinal artery

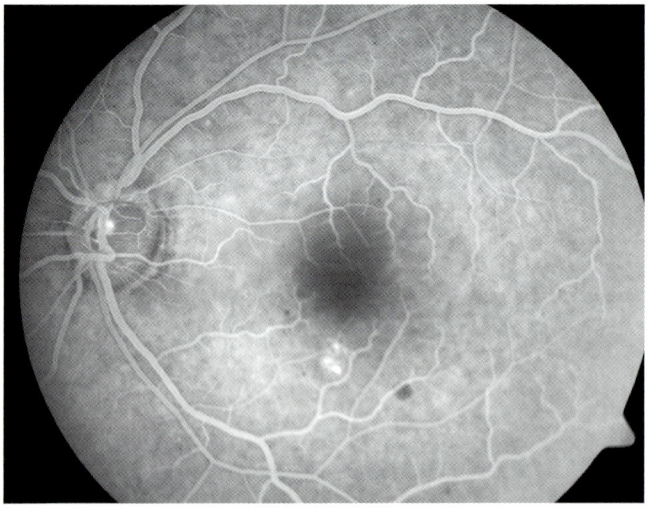

Late arteriovenous phase showing some blurring of the capillary details in the region of the retinal whitening

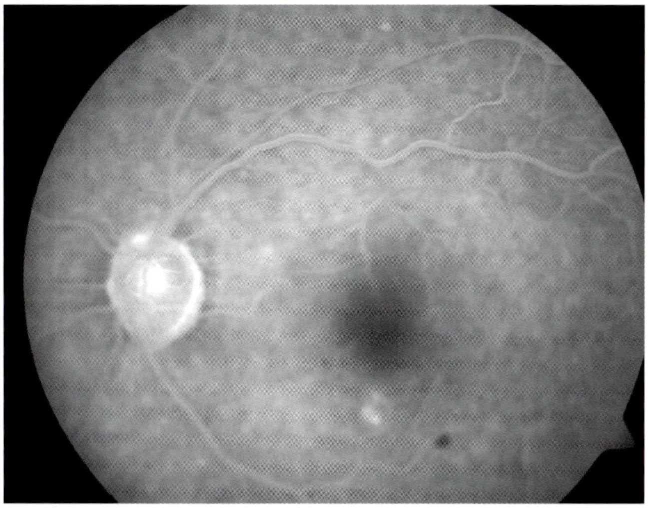

Late phase angiogram shows minimal fuzziness in the area of retinal whitening

COMMENT

This patient has a cilioretinal artery occlusion with reopening of the cilioretinal artery. However, despite reopening, permanent closure of the capillary bed in the region of the affected cilioretinal artery is seen.

CASE 7

A 38-year-old female presented with sudden onset reduced vision in the right eye of three weeks duration. Visual acuity was 6/9; N6.

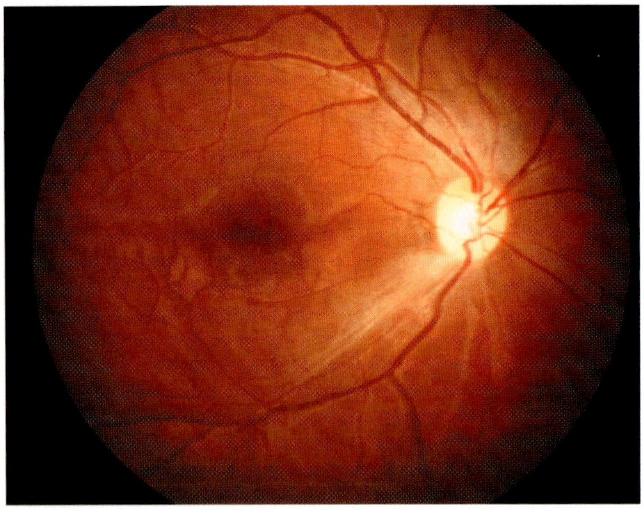

Fundus photograph of the right eye showing retinal whitening in the inferior part of the fovea

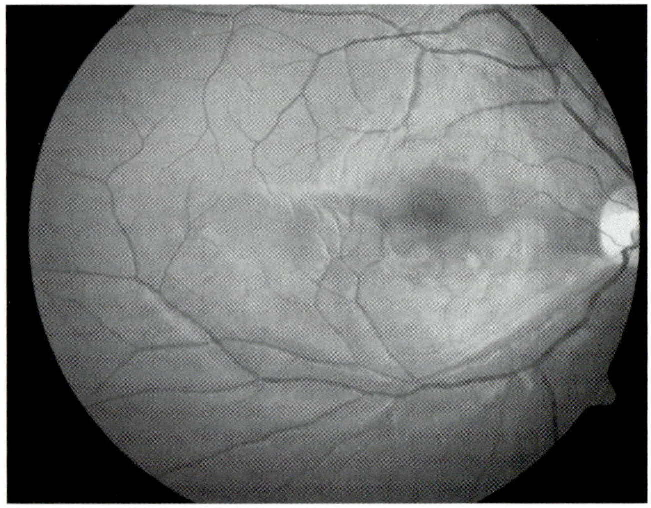

Red free photograph showing the retinal whitening inferior to the fovea

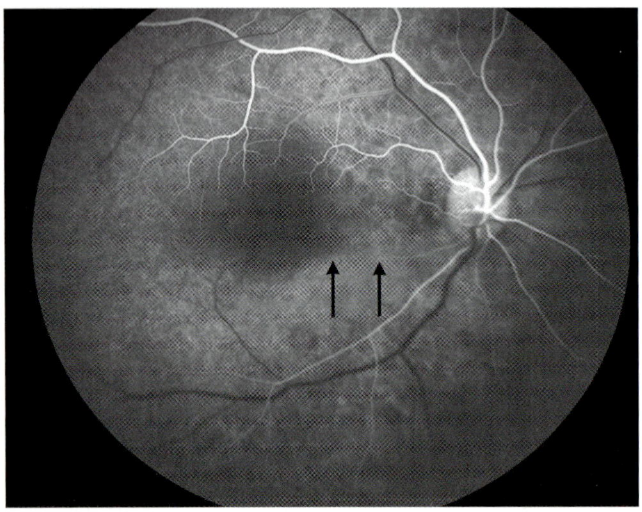

Arterial phase showing delayed filling of the arteriole exiting from the inferotemporal part of the disc (arrows). The arterioles superior to the fovea have filled up

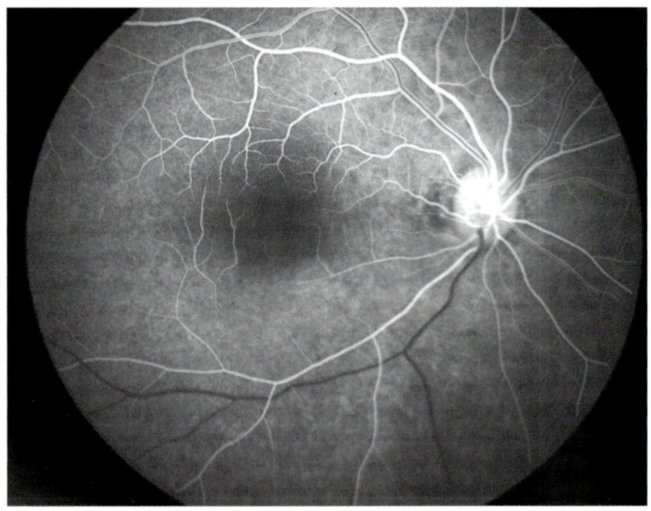

Early arteriovenous phase showing normal filling of the arteriole in the upper part of the macula. In contrast those in the lower half have not filled

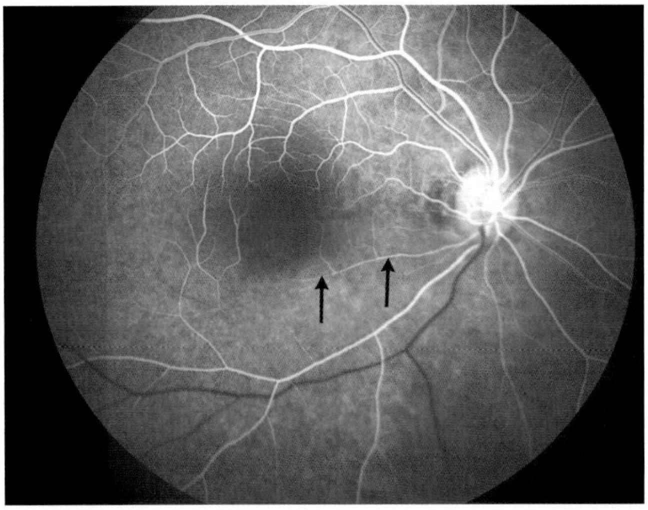

Midarteriovenous phase showing absence of capillary details in the lower part of the macula. There is some progression of the dye column in the inferotemporal macular arteriole (arrows)

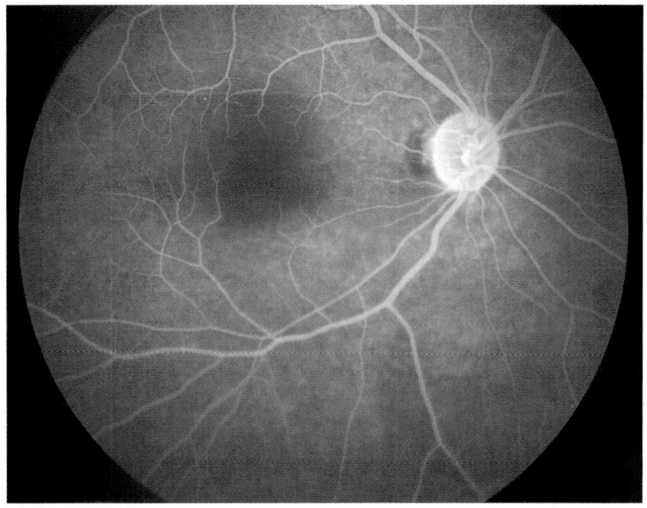

Arterioles in the lower part of the macula have not filled up completely even in the late phase of the angiogram

CASE 8

A 36-year-old gentleman reported with sudden visual loss in left eye. BCVA was 6/6 in right eye and no perception of light in left. Anterior segment examination was normal.

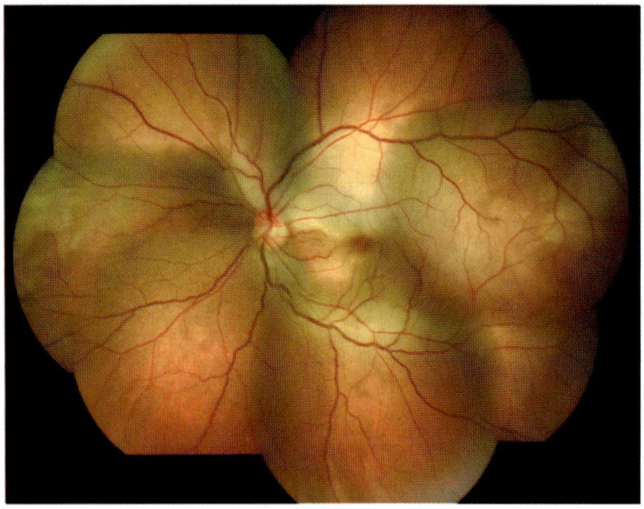

Color fundus montage of the left eye reveals marked retinal edema in the superior hemispheric distribution with an accentuated foveal reflex

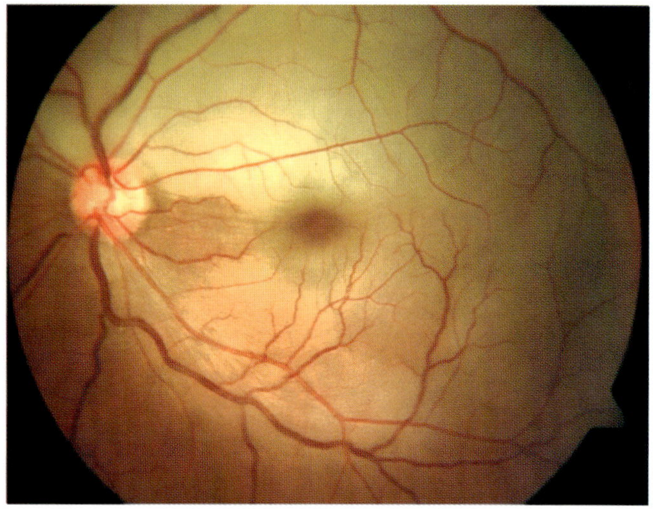

Color fundus photograph of the left eye reveals two separate central retinal artery hemi-trunks emerging from the optic disc. Marked retinal edema in the superior hemispheric distribution is made out. Generalized arteriolar attenuation, box-carring of vessels and cherry red spot at fovea were seen

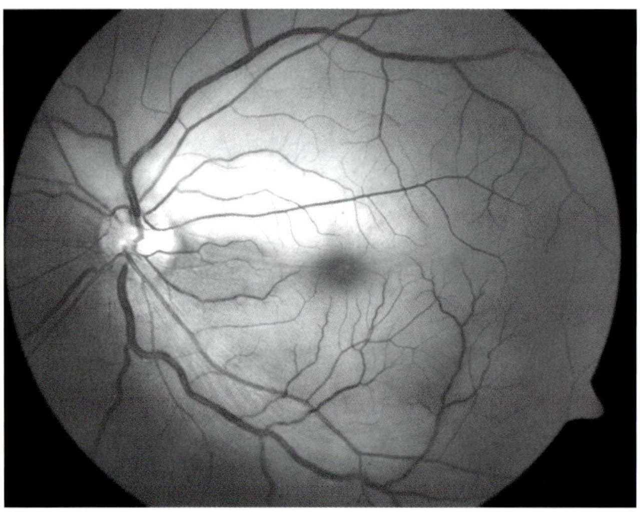

Red free photograph of the left eye highlights the retinal edema in the superior quadrant

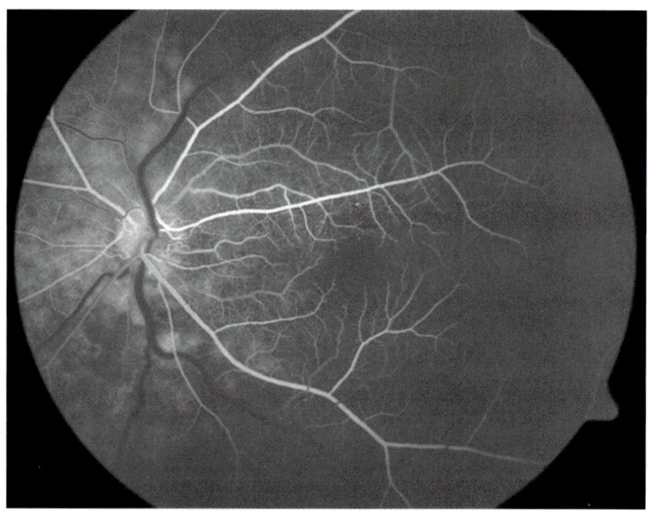

Early A-V phase angiogram reveals recanalization of the superior central retinal artery hemi-trunk

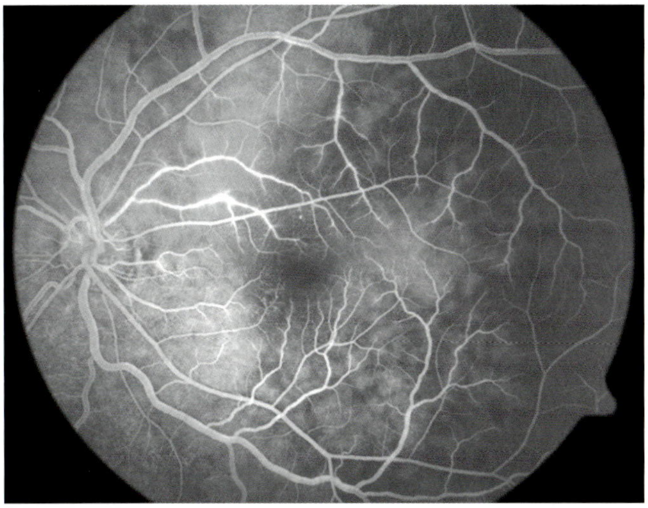

Late A-V phase reveals staining of the superior central retinal artery hemi-trunk

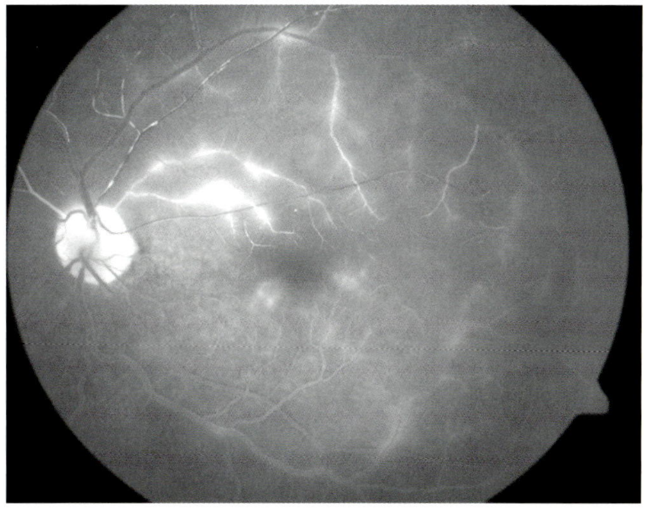

Late phase angiogram reveals staining of the disc and the superior central retinal artery hemi-trunk

COMMENT

This patient was investigated and found to have polycythemia vera and malignant hypertension. The patient was referred to the physician and was treated with antihypertensive agents and serial phlebotomies.

CLINICAL NUGGETS

1. A cilioretinal artery is normally present in 20 percent of the eyes.
2. Neovascularization of iris can develop in 80 percent of eyes with combined central retinal artery and vein occlusion.
3. Posterior ophthalmic artery occlusion is usually not associated with a cherry red spot.
4. Electroretinogram shows a reduction in the b-wave (negative waveform) in eyes with central retinal artery occlusion.

BIBLIOGRAPHY

1. Brown GC, Magargal LE. Central retinal artery obstruction and visual acuity. Ophthalmology 1982;89:14-9.
2. David NJ, Gass JDM, Beauchamp J. Fluorescein angiography in central retinal artery occlusion. Arch Ophthalmol 1967;77:619-29.
3. Eagling EM, Sanders MD, Miller SJH. Ischemic papillopathy: clinical and fluorescein angiographic review of forty cases. Br J Ophthalmol 1974;58:990-1008.
4. Rishi P, Rishi E, Sharma T, Mahajan S. Hemi-central retinal artery occlusion in young adults. Indian J Ophthalmol 2010; 58(5): 425-32.

27 Chapter

Coats' Disease

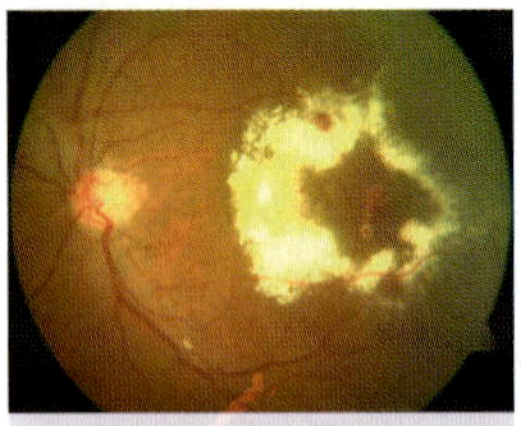

- Coats' disease is an idiopathic condition occurring predominantly in males with no racial predilection.
- It is unilateral in 80 percent of the cases.
- The common changes seen in the fundus include vascular abnormalities such as retinal telangiectasia and aneurysmal dilations, and zones of capillary nonperfusion.
- The extent of vascular abnormalities can range from minimal to very extensive.
- It is associated with intraretinal and subretinal lipid deposits.
- Leber's miliary aneurysm is considered to be a localized form of Coats' disease.

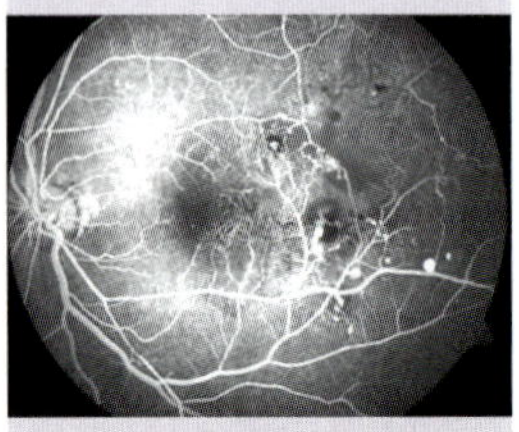

- Fluorescein angiogram shows numerous localized anomalies of the retinal vasculature.
- Telangiectasia, aneurysms, beading of vessel walls and vascular communicating channels are seen.
- These are very well-made out in the early and midarteriovenous phases of the angiogram.
- The retinal capillary bed shows marked dilation and tortuosity with multiple saccular and aneurysmal outpouchings simulating a 'light bulb appearance'.
- Leakage from the vascular abnormalities is seen in the late films.
- Areas of diffuse capillary nonperfusion may be seen in the midperiphery.

CASE 1

A 27-year-old male presented with history of decreased vision in the left eye of ten days duration. Visual acuity was 6/9; N6. He was found to have extensive exudation at the posterior pole with vascular abnormalities seen in the periphery. The right eye was normal.

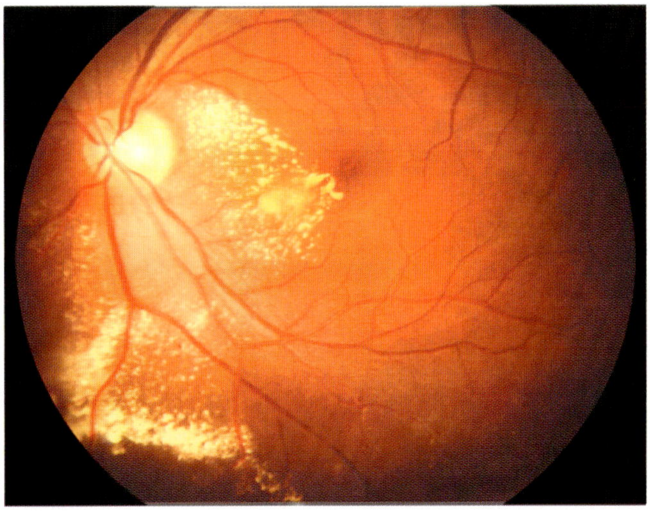

Fundus photograph showing hard exudates at the macula and inferiorly

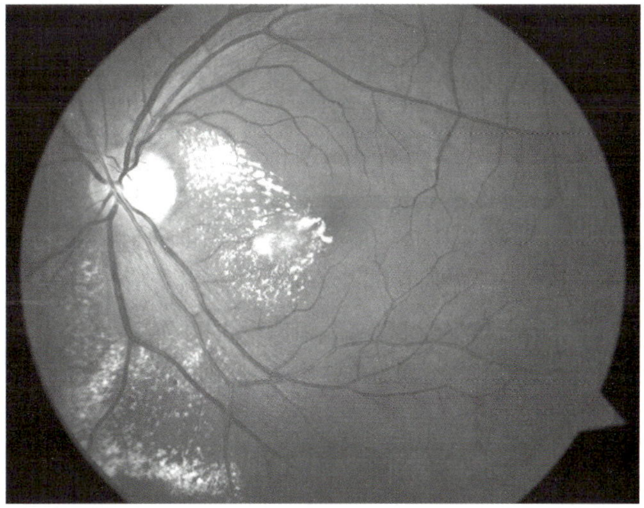

Red free photograph highlights these features

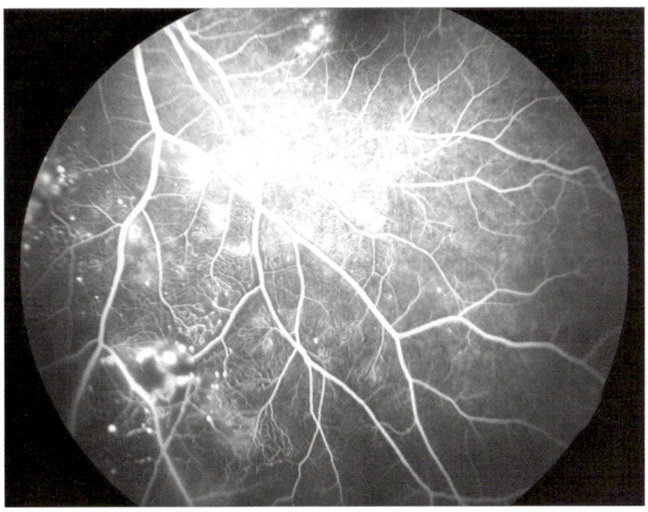

Dilated retinal capillaries and telangiectasias are clearly made out in the arteriovenous phase. Vascular abnormalities are also noted close to the fovea. Aneurysmal dilatations are seen inferiorly

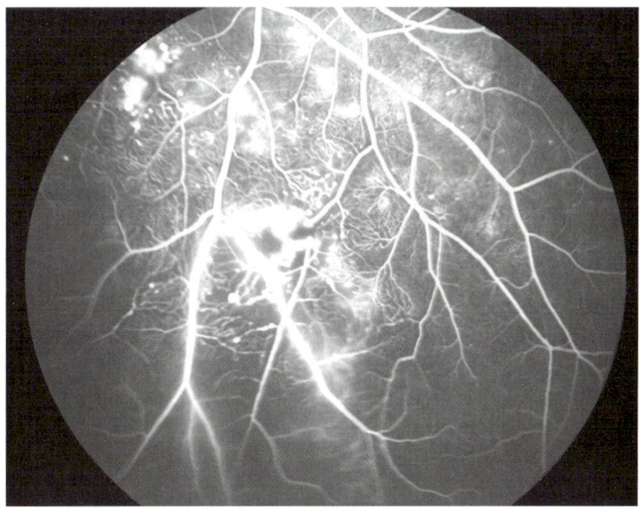

Leakage of dye is noted from the dilated capillaries and the aneurysmal dilatations. Areas of capillary non-perfusion are also seen

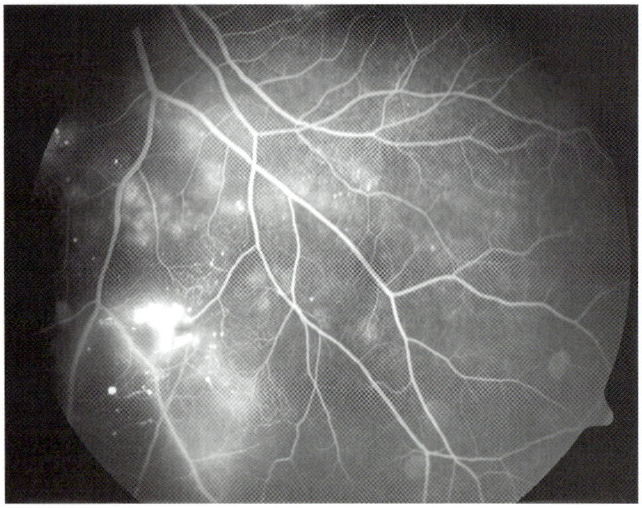

Late phase shows leakage of the dye from the vascular abnormalities

COMMENT

Retinal capillary telangiectasias, capillary dilatations, aneurysmal dilatations and areas of capillary nonperfusion are hallmarks of Coats' disease.

CASE 2

A 43-year-old male was referred with a diagnosis of CRVO in the left eye. The visual acuity in the left eye was 6/60; N36. Right eye was normal. Examination revealed changes suggestive of Coats' disease.

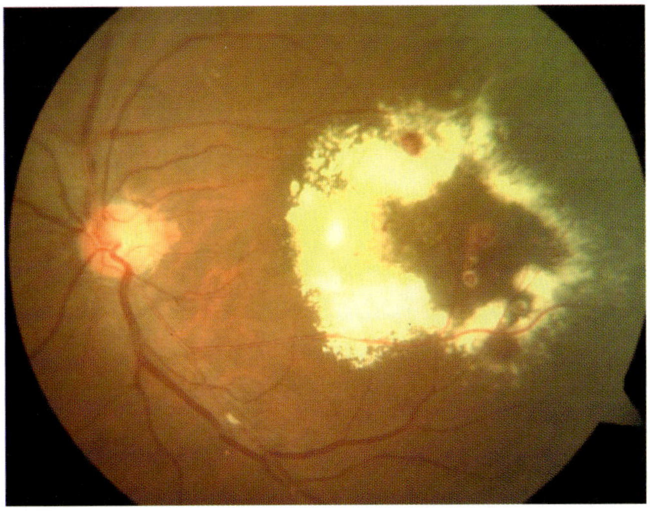

Fundus photograph showing severe exudation arranged in a circinate. Large aneurysmal dilation of the retinal vessels are noted in the center of the circinate

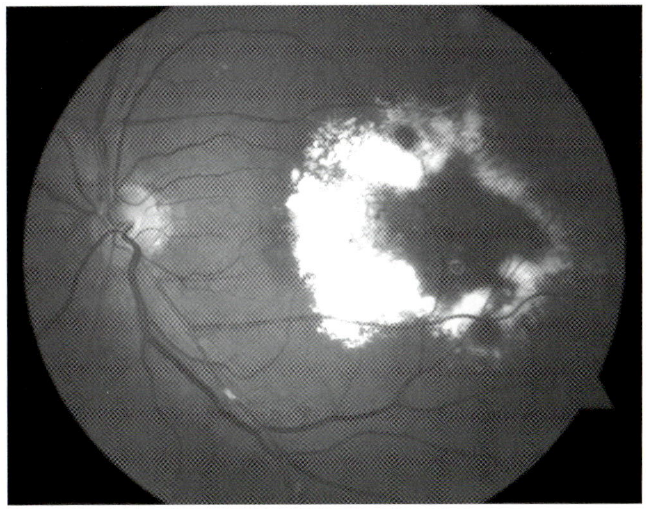

Red free photograph showing the circinate with vascular abnormalities in the center

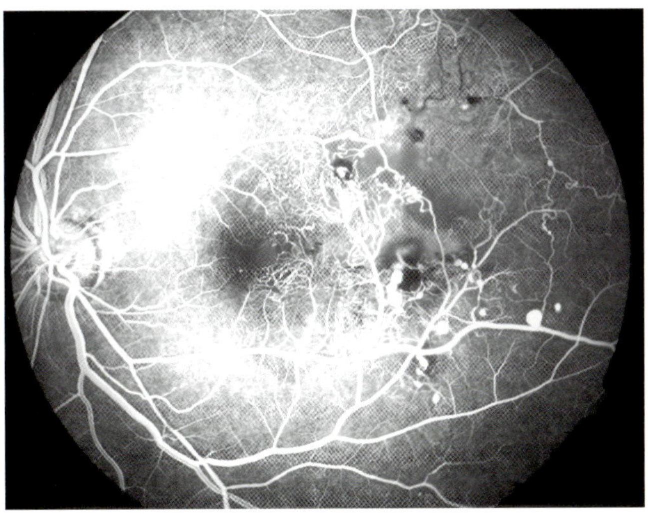

The aneurysmal dilatations are clearly seen in the arteriovenous phase. A large area of capillary non-perfusion is seen temporally. Note the telangiectatic vessels in the temporal parafoveal region

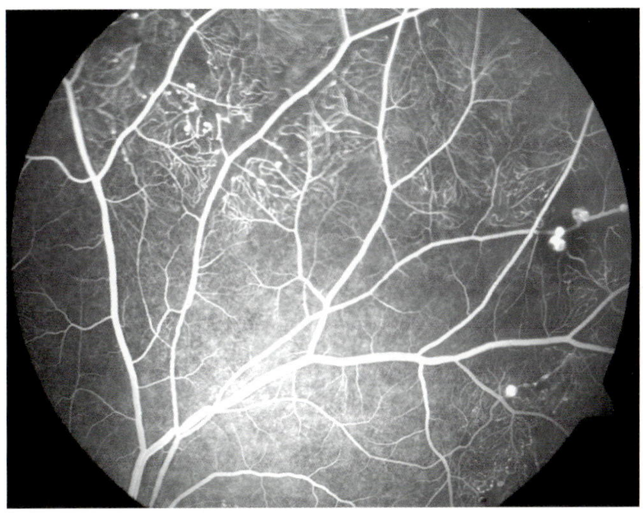

Extensive telangiectasias with areas of capillary non-perfusion and aneurysmal dilatation is seen in the supero-temporal periphery

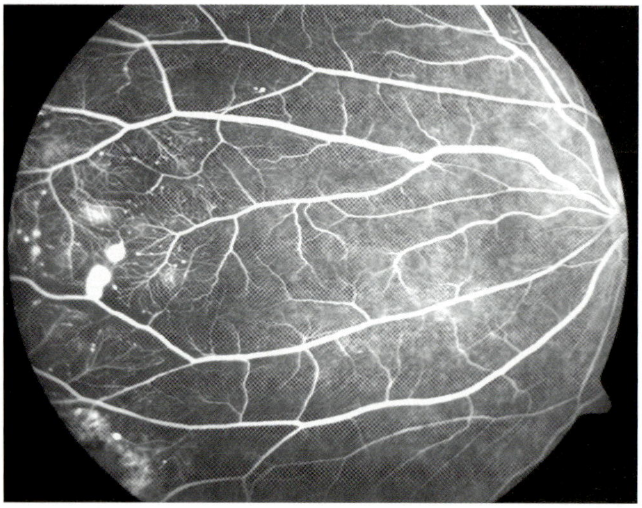

Similar changes are seen in the nasal periphery

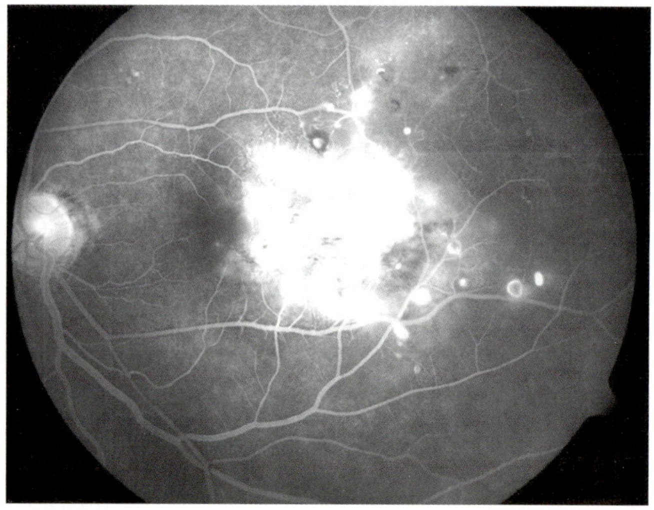

Late phase picture showing leakage of the dye from the vascular abnormalities

CLINICAL NUGGETS

1. Early treatment of the vascular abnormalities in Coats' disease provides the best control of leakage and prevents severe visual loss.
2. Laser or cryotherapy can be used to treat the vascular abnormalities.
3. Multiple treatment sessions may be required.
4. Coats' disease with severe exudative retinal detachment may present with leukocoria.

BIBLIOGRAPHY

1. Gass JDM. A fluorescein angiographic study of macular dysfunction secondary to retinal vascular disease. V. Retinal telangiectasias. Arch Ophthalmol 1968;80:592-605.
2. Chopdar A. Retinal telangiectasis in adults: fluorescein angiographic findings and treatment by argon laser. Br J Ophthalmol 1978;62:243-50.
3. Egerer I, Tasman W, Tomer TL. Coats' disease. Arch Ophthalmol 1974;92:109-12.
4. Gass JDM, Oyakawa RT. Idiopathic juxtafoveal retinal telangiectasias. Arch Ophthalmol 1982;100:769-80.
5. Panleikhoff D, Kruger K, Heinreich T, Wessing A. Epidemiological features and therapeutic result in Coats' disease. Invest Ophthalmol 1988;29:335.
6. Rishi P, Rishi E, Uparkar M, Sharma T, Gopal L, Bhende P, Bhende M, Sen PR, Sen P. Coats' disease: an Indian perspective. Indian J Ophthalmol 2010;58(2):119-24.

28 Chapter

Diabetic Retinopathy

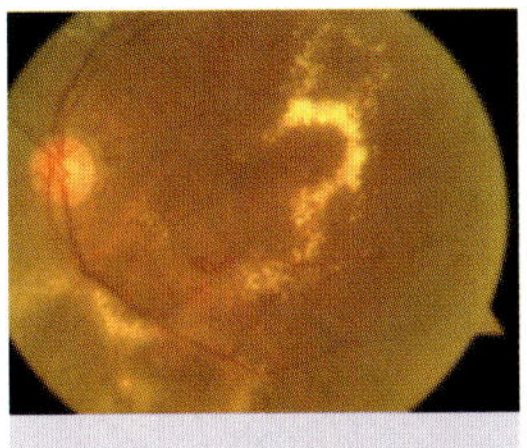

- Diabetic retinopathy is classified as:
  - Nonproliferative diabetic retinopathy (NPDR): Mild/moderate/severe
  - Proliferative diabetic retinopathy (PDR)
- Diabetic maculopathy can be either
  - *Focal:* Microaneurysms leaking fluid into the retina.
  - *Diffuse:* Dilated retinal capillaries leaking fluid into the retina.
  - *Ischemic:* Capillary nonperfused area in the macula.
  - *Mixed:* Combination of any of the above.
- Clinically significant macular edema
  - Thickening of the retina located < 500 microns from the center of the macula.
  - Hard exudates with thickening of the adjacent retina located < 500 microns from the center of the macula.
  - A zone of retinal thickening, 1 DA or larger in size, located < 1DA from the center of the macula.
- Basic pathology involves
  - Increased permeability of the retinal capillaries.
  - Closure of the retinal capillaries.

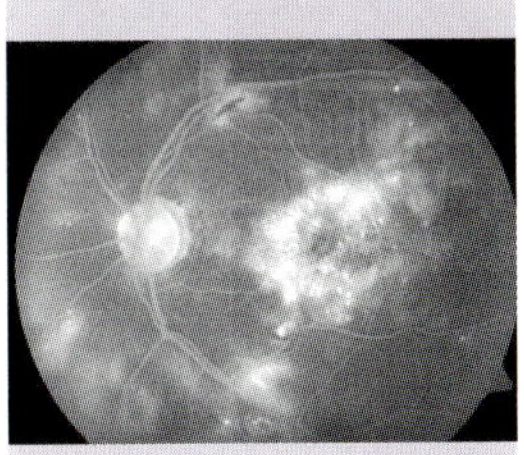

- Microaneurysms: Appear as hyperfluorescent dots which leak dye in the later phases.
- Dilation of the retinal capillaries may occur.
- Capillary closure appears as areas of hypofluorescence due to nonfilling; they are usually bordered by dilated capillaries and microaneurysms.
- Intraretinal microvascular abnormalities (IRMA): Irregular segmental dilatation of the retinal capillary bed. They usually occur in areas of capillary nonperfusion and usually appear to originate and drain into the venous side of the circulation. They remain within the confines of the retina and do not leak fluorescein except minimally at their growing tips. They probably represent intraretinal neovascularization or dilatation of existing retinal channels.
- Superficial and deep retinal hemorrhages cause blocked choroidal fluorescence.
- Venous abnormalities in the form of venous dilation, beading, loops and reduplication may be seen.
- Neovascularization on the disc or the retinal surface appears as irregularly branching vessels which freely leaks the dye.

CASE 1

A 56-year-old male presented with history of decreased vision in both eyes for the past 6 months. He was a known diabetic for the past 6 years and a hypertensive for the last 1 year. Visual acuity was 6/9; N6 in both eyes.

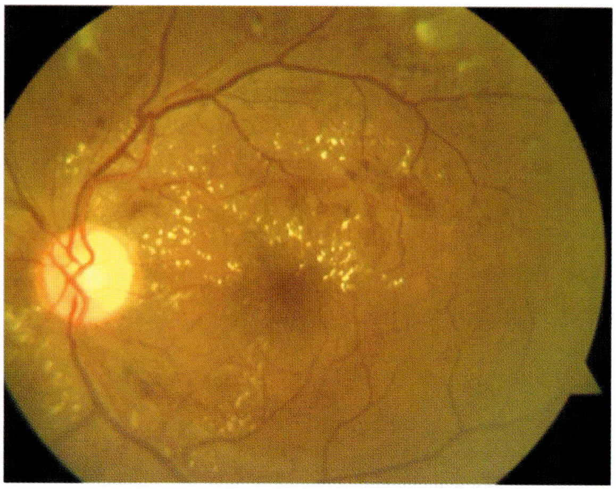

Fundus photograph of the left eye showing hard exudates arranged in a loose circinate pattern in the superior part of the macula

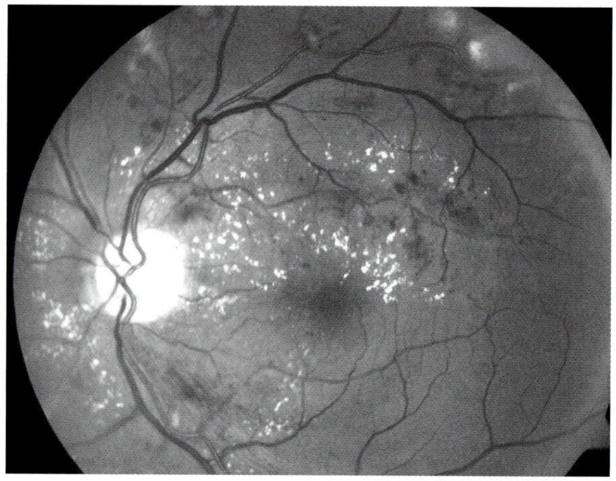

Red free photograph highlights the scattered hard exudates and the retinal hemorrhages

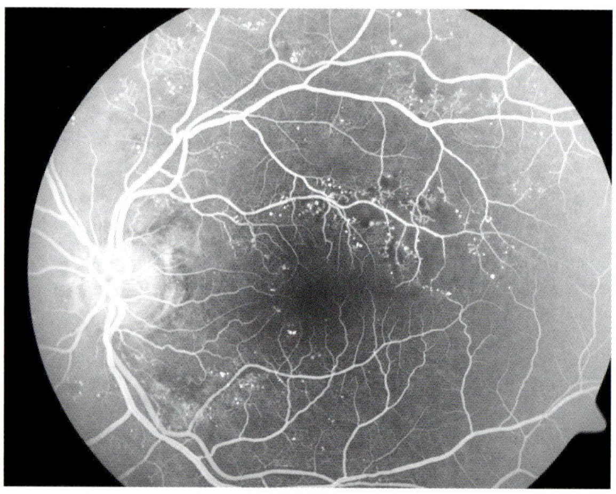

Arteriovenous phase showing the multiple hyperfluorescent points caused by microaneurysms. These are seen bordering the areas of capillary nonperfusion

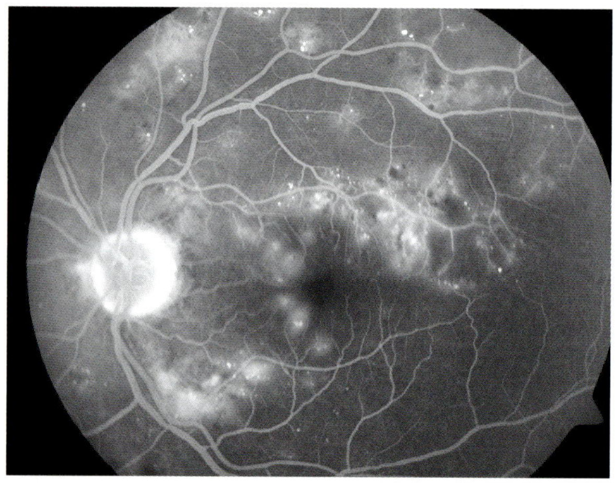

Increased fuzziness is seen around the microaneurysms due to leakage of the dye in the late phase. The areas of capillary nonperfusion remain hypofluorescent

COMMENT

- Focal maculopathy is characterized by presence of leaking microaneurysms. Fluorescein angiography can be used to guide laser photocoagulation of these microaneurysms.
- Direct laser treatment is done to all focal points of leakage located between 500 and 3,000 μm from the center of the macula.
- At the follow-up session, lesions located between 300 and 500 μm from the macular center could be optionally treated if visual acuity is 20/40 or worse, and if treatment would not destroy the remaining perifoveal capillary network.

CASE 2

A 54-year-old male with diabetes for the past ten years presented with history of reduced vision in both eyes for the last one month. Visual acuity was 6/12; N8 in the right eye and 6/9; N10 in the left eye.

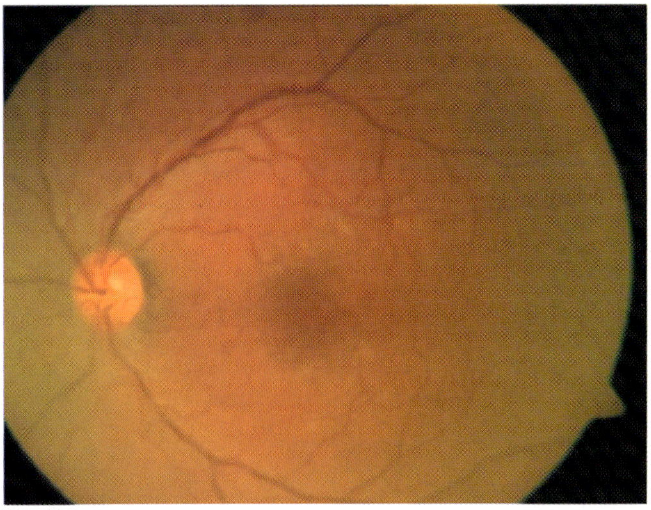

Fundus photograph of the left eye. Retinal thickening was noted in the macular region. Note the absence of hard exudates or retinal hemorrhages

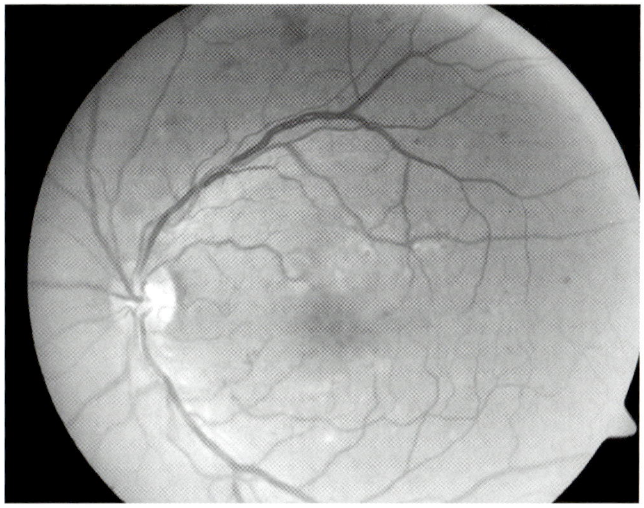

Red free photograph highlighting the cystoid changes in the foveal region

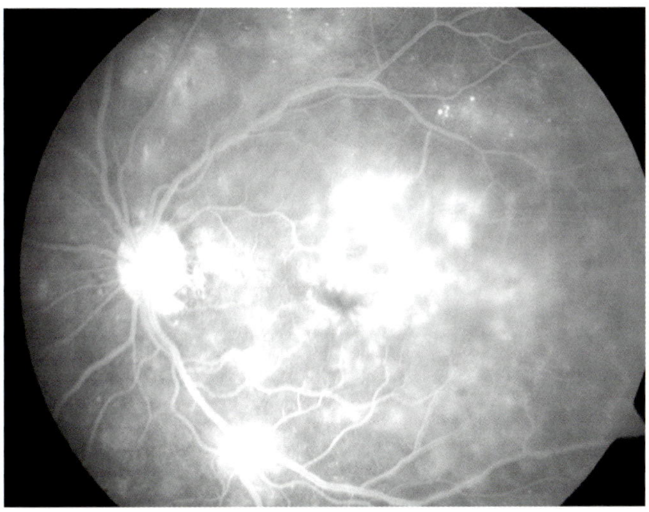

Midarteriovenous phase shows leakage of dye from the dilated capillaries throughout the macula. A fuzzy hyperfluorescence is seen along the inferotemporal arcade indicative of a small neovascular frond. Few microaneurysms are noted superiorly

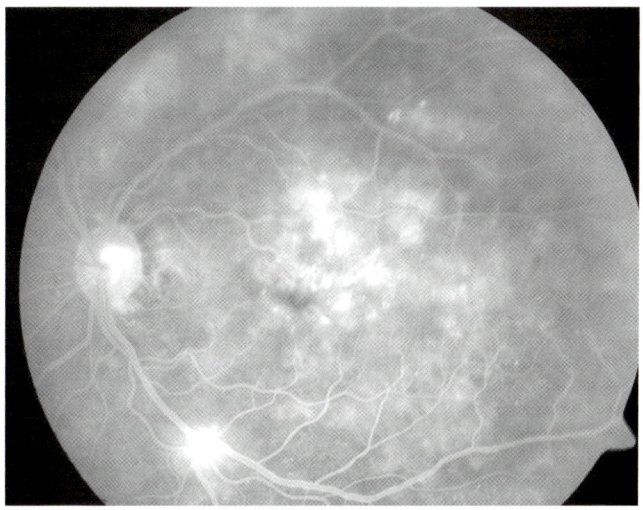

The leakage from the capillaries has increased and the dye is seen to be collecting in cystoid spaces around the fovea

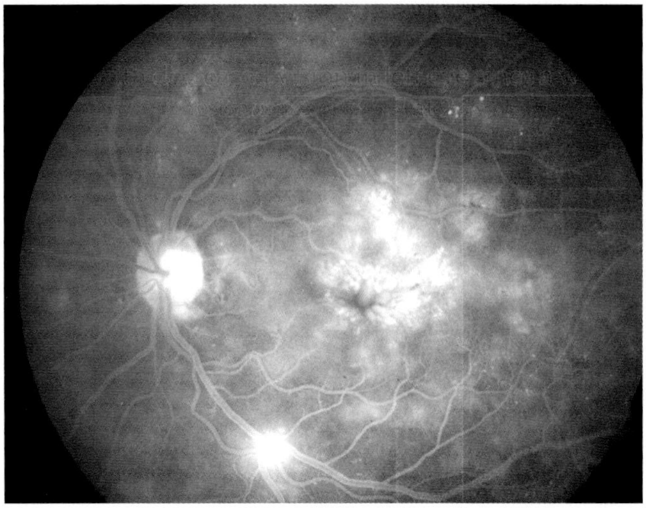

Late film shows accumulation of the dye in cystoid spaces around the fovea. Noncystoid collection of the dye is also noted in the other parts of the macula. The leakage from the neovascular frond has also increased

CASE 2 (*Continued*)

Right Eye of the Patient

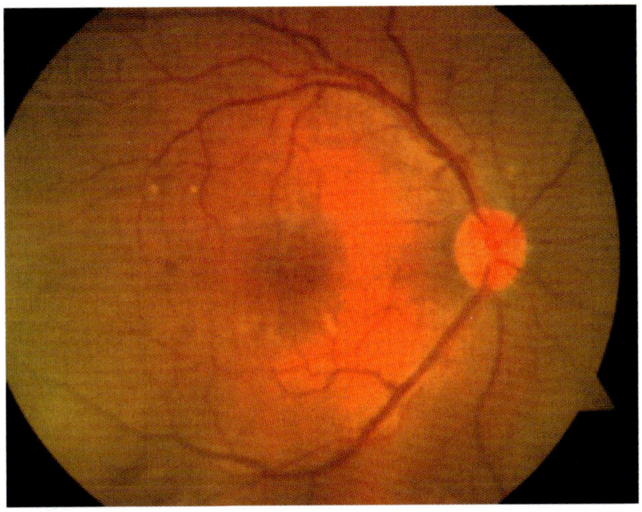

Fundus photograph of the right eye of the same patient showing cystoid changes at the fovea. Few hard exudates are seen superotemporal to the fovea

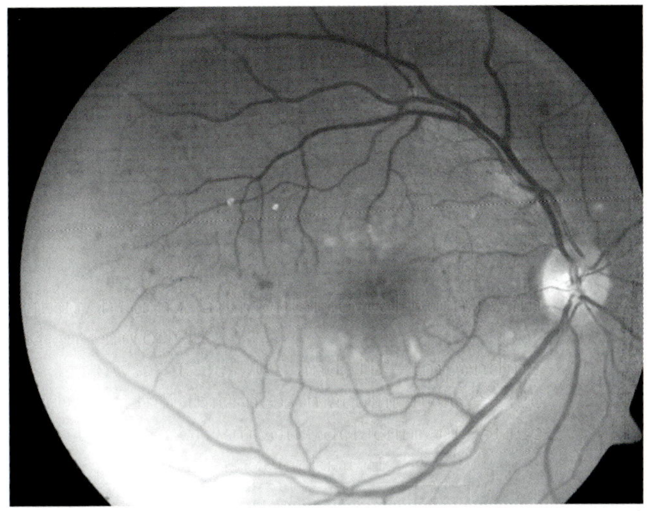

Red free photograph highlights the cystoid changes at the fovea

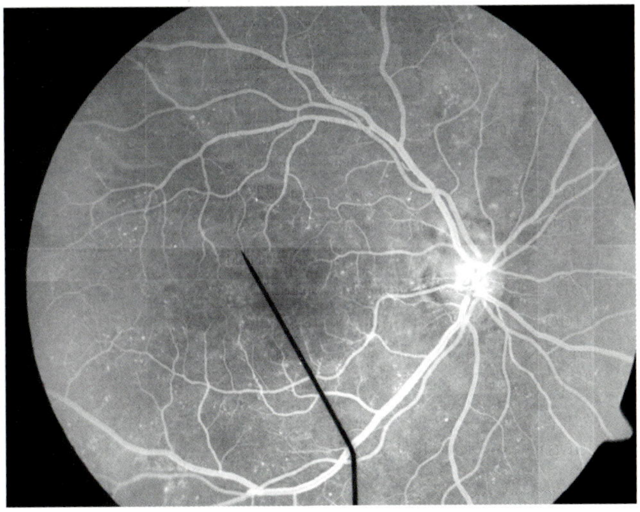

Midarteriovenous phase showing the dilated capillary network in the perifoveal region

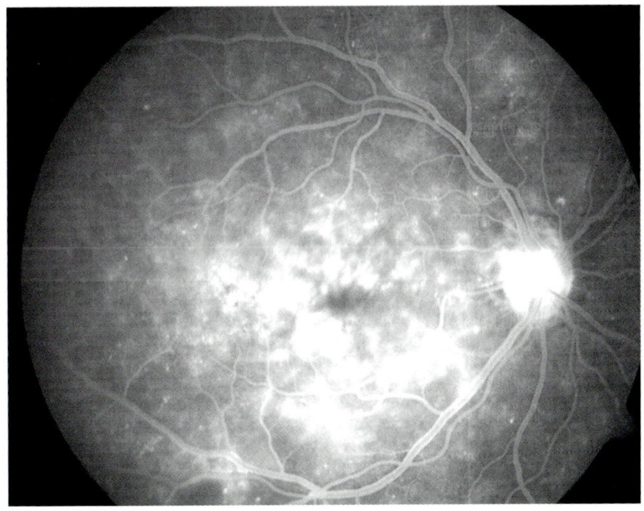

Significant leakage of the dye is seen from the dilated capillaries

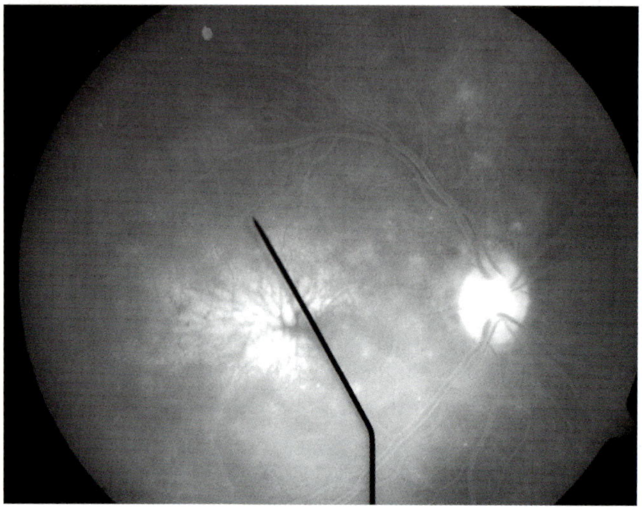

The petalloid pattern of cystoid macular edema is well seen in the late phase

COMMENT

- Diffuse maculopathy is characterized by dilated capillaries which leak fluorescein dye.
- Hard exudates are not usually associated with diffuse type of diabetic maculopathy.
- The grid technique of laser is applied to treat areas of diffuse leakage, including MA's, IRMA's, leaking capillary segments, and areas of nonperfusion.
- Patients who develop macular edema during pregnancy frequently have different prognosis than nonpregnant patients. Spontaneous resolution after pregnancy is a common occurrence and is associated with improvement of visual acuity more frequently than in nonpregnant patients.

CASE 3

A 44-year-old male diabetic patient presented with marked reduction in vision in both eyes for the past one year. Visual acuity was 2/60 in the right eye and 1/60 in the left eye.

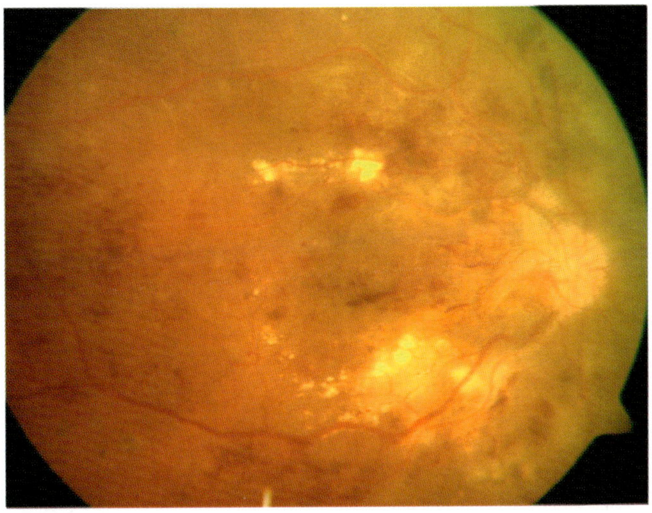

A large neovascular frond is seen at the disc. Hard exudates are seen in the upper and lower part of the macula while the foveal area has a dull washed out appearance

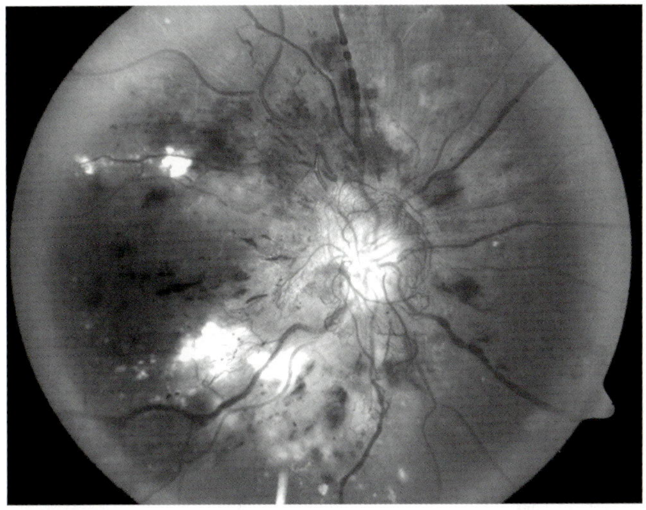

The red free photograph highlights the features seen in the fundus photograph

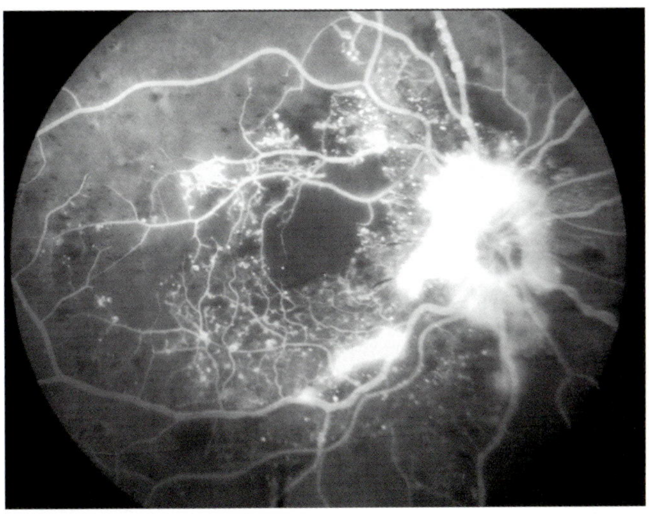

Marked leakage of the dye is seen from the NVD. A large area of capillary nonperfusion is seen in the upper part of the macula involving the fovea; dilated capillaries are seen around this

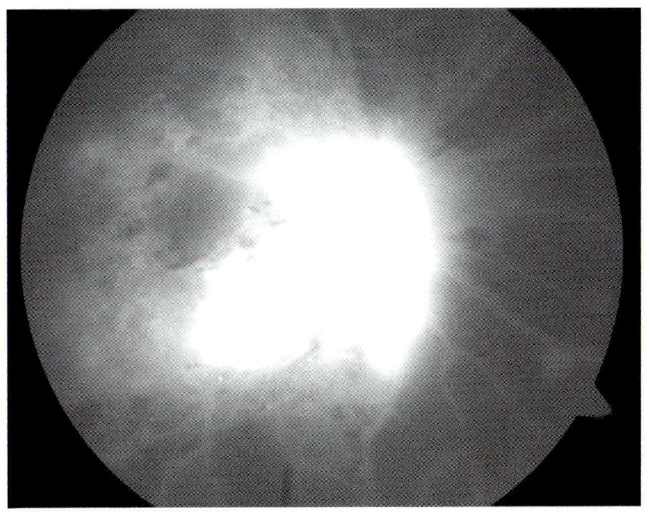

Marked leakage of the dye is seen from the NVD. Increased staining of the retinal tissue in the macula is seen except in the region of the capillary dropout which remains hypofluorescent

COMMENT

Ischemic maculopathy is characterized by areas of capillary dropout at the macula. They have a very poor visual prognosis.

CASE 4

A 65-year-old male, who was a known diabetic and hypertensive for the past 8 years presented with decreased vision in the left eye. Visual acuity was 3/60 in the left eye.

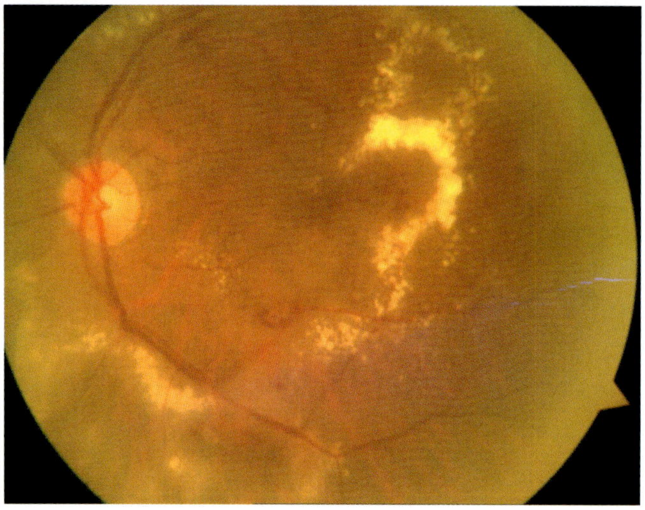

Fundus photograph of the left eye showing extensive hard exudate deposition in the form of incomplete circinate. Vascular abnormalities are seen within the circinate

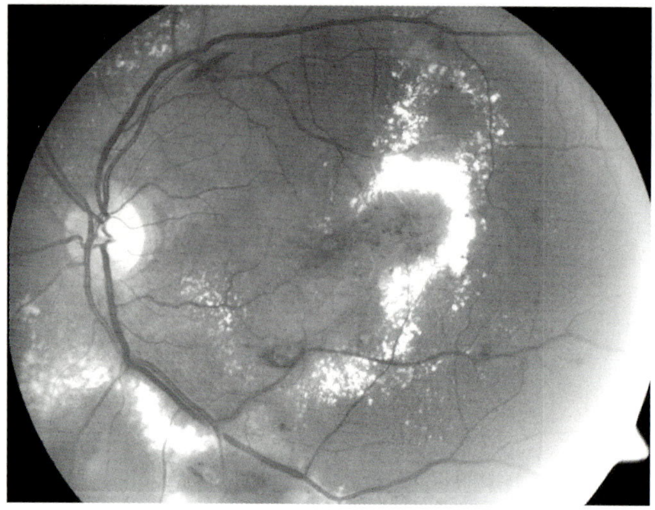

The vascular abnormalities are well made out within the circinates in the red free photograph

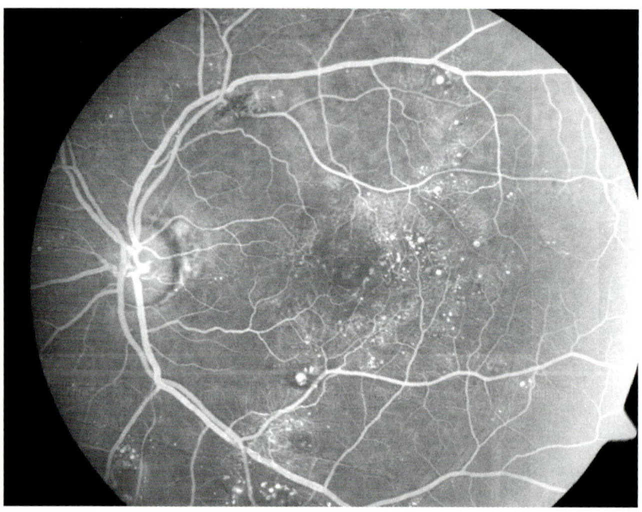

Numerous microaneurysms are made out as hyperfluorescent dots. Note the dilated perifoveal capillaries

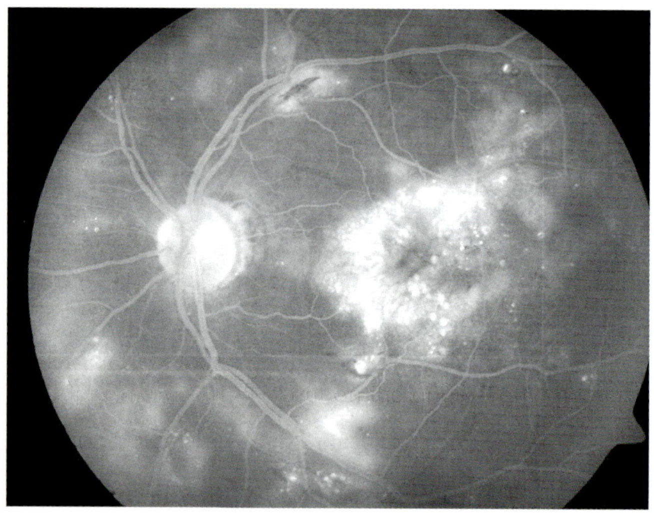

Marked leakage of the dye is seen from the micro-aneurysms and the dilated capillaries. Cystoid pattern of dye accumulation is clearly evident

COMMENT

Patient is having both focal and diffuse type of maculopathy. Mixed type of maculopathy is quite common.

CASE 5

A 48-year-old male patient with a history of diabetes for the past 20 years presented with decreased vision in the left eye of one week duration. Visual acuity was 6/18; N36.

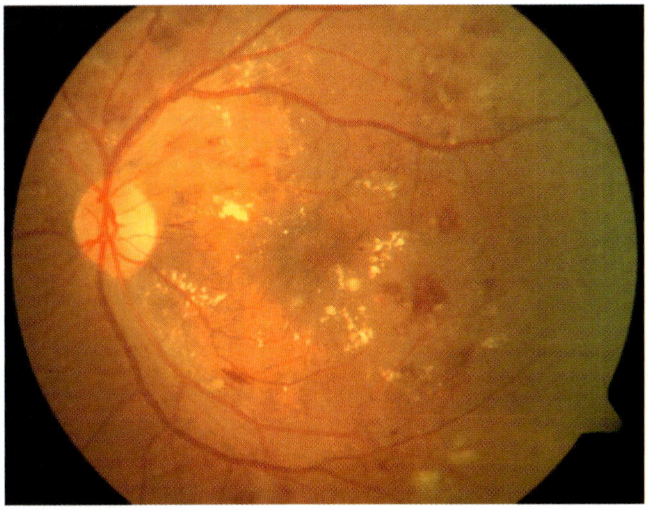

Fundus photograph of the left eye showing scattered hard exudates and hemorrhages in the macula

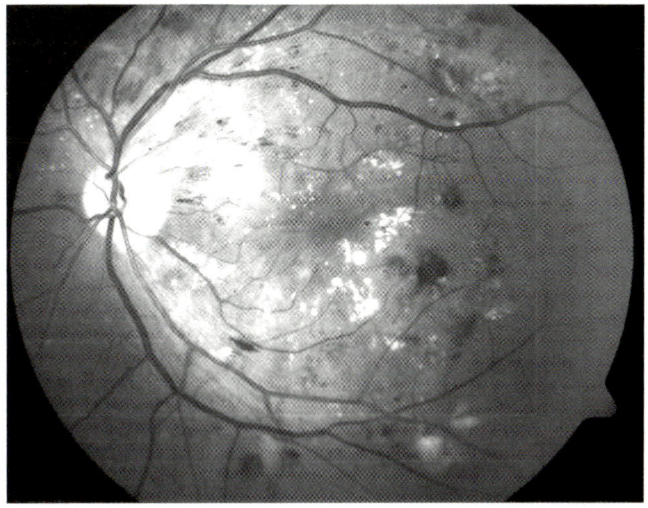

Red free photograph highlights these retinal changes

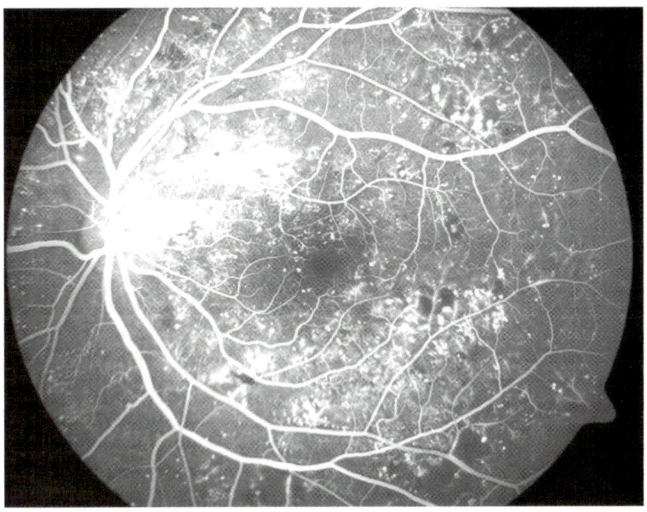

Innumerable microaneurysms are seen as hyperfluorescent dots. The perifoveal capillary network is broken superotemporally

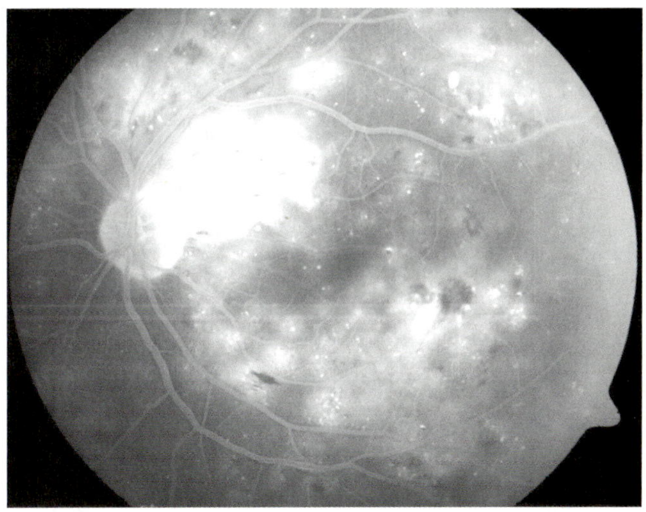

Marked leakage of the dye into the retinal tissue is seen from the microaneurysms

COMMENT

Fluorescein angiography is very useful to assess the para- and perifoveal capillary network.

CASE 6

A 50-year-old male presented with decreased vision in the right eye of two months duration. He was a known diabetic for the last three years. Visual acuity was 6/12; N36 in the right eye.

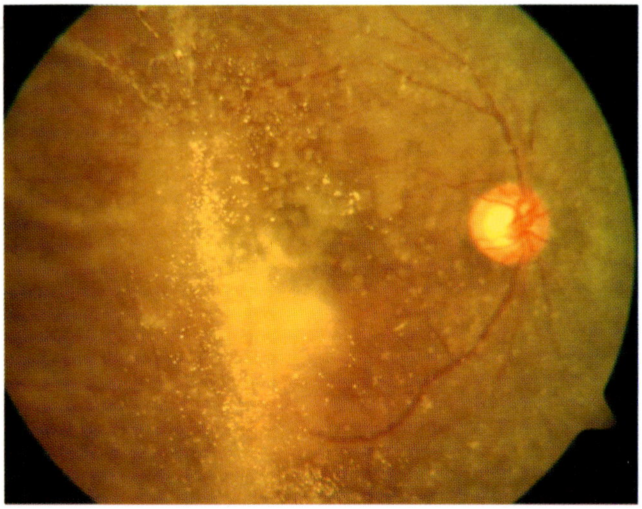

Fundus photograph of the right eye showing asteroid hyalosis which is obscuring the view of the fundus. Gliosis is seen in the temporal macular region

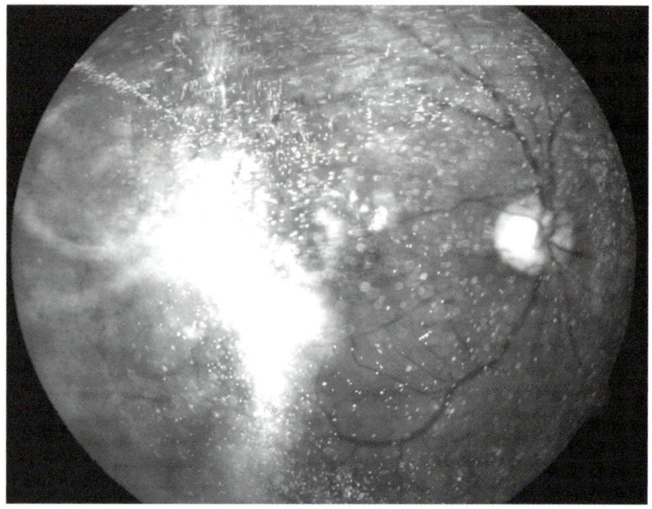

The view of the retina is obscured by the asteroid hyalosis even in the red free photograph

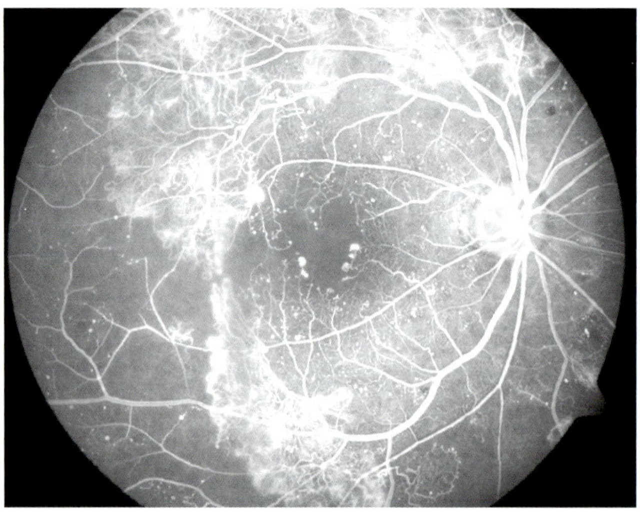

Midarteriovenous phase showing the large neovascular network. Area of capillary nonperfusion is seen involving the parafoveal capillary network. Microaneurysms are noted bordering this

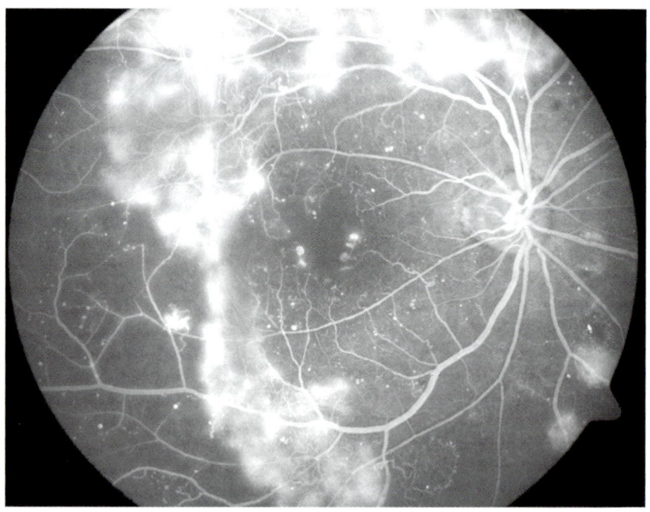

Increased leakage of the dye is seen from the neovascular network. Areas of capillary nonperfusion are seen temporally

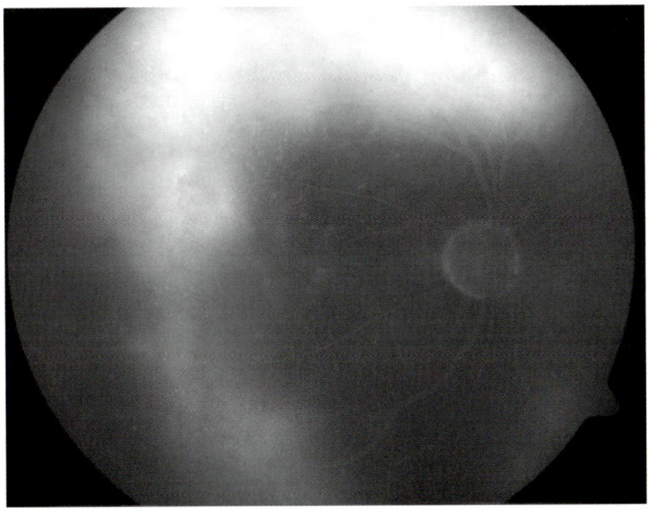

Marked leakage of the dye is evident in the late phase

COMMENT

- Fluorescein angiography is extremely useful to evaluate the retina in patients with asteroid hyalosis.
- The presence of a barrier filter prevents the blue light reflected from the asteroids to enter the camera. Only the green light from the retina is allowed to enter. Hence, the retinal details are very well-seen in the angiogram despite the presence of asteroid hyalosis.

CASE 7

A 51-year-old male diabetic presented with history of panretinal photocoagulation done for both eyes in the past. Visual acuity was 6/6; N6 in both eyes.

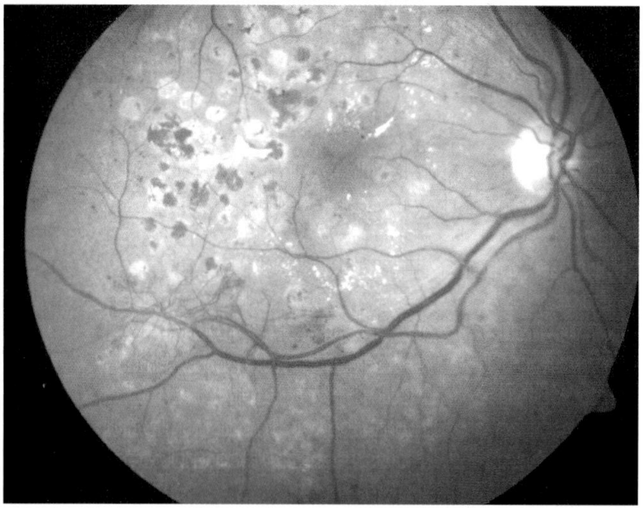

Red free photograph of the right eye showing old laser photocoagulation marks temporally. A neovascular frond is seen along the inferotemporal arcade

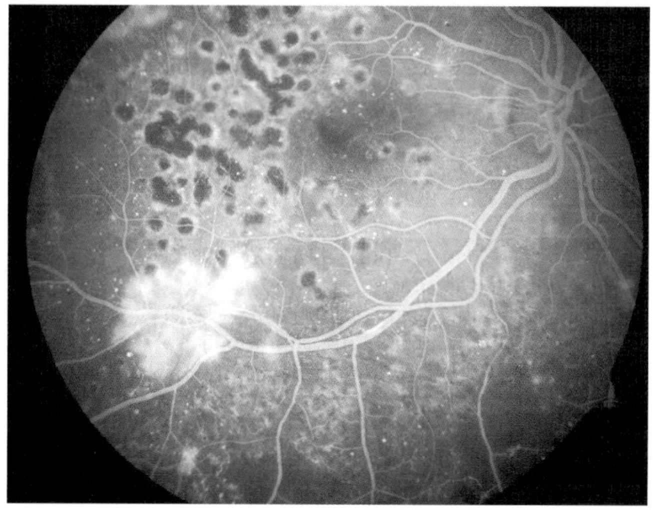

Hyperfluorescence due to leakage of dye from the neovascular frond is seen in the midarteriovenous phase. The laser marks appear as central hypofluorescence surrounded by a rim of hyperfluorescence

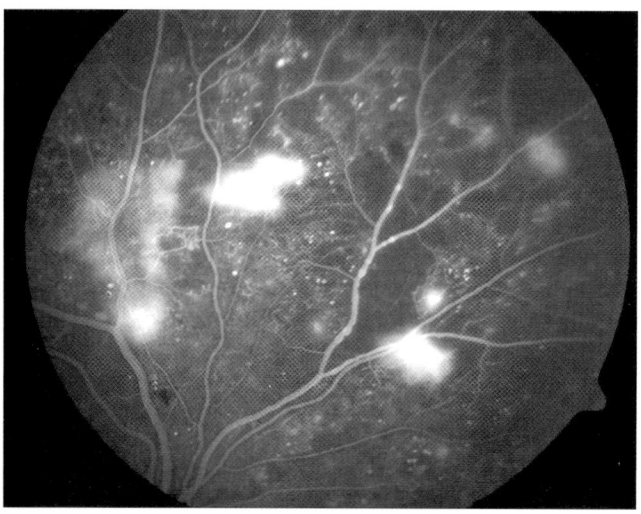

Multiple areas of intense hyperfluorescence due to leakage of the dye from the neovascular fronds are seen. Large areas of capillary dropout are also seen

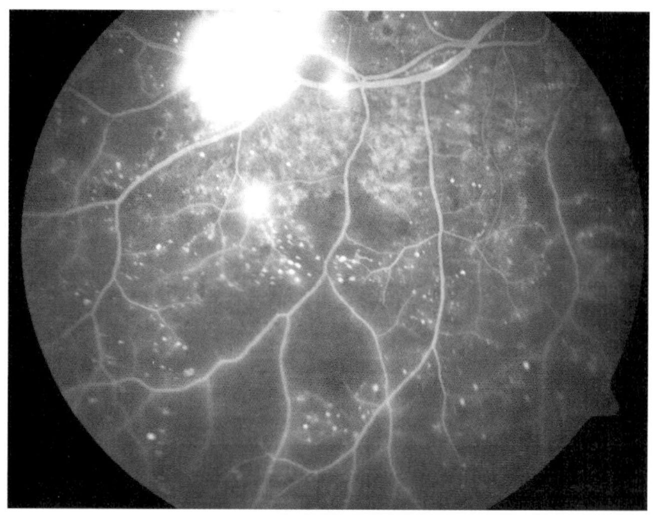

The leakage of dye from the inferotemporal frond has increased in the recirculation phase. Extensive areas of capillary nonperfusion are seen inferiorly

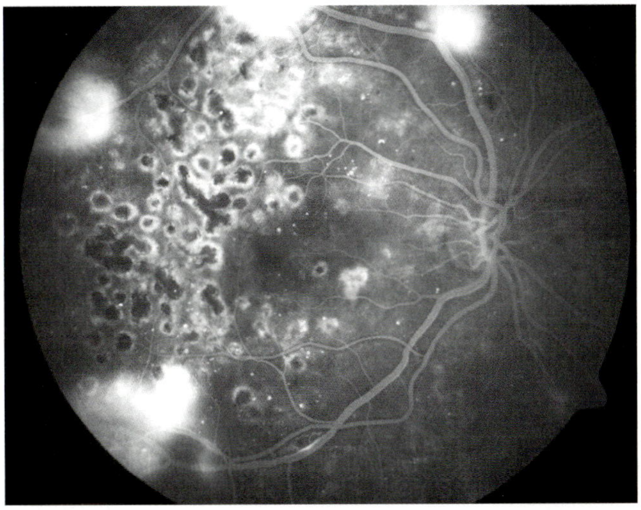

Increased leakage from the neovascular fronds is seen in the late phase. The rim of hyperfluorescence around the laser marks is more prominent

COMMENT

Flat, subtle NVEs which may be difficult to appreciate clinically in a heavily ablated eye can be picked up quite well in the fluorescein angiogram.

CLINICAL NUGGETS

1. Close follow-up of patients with severe NPDR is needed, as the risk of progression to PDR is high.
2. In eyes requiring laser for PDR and CSME, it is better to do the treatment for the CSME first followed by a panretinal photocoagulation 2 to 3 weeks later. This is to avoid the aggravation of the macular edema that may follow panretinal photocoagulation.
3. It is not unusual to have a transient mild increase in macular edema immediately following focal laser photocoagulation. There is often migration of lipids towards the center of the fovea during resolution of macular edema.
4. Systemic hypertension can accelerate the progression of diabetic retinopathy.
5. Optical coherence tomography is an important tool to identify vitreomacular traction in macular edema. These cases do not respond to laser photocoagulation and need vitreoretinal surgery.

BIBLIOGRAPHY

1. Diabetic Retinopathy Study Research Group: Photocoagulation treatment of proliferative diabetic retinopathy. Ophthalmology 1981; 88: 583-600.
2. Early Treatment Diabetic Retinopathy Study Research Group: Focal photocoagulation treatment of diabetic macular edema: relationship of treatment effect to fluorescein angiographic and other retinal characteristics at baseline. ETDRS report no.19. Arch Ophthalmol 1995; 113:1144-55.
3. Early Treatment Diabetic Retinopathy Study Research Group: Fundus photographic risk factors for the progression of diabetic retinopathy. ETDRS report no 12. Ophthalmology 1991;98:23-33.
4. Early Treatment Diabetic Retinopathy Study Research Group–Report no 11, classification of diabetic retinopathy from fluorescein angiograms. Ophthalmology 1991; 98:807-22.
5. Kohner EM, Dollery CT, Peterson JW, Oakley NW. Arterial fluorescein studies in diabetic retinopathy. Diabetes, 1967;16:1-10.
6. Norton EW, Gutman F. Diabetic retinopathy studied by fluorescein angiography. Ophthalmologica 1965;150: 5-17.
7. Stoessel KM, Liao PM, Thompson JT, et al. Diabetic retinopathy and macular edema in pregnancy. Ophthalmology 1991; 98:146.
8. Takeshi N, Mukara K, Shimuzi K. Distribution of capillary non-perfusion in early stage of diabetic retinopathy. Ophthalmology 91: 1984;1431-39.

29

Chapter

Venous Occlusion

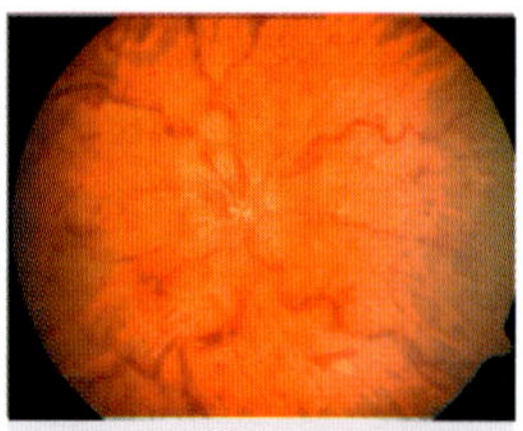

CENTRAL RETINAL VEIN OCCLUSION

- Central retinal vein occlusion (CRVO) is characterized by diffuse retinal hemorrhages in all quadrants and dilated and tortuous retinal veins.
- The clinical appearance may vary from a few scattered retinal hemorrhages with a few cotton-wool spots to very extensive retinal hemorrhages occurring throughout the fundus.
- Macular edema is present in most cases.
- Based on the visual acuity, presence or absence of an afferent pupillary defect, ophthalmoscopic findings, fluorescein angiographic findings, visual fields and electroretinographic findings, central retinal vein occlusion is divided into two groups:
    1. Nonischemic/perfused CRVO (NICRVO)
    2. Ischemic/nonperfused CRVO (ICRVO).

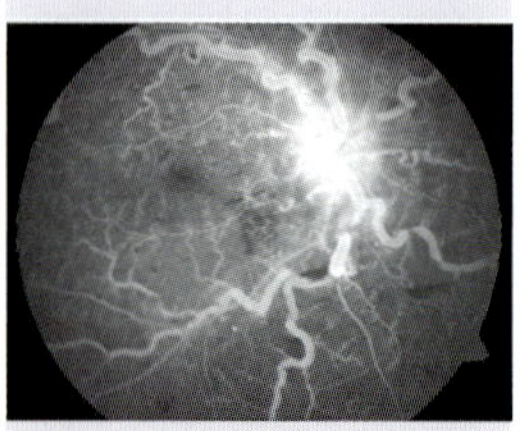

Nonischemic Central Retinal Vein Occlusion (NICRVO)

- The superficial retinal hemorrhages cause blocked retinal and choroidal fluorescence through all the phases of the angiogram.
- There is a delay in the filling of the veins.
- Veins are markedly engorged, tortuous and appear disrupted because of hemorrhage and retinal edema masking their view.
- The disc capillaries are also dilated and engorged.
- Venous return is severely delayed.
- Capillaries are dilated, tortuous and may show microaneurysmal changes. Perifoveal arcade may show marked congestion and dilatation.
- Few areas of capillary nonperfusion may be seen in the midperipheral retina. However, this is not as extensive as in ischemic CRVO.
- Late phase shows considerable staining of the vein walls and leakage of dye into the surrounding retina. In the macula this leads to cystoid macular edema.

Ischemic Central Retinal Vein Occlusion (ICRVO)

- In addition to the above changes, extensive areas of capillary closure are seen throughout the fundus.
- There is marked delay in the filling of the veins.
- Ischemic changes usually extend to the macular region.

CASE 1

A 41-year-old patient presented with history of blurring of vision in the right eye for the past three months. Patient was a hypertensive. Visual acuity was 6/6; N6 in both eyes.

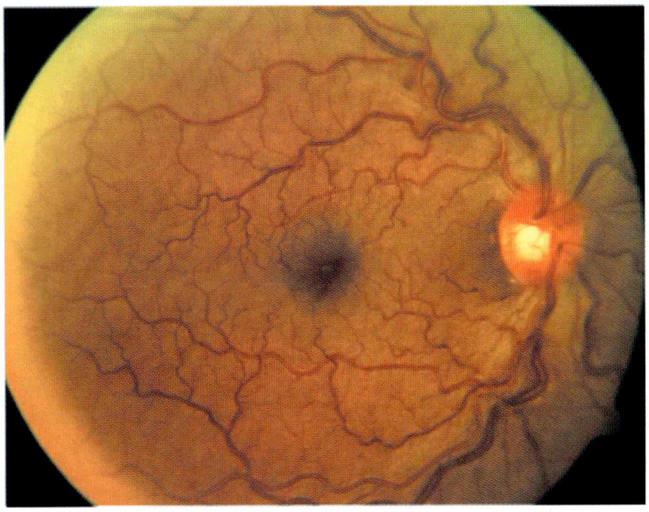

Fundus photograph of the right eye showing dilation and tortuosity of the veins

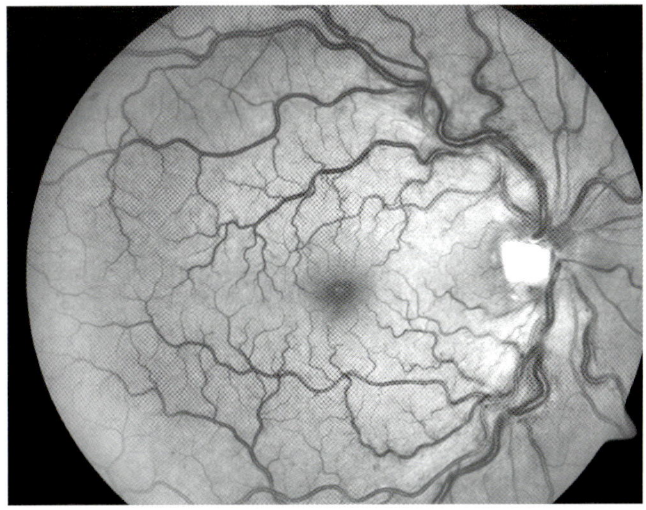

Red free photograph of the right eye showing the tortuosity of the veins. A superficial retinal hemorrhage is seen along the superotemporal vein

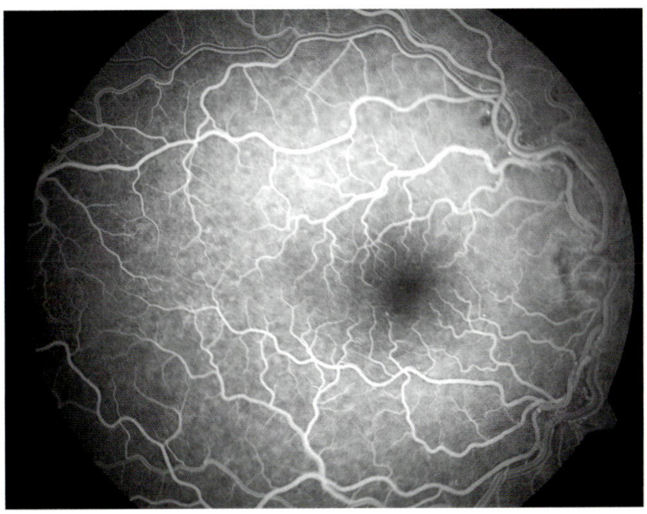

Laminar flow is seen at 28 seconds indicating a delay in the filling of the veins. The choroid is brightly fluorescent in the background

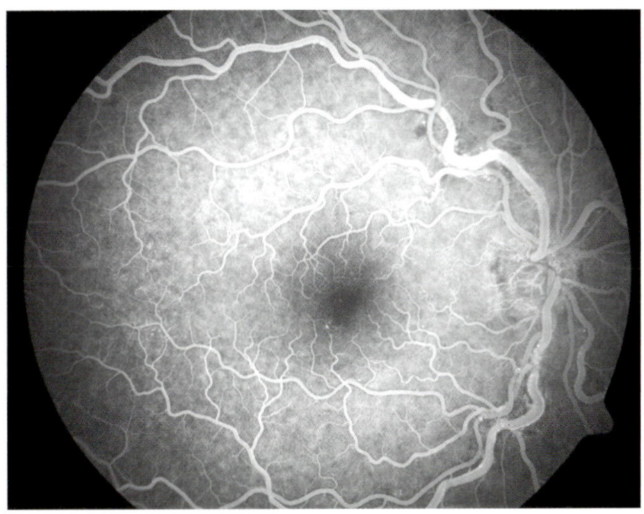

Complete filling of the veins is seen at 36 seconds

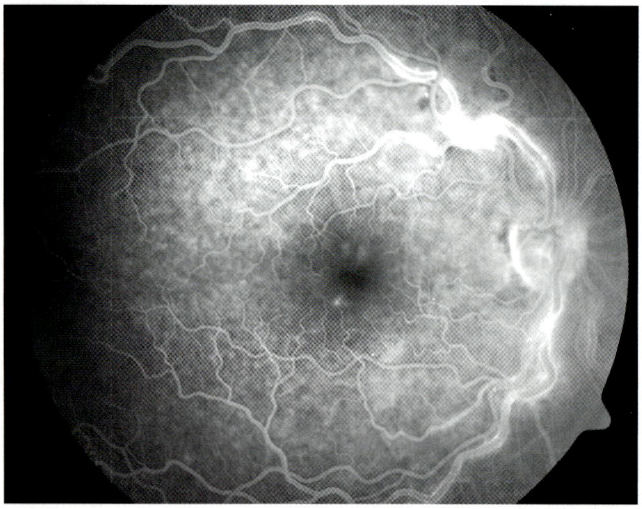

Late phase shows prominent staining of the walls of the veins close to the disc. Minimal hyperfluorescence is seen in the parafoveal region

COMMENT

Patient is having a NICRVO with very minimal macular edema suggesting a lesser degree of occlusion of the central retinal vein.

CASE 2

A 47-year-old patient presented with a history of decreased vision in the right eye of one day duration. Visual acuity was 6/6; N10 in the right eye. Left eye was normal.

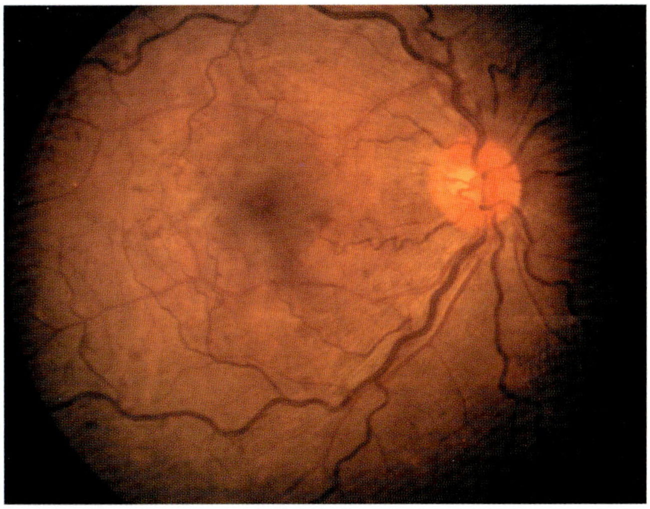

Fundus photograph of the right eye showing mild dilation and tortuosity of the veins and scattered superficial and deep retinal hemorrhages

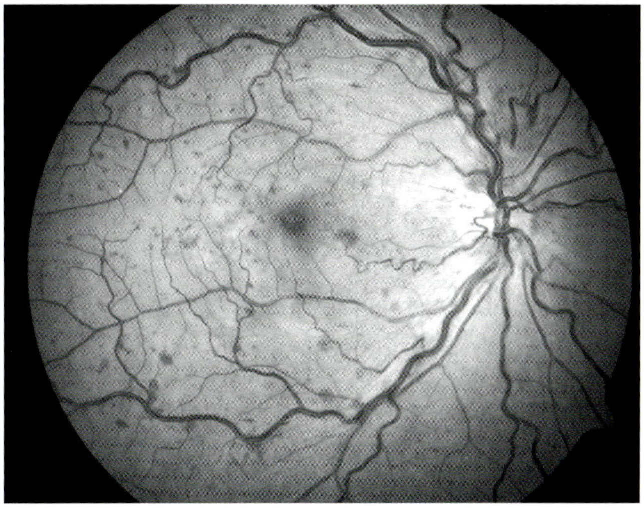

Red free photograph of the right eye

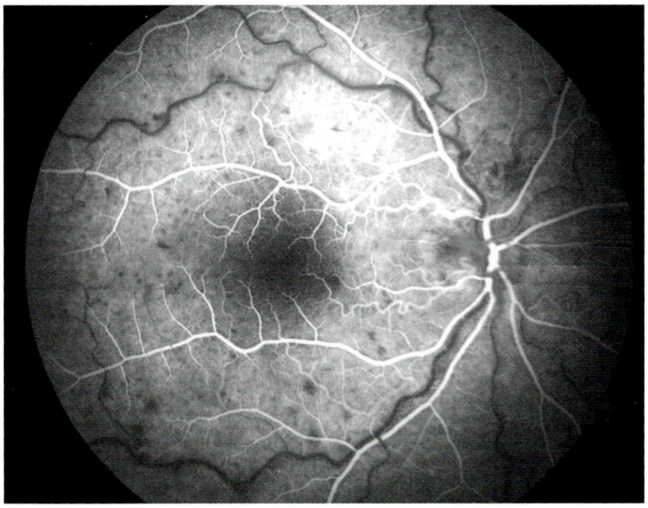

Marked delay in the filling of the veins is seen; no filling is seen even at 30 seconds

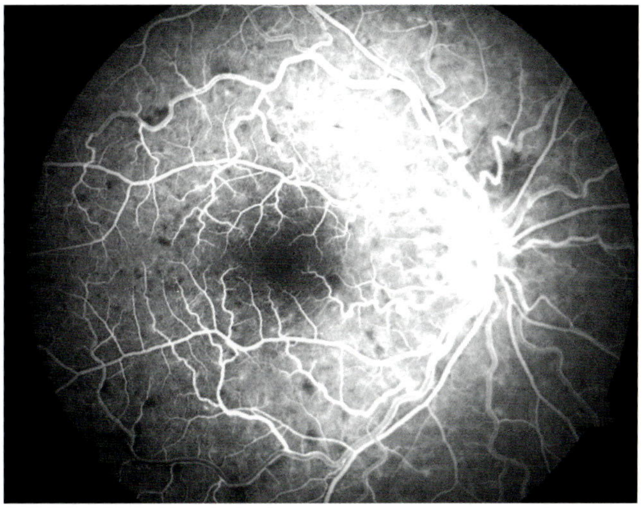

Fluorescein dye has filled the vein completely. The tortuosity of the venules in the macula is well made out

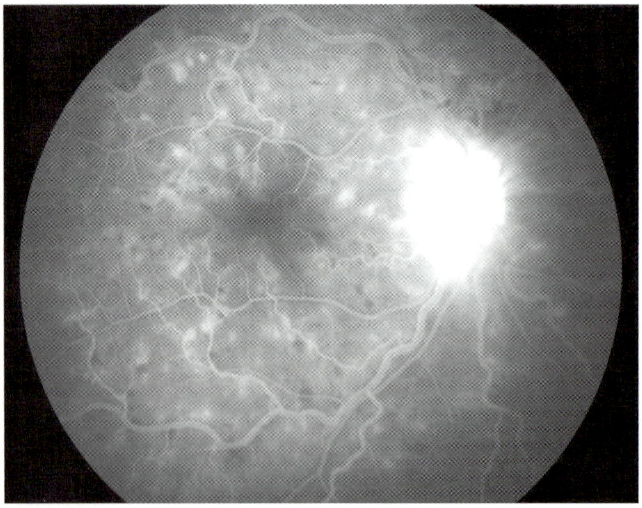

Late stage shows extensive staining of the vessel wall throughout the macula

COMMENT

Patient is having a NICRVO. There is delayed filling of the veins. No significant capillary dropout areas are seen.

CASE 2 (*Continued*)

At two months follow-up visit the visual acuity in the right eye was 6/9; N6.

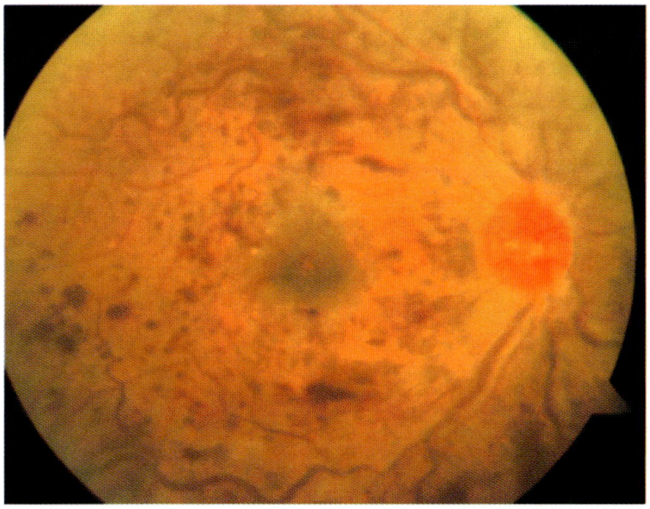

Fundus photograph of the right eye showing increase in the amount of retinal hemorrhages

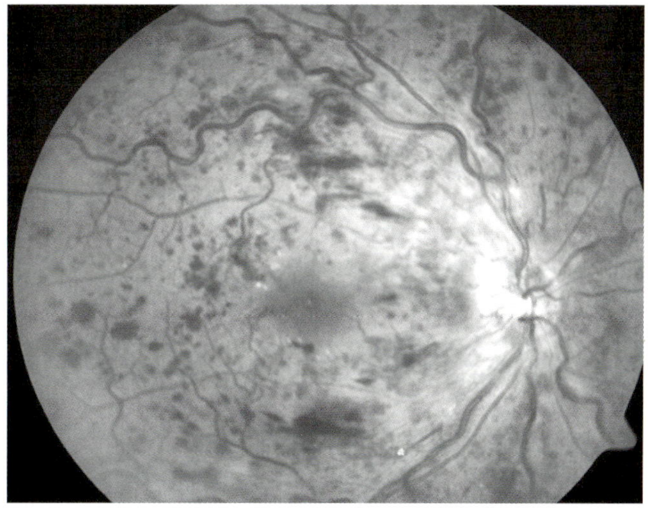

Red free photograph of the right eye

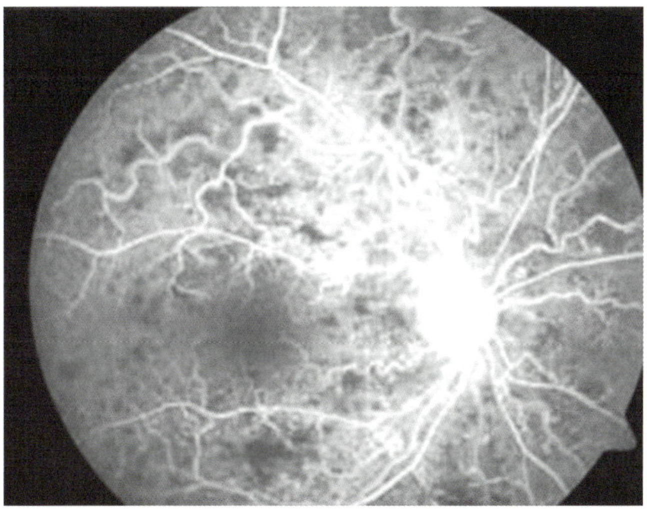

The filling of the vein is better with the vein completely filled by 32 seconds. Scattered areas of blocked fluorescence is seen due to the retinal hemorrhages

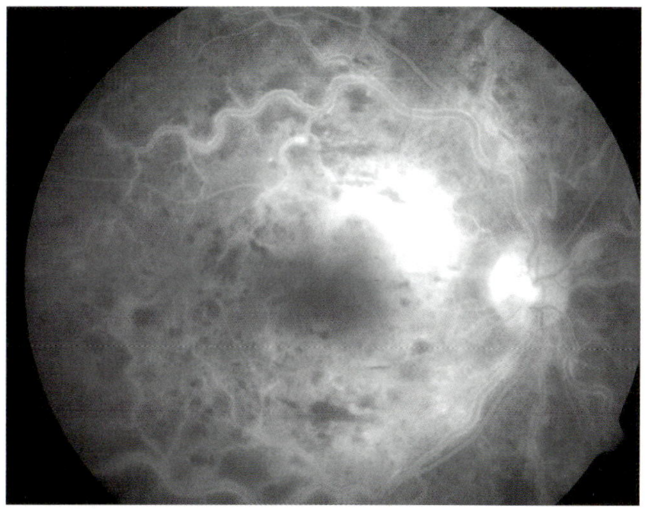

Late phase angiogram shows increased staining of the retina at the macula. No cystoid changes are seen

COMMENT

Increased tortuosity of the veins and more delayed emptying of the veins is seen in the follow-up angiogram. This suggests progression of the CRVO.

CASE 3

A 39-year-old male presented with a history of sudden reduction of vision in the left eye two months back. Visual acuity was 6/9; N6. He was found to have a NICRVO.

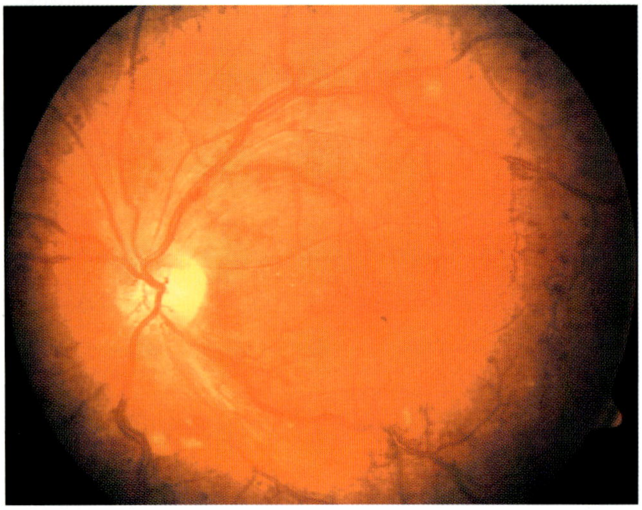

Fundus photograph of the left eye showing scattered retinal hemorrhages. Few cotton-wool spots are seen

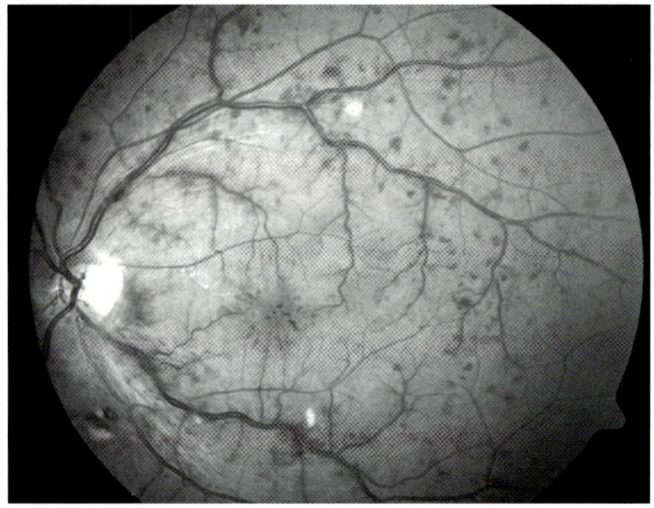

Red free photograph of the left eye

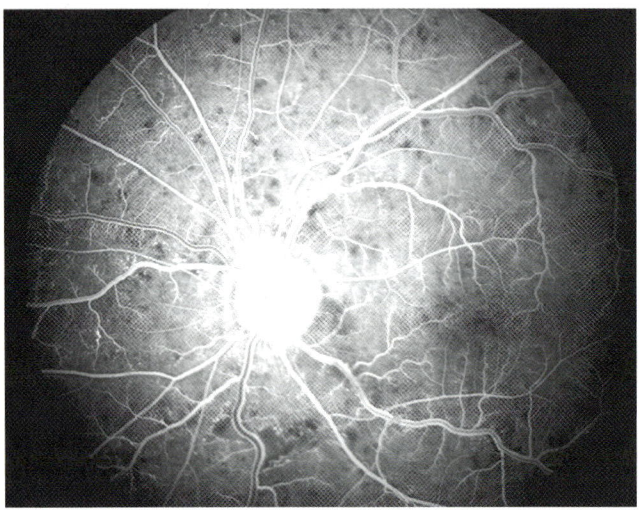

Dilation of the disc capillaries is seen. Scattered blocked fluorescence due to the retinal hemorrhage is evident

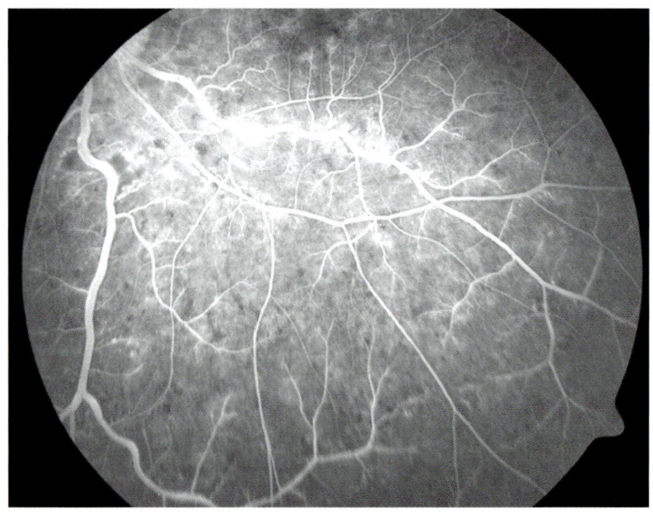

No significant area of capillary nonperfusion is seen in the inferotemporal periphery

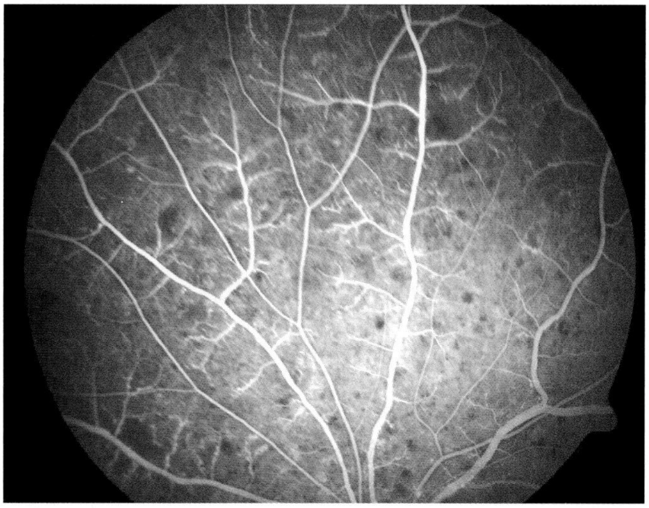

Few areas of capillary nonperfusion are seen in the superior midperiphery

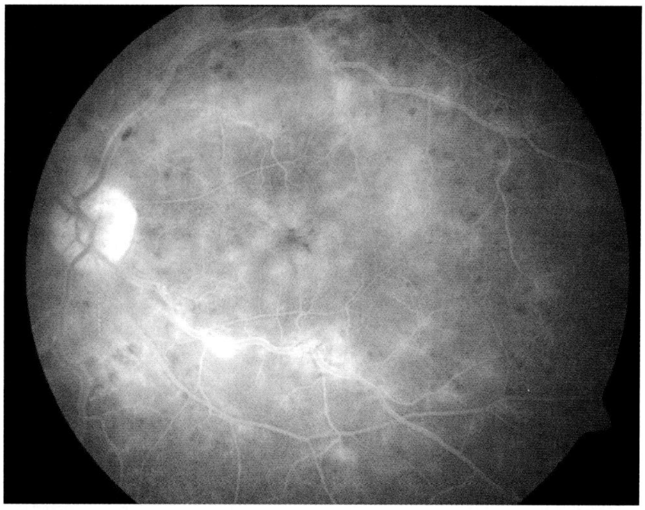

Late phase angiogram showing accumulation of the dye at the macula

CASE 4

A 32-year-old male presented with a history of decreased vision in the right eye of six months duration. Visual acuity was 6/60; N18 in the right eye. Left eye was normal. Detailed laboratory investigations did not reveal any abnormality.

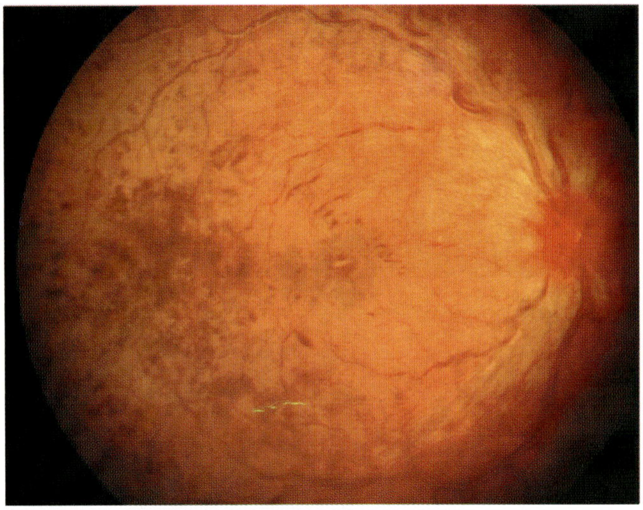

Hyperemia and swelling of the disc with dilation of the veins and superficial retinal hemorrhages are seen in the right eye

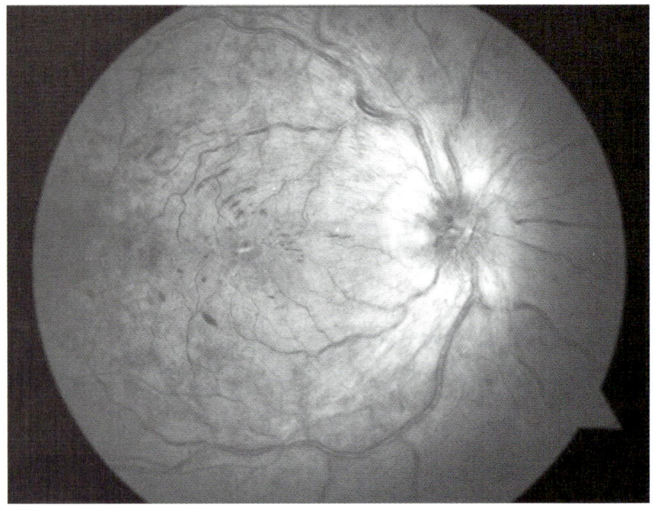

Red free photograph of the right eye. Cystoid changes are seen at the fovea

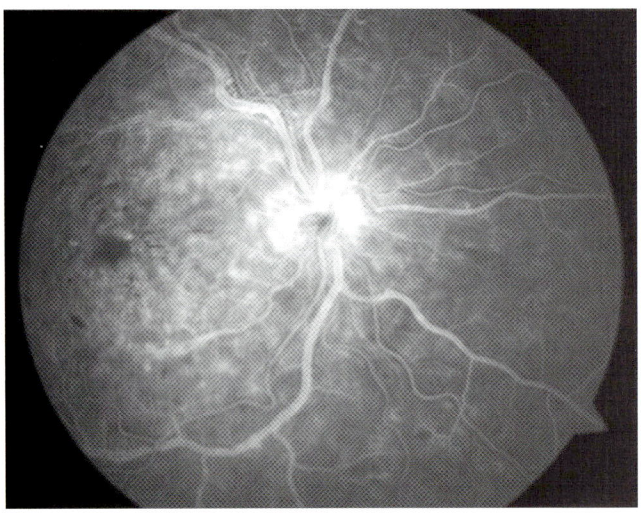

Dilation of the capillaries at the disc and in the macula is seen. Early leakage of the dye from the smaller vessels is seen in the macula

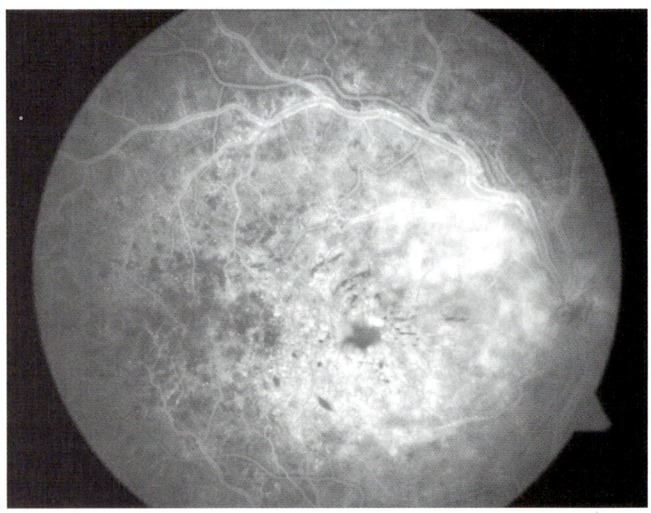

Further leakage of the dye from the vessels is seen at the macula

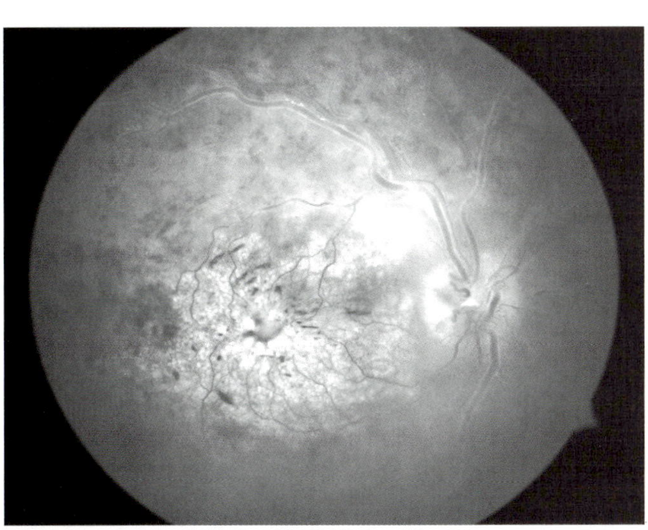

Late phase shows accumulation of the dye in a honeycomb pattern in the macula

COMMENT

Patient has a NICRVO with gross macular edema as indicated by the cystoid accumulation of dye in the late phase.

CASE 5

A 55-year-old male presented with a history of decreased vision in both eyes for the past fifteen days. He was a known hypertensive for the past ten years on treatment. Visual acuity was 6/60; N36 in the right eye and 3/60 in the left eye. Investigations showed the patient to have hypergammaglobulinemia.

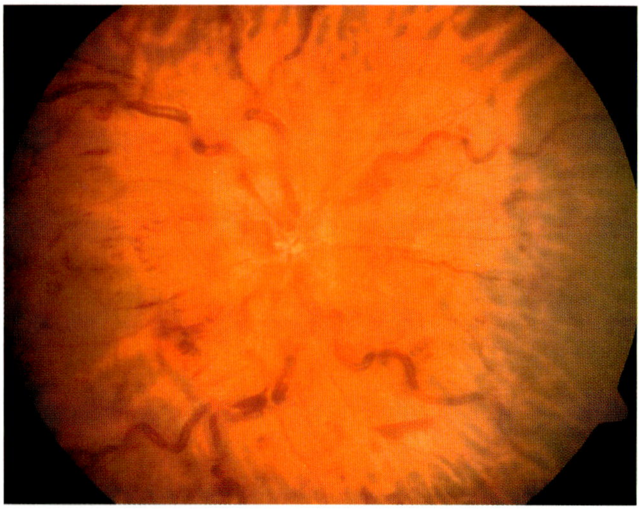

Fundus photograph of the right eye showing swelling of the disc with marked dilation and tortuosity of the veins

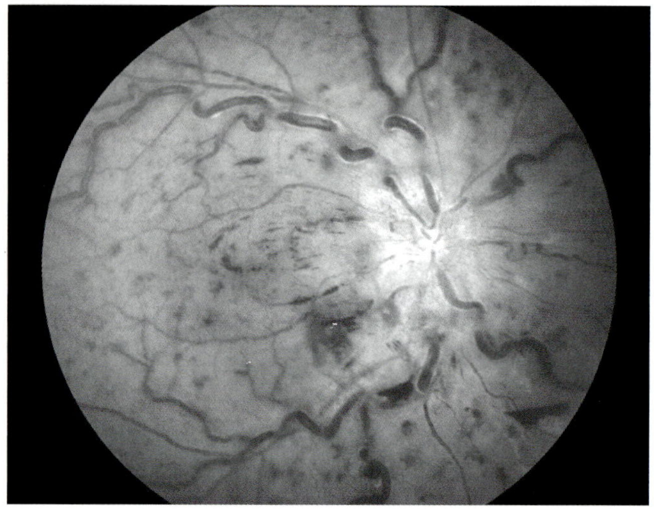

Red free photograph of the right eye

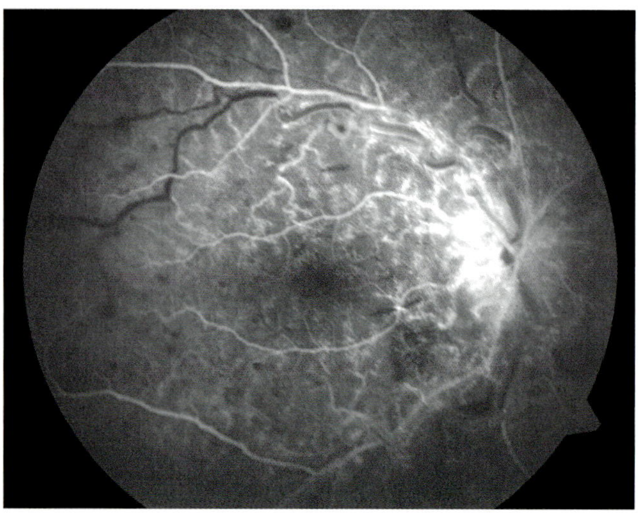

Marked delay in the filling of the veins is noted. Dilation of the capillaries is seen in the macula

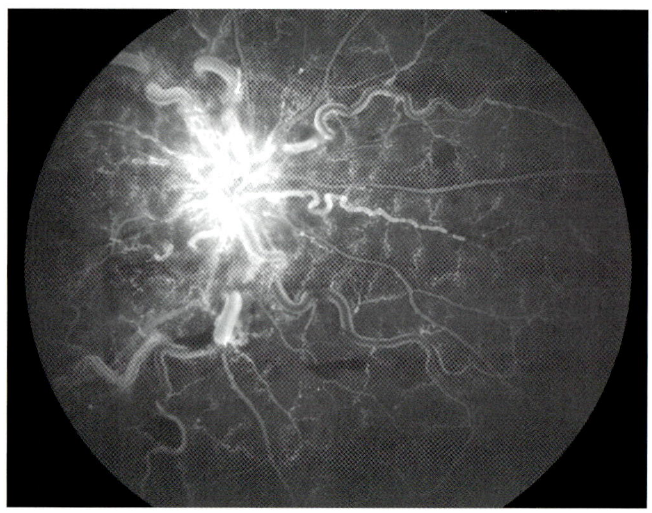

Dilation of the disc capillaries is seen. Extensive areas of capillary nonperfusion are seen in the midperiphery

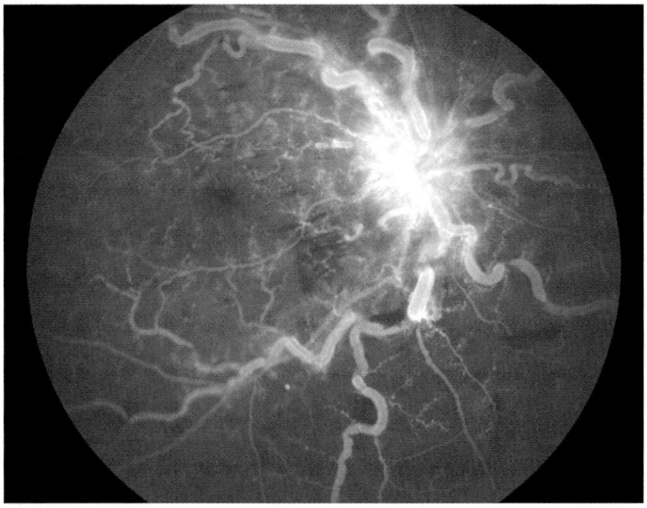

Extensive areas of capillary nonperfusion are seen. The parafoveal capillary network is affected

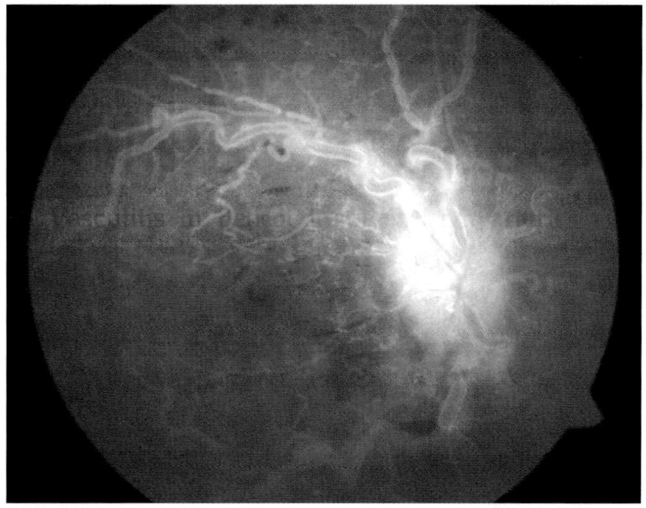

Increased staining of the disc and the walls of the veins is seen. The fovea remains hypofluorescent

CASE 5 (*Continued*)

Left Eye of the Patient

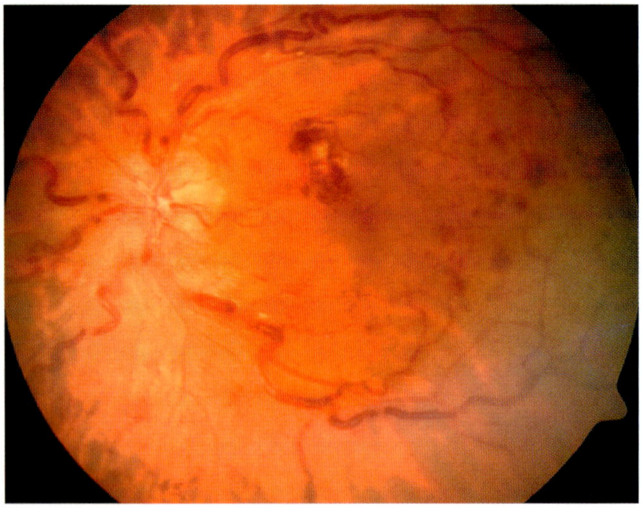

Fundus photograph of the left eye showing a similar picture as that in the right eye

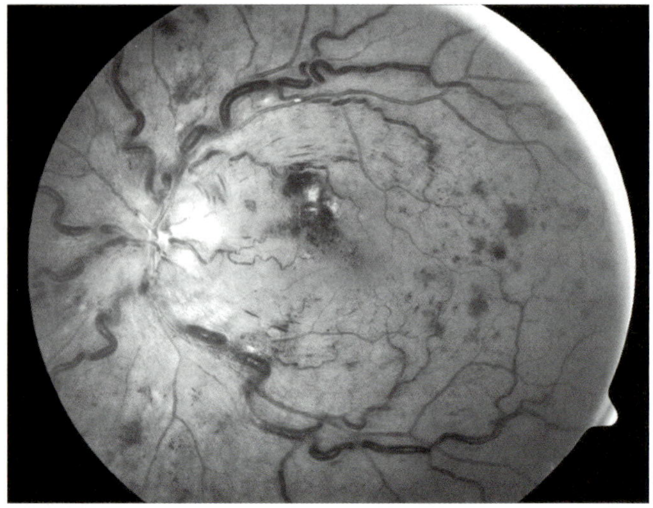

Red free photograph of the left eye

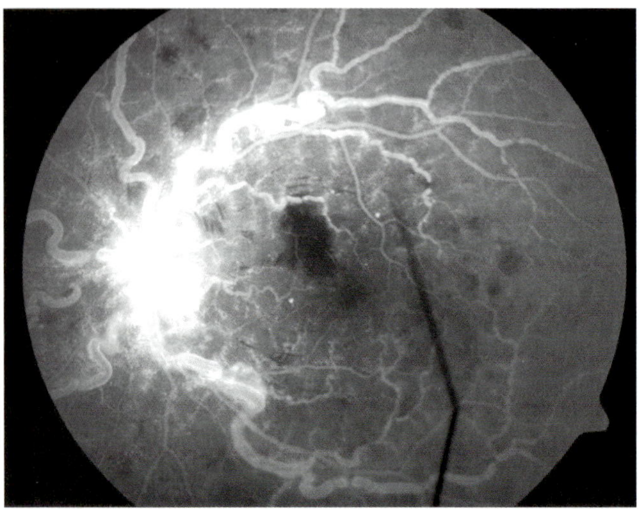

Marked dilation of the disc capillaries is seen. Extensive areas of capillary nonperfusion including the fovea are seen

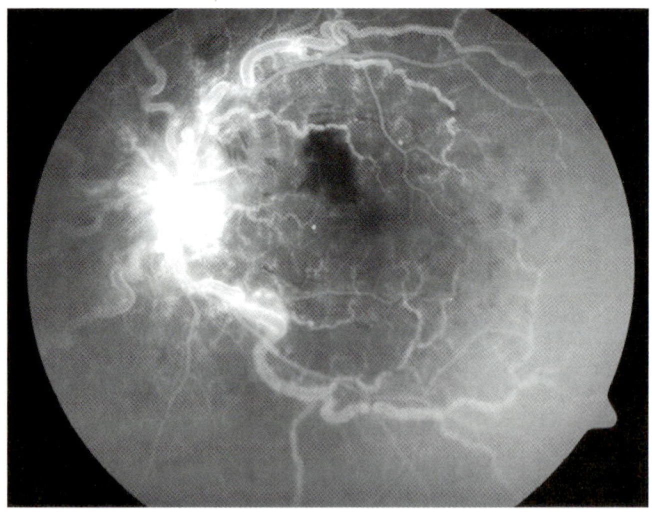

Staining of the disc and the walls of the veins is seen. The fovea remains hypofluorescent

COMMENT

- Patient has an ICRVO in both eyes with extensive areas of capillary non-perfusion seen in the midperiphery.
- Patients presenting with simultaneous bilateral CRVO should always be investigated for hematological disorders.

CASE 6

A 32-year-old male presented with reduced vision in the right eye of one month duration. Visual acuity was 3/60 in the right eye. Left eye was normal. Laboratory investigations were within normal limits.

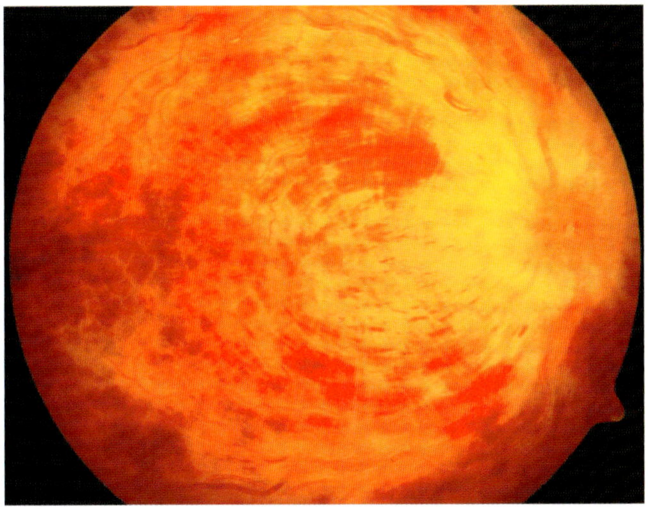

Fundus photograph of the right eye showing extensive superficial retinal hemorrhages

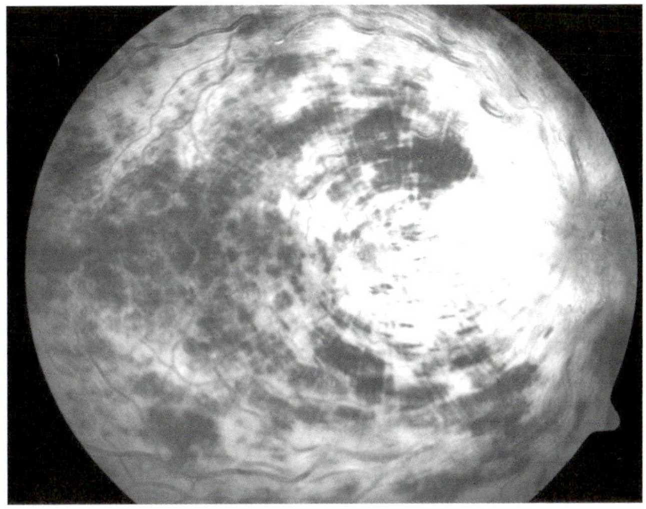

Red free photograph of the right eye

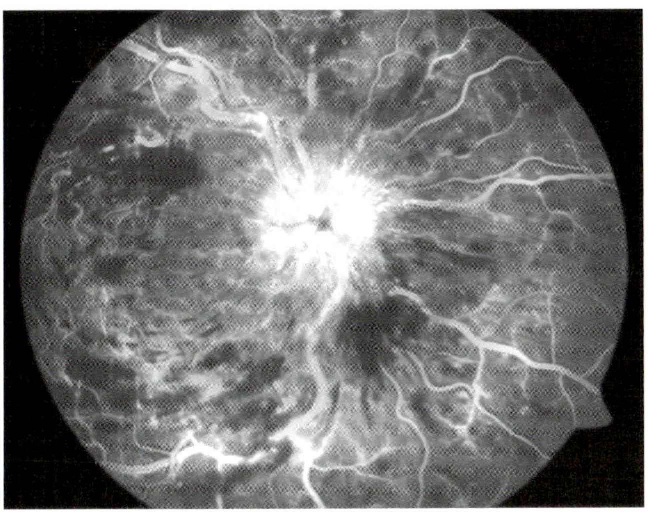

Dilation of the disc capillaries is seen. Areas of blocked fluorescence due to the retinal hemorrhages are seen

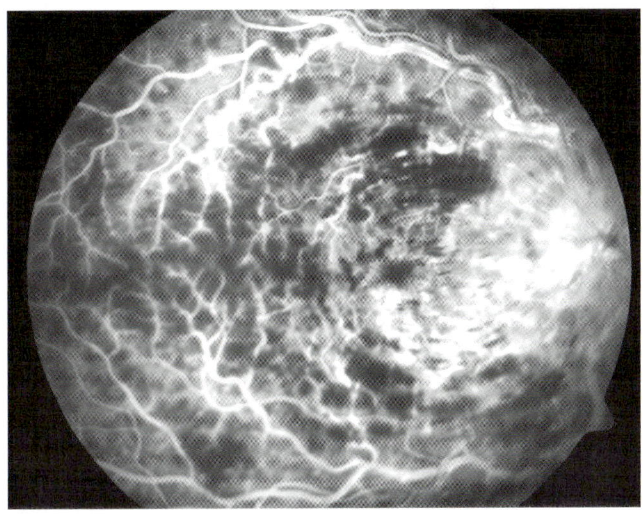

Extensive areas of blocked fluorescence due to retinal hemorrhages are seen

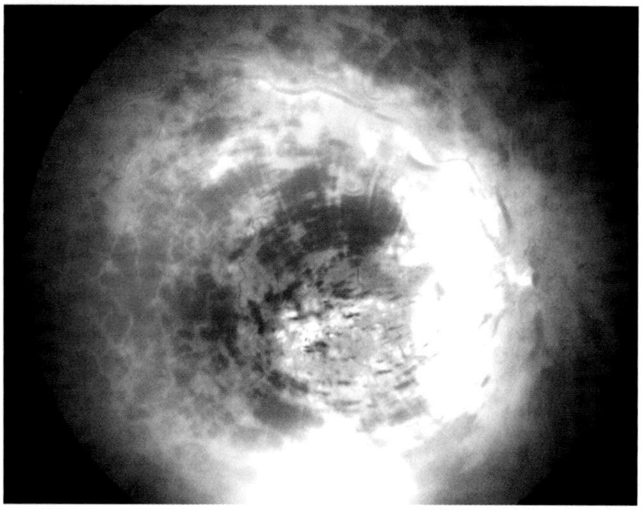

Marked staining of the retina throughout the posterior pole is seen

COMMENT

Fluorescein angiography is not very informative in the presence of extensive retinal hemorrhage as it blocks the underlying fluorescence.

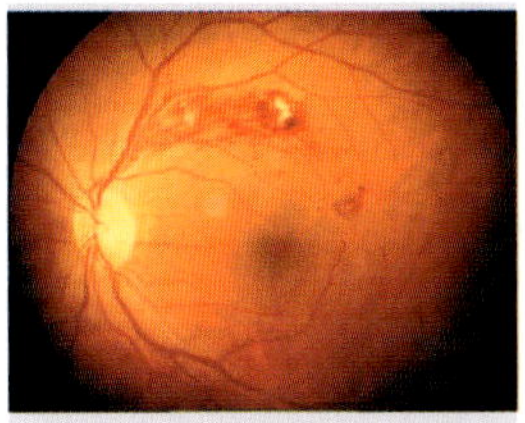

BRANCH RETINAL VEIN OCCLUSION

- Branch retinal vein occlusion (BRVO) is characterized by dilation and tortuosity of the affected vein associated with retinal hemorrhages, cotton-wool spots and edema in the area drained by the vein.

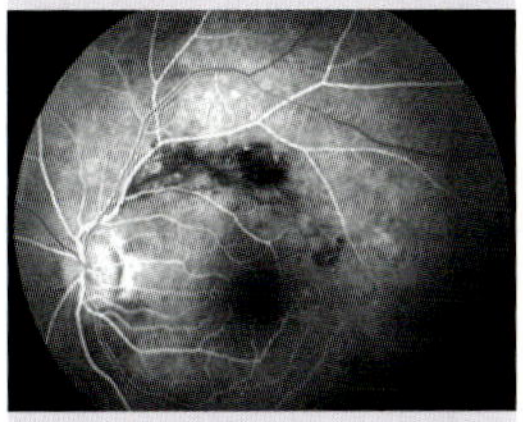

- Blocked fluorescence due to the retinal hemorrhages is seen through all phases of the angiogram.
- There is delayed filling and emptying of the affected vein.
- Dilated capillaries, microaneurysms and telangiectatic changes are well-made out on the angiogram.
- Areas of capillary closure may be present in the involved segment.
- Perfused BRVO—area of capillary closure is less than five disc areas.
- Nonperfused BRVO—area of capillary closure is more than five disc areas.
- Macular edema may be perfused, nonperfused or mixed.
  - Perfused macular edema—an intact parafoveal capillary network is seen during the arteriovenous phase, followed by late accumulation of the dye involving the foveal center.
  - Nonperfused macular edema—areas of parafoveal and perifoveal capillary nonperfusion are seen with no accumulation of the dye in the late phase.
  - Mixed macular edema—a combination of capillary dilation and leakage and areas of capillary nonperfusion in the parafoveal region. Late phase shows some degree of accumulation of the dye.
- Late staining and leakage from the affected veins is seen.

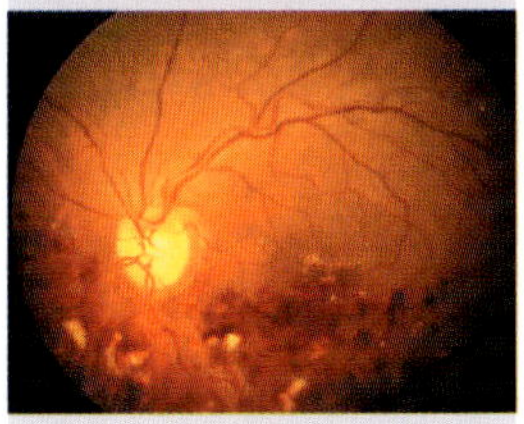

HEMICENTRAL RETINAL VEIN OCCLUSION (HCRVO)

- The two venous channels that develop during the third month of intrauterine life may fail to join in front of the lamina cribrosa—the two trunks travel inside the optic nerve independently for a considerable distance before joining. They are usually seen entering the optic nerve separately. Occlusion of one of the channels leads to a hemicentral retinal vein occlusion.

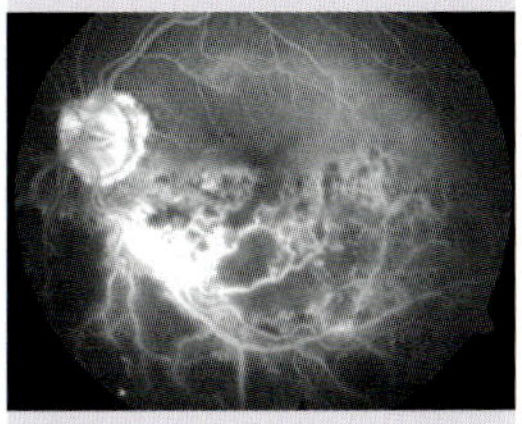

- Pattern is similar to CRVO except that only half the fundus area is involved.

CASE 7

A 56-year-old male hypertensive presented with mild blurring of vision in the right eye. Visual acuity was 6/6; N6 in both eyes.

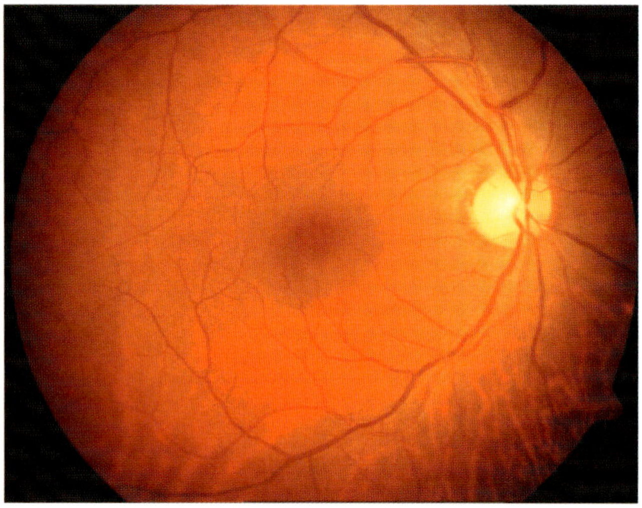

Fundus photograph of the right eye

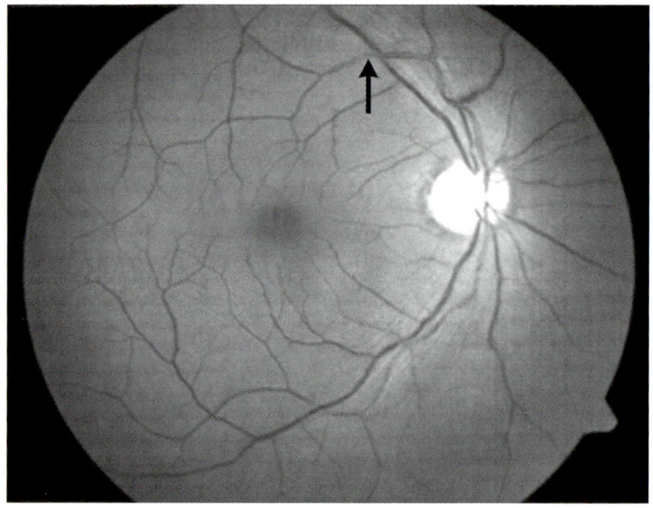

Red free photograph of the right eye. Note the small deflection of the vein seen at the first A-V crossing (arrow) superotemporal to the disc

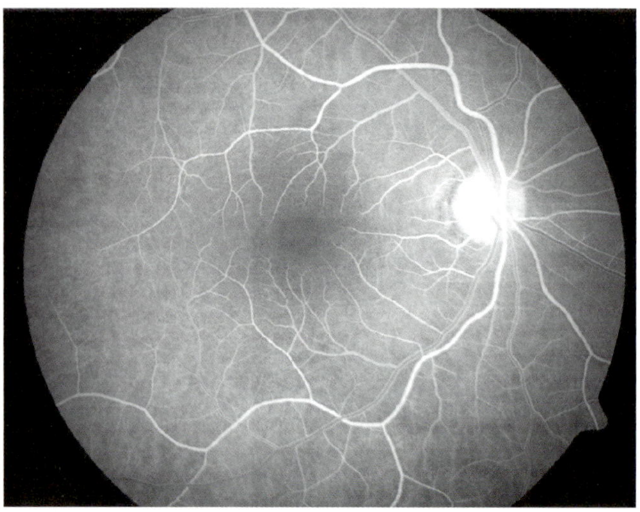

Early arteriovenous phase of the angiogram. Laminar flow is seen in the superotemporal vein up to the A-V crossing only

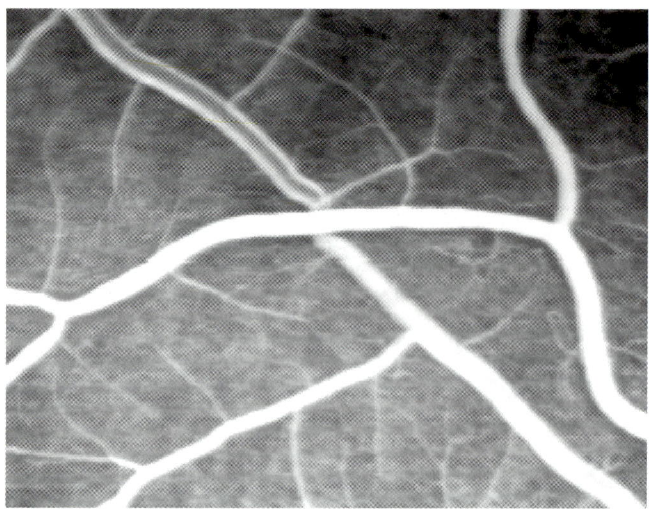

Magnified view of the A-V crossing. Note the absence of laminar flow proximal to the A-V crossing indicating turbulence of flow due to compression of the vein at the crossing

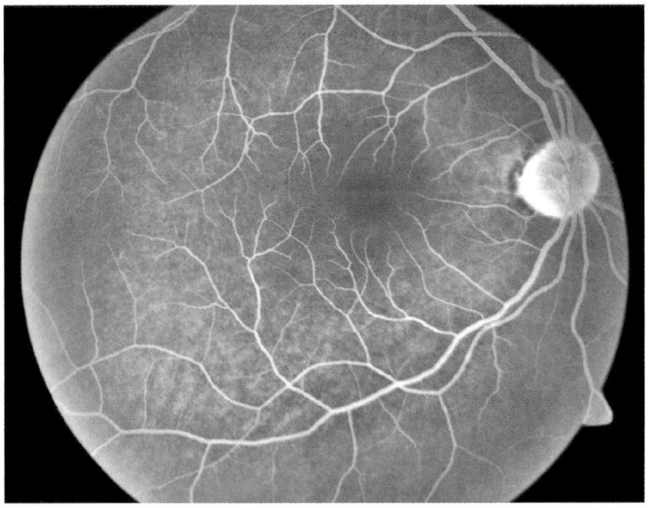

Late phase angiogram picture of the right eye

COMMENT

Disturbance of the laminar flow in the vein at the AV crossing indicates turbulence of flow due to vein compression at the crossing.

CASE 8

A 48-year-old male presented with a history of disturbance of vision in the left eye of 3 days duration. He was on medication for systemic hypertension for the past two years and was noted to have raised serum cholesterol. Visual acuity was 6/6; N6 in the left eye. The right eye was normal.

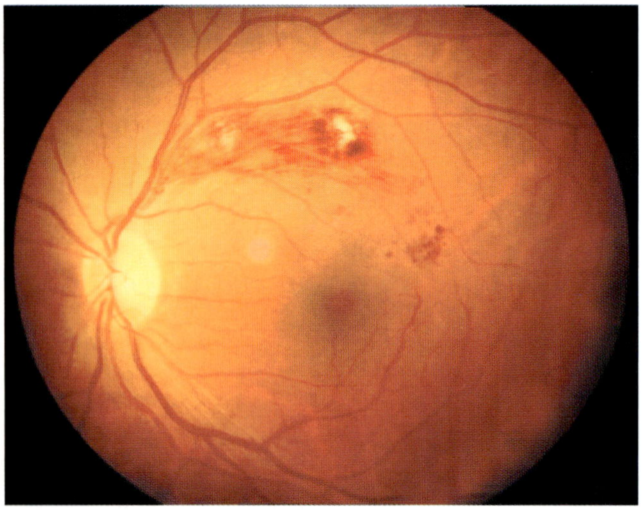

Fundus photograph of the left eye showing a small tributary vein occlusion superotemporal to the disc

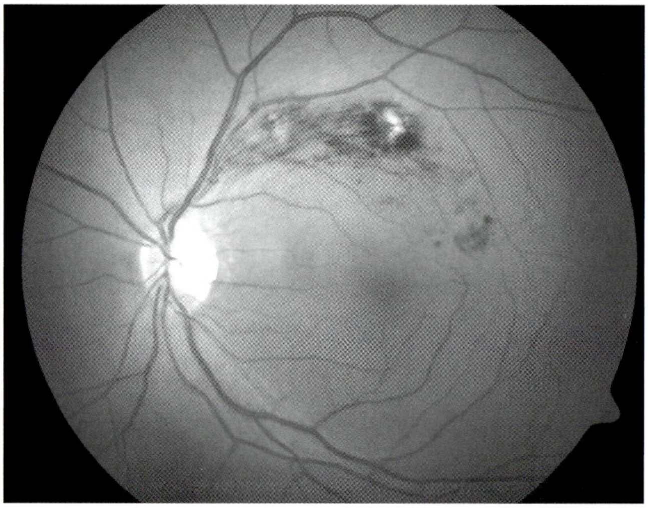

Red free photograph showing superficial retinal hemorrhages and cotton-wool spots along the affected segment

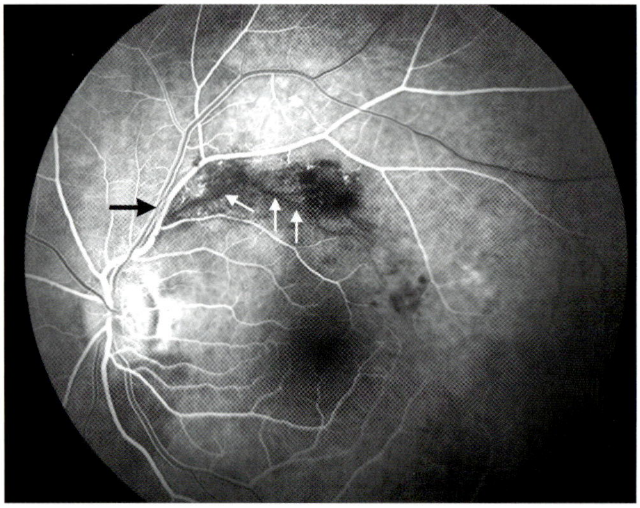

Early arteriovenous phase showing delayed filling of the affected vein (white arrows). The site of occlusion at the AV crossing is well seen (black arrow)

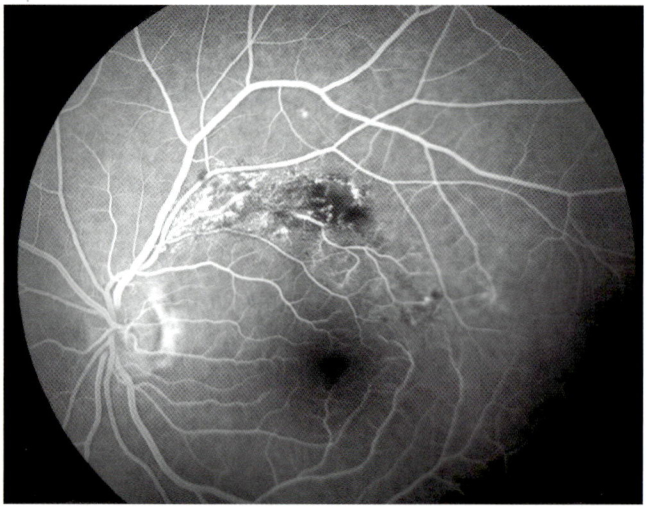

The affected vein has filled up. Blocked fluorescence is seen due to the retinal hemorrhages

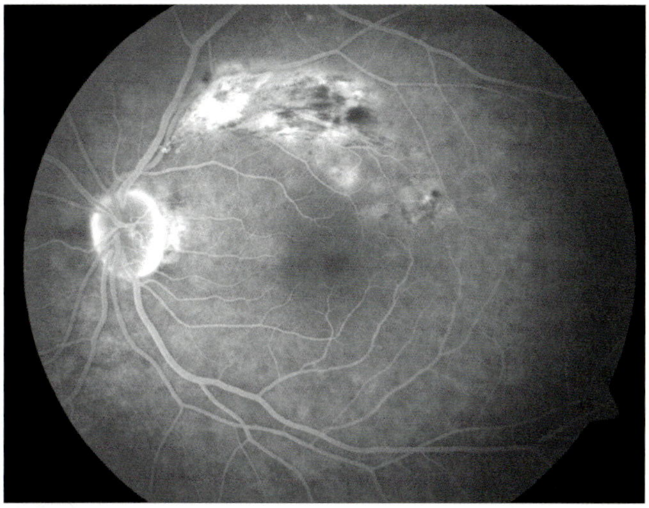

Late phase angiogram showing staining of the retina in the affected segment

COMMENT

A macular tributary vein occlusion involves a small segment of the retina and does not give rise to significant ischemic changes. Vision however, is compromised if the FAZ is involved. Fluorescein angiogram is useful to assess the status of the FAZ.

CLINICAL NUGGETS

1. Bilateral simultaneous central retinal vein occlusion is more common in patients with underlying systemic disorders.
2. Laser photocoagulation has not been found to be useful for the treatment of macular edema secondary to a central retinal vein occlusion.
3. Patients with CRVO should be followed up on a monthly basis to look for the development of ocular neovascularization; if so, panretinal photocoagulation is performed.

VENOUS OCCLUSIONS

Practice since 2 decades

Until recently, the options for retinal vein occlusion therapy were limited. The standard of care was defined by two twenty-year-old clinical studies, BVOS (Branch Vein Occlusion Study) and CVOS (Central Vein Occlusion Study).

Studies which would change the practice

Overview of these studies

SCORE Study

- The SCORE study showed that for CRVO, triamcinolone was superior to observation both initially and at one and two years.[4]
- The SCORE study also showed that for BRVO, laser was better than triamcinolone at one, two, and three years.[5]
- In terms of IOP effects, in the CRVO study 7 percent of the standard care group, 18 percent of the 1 mg group, and 32 percent of the 4 mg group required IOP medicines.[4]
- In the BRVO study 3 percent of the standard care group, 11 percent of the 1 mg group, and 57 percent of the 4 mg group needed IOP medicines.[5]

Ozurdex Study

- The Ozurdex/Geneva study compared a 700 μg biodegradable implant injected intravitreally versus a sham in both CRVO and BRVO patients. This six-month study was followed by a six-month open-label follow-up.[6]
- The data showed significance in terms of mean visual acuity versus sham, and more patients gained 15 letters with Ozurdex versus sham, and Ozurdex patients lost fewer letters versus sham.
- The Ozurdex group had a peak gain in vision at day 60 and, although this later dipped, maintained an increase of mean visual acuity versus sham for six months.
- When patients were reinjected, they achieved the same increase or better gain in visual acuity in the second six months as they did in the first six months
- In addition, in 20 percent of patients only one injection was needed to get to 20/20 vision and OCT<250 microns, and no other injections were needed for the entire course of the one-year study.
- In terms of IOP, 15 percent had an IOP elevation over 25 at day 60; this was reduced to 1.2 percent by day 180.

CRUISE and BRAVO Study

- The BRAVO[7] and CRUISE[8] studies were 12-month studies to observe the effectiveness of intravitreal injections of ranibizumab to treat retinal vein occlusion.
- The BRAVO[7] data showed at six months that the mean visual improvement was 18.3 letters in the 0.5 mg group, 16.6 in the 0.3 mg group vs 7.3 letters in the sham group.
- In addition approximately 60% of patients in the 0.5 mg group gained 3 lines of vision as opposed to 7.3 in the sham group.
- The CRUISE[8] study had similar six-month results, with patients gaining 14.9 letters in the 0.5 mg group, 12.7 letters in the 0.3 mg group vs 0.8 letters in the sham group, with 47% of patients in the 0.5 and 0.3 mg groups gaining 3 lines of vision vs 16.9% in the sham cohort.
- In both the BRAVO and CRUISE studies patients had monthly injections in the first six months. The twelve-month data showed that these effects were sustained with an average of approximately three additional injections.
- There were no cases of IOP elevation in either the BRAVO or the CRUISE studies.

Results (Tables 1 and 2)

- The SCORE Study showed that Trivaris is better than observation for CRVO.
- For BRVO, although Trivaris showed better results initially, the laser (standard-care) group caught up, and by one year laser treatment was superior to steroids. This superiority continued in years two and three.
- The 12-month Ozurdex/Geneva data showed that patients randomized to the sham group never achieved visual results that were as good as those who had treatment early, even after they crossed over from sham to active treatment.
- In the BRAVO and CRUISE studies patients had excellent results with monthly injections in the first six months. The patients randomized to sham although they improved when they were given ranibizumab during the second six months never achieved the same level of visual improvement as the initially treated patients.
- This finding, which is seen in both the Ozurdex/Geneva and the BRAVO/CRUISE studies, suggests that chronicity of disease has an effect on final visual prognosis. What is not known in all of these studies is how long you have to continue these therapies, and how does laser fit into the equation?

Table 1: Summary of functional and anatomical outcome in treatment of CRVO

	*Functional outcome (%)**	*Anatomical outcome***
SCORE -Standard care	7	304 μ
IVTA (1 mg)	27	286 μ
IVTA (4 mg)	26	236 μ
OZURDEX (0.75 mg)	22	119 μ
CRUISE (0.5 mg)	46.2	452 μ

SCORE: The Standard Care Versus Corticosteroid for Retinal Vein Occlusion
IVTA: Intravitreal Ttrimacinolone Acetonide
CRUISE: Central Retinal Vein Occlusion Study: Evaluation of Efficacy and Safety
Functional outcome: Percentage of patients gaining 15 letters in BCVA at final fo up*
*Anatomical outcome**: Mean decrease in central foveal thickness at final fo up*

Table 2: Summary of functional and anatomical outcome in treatment of BRVO

	*Functional outcome (%)**	*Anatomical outcome***
SCORE -Standard care	28.9	113 μ
IVTA (1 mg)	25.6	77 μ
IVTA (4 mg)	27.2	142 μ
OZURDEX (0.75 mg)	22	119 μ
BRAVO (0.5 mg)	61.1	345 μ

SCORE: The Standard Care versus Corticosteroid for Retinal Vein Occlusion
IVTA: Intravitreal Ttrimacinolone Acetonide
BRAVO: Ranibizumab for the treatment of macular edema following Branch Retinal Vein Occlusion: Evaluation of Efficacy and Safety
Functional outcome: Percentage of patients gaining 15 letters in BCVA at final fo up*
*Anatomical outcome**: Mean decrease in central foveal thickness at final fo up*

BIBLIOGRAPHY

1. A randomized clinical trial of early panretinal photocoagulation for ischemic central vein occlusion: the Central Vein Occlusion Study Group N Report. Ophthalmology 1995;102:143-4.
2. A randomized trial comparing the efficacy and safety of intravitreal triamcinolone with *standard care* to treat vision loss associated with macular Edema secondary to branch retinal vein occlusion: the Standard Care vs Corticosteroid for Retinal Vein Occlusion (SCORE) study report 6. Scott IU, Ip MS, VanVeldhuisen PC, Oden NL, Blodi BA, Fisher M, Chan CK, Gonzalez VH, Singerman LJ, Tolentino M; SCORE Study Research Group. Arch Ophthalmol. 2009 Sep;127(9):1115-28.
3. Ip MS, Oden NL, Scott IU, et al. SCORE Study Report 3: study design and baseline characteristics [published online July 21, 2009]. Ophthalmology. doi:10.1016/j. ophtha.2009.03.022.
4. Randomized, sham-controlled trial of dexamethasone intravitreal implant in patients with macular edema due to retinal vein occlusion. Haller JA, Bandello F, Belfort R Jr, Blumenkranz MS, Gillies M, Heier J, Loewenstein A, Yoon YH, Jacques ML, Jiao J, Li XY, Whitcup SM; OZURDEX GENEVA Study Group. Ophthalmology. 2010 Jun; 117(6):1134-1146.e3. Epub 2010 Apr 24
5. Ranibizumab for macular edema following branch retinal vein occlusion: six-month primary end point results of a phase III study. Campochiaro PA, Heier JS, Feiner L, Gray S, Saroj N, Rundle AC, Murahashi WY, Rubio RG; BRAVO Investigators. Ophthalmology. 2010 Jun;117(6):1102-1112.e1. Epub 2010 Apr 15.
6. Ranibizumab for macular edema following central retinal vein occlusion: six-month primary end point results of a phase III study. Brown DM, Campochiaro PA, Singh RP, Li Z, Gray S, Saroj N, Rundle AC, Rubio RG, Murahashi WY; CRUISE Investigators. Ophthalmology. 2010 Jun;117(6):1124-1133.e1. Epub 2010 Apr 9.
7. The Branch Vein Occlusion Study Group Argon laser photocoagulation for macular edema in branch vein occlusion. Am J Ophthalmol. 1984; 98271–282.
8. The Central Vein Occlusion Study Group Evaluation of grid pattern photocoagulation for macular edema in central vein occlusion. Ophthalmology. 1995; 102: 1425–33.
9. The SCORE Study Research Group. A randomized trial comparing the efficacy and safety of intravitreal triamcinolone with observation to treat vision loss associated with macular edema secondary to central retinal vein occlusion: The Standard Care vs Corticosteroid for Retinal Vein Occlusion (SCORE) Study Report 5. Arch Ophthalmol. 2009;127(9):1101-14.

30 Chapter

Ocular Ischemic Syndrome

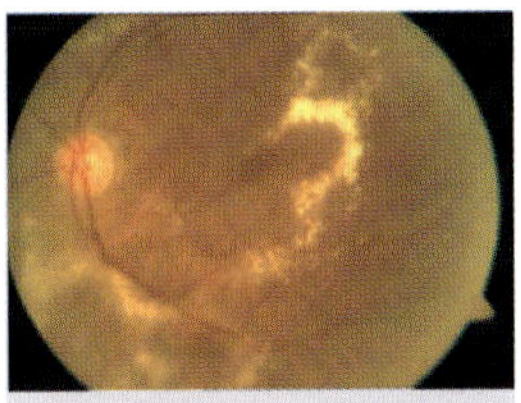

- Ocular ischemic syndrome occurs in 5 percent of patients with severe carotid artery insufficiency or thrombosis. Either eye can be affected, and in approximately 20 percent of patients, ocular involvement is bilateral.
- It has been shown that a 90 percent carotid stenosis reduces the ipsilateral central retinal artery perfusion pressure by about 50 percent. Greater than 90 percent of patients with ocular ischemic syndrome relate a history of visual loss in the affected eye(s). Dull aching pain is present in the affected eye or orbital region in about 40 percent of cases
- Anterior segment signs include rubeosis. However, intraocular pressure rise occurs in only half of them, despite angle occlusion by fibrovascular tissue. This is due to ciliary body hypoperfusion. There may be anterior segment reaction and a variable amount of asymmetric cataract depending on the site of involvement.
- The retinal arteries are usually narrowed and the retinal veins are most often dilated, but not tortuous. Retinal hemorrhages mostly dot and blot, are seen in about 80 percent of affected eyes. They are most commonly present in the midperiphery area. Microaneurysms are frequently observed outside the posterior pole, but can be seen in the macular region also. Posterior segment neovascularization can occur at the optic disc or on the retina.

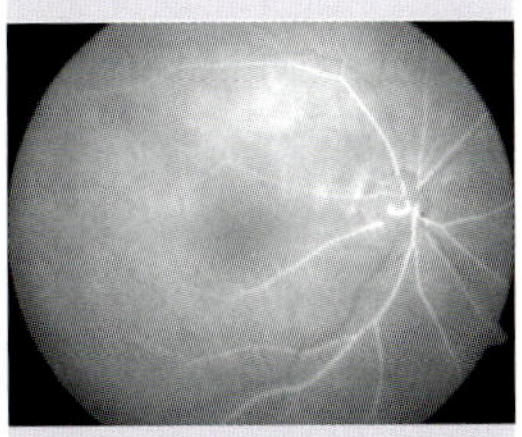

- Delayed arm to retina circulation time is frequently seen in OIS
- The observation of a well-demarcated, leading edge of fluorescein dye within a retinal artery after an intravenous injection is a distinctly unusual finding. It can be seen in eyes with the ocular ischemic syndrome, secondary to hypoperfusion
- Sixty percent of eyes with the ocular ischemic syndrome demonstrate patchy and/or delayed choroidal filling. In late phases, staining of retinal vessels (both arteries and veins) is seen due to chronic hypoxic damage to endothelial cells.
- Infrequently, there is also a presence of macular edema. Retinal capillary nonperfusion can be seen in some eyes.

CASE 1

A 23-year-old male (known case of Takayasu's arteritis with hypertension) presented with defective vision in the right eye since 2 months. Visual acuity was CF in the right eye and 6/36 in the left. Anterior segment evaluation revealed rubeosis iris, neovascularization of angles and elevated IOP. The patient underwent 3 sessions of panretinal photocoagulation and was initiated on topical antiglaucoma treatment.

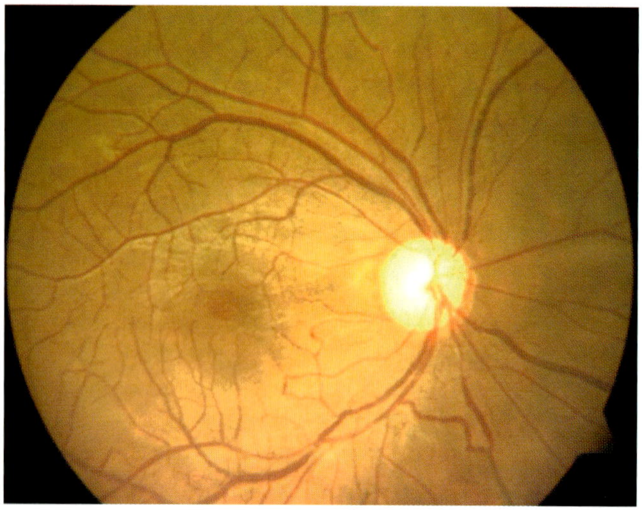

Right color fundus photograph shows dilated retinal veins and arteriovenous anastomotic channels (inferior to the disc)

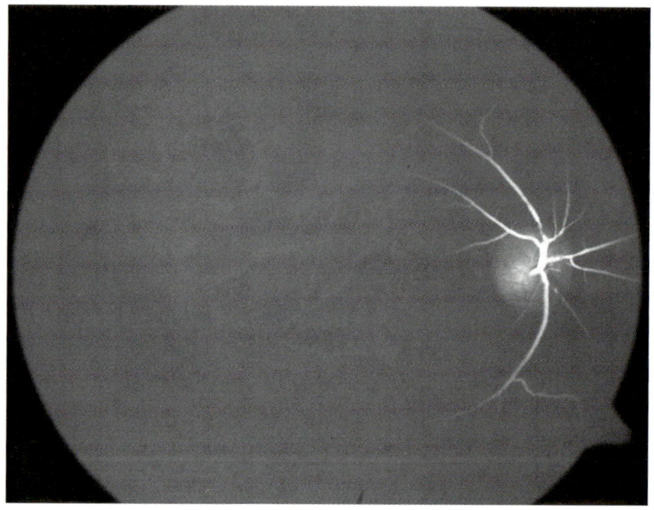

FA (early phase) shows increased arm to retina circulation (normal-10 sec) time and absence of choroidal filling

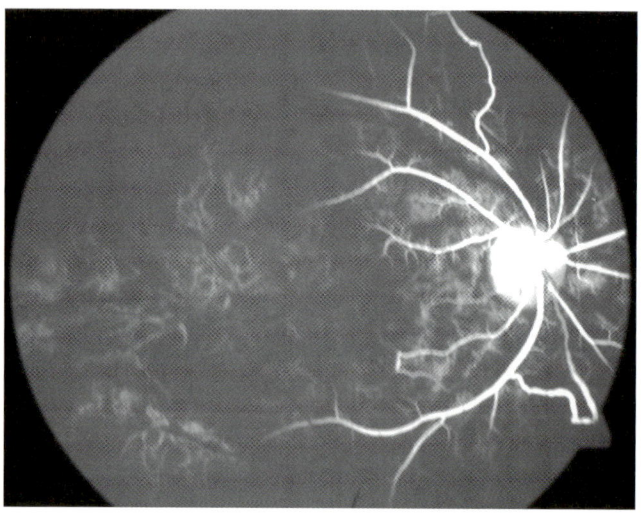

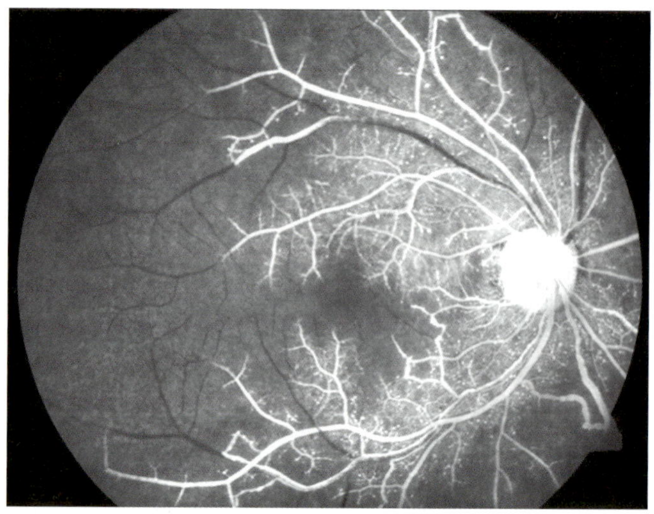

FA (early and midphases) show patchy choroidal filling, delayed A-V transit with classic sign of leading edge of fluorescein dye in the retinal arterioles and macular ischemia

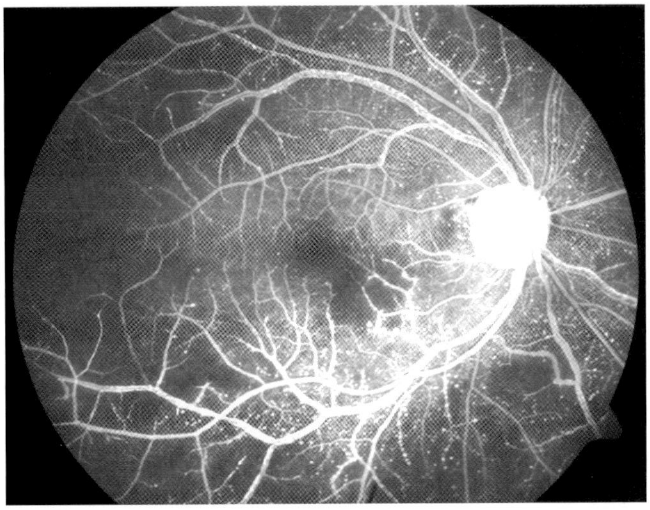

FA (late A-V phase) shows multiple pinpoint hyperfluorescent spots suggestive of microaneurysms

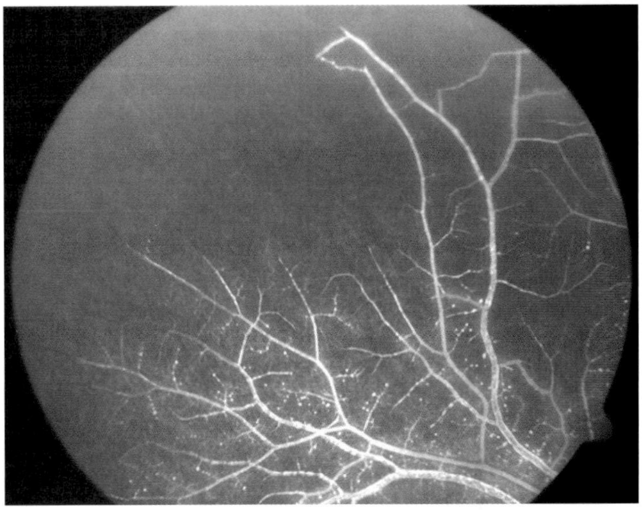

Peripheral fundus shows capillary nonperfusion areas distal to arteriovenous anastomotic channels

BIBLIOGRAPHY

1. Brown GC, Magargal LE. The ocular ischaemic syndrome. Clinical, fluorescein angiographic and carotid angiographic features. Int Ophthalmol 1988; 11:239.
2. Costa VP, Kuzniec S, Molnar LJ, et al. Clinical findings and hemodynamic changes associated with severe occlusive carotid artery disease. Ophthalmology 1997; 104: 1994-02.
3. Mizener JB, Podhajsky P, Hayreh SS. Ocular ischemic syndrome. Ophthalmology 1997; 104:859-64.
4. North American Symptomatic Carotid Endarterectomy Trial Collaborators. Beneficial effect of carotid endarterectomy in symptomatic patients with high-grade carotid stenosis. N Engl J Med 1991; 325: 445-53.
5. Riordan-Eva P, Restori M, Hamilton AM, et al. Orbital ultrasound in ocular ischaemic syndrome. Eye 1994; 8: 93-6.
6. Ros MA, Margargal LE, Hedges Jr TR, et al. Ocular ischaemia: long term complications. Ann Ophthalmol 1987; 19:270-2.
7. Sharma T, Khare B, Sharma R, Shanmugam MP, Gopal L. Vitrectomy in takayasu's disease. Indian J Ophthalmol 1999; 47: 126-9.
8. Sivalingam A, Brown GC, Magargal LE. The ocular ischaemic syndrome. Visual prognosis and the effect of treatment. Int Ophthalmol 1991; 15: 15-20.
9. Uyama M, Asayama K. Retinal vascular changes in Takayasu disease (pulseless disease), occurrence and evaluation of the lesion. Doc Ophthalmol Proc Ser 1976; 9: 549-54.

Chapter 31

Eales' Disease

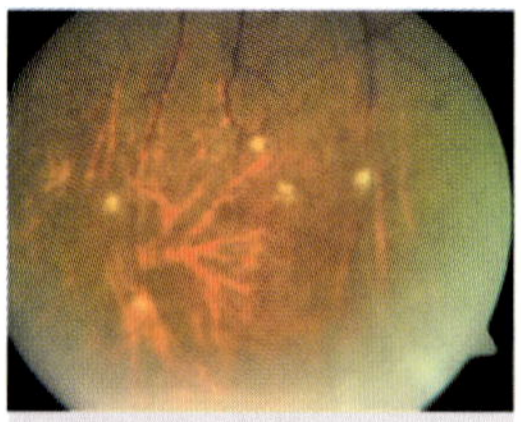

- Common clinical condition in the Indian subcontinent typically affecting young healthy males.
- Idiopathic retinal periphlebitis in the active stage is more commonly seen in the periphery. This leads to areas of capillary nonperfusion which may lead to the development of neovascularization.
- Recurrent vitreous hemorrhage is common.
- Rarely the larger posterior veins are involved and the patient may present with a branch retinal vein or a central retinal vein occlusion.

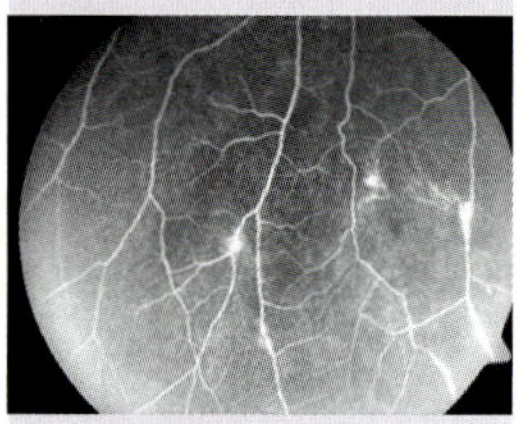

- Narrowing of the lumen may be seen in the areas of active periphlebitis.
- The wall of the vein in the affected part stains and leaks dye in the late phase of the angiogram.
- Areas of capillary nonperfusion are seen in the periphery. Associated vascular abnormalities like collaterals are also common.
- Neovascularization is commonly seen in the periphery.

CASE 1

A 33-year-old male presented with a history of reduced vision in the left eye for the past one year. Visual acuity was 3/60. The right eye had 6/5; N6 visual acuity and showed few areas of peripheral vascular sheathing.

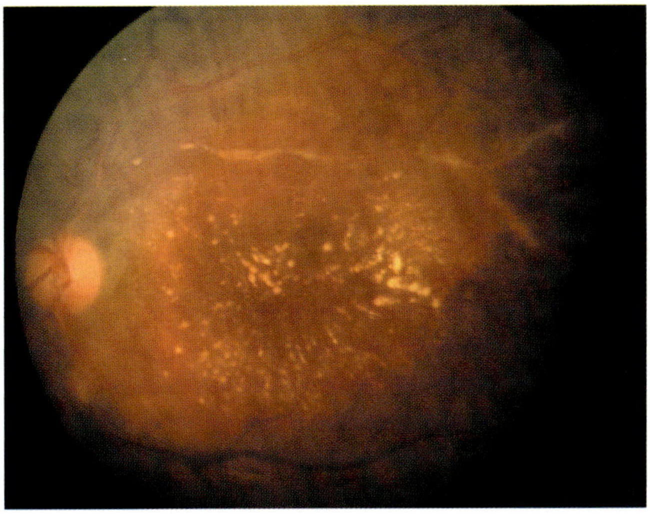

Fundus photograph of the left eye showing a sheathed superotemporal vessel. Hard exudates are seen in the macula

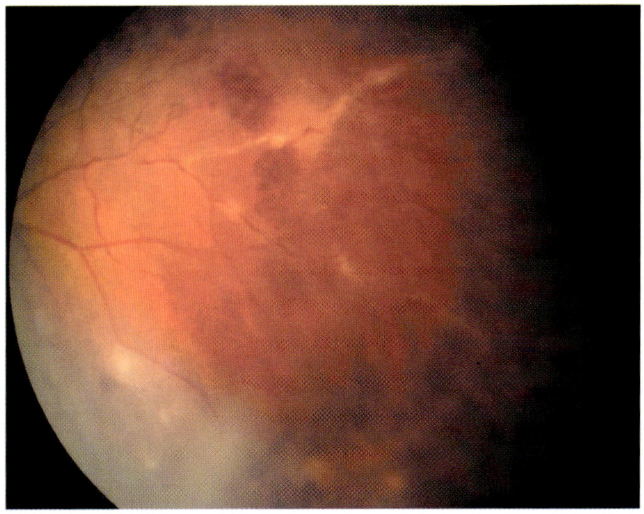

Fundus photograph of the temporal periphery showing areas of resolving periphlebitis

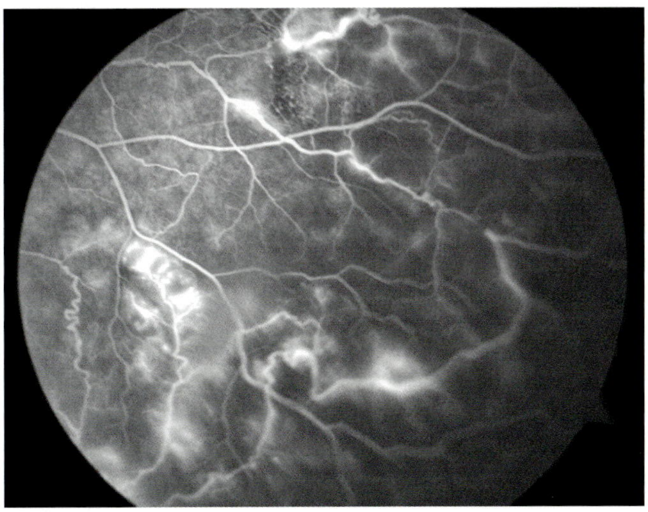

Arteriovenous phase showing leakage of the dye from the vessel walls. Areas of capillary nonperfusion are seen

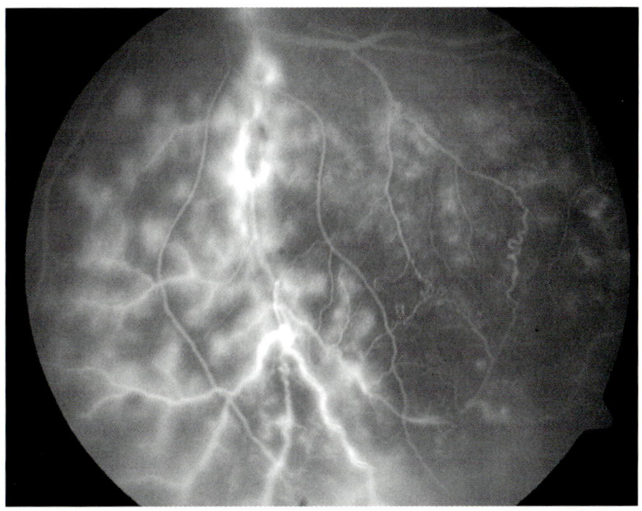

Extensive leakage of the dye from the walls of the veins and its draining channels is seen. The arterioles are unaffected

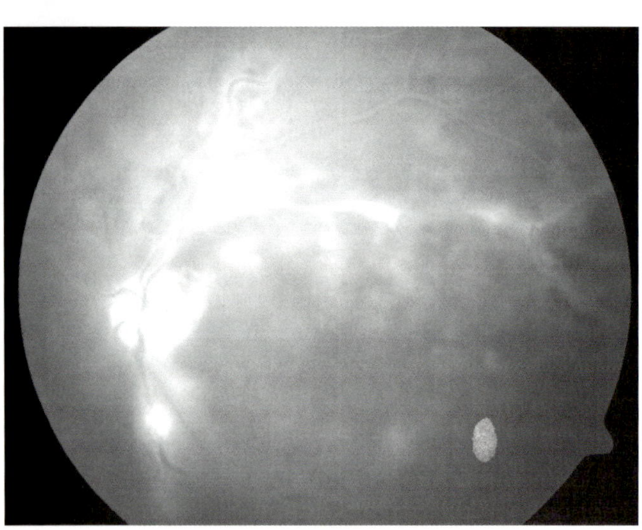

Late phase shows extensive staining of the vessel walls and the adjacent retina

COMMENT

Active stage of Eales' disease is characterized by periphlebitis which causes leakage of dye and staining of the walls of the vein.

Eales' disease predominantly affects the peripheral veins but can also involve the larger posterior veins.

CASE 2

A 30-year-old male presented with minimal blurring of vision in the left eye. Visual acuity was 6/5; N6 in both eyes. Vitreous cells were seen in both eyes.

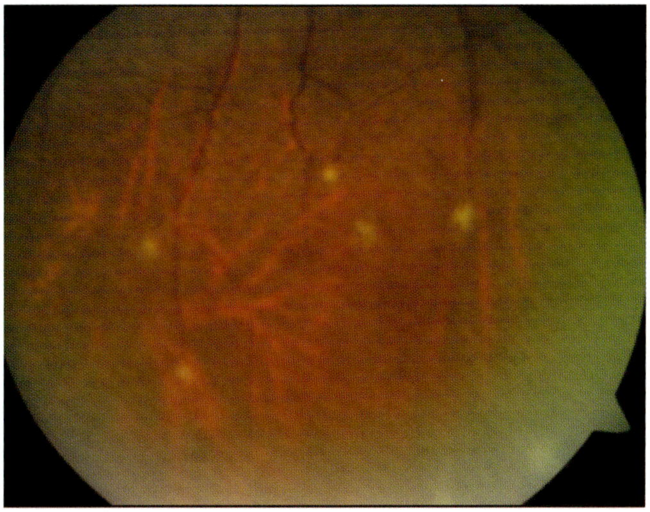

Fundus photograph of the right eye showing multiple foci of active periphlebitis in the inferior periphery

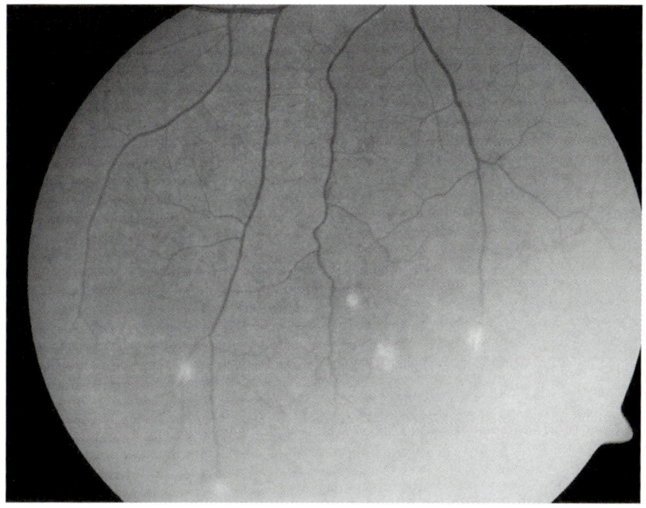

Red free photograph shows the active cuffs of periphlebitis

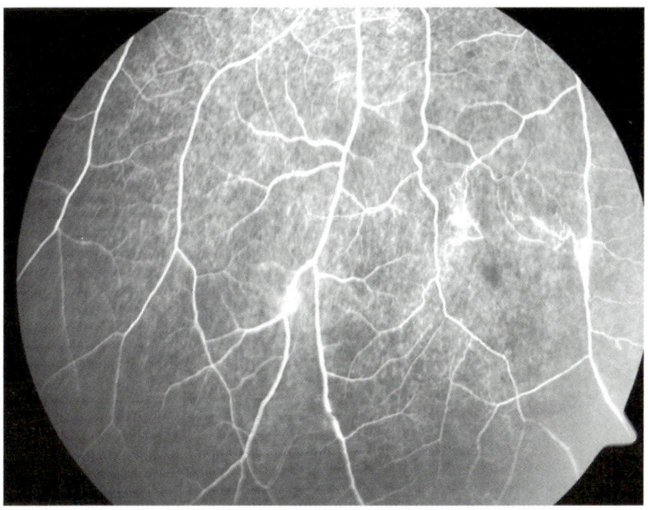

Minimal leakage of the dye is noted through the walls of the vein in the areas of perivasculitis. Areas of capillary nonperfusion are seen

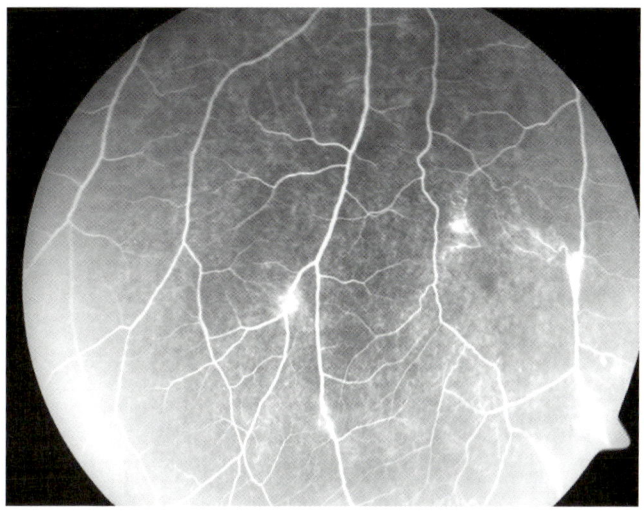

The leakage of dye in the areas of perivasculitis has increased

CASE 2 (*Continued*)

Left Eye of the Patient

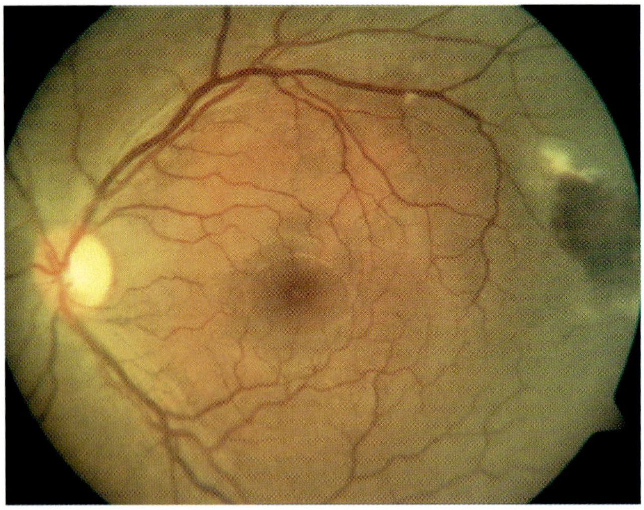

Fundus photograph of the left eye of the same patient showing an area of superficial retinal hemorrhage temporally with areas of active periphlebitis

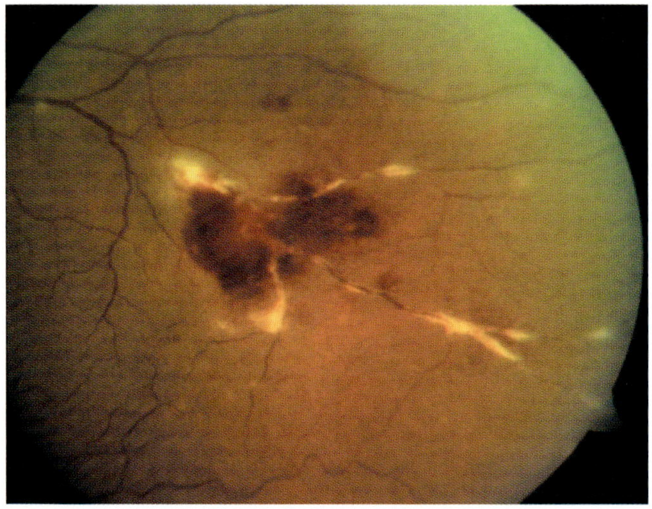

The active periphlebitis is well seen in this fundus photograph

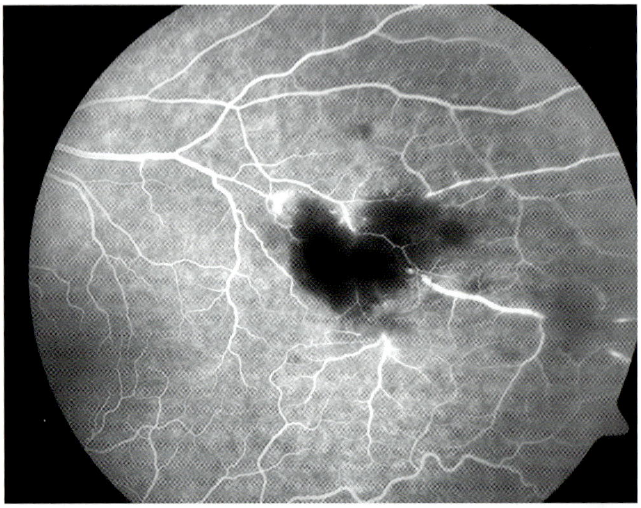

Arteriovenous phase shows blocked retinal and choroidal fluorescence in the region of the retinal hemorrhage. The vessel wall in the areas of active perivasculitis appears more hyperfluorescent. Areas of capillary nonperfusion are noted peripheral to the areas of periphlebitis

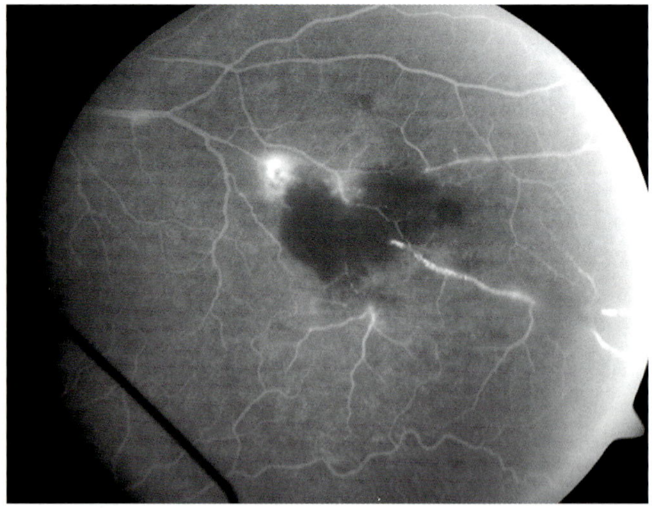

Increased staining of the vessel wall is seen in the late phase

COMMENT

Periphlebitis can lead to retinal hemorrhages and can even cause a vitreous hemorrhage.

CASE 3

A 41-year-old male was examined for floaters noticed in front of both eyes for the past two years. Visual acuity was 6/6; N6 in both eyes.

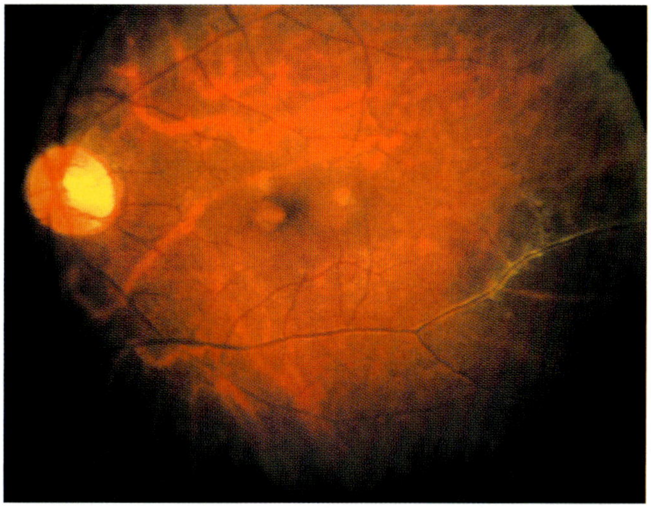

Fundus photograph of the left eye showing small patches of RPE atrophy around the foveal center. Sheathing of the inferotemporal vein is seen in the periphery

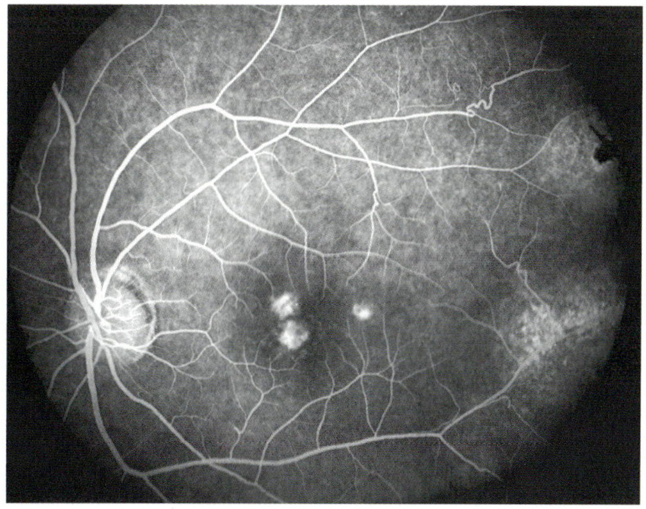

Arteriovenous phase showing hyperfluorescence in the areas of atrophy due to transmission window defect. Stippled hyperfluorescence is seen around the vein temporally

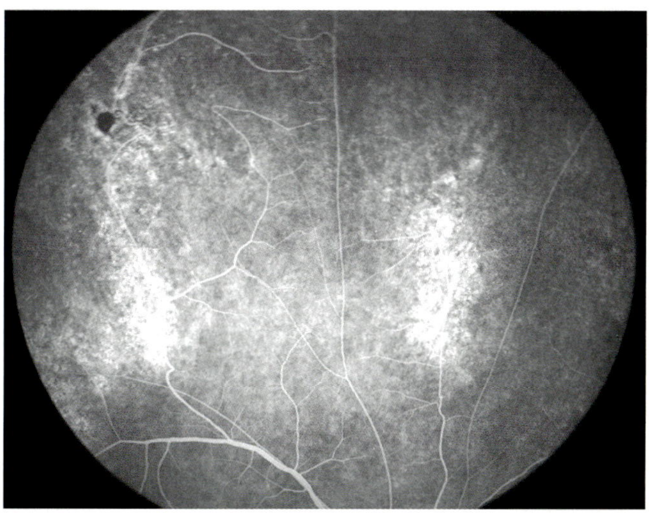

Stippled hyperfluorescence is seen along the veins in the superior periphery

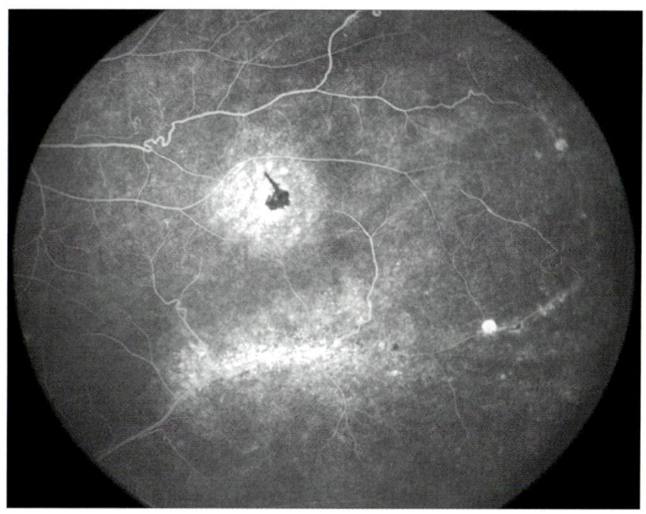

Similar changes are seen temporally. Aneurysmal dilatation is seen peripherally. An area of blocked fluorescence is seen due to RPE hypertrophy

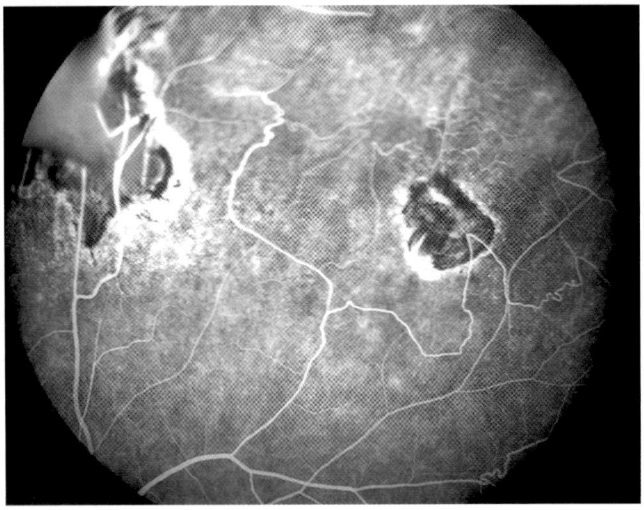

Areas of hypofluorescence surrounded by a ring of hyperfluorescence are seen superiorly corresponding to the 'sun-burst' like lesion seen clinically

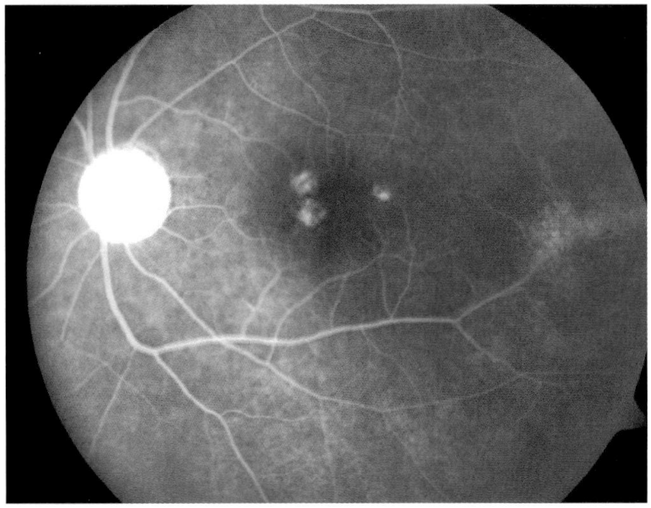

Late phase photograph showing fading of the hyperfluorescence in the atrophic patches at the fovea

CASE 4

A 36-year-old patient presented with an episode of decreased vision one year back following which the vision had cleared. Visual acuity was 6/6; N6 in both eyes.

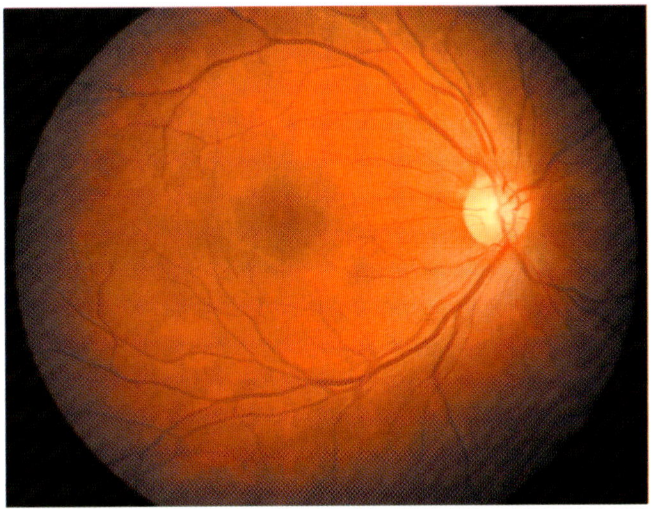

Fundus photograph of the right eye showing the normal posterior pole

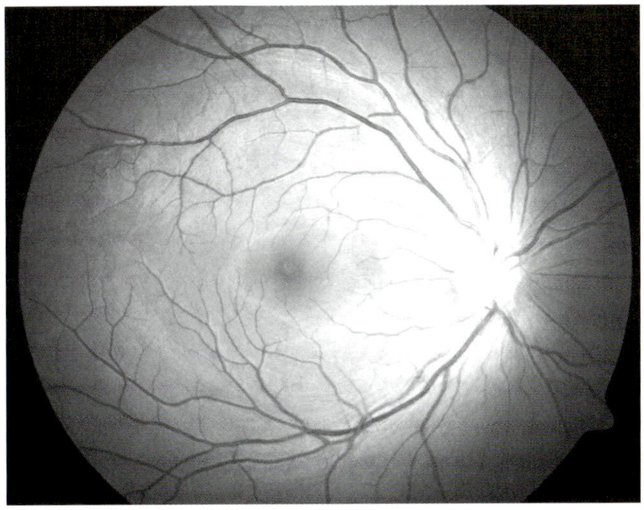

Red free photograph of the right eye

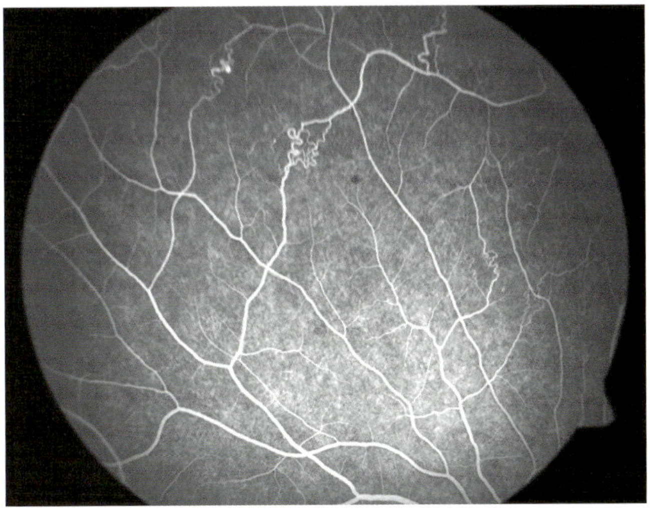

Arteriovenous phase showing collateral channels in the superotemporal periphery. Areas of capillary nonperfusion are seen peripherally

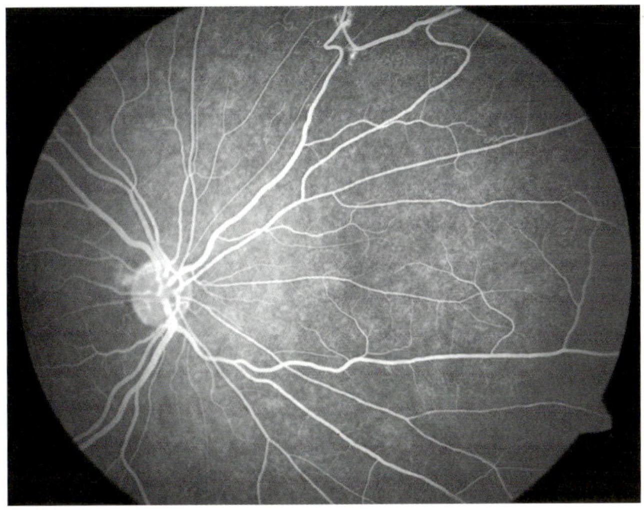

Nasal periphery showing similar changes

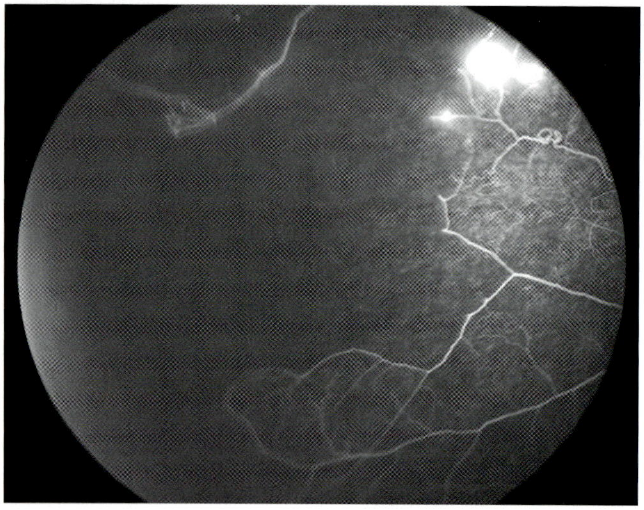

Temporal periphery shows extensive areas of capillary nonperfusion. Few foci of intense fuzzy hyperfluorescence are seen indicative of neovascularization

COMMENT

In most cases of Eales' disease, the changes are restricted to the peripheral fundus.

CASE 5

A 38-year-old male presented with a history of floaters in front of both eyes for the past three months. Visual acuity was 6/6; N6 in both eyes.

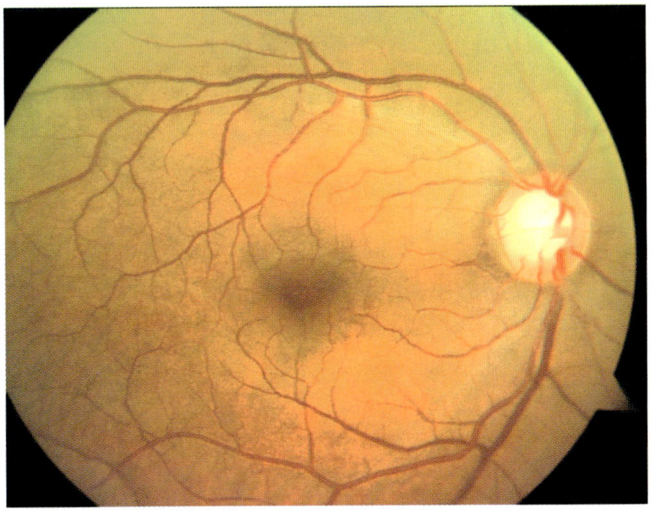

Fundus photograph of the right eye showing the normal posterior pole

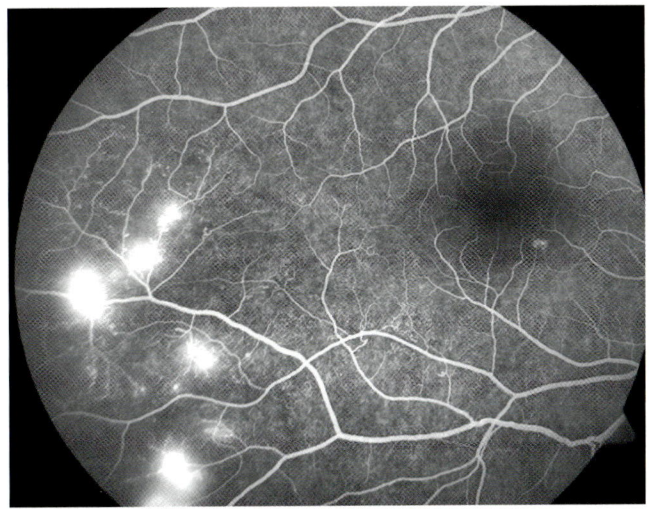

Arteriovenous phase showing multiple foci of fuzzy hyperfluorescence indicative of neovascularization

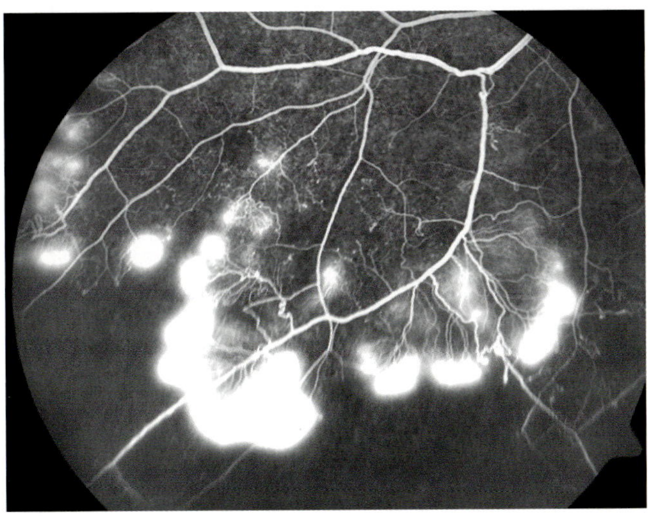

Extensive fan-shaped neovascular fronds are seen in the inferotemporal quadrant with leakage of the dye. Areas of capillary nonperfusion are seen peripherally

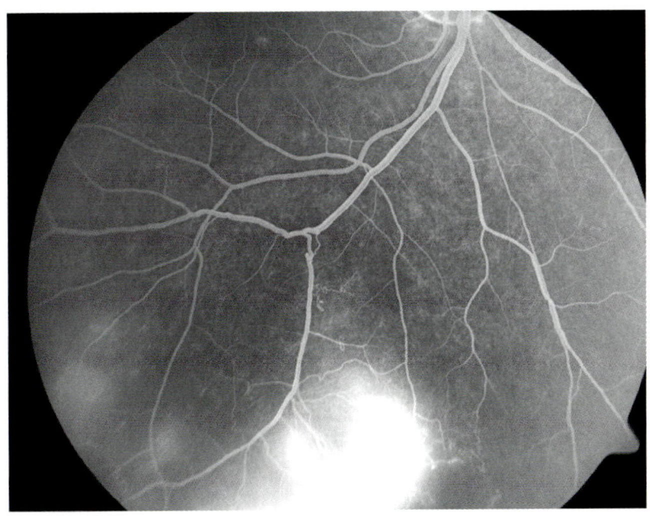

Leakage of the dye from the neovascular fronds into the vitreous is seen in the late phase

COMMENT

NVE at the junction of the perfused and nonperfused retina is common in Eales' disease and usually occurs in the mid periphery of the fundus.

CLINICAL NUGGETS

1. Eales' disease is common in young, healthy, males, usually occurring in the third decade of life.
2. Macula is usually spared in Eales' disease.
3. Patients with active periphlebitis are treated with systemic steroids.
4. Laser photocoagulation is required in eyes that develop neovascularization.
5. Intravitreal antivascular endothelial growth factor (VEGF) agents have been tried for regression of retinal neovascularization.

BIBLIOGRAPHY

1. Karel I, Votoková J, Peleka M. Fluorescein angiography in unusual forms of idiopathic retinal vasculitis. Ophthalmologica 1974;168:446-61.
2. Malik SR, Patnaik B. Fluorescein angiography in Eales' disease. Indian J Ophthalmol 1973;21:5-15.
3. Theodossiadis G. Fluorescein angiography in Eales' disease. Am J Ophthalmol 1970;69:271-7.

32

Chapter

Familial Exudative Vitreoretinopathy

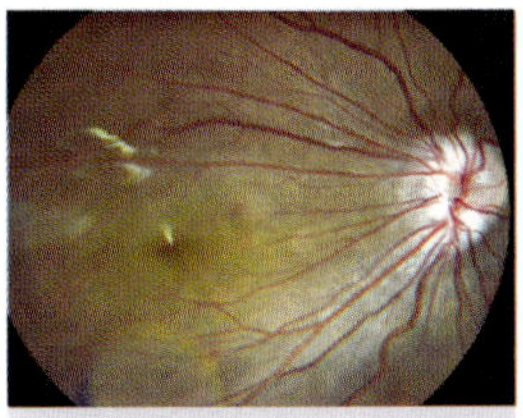

- Familial exudative vitreoretinopathy (FEVR) is an autosomal dominant condition characterized by failure of peripheral retinal vascularization.
- FEVR is associated with variable phenotypes. It is characterized by:
  - Bilaterality (may be asymmetric)
  - Peripheral avascular retina (usually temporal periphery) with retinal vascular anomalies (peripheral brush border anastomoses)
  - Straightening of vessels at the posterior pole due to retinal traction
  - Macular ectopia
  - Acute-angle vascular branching
  - Falciform retinal folds
  - Retinal breaks and retinal detachment.
- The visual problems with FEVR result from secondary complications caused by retinal ischemia *viz* retinal neovascularization and exudation. Risk factors for progression have not yet been elucidated, but genetic factors have been postulated to play a role. Family screening is recommended.
- Differential diagnosis: Retinopathy of prematurity is seen in premature infants or in those with very low birth weight. It does not have an associated family history. Progress of retinal vascularization towards the periphery can be observed. In contrast, the avascular periphery in eyes with FEVR never undergoes vascularization.
- Treatment: Laser photocoagulation/cryotherapy to peripheral avascular retina in case of neovascular/exudative complications. Rhegmatogenous retinal detachments require surgery. Regular fundus examination in children for detecting these complications at the earliest is recommended.

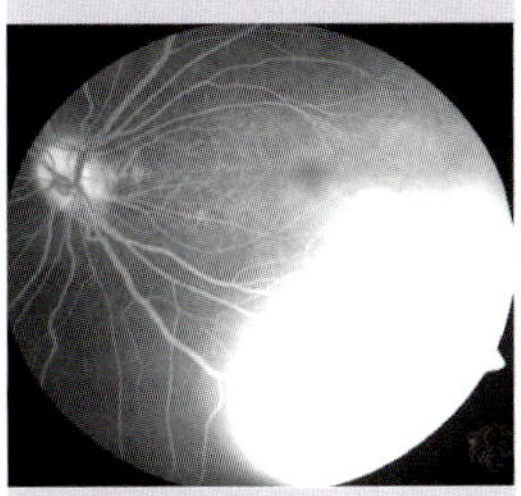

Fluorescein angiography can delineate peripheral avascular retina with brush border anastomoses. Profuse leakage from fibrovascular proliferations is noteworthy. Straightening of vessels at the posterior pole and acute-angle vascular branching is highlighted.

CASE 1

A 3-year-old healthy male child presented with history of deviation of the right eye since childhood. He was a child born at term. There was no family history of childhood onset visual loss or heredomacular degeneration, nor was there consanguinity amongst the parents. He was found to fixate and follow light well and had a myopic refraction of -6 D sphere in both eyes.

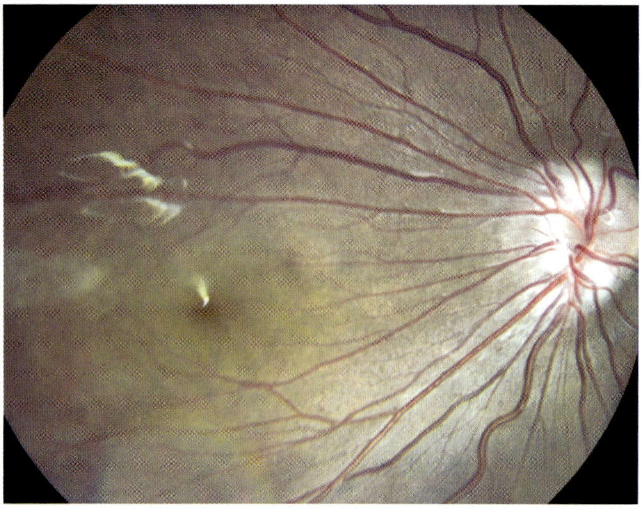

Color fundus photograph of the right eye reveals macular ectopia, straightening of the retinal vessels at the posterior pole and acute-angle vascular branching

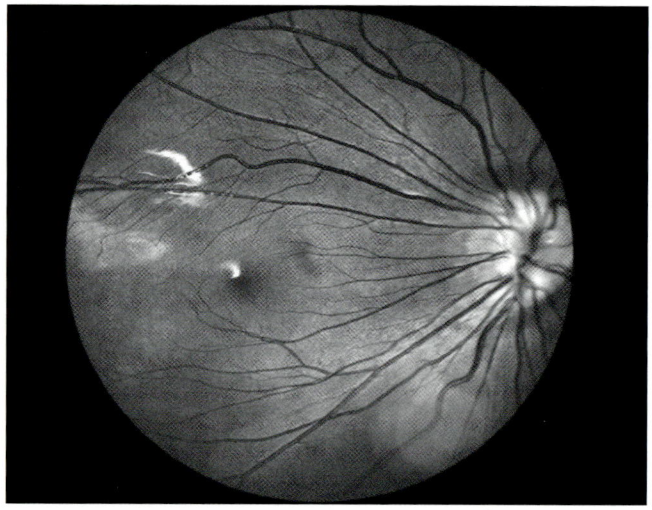

Red free photograph of the right eye highlights the typical fundus features

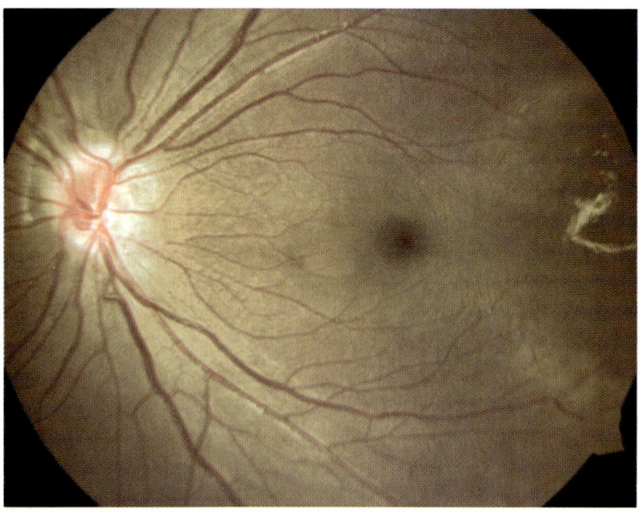

Color fundus photograph of the left eye reveals macular ectopia, straightening of the retinal vessels at the posterior pole and acute-angle vascular branching

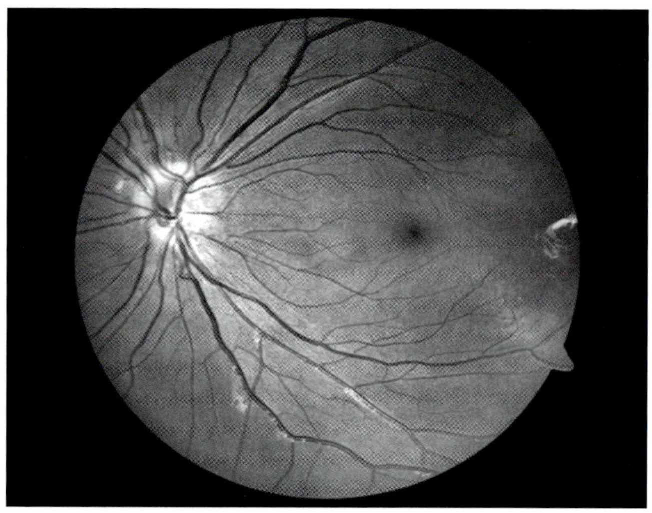

Red free photograph of the left eye highlights the typical fundus features

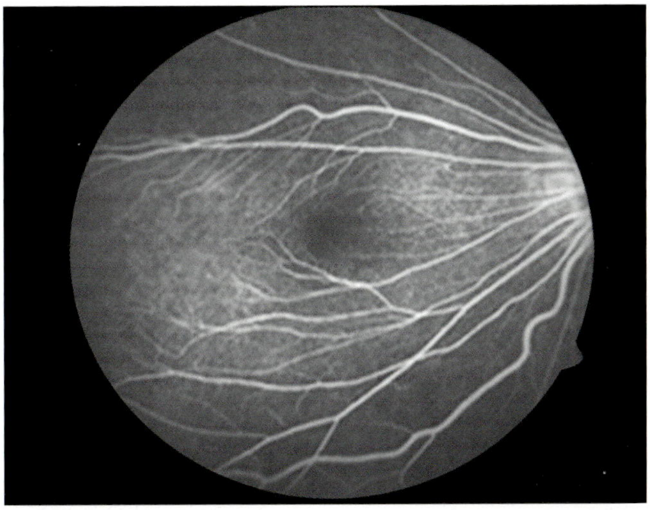

Mid A-V phase of the right eye shows straightening of the retinal vessels at the posterior pole and acute-angle vascular branching

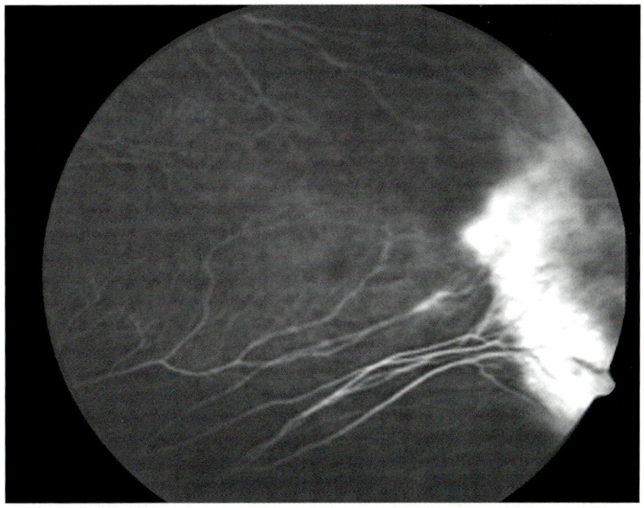

Late A-V phase angiogram of the left superotemporal periphery reveals intense hyperfluorescence due to leakage from the fibrovascular proliferation

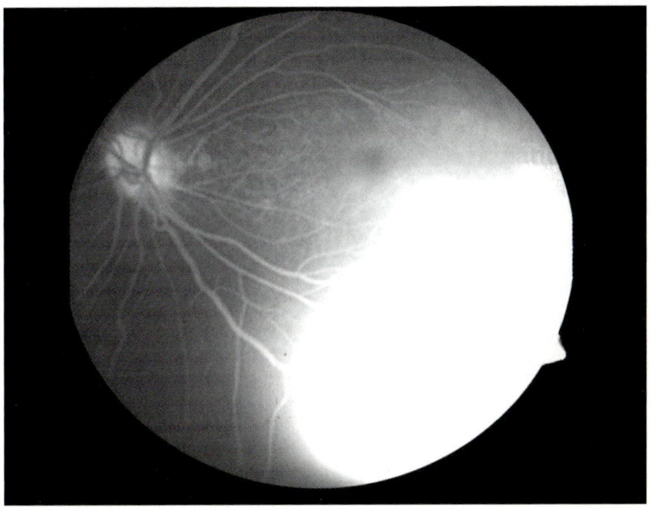

Late A-V phase angiogram of the left inferotemporal mid-periphery reveals intense hyperfluorescence due to leakage from the fibrovascular proliferation

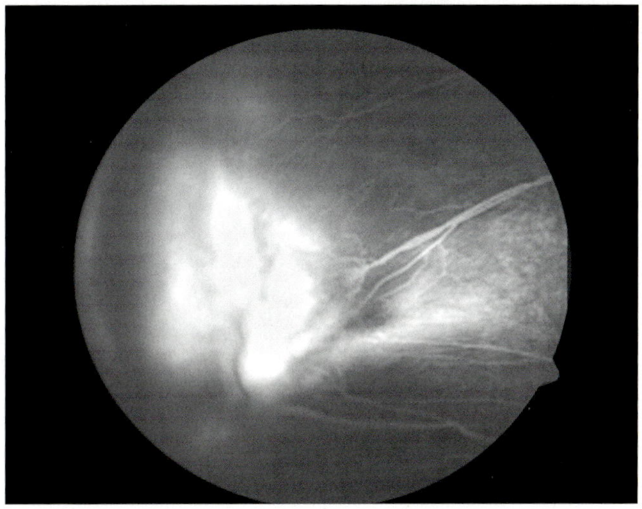

Late phase angiogram of the right inferotemporal mid-periphery reveals intense hyperfluorescence due to leakage from the fibrovascular proliferation

COMMENT

The patient underwent laser photocoagulation to the avascular retina in both eyes. Fundus remained stable till the last follow-up.

BIBLIOGRAPHY

1. Benson WE. Familial exudative vitreoretinopathy. Trans Am Ophthalmol Soc. 1995; 93:473-521.
2. de Crecchio G, Simonelli F, Nunziata G, Mazzeo S, Greco GM, Rinaldi E, et al. Autosomal recessive familial exudative vitreoretinopathy: evidence for genetic heterogeneity. Clin Genet 1998; 54:315-20.
3. Jiao X, Ventruto V, Trese MT, Shastry BS, Hejtmancik JF. Autosomal recessive familial exudative vitreoretinopathy is associated with mutations in LRP5. Am J Hum Genet 2004; 75:878-84.

33

Chapter

Hypertensive Retinopathy

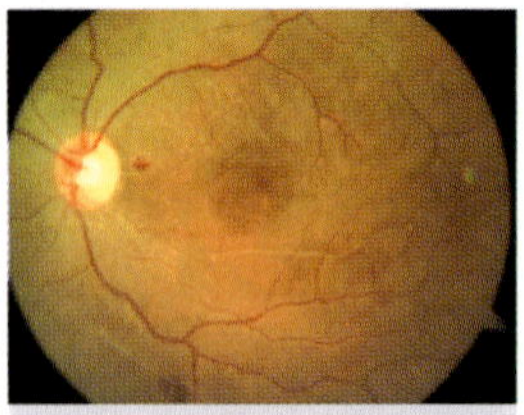

- Features seen clinically are those associated with hypertensive retinopathy, hypertensive choroidopathy or hypertensive optic neuropathy.
- Hypertensive retinopathy is characterized by retinal arteriolar attenuation, changes in the arteriolar reflex, arteriovenous crossing changes, cotton wool spots, flame shaped hemorrhages and vascular occlusion.
- Hypertensive choroidopathy is characterized by Elschnig's spot at the posterior pole and Siegrist's streak peripherally. Both these occur as a result of choroidal infarction.
- Hypertensive optic neuropathy is characterized by disc swelling, associated with retinal edema and exudation.

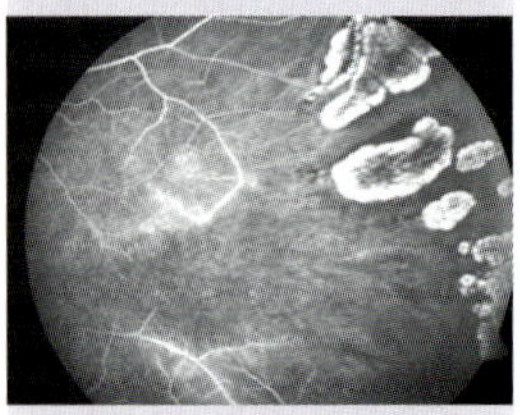

- Arteriovenous crossing changes with evidence of vein compression may be seen.
- Areas of cotton wool spots show up as areas of capillary nonperfusion.
- Dilation and at times, occlusion of the terminal arterioles may be seen.
- In acute stage, Elschnig's spot shows up as hyperfluorescence in the early phase of the angiogram with leakage of the dye seen in the later phases. Healed Elschnig's spots block fluorescence in the region of the central hyperpigmentation with a halo of surrounding hyperfluorescence due to transmission defect.
- Siegrist's streak shows areas of blocked fluorescence in the region of hyperpigmentation and nonfilling in the region of atrophy. Late staining of the underlying sclera is seen.

CASE 1

A 56-year-old hypertensive female, presented with a history of reduced vision in the left eye for six months. Visual acuity was 6/12; N8 in the left eye.

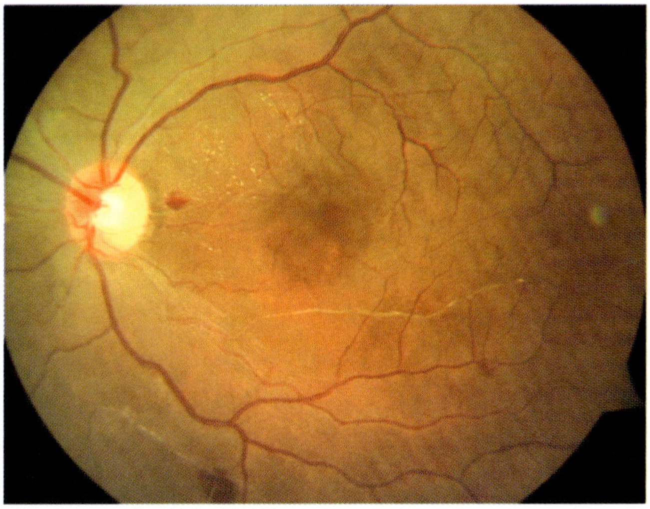

Fundus photograph of the left eye showing a sclerosed vessel in the inferior macular region. Superficial retinal hemorrhage is seen temporal to the disc

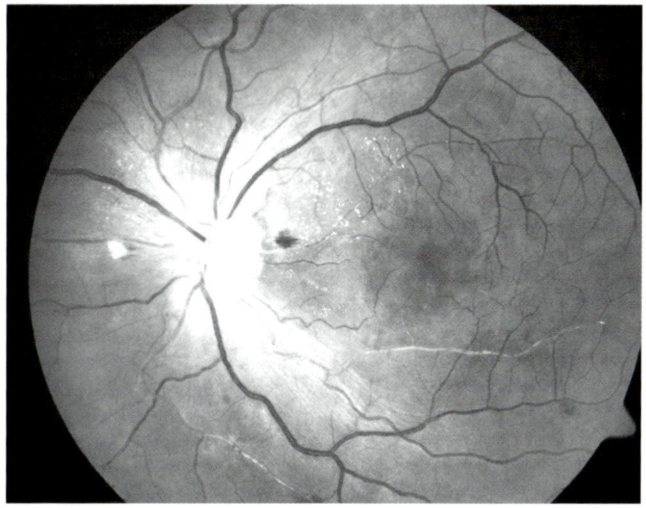

Red free photograph of the left eye

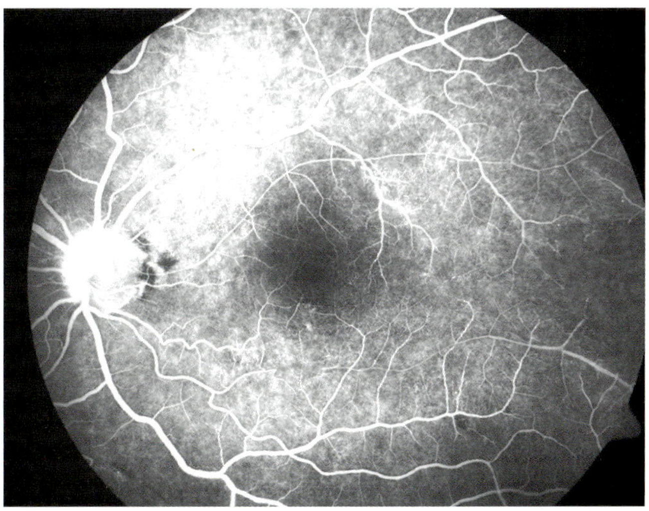

Arteriovenous phase shows area of capillary nonperfusion temporally suggestive of an old branch vein occlusion. The arterioles appear narrowed. The sclerosed arteriole in the inferior macular region shows very minimal filling with dye

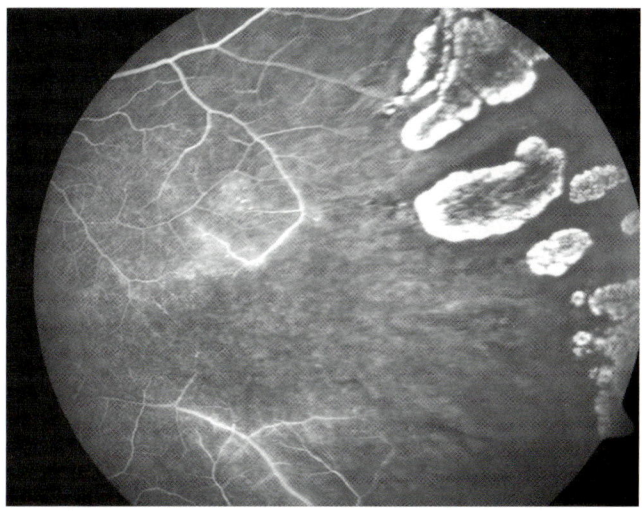

Tongue shaped areas of hypofluorescence with a rim of hyperfluorescence is seen in the temporal periphery

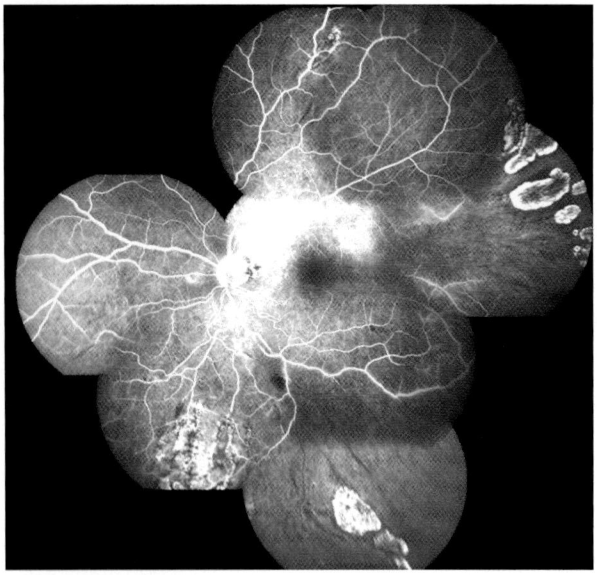

Montage picture shows Siegrist's streaks in the temporal, inferior and inferotemporal periphery

COMMENT

Siegrist's streaks are tongue shaped atrophic patches seen in the periphery of the fundus. They result from small choroidal infarcts which leads to atrophy of the overlying RPE.

CASE 2

A 37-year-old male, presented with decreased vision in left eye for 5 days. Visual acuity was 6/9; N8. His blood pressure at the time of presentation was 220/120 mm Hg.

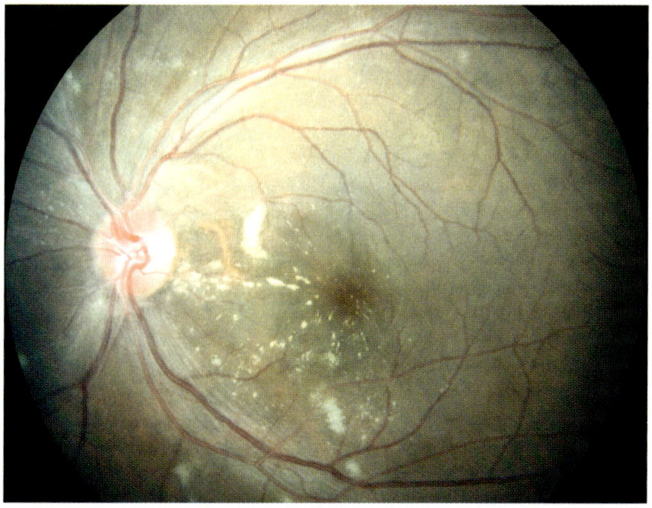

Fundus photograph of left eye showing slight hyperemic disc with blurred nasal margin, cotton wool spots and hard exudates

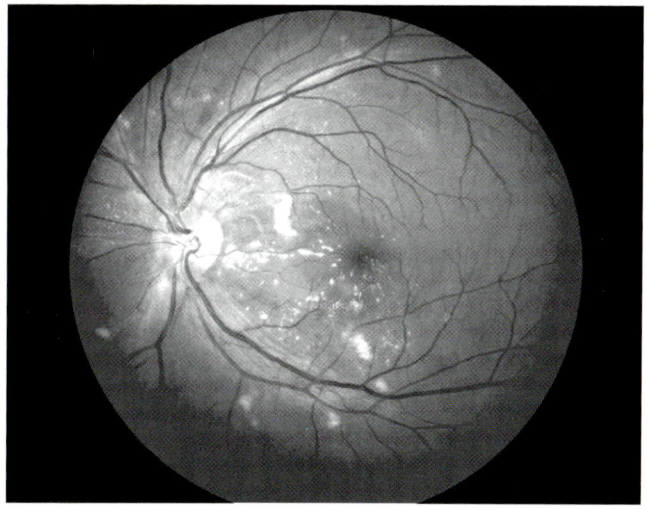

Red free photograph of left eye

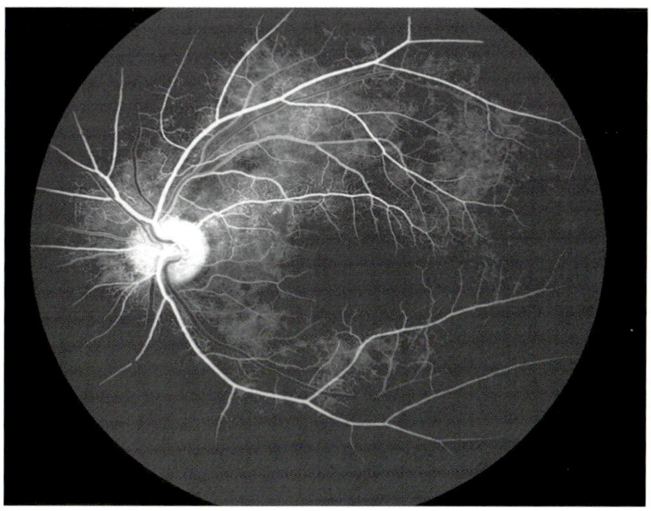

Early phase showing narrowed, straightened arterioles and capillary nonperfusion areas corresponding to the cotton wool spots

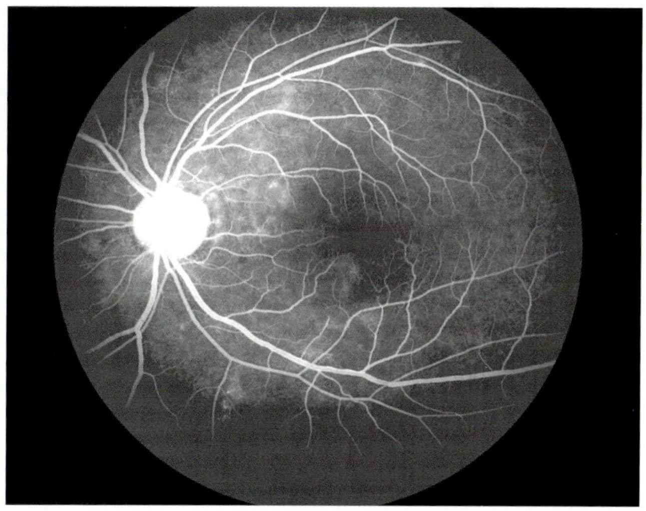

Arteriovenous phase showing venous beading

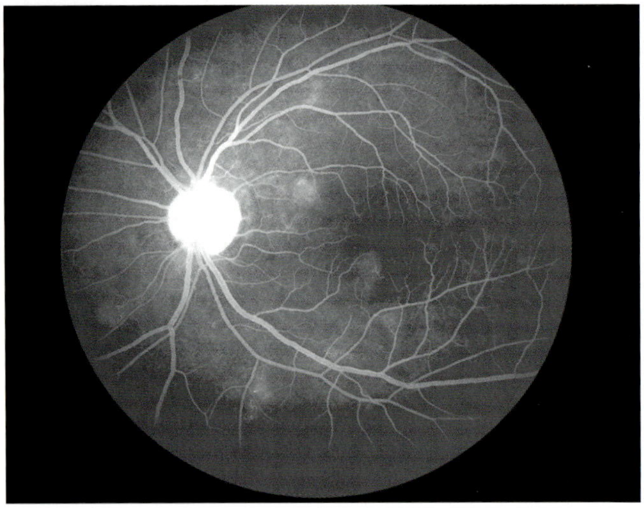

Late phase shows staining of disc and cotton wool spots

COMMENT

Accelerated hypertension leads to target organ damage. Immediate control of blood pressure leads to reversal of fundus changes.

CLINICAL NUGGETS

1. Elevated high blood pressure causes both focal and generalized constriction of the retinal arterioles due to autoregulation.
2. Elschnig's spots occur at the posterior pole and are seen as white spots in the acute stage.
3. Siegrist's streaks occur as tongue shaped lesion in the retinal periphery.
4. Malignant hypertension is associated with disc swelling and retinal hemorrhages around the disc.

BIBLIOGRAPHY

1. Dollery CT, Hodge JV. Hypertensive retinopathy studied with fluorescein. Trans Ophthalmol Soc UK. 1963; 83:115-32.
2. Gass JDM. Fluorescein angiographic study of macular dysfunction secondary to retinal vascular disease III. Hypertensive retinopathy. Arch Ophthalmol 1968;80: 569-82.
3. Scheie HG. Evaluation of ophthalmoscopic changes of hypertension and arteriolar sclerosis. Arch Ophthalmol 1953;49:117.

Chapter 34

Retinal Artery Macroaneurysm

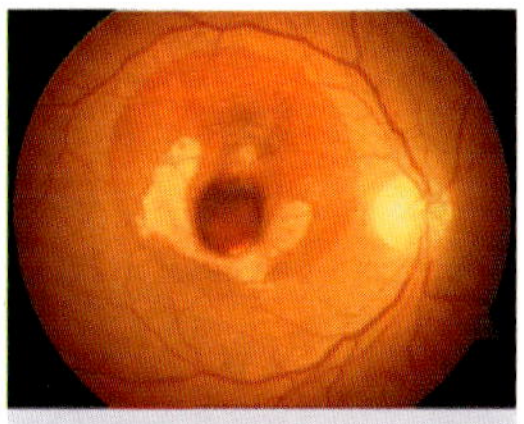

- A retinal arterial macroaneurysm is a round or fusiform dilation occurring in arterioles within the first three orders of the arteriolar bifurcation.
- It is usually unilateral, more common in females and occurs in the fifth to sixth decades of life.
- It usually occurs unrelated to other ocular disorders, but has been described in Eales' disease, angiomatosis retinae, hypertensive retinopathy and retinal vascular occlusions.
- It is often located at the site of an arteriolar bifurcation or an AV crossing.
- Bleeding from a macroaneurysm can occur in the subretinal space, into the retina, beneath the internal limiting membrane or into the vitreous.

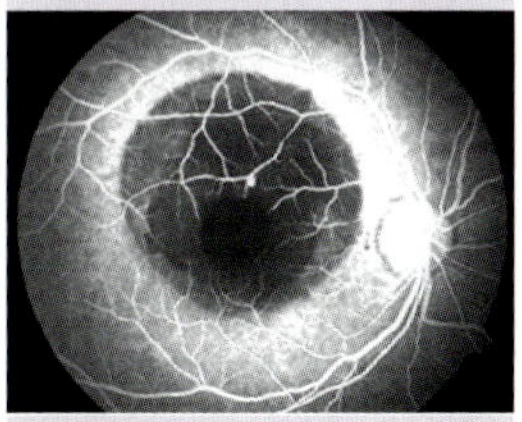

- Typically, a macroaneurysm fills in the early arterial phase of the angiogram.
- Occasionally, it may be hypofluorescent in the early films, probably due to the slow filling of the macroaneurysm.
- The appearance in the late phase varies, ranging from minimal staining of the vessel wall to marked leakage.
- Dilation of surrounding capillaries, adjacent areas of capillary nonperfusion and microaneurysms may be seen in some cases.
- If retinal hemorrhage overlies the macroaneurysm, it may not be seen on a fluorescein angiogram.

CASE 1

A 63-year-old hypertensive male, presented with sudden onset of decreased vision in the right eye of six weeks duration. The visual acuity was 1/60 in the right eye.

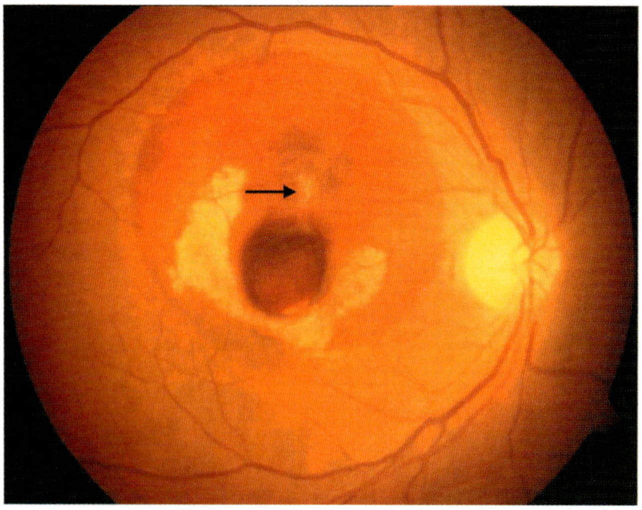

Fundus photograph of the right eye showing subretinal dark and altered hemorrhage. The macroaneurysm is seen as a white round lesion (arrow) superior to the fovea, along the retinal arteriole

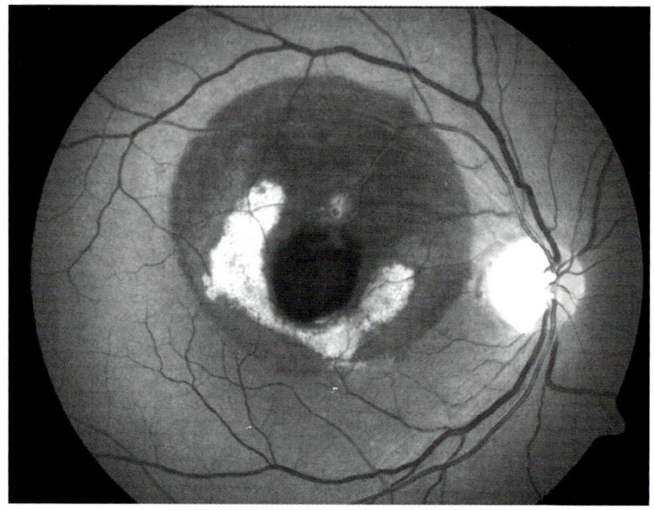

Red free photograph of the right eye

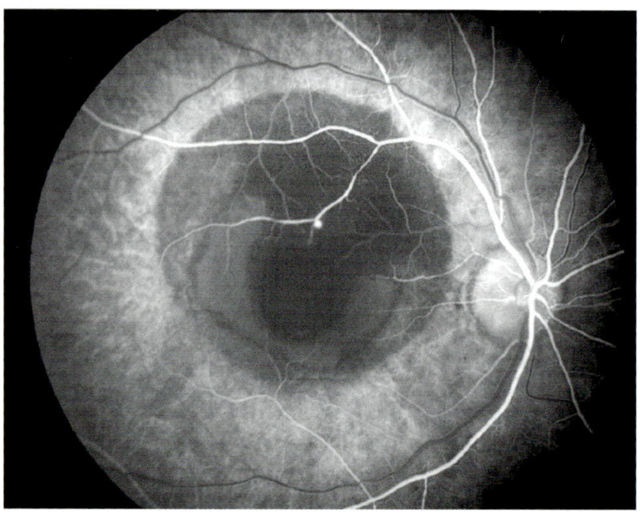

Early arteriovenous phase showing blocked choroidal fluorescence caused by the hemorrhage. The macroaneurysm is seen as a hyperfluorescent spot along the retinal arteriole

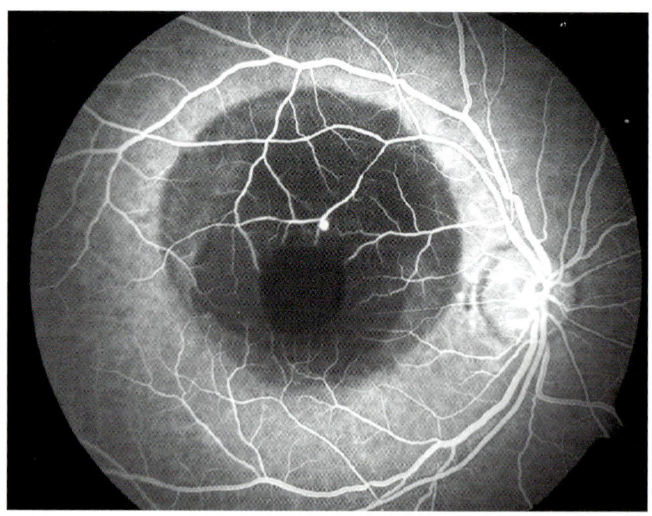

Arteriovenous phase shows increased hyperfluorescence of the macroaneurysm

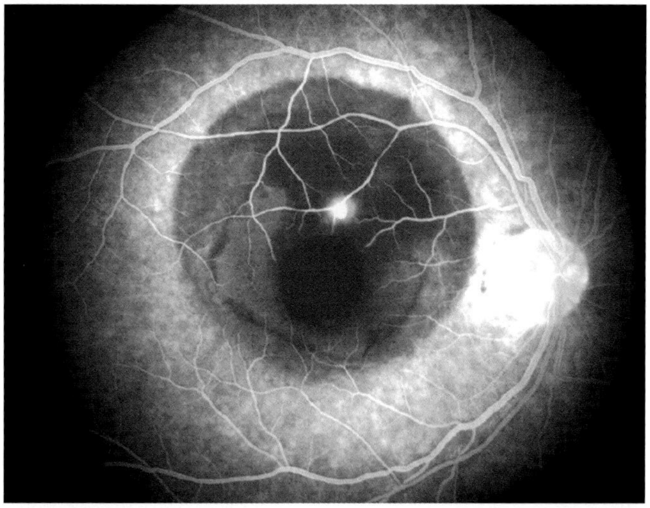

Late phase angiogram shows some fuzziness around the borders of the macroaneurysm due to leakage of the dye through its wall

COMMENT

Macroaneurysm appears as a hyperfluorescent spot along the arteriole with increasing intensity of fluorescence in later phases.

CASE 2

A 54-year-old hypertensive male presented with reduced vision in the right eye for the past four months. Visual acuity was 6/60; N36 in the right eye.

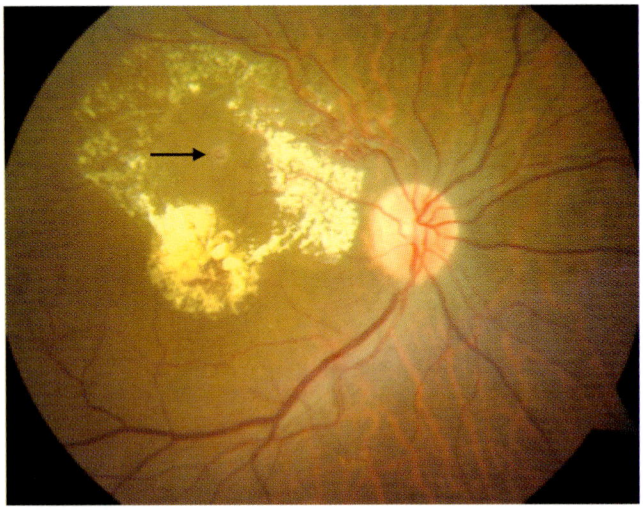

Fundus photograph of the right eye showing a large circinate of hard exudates. A macroaneurysm is seen in the center (arrow) as a whitish globular lesion along the arteriole

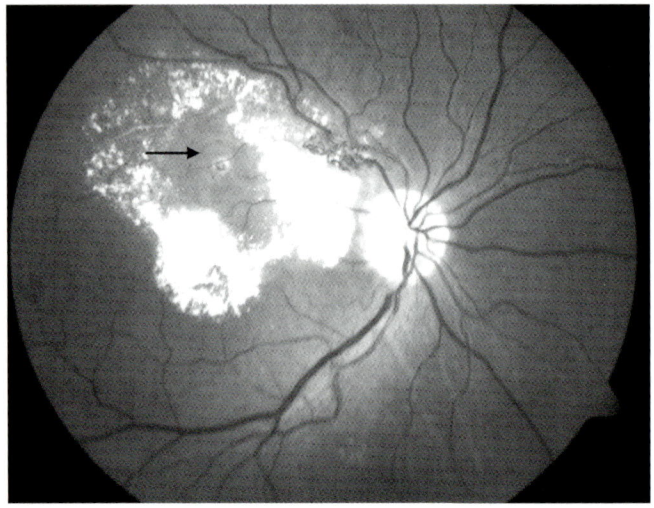

Red free photograph showing the macroaneurysm (arrow) at the center of the circinate. Collateral vessels are seen at the A-V crossing just superotemporal to the disc

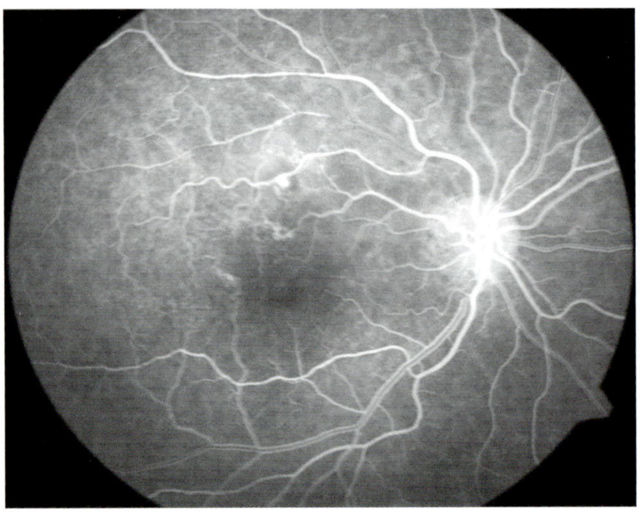

Early arteriovenous phase showing the filling up of the macroaneurysm. It appears as a saccular outpouching from the walls of the arteriole

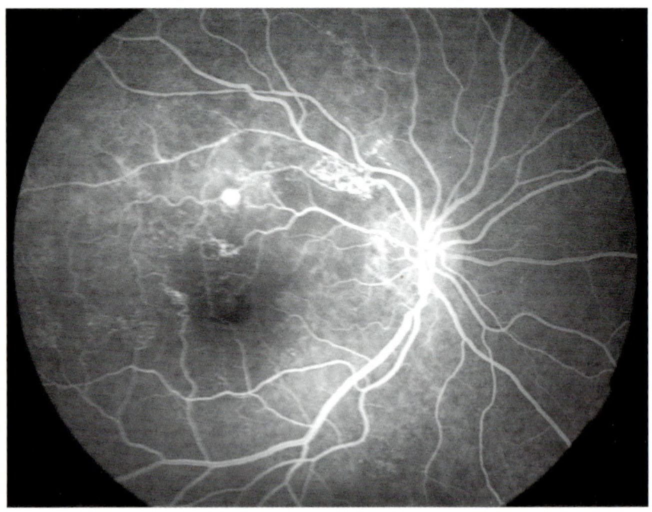

Increased hyperfluorescence is seen at the macroaneurysm. Collateral channels are seen superotemporal to the disc. Areas of capillary nonperfusion is seen in the superior macula

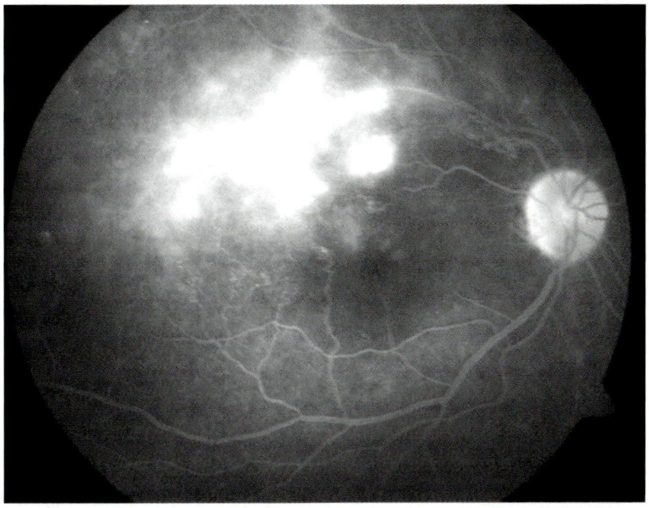

Late phase of the angiogram showing leakage through the walls of the macroaneurysm. Staining of the vessel wall in the region of the vein occlusion is seen. No leakage is seen from the collateral vessels

COMMENT

Macroaneurysm could be associated with vein occlusion as seen in this case.

CASE 3

A 36-year-old male came to us with a history of sudden drop in the vision in the left eye. He was a known hypertensive on 3 antihypertensive drugs. His visual acuity was HM close to face in the left eye.

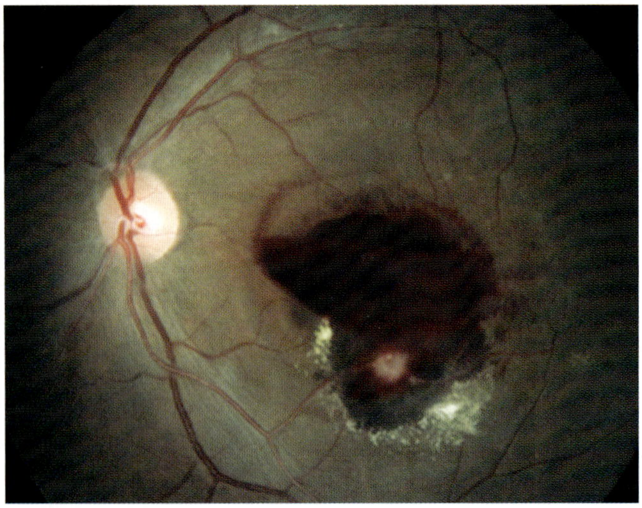

Fundus photograph of the left eye showing subretinal blood with hard exudates. Macroaneurysm is seen as a yellowish lesion along the inferotemporal arteriole

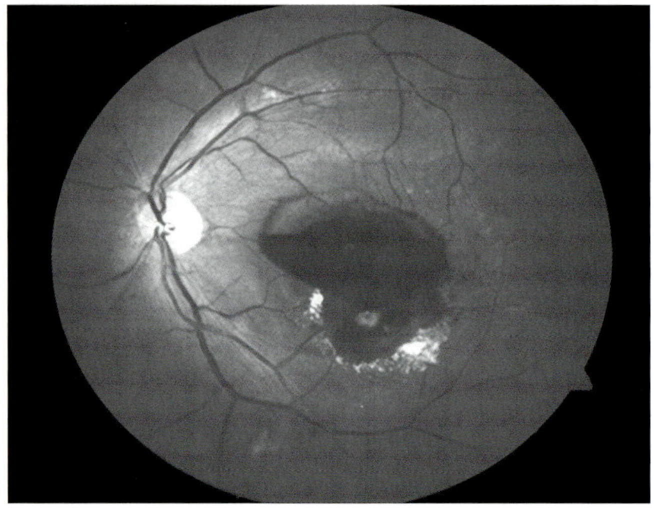

Red free photograph of the left eye

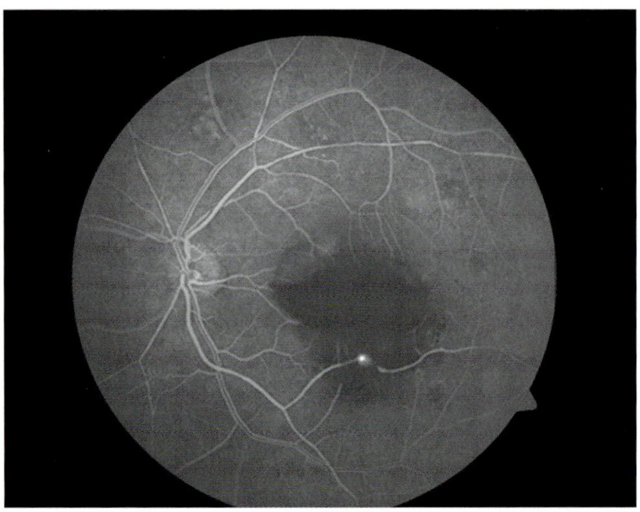

Early AV phase showing early hyperfluorescence of the macroaneurysm

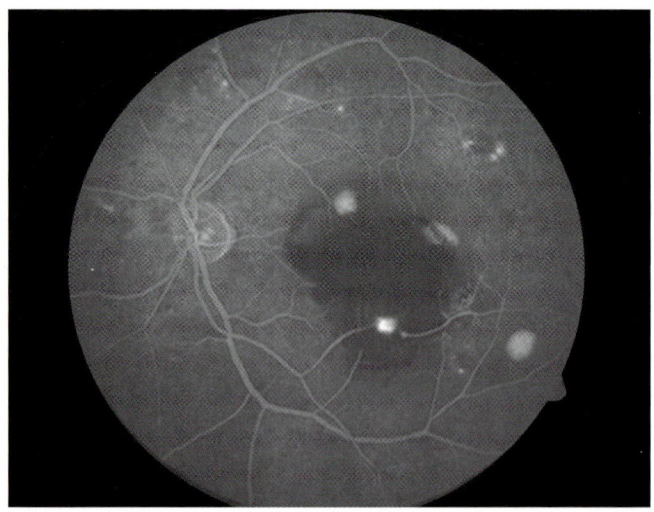

Increased hyperfluorescence seen in the midphase with the subretinal heme showing blocked fluorescence. Late filling of the PED's is seen superonasal and inferotemporal to fovea because of coexisting changes secondary to CSR

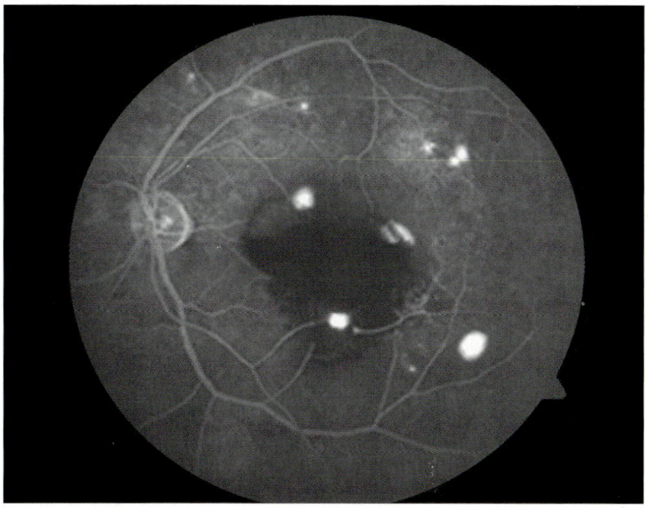

Late phase FFA

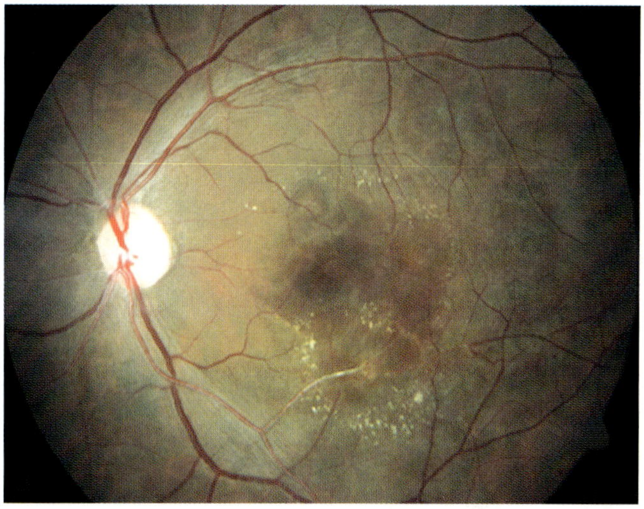

Fundus photo after laser photocoagulation to the macroaneurysm showing resolution of the heme. His visual acuity improved to 6/12; N10 following treatment

CLINICAL NUGGETS

1. The superotemporal artery is more commonly involved.
2. Macroaneurysms are more common in females and generally occur in the 6th and 7th decade of life.
3. Patients with macroaneurysm may be asymptomatic if the fovea is not involved.
4. Macroaneurysms with exudation can be treated with direct and mild photocoagulation; a heavy burn might cause arterial occlusion.

BIBLIOGRAPHY

1. Abdel-Khalek MN, Richardson J. Retinal macroaneurysm: natural history and guidelines for management. Br J Ophthalmol; 1986;70:2-11.
2. Cleary PE, Kohner EM, Hamilton AM, et al. Retinal macroaneurysms. Br J Ophthalmol; 1975;59:355-61.
3. Panton RW, Goldberg MF, Farber MD. Retinal arterial macroaneurysm: Risk factors and natural history. Br J Ophthalmol 1990;74:595-600.

Chapter 35

Parafoveal Telangiectasia

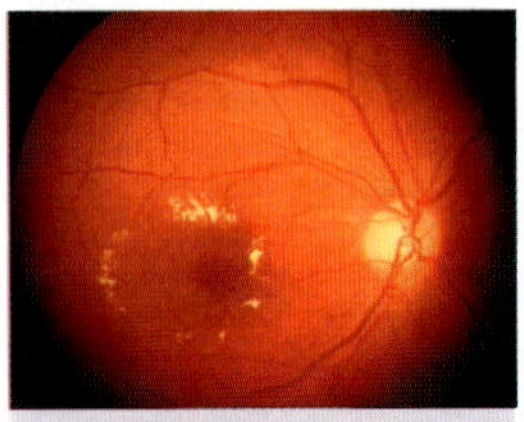

- Parafoveal telangiectasia is characterized by the presence of focal microaneurysmal or saccular dilatation of some portion of the parafoveal capillary network.
- Three types have been described:

Group 1

1 A—*Unilateral Congenital Parafoveal Telangiectasia*
It is more common in men, with a mean age of onset at 40 years of age. It is unilateral with the temporal 1 to 2 disc diameter of the parafoveal capillary network involved. Macular edema and hard exudation is common. This could be a variant of Coats' disease.

1 B—*Unilateral Idiopathic Parafoveal Telangiectasia*
Found in middle aged men with a very small area of capillary telangiectasia confined to 1 clock hour. Exudation is not very common.

Angiographic pattern: Fluorescein angiography shows microaneurysmal and saccular dilatation of the temporal parafoveal capillaries with staining of the retina seen in the late phase.

Group 2

Bilateral Acquired Parafoveal Telangiectasia
Bilateral, symmetric and involving the area temporal to the fovea, may involve the entire parafoveal capillary network. Right-angled retinal venules are commonly seen. Lipid exudation is uncommon. RPE hyperplasia may develop along the right angled venule.

Angiographic pattern: Fluorescein angiography shows dilated parafoveal capillaries with staining of the adjacent retina in the mid and late phases. This does not extend to the center of the fovea and no cystoid changes are seen. The area of RPE hyperplasia blocks fluorescence. The right angled venules are better visualized on the angiogram. They appear as abruptly ending vessels in the parafoveal venules. Presence of a neovascular membrane is associated with increased leakage of the fluorescein dye and its accumulation in cystoid spaces in the late films.

Group 3

Bilateral Idiopathic Perifoveal Telangiectasia and Capillary Obliteration
Telangiectasia with progressive obliteration of the perifoveal network is seen. These changes are very well seen on the fluorescein angiogram.

CASE 1

A 48-year-old male patient was referred with a diagnosis of a branch retinal vein occlusion in the right eye. He complained of reduced vision in that eye for the past eight months. Visual acuity was 6/24; N36. Left eye was normal.

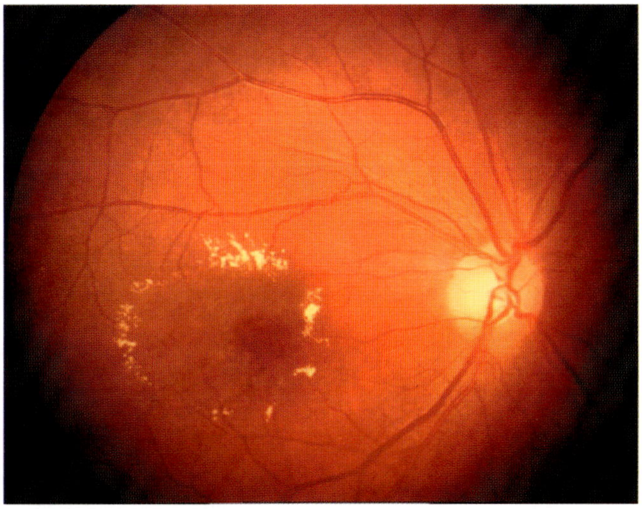

Fundus photograph of the right eye showing hard exudates arranged in a circinate pattern temporal to the fovea. Vascular abnormalities are seen within

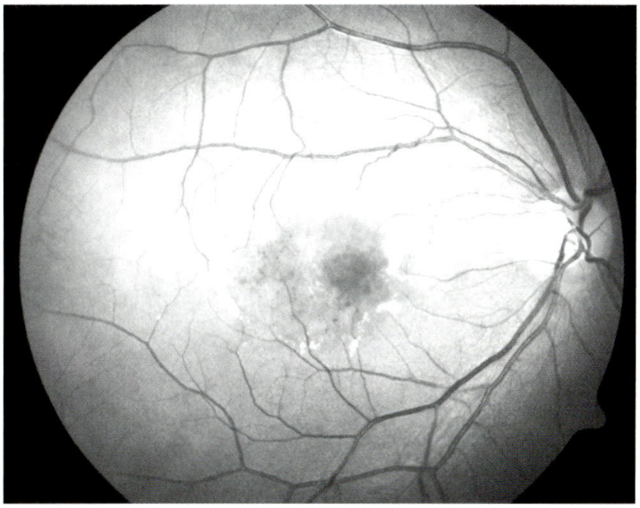

Red free photograph shows vascular abnormalities within the circinate

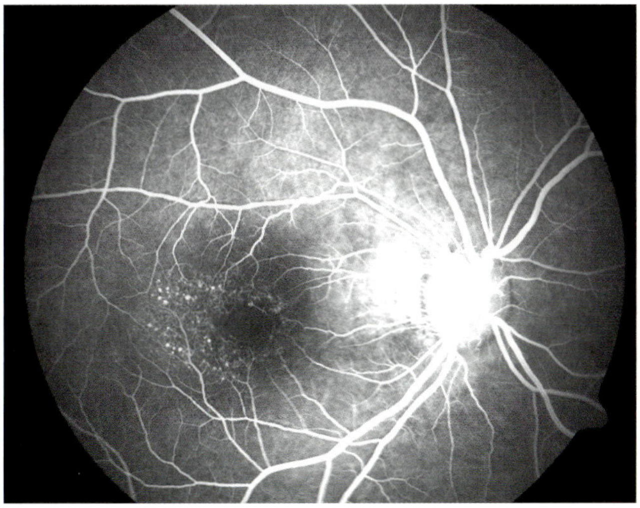

Arteriovenous phase showing vascular abnormalities including capillary dilation and microaneurysmal dilation of the parafoveal capillary network, more marked temporally

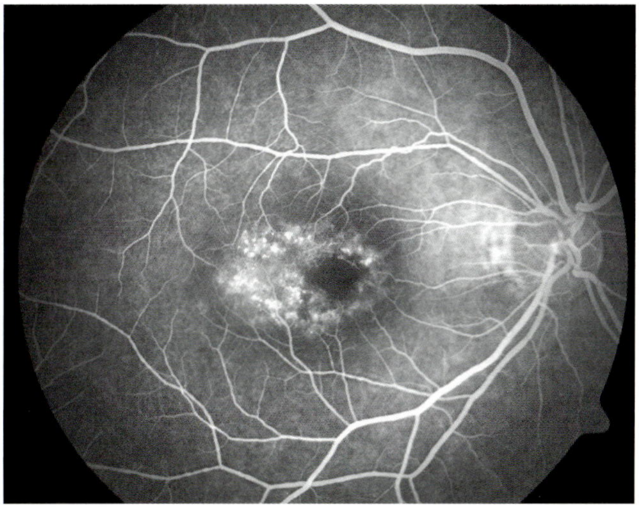

Increased leakage of the dye is seen from the vascular abnormalities

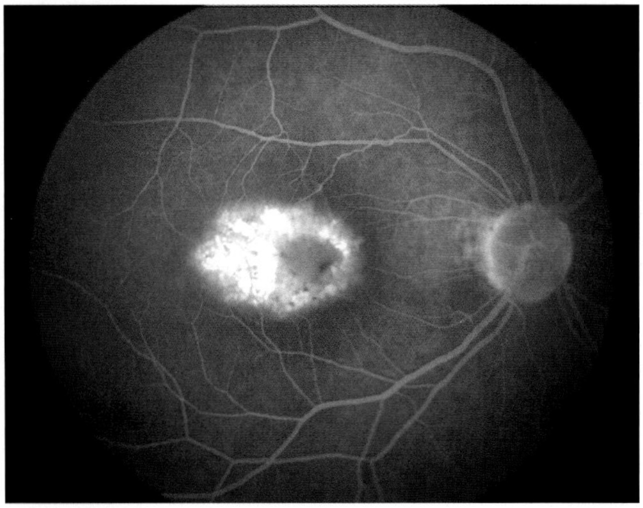

Late staining of the parafoveal retina is seen. Note that the foveal center remains hypofluorescent

COMMENT

This case represents Group 1A type of parafoveal telangiectasia. Hard exudates are common in this type.

Involvement of the entire parafoveal network differentiates this from a small tributary vein occlusion in which the changes would be restricted to the affected segment.

CASE 2

A 47-year-old male presented with history of noticing reduced vision in both eyes for the past two months. Visual acuity was 6/9; N8 in the right eye and 6/6; N6 in the left eye.

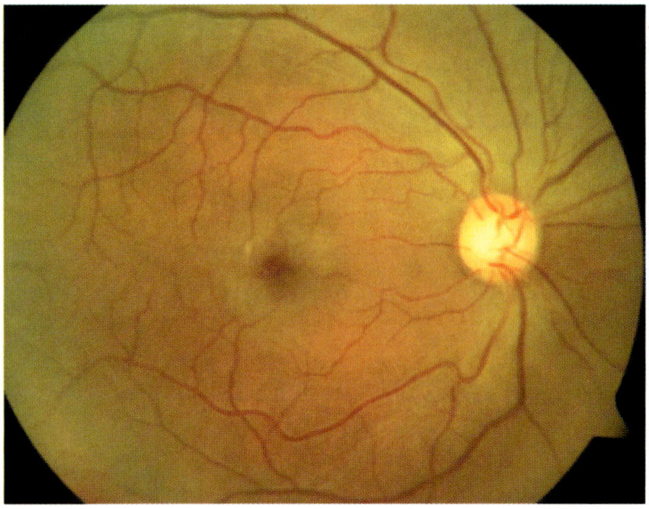

Fundus photograph of the right eye showing a zone of retinal whitening in the parafoveal region

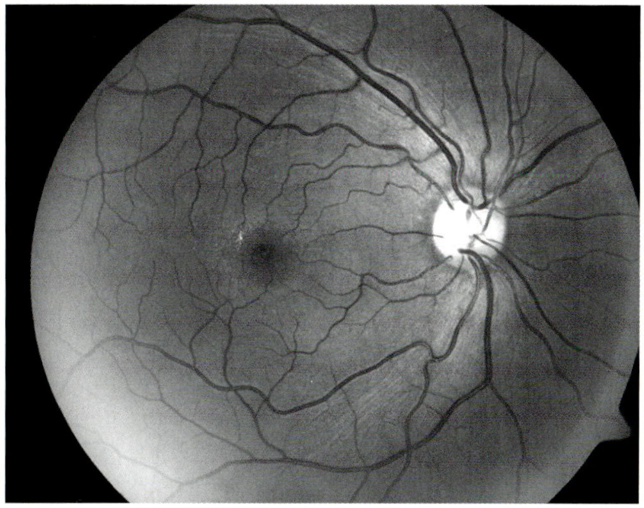

Red free photograph of the right eye

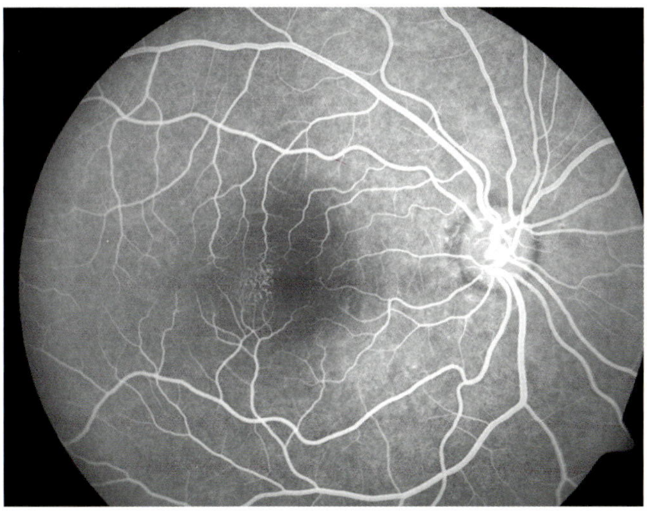

Arteriovenous phase shows capillary dilation and telangiectasia especially in the temporal parafoveal region

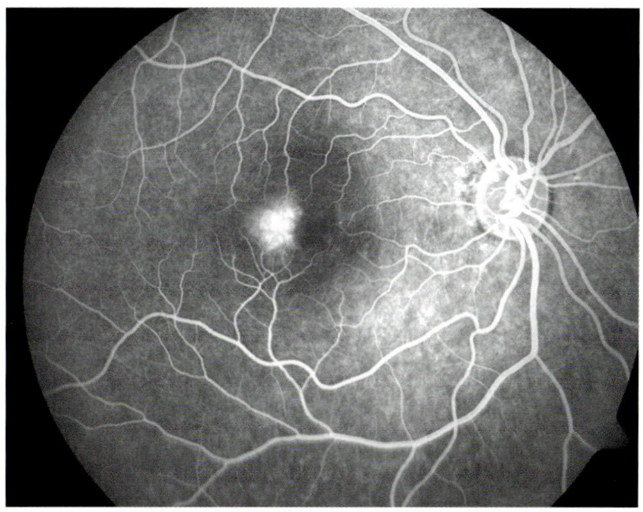

Increased intensity of hyperfluorescence is seen in the temporal parafoveal region

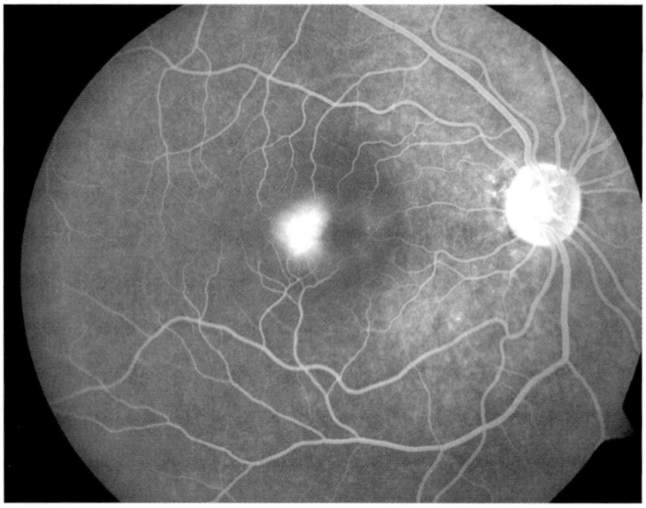

Late staining of parafoveal retina is seen, much more prominent on the temporal aspect

CASE 2 (*Continued*)

Left Eye of the Patient

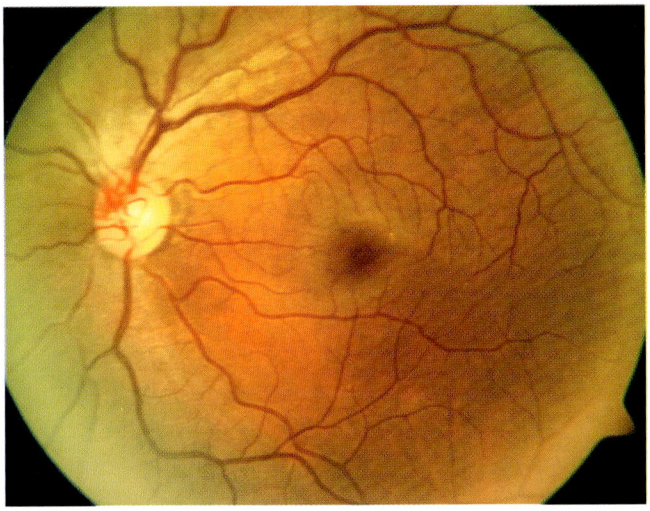

Fundus photograph of the left eye showing the retinal whitening in the parafoveal region

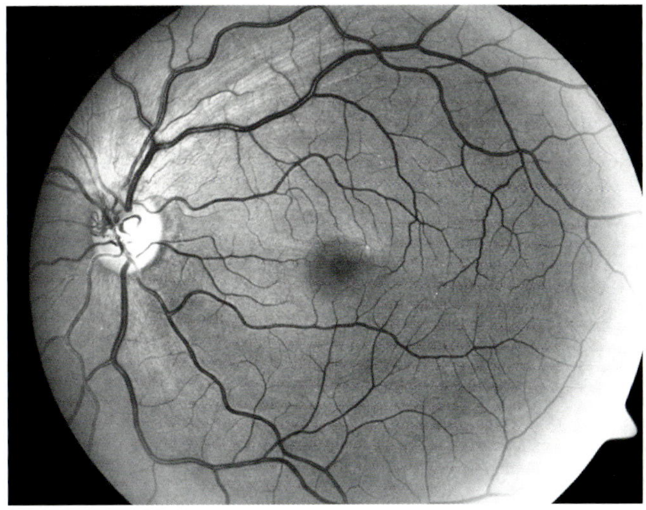

Red free photograph of the left eye

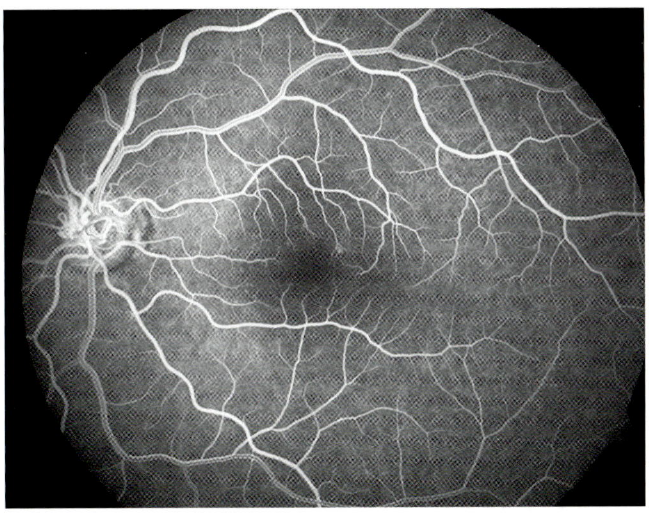

Very subtle vascular abnormality is seen at the superotemporal edge of the foveal avascular zone

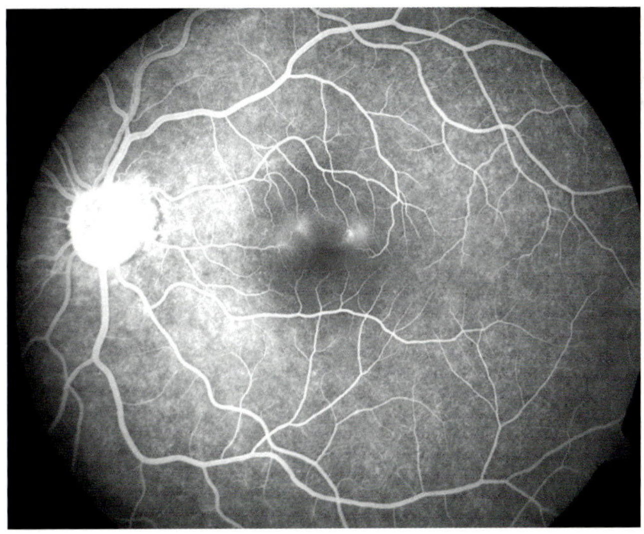

Late minimal staining of the superior parafoveal region is seen

COMMENT

The temporal parafoveal capillary network is more commonly involved in the initial stages. Note that no cystoid changes are seen and the center of the FAZ remains hypofluorescent even in the late phase.

CASE 3

A 52-year-old female presented with history of reduced vision in both eyes for the past one month. Patient had recently been diagnosed to have diabetes. Visual acuity was 6/18; N6 in both eyes.

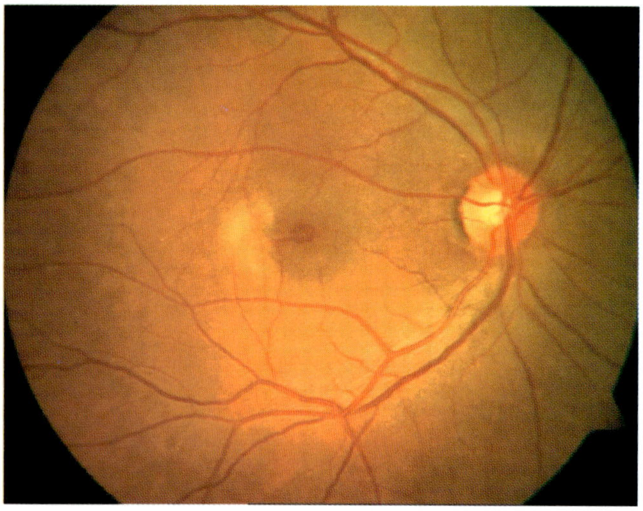

Fundus photograph of the right eye showing a dull white subretinal lesion with adjacent hemorrhage on the foveal side

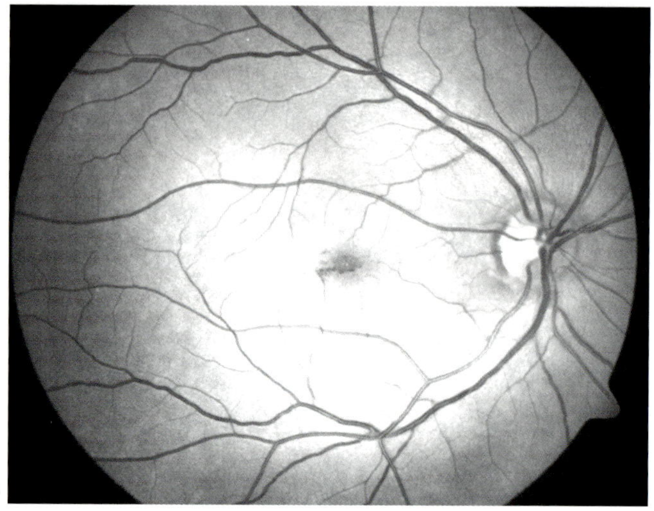

Red free photograph of the right eye

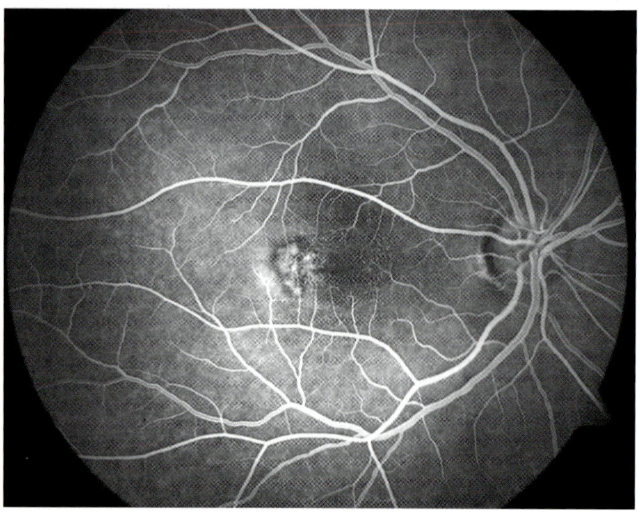

Midarteriovenous phase shows intense irregular hyperfluorescence in the temporal parafovea. Dilation of the parafoveal capillary network is seen

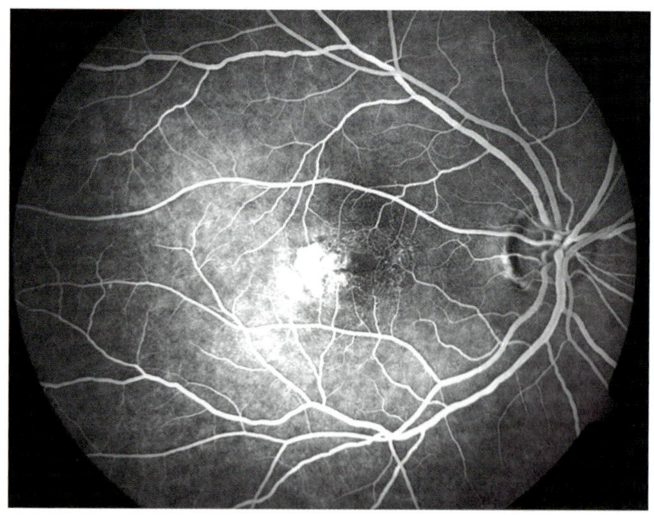

Hyperfluorescence in the temporal parafoveal lesion has increased. The vascular abnormalities are better made out

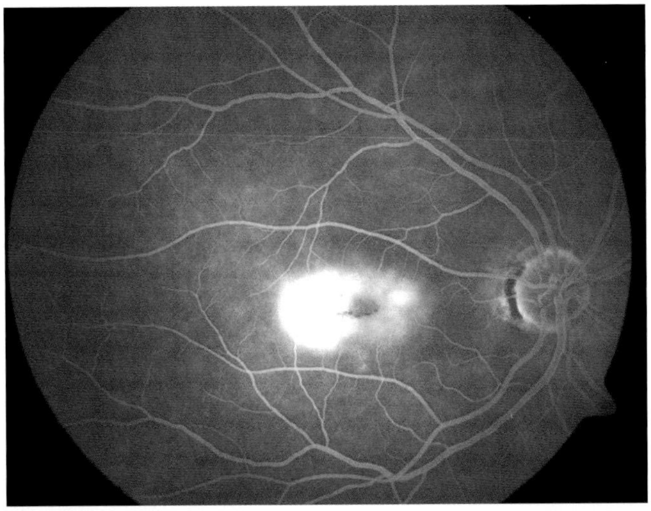

Intense hyperfluorescence is seen in the temporal neovascular lesion. Staining of the parafoveal area is seen. Central blocked fluorescence caused by the hemorrhage is seen

COMMENT

Occurrence of subretinal hemorrhage or fluid, cystoid macular edema and presence of focal, intense hyperfluorescent lesion in the angiogram are suggestive of development of neovascular membrane in eyes with parafoveal telangiectasia.

CASE 3 (*Continued*)

Left Eye of the Patient

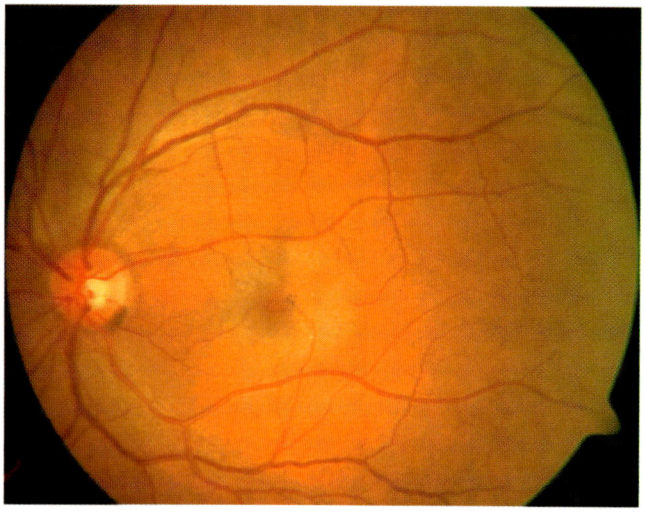

Annular zone of whitening is seen in the parafoveal region in the left eye

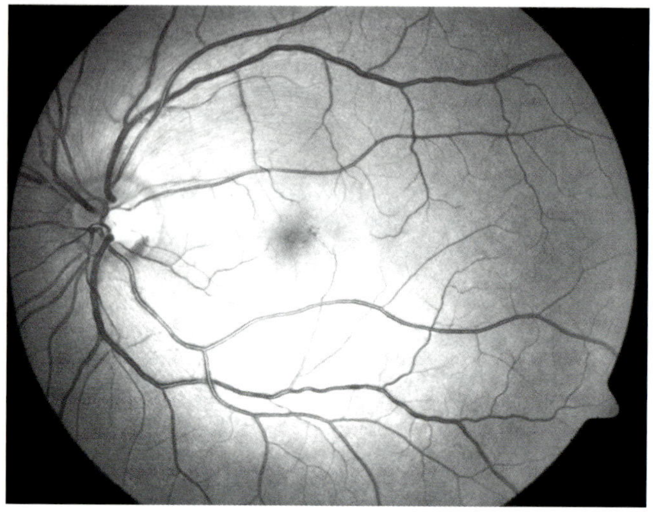

Red free photograph of the left eye

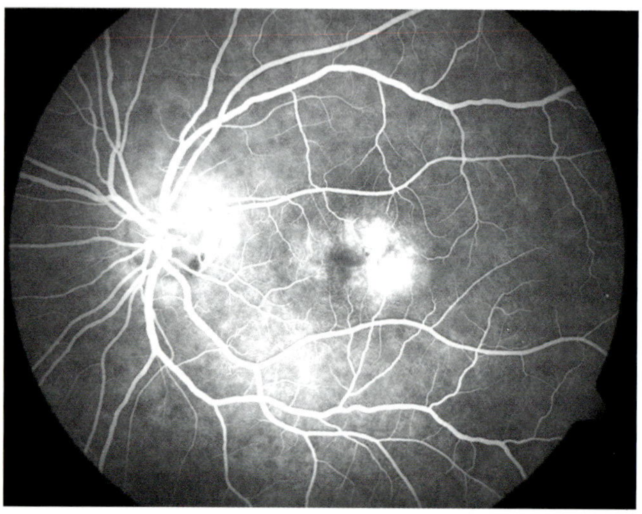

Leakage of dye from the vascular abnormalities in the parafoveal region is seen

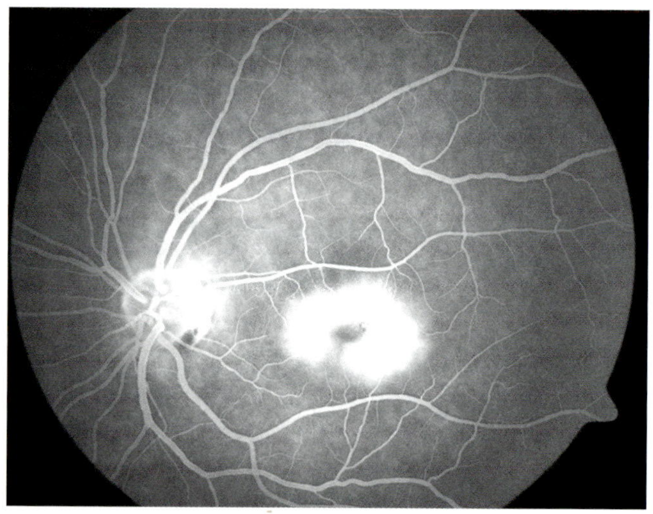

Intense staining of the parafoveal region is seen in the late film. The foveal center remains hypofluorescent

CASE 4

A 56-year-old lady presented with diminution of vision in the right eye since the last 4 weeks. Her visual acuity in the right eye was 6/36; N36 in the right eye and 6/12; N6 in the left eye. She had a history of diabetes mellitus over the last 12 years with good glycemic control. No prior laser photocoagulation was done.

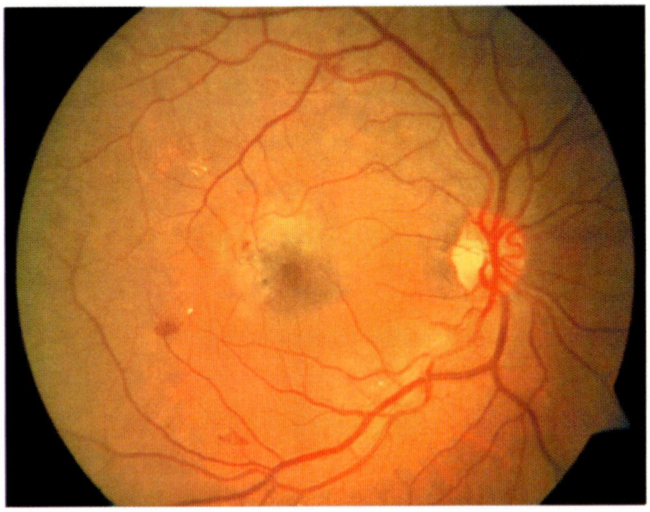

Color fundus photograph of the right eye reveals an area of retinal opacification in the perifoveal area with subretinal hemorrhage and a right angled venule temporal to the fovea. A yellowish-gray subretinal lesion superior to the fovea is suggestive of subretinal neovascular membrane (SRNV). Other macular changes suggestive of moderate NPDR (hard exudates and blot hemorrhages) are also noted

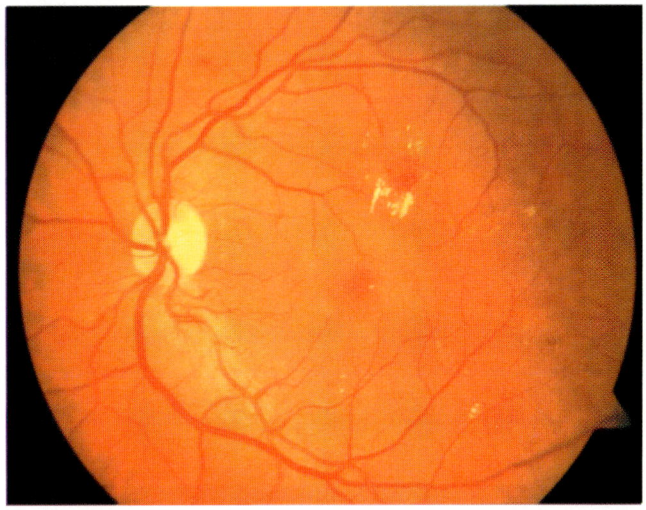

Color fundus photograph of the left eye reveals an area of retinal opacification in the perifoveal area. Circinate hard exudates and microaneurysms suggestive of moderate NPDR are noted away from the fovea

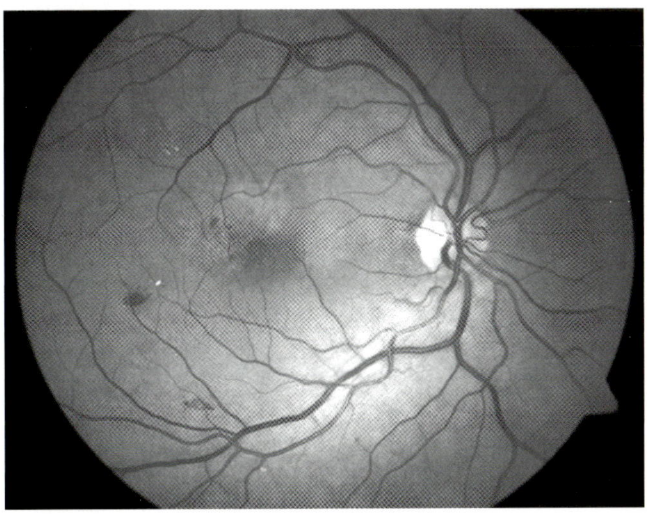

Red free photograph of the right eye highlights the microvascular changes better. Area of perifoveal opacification is better appreciated

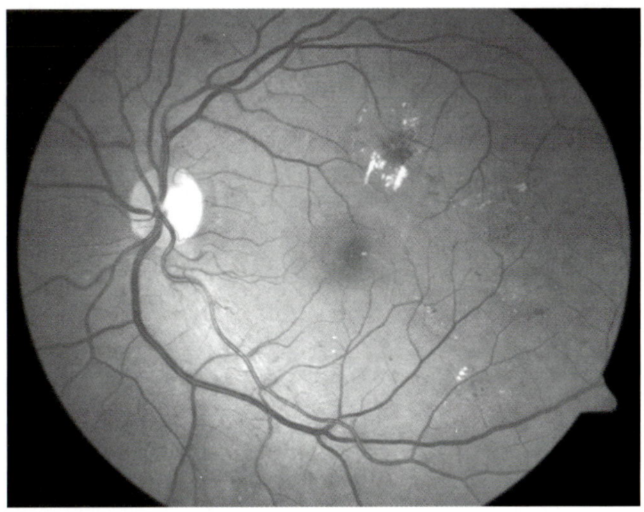

Red free photograph of the left eye highlights the microvascular changes better. Area of perifoveal opacification is better appreciated

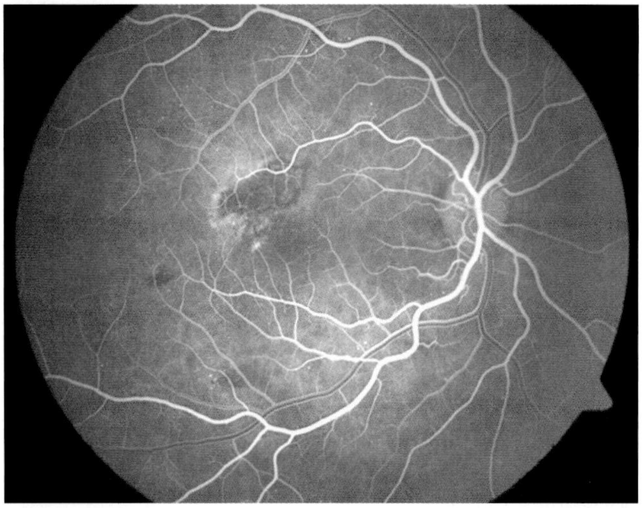

Early AV phase angiogram reveals early diffuse leakage in the perifoveal area along with blocked fluorescence secondary to hemorrhage and pigmentation

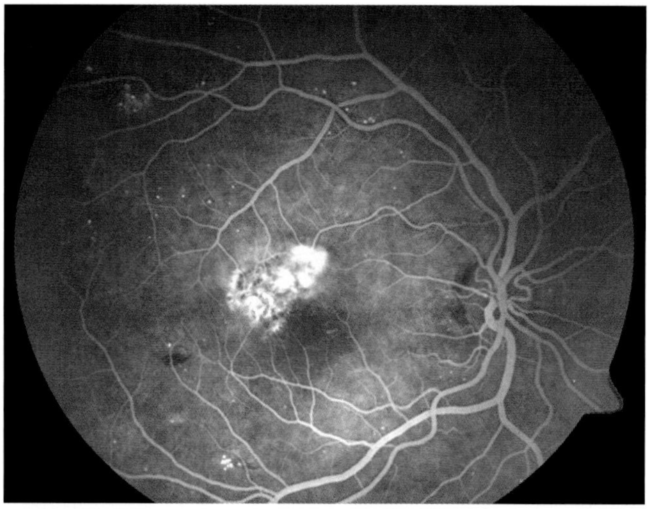

Mid AV phase angiogram reveals increased hyperfluorescence superior to the fovea delineating a SRNV. Diffuse leakage has increased in the background

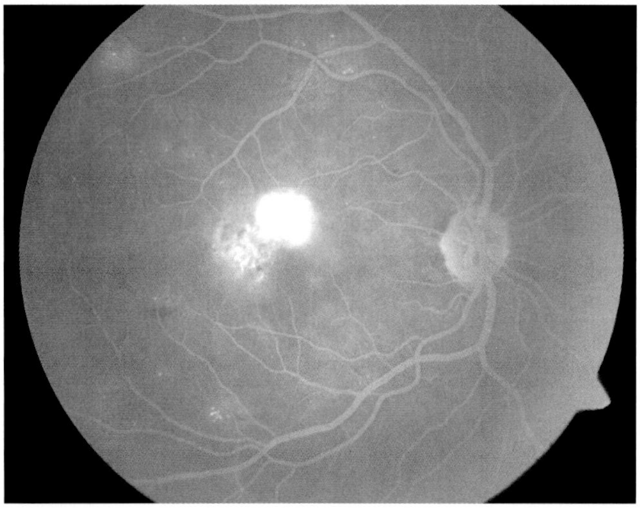

Late AV phase angiogram reveals intense hyperfluorescence associated with leakge from the SRNV. Diffuse leakage has increased further in the background

The patient underwent combined PDT and intravitreal Ranibizumab in the right eye. The laser spot size was kept equal to the greatest linear dimension of the SRNV.

Visit 1

Eight weeks after the initial treatment, visual acuity improved to 6/18; N12 in the right eye with regression of SRNV. Clinical findings were confirmed on FFA and OCT. Fundus remained stable till the last visit, 20 months following treatment.

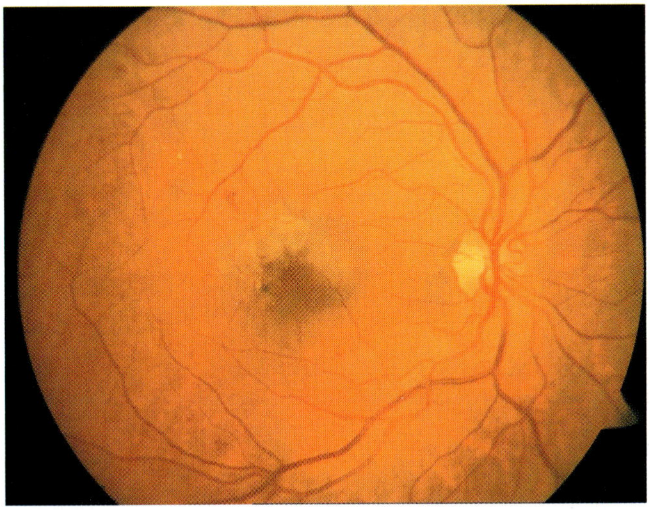

Clinically, SRNV appeared regressed with resolution of subretinal fluid and hemorrhage

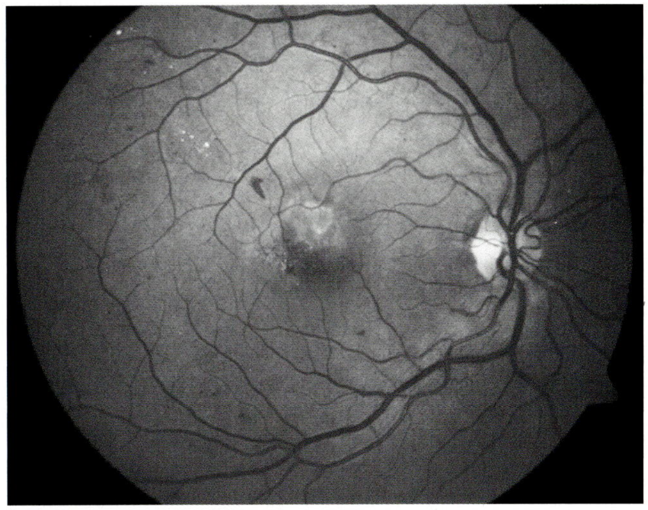

Red free photograph of the right eye highlights the regressed SRNV

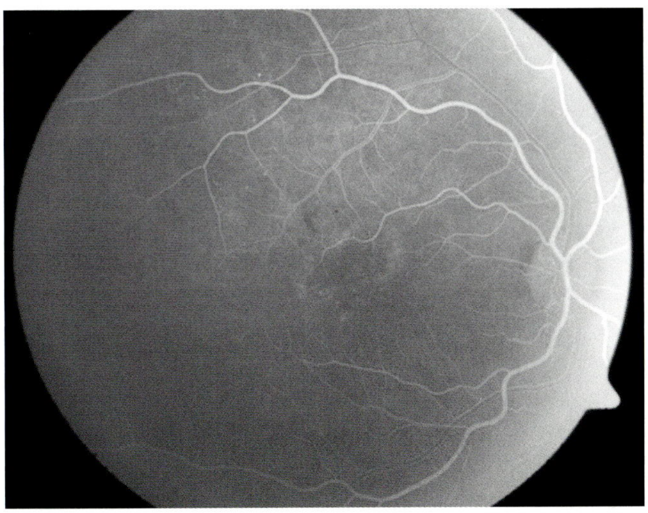

Arterial phase of angiogram outlines the regressed SRNV with stippled fluorescence and no leakage

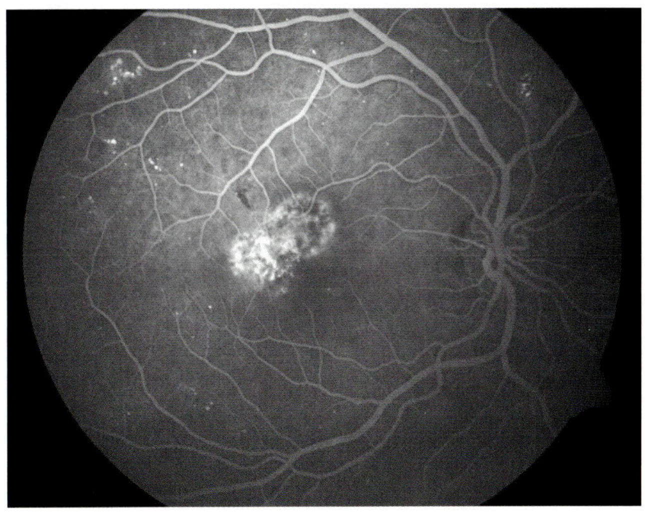

Mid AV phase angiogram reveals staining of SRNV

CLINICAL NUGGETS

1. Group 2 is the most common from of parafoveal telangiectasia.
2. Abnormal glucose tolerance test is seen in 35 percent of patients with unilateral disease and 60 percent of patients with bilateral disease.
3. Patients with parafoveal telangiectasia should be followed up to look for the development of subretinal neovascular membrane.
4. Treatment of parafoveal telangiectasia with laser photocoagulation is controversial.
5. Intravitreal anti-VEGF agents with or without PDT may help in regression of SRNV associated with PFT.

BIBLIOGRAPHY

1. Chopdar A. Retinal telangiectasias in adults: Fluorescein angiographic findings and treatment by argon laser.Br J Ophthalmol; 1978;62:243-50.
2. Gass JDM, Oyakawa RT. Idiopathic juxtafoveolar retinal telangiectasia. Arch Ophthalmology; 1982;100: 769-80.
3. Gass JDM. A fluorescein angiographic study of macular dysfunction secondary to retinal vascular diseases vs retinal telangiectasia. Arch Ophthalmol 1968;80:592-605.
4. Gass JDM. Stereoscopic atlas of macular diseases: diagnosis and treatment. 4th edition Vol. 1, Mosby, St Louis, Chapter 6 – Macular dysfunction caused by retinal vascular diseases 1997;506-11.
5. Rishi P, Rishi E, Shroff D. Combined photodynamic therapy and intravitreal bevacizumab as primary treatment for subretinal neovascularization associated with type 2 idiopathic macular telangiectasia. Indian J Ophthalmol. 2009;57(3):241-2.
6. Rishi P, Shroff D, Rishi E. Combined photodynamic therapy and intravitreal ranibizumab as primary treatment for subretinal neovascular membrane (SRNVM) associated with type 2 idiopathic macular telangiectasia. Graefes Arch Clin Exp Ophthalmol 2008; 246(4):619-21.
7. Yannuzzi, LA, Bardal AMC, Freund KB, Chen K, Eandi CM, Blodi B. Idiopathic Macular Telangiectasia. Arch Ophthalmol. 2006; 124:450-60.

36 Chapter

Purtscher's Retinopathy

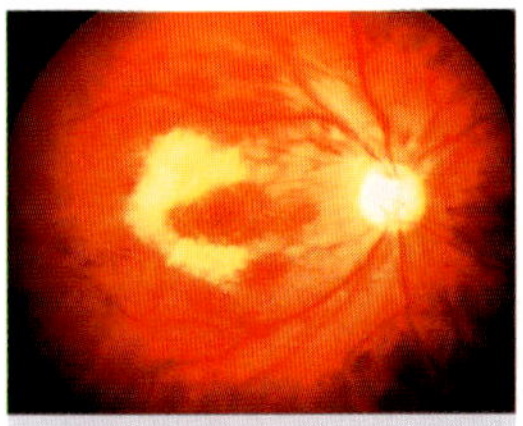

- It is characterized by the presence of multiple patches of retinal whitening and retinal hemorrhages at the posterior pole.
- It usually follows compressive injuries of the head and trunk.
- It has also been reported in cases of pancreatitis, chronic renal failure, following child birth, in connective tissue disorders, etc.
- It is possibly due to complement induced leukocyte aggregation and leukoembolism.

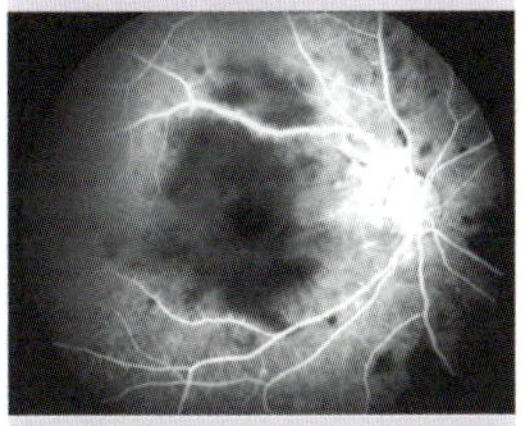

- Areas of capillary nonperfusion is seen in the affected areas.
- Minimal leakage of the dye from the retinal vasculature and perivascular staining may be seen.

CASE 1

A 35-year-old male presented with loss of vision noted in both eyes following a road traffic accident. Visual acuity was hand movements close to face in both eyes.

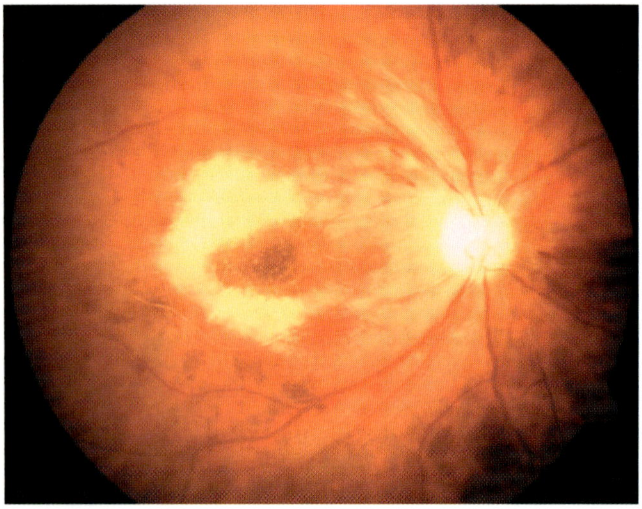

Fundus photograph of the right eye showing patches of retinal whitening and retinal hemorrhages at the posterior pole

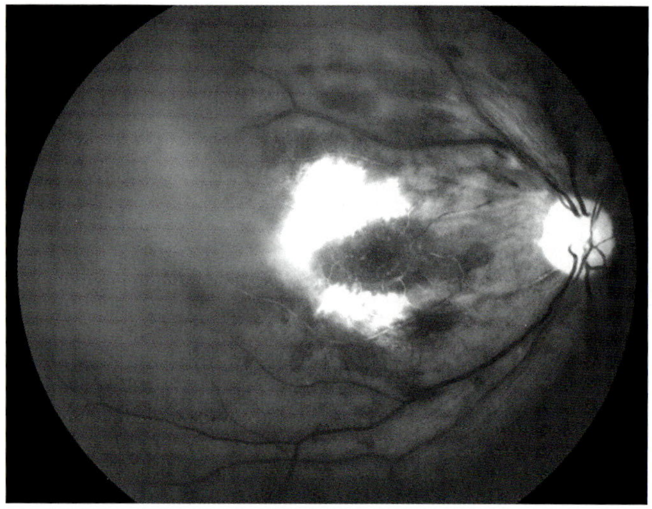

Red free photograph of the right eye

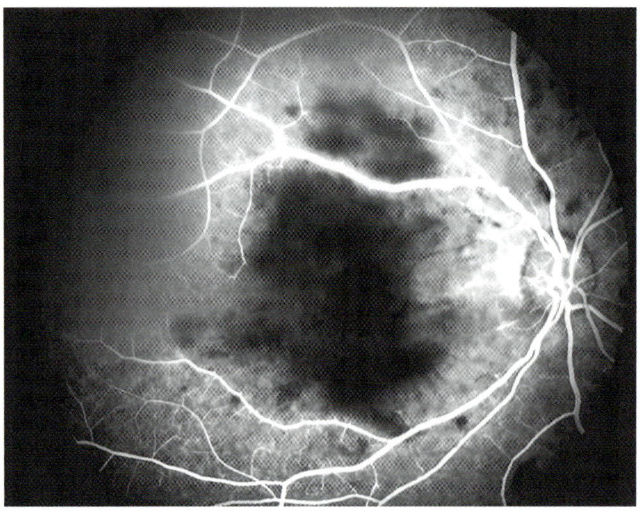

Arteriovenous phase of the right eye showing a large hypofluorescent patch in the macula due to a combination of blocked fluorescence and nonfilling of the vasculature

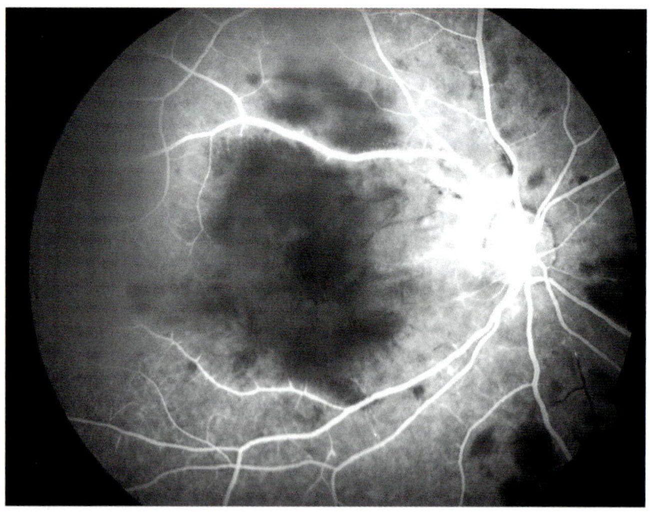

The hypofluorescence is persisting in the later arteriovenous phase. Note there is no filling of the vessels in the macula. Minimal leakage of the dye is seen through the walls of the larger vessels

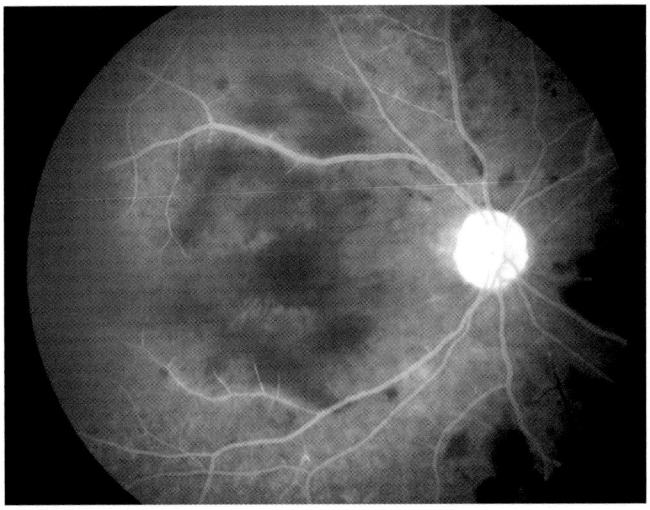

Late phase angiogram showing persistent hypofluorescence at the macula. Perivascular and disc staining is also seen

COMMENT

Occlusion of the arterioles possibly due to leukoembolization, results in closure of the capillaries in the macula resulting in visual impairment.

CASE 1 (*Continued*)

Left Eye of the Patient

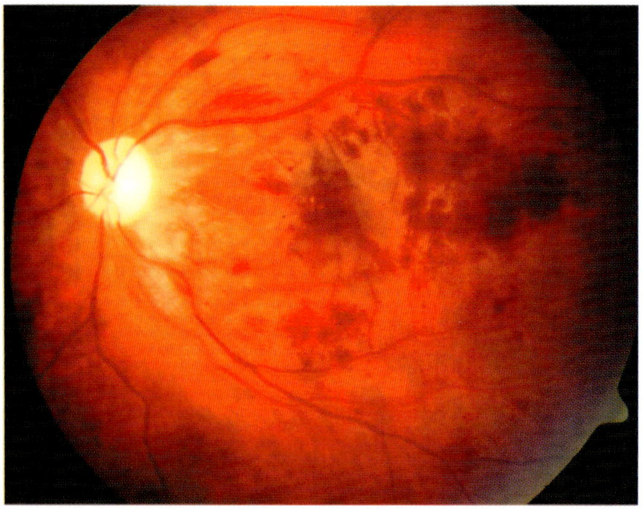

Fundus photograph of the left eye showing patches of retinal whitening and retinal hemorrhages at the posterior pole

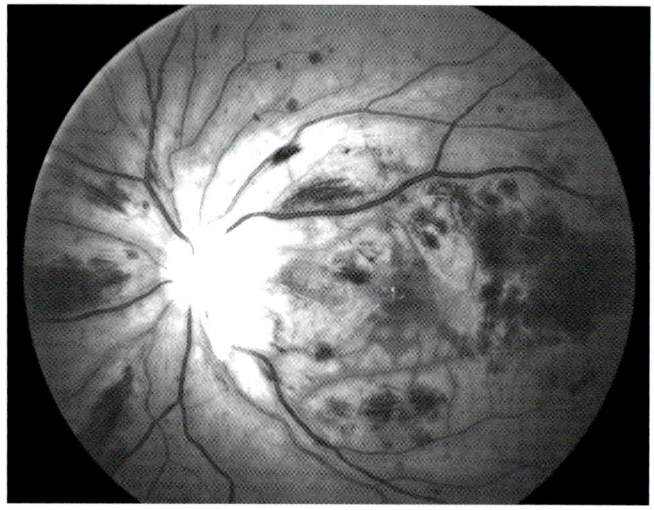

Red free photograph of the left eye

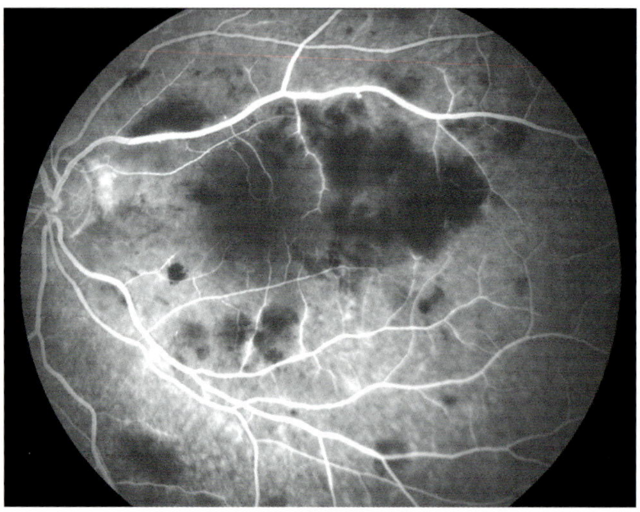

Arteriovenous phase shows areas of blocked fluorescence due to hemorrhage and areas of hypofluorescence due to nonfilling of the vasculature

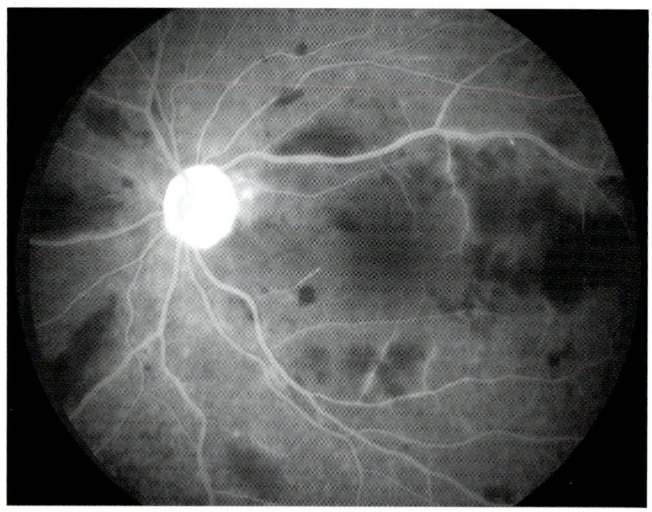

Late perivascular and disc staining is noted. The macula remains hypofluorescent

COMMENT

Purtscher's retinopathy is characterized by the presence of areas of nonperfusion at the macula.

CLINICAL NUGGETS

1. Leukocyte aggregation resulting from activation of the complement system due to varied etiology, leads to leukoembolization resulting in Purtscher's retinopathy.
2. Visual prognosis is poor in patients with Purtscher's retinopathy.
3. There is no specific treatment for Purtscher's retinopathy.

BIBLIOGRAPHY

1. Burton TC. Unilateral Purtscher's retinopathy. Ophthalmology 1980;87:1096-1105.
2. Kelley JS. Purtscher's retinopathy related to chest compression by safety belts. Fluorescein Angiographic findings, Am J Ophthalmol 1972;74:278-83.

37

Chapter

Valsalva Retinopathy

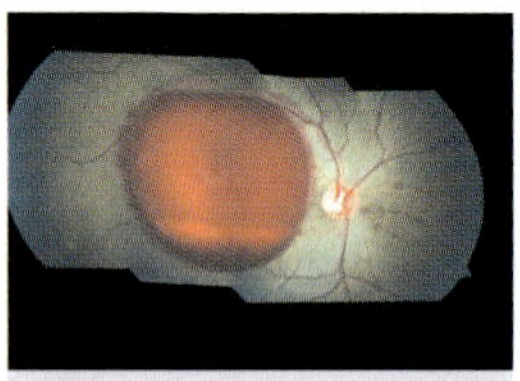

- Valsalva retinopathy is a form of retinopathy with preretinal hemorrhages and sometimes intra- and subretinal hemorrhages resulting from increased intrathoracic pressure.
- Rapid rise in intraocular venous pressure may cause spontaneous rupture of perifoveal capillaries, causing sudden, painless decrease in vision or scotoma in an otherwise healthy eye.
- Usually it is a self-resolving condition, which resolves in few weeks to months.

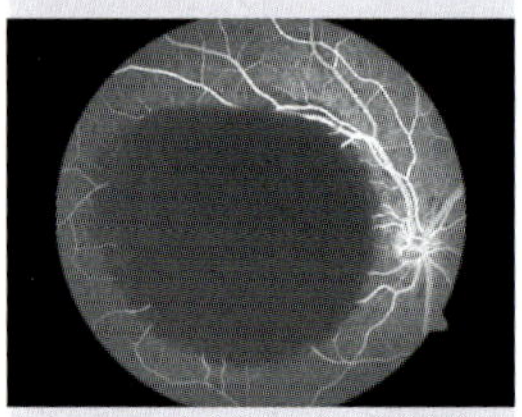

- Fundus fluorescence angiography (FFA) and ICG are done to rule out any underlying vascular pathology.
- OCT is helpful in exact localization of the plane of the hemorrhage.

CASE 1

A 25-year-old healthy male came with a complaint of sudden loss of vision in the right eye after a session of strenuous physical exercise. Visual acuity was counting fingers close to face. Left eye was normal.

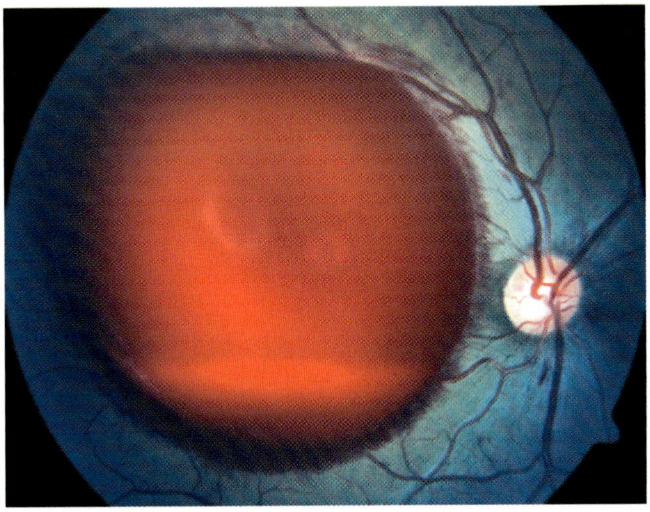

Color fundus photograph of the right eye reveals fresh subhyaloid hemorrhage over the posterior pole obscuring macular details

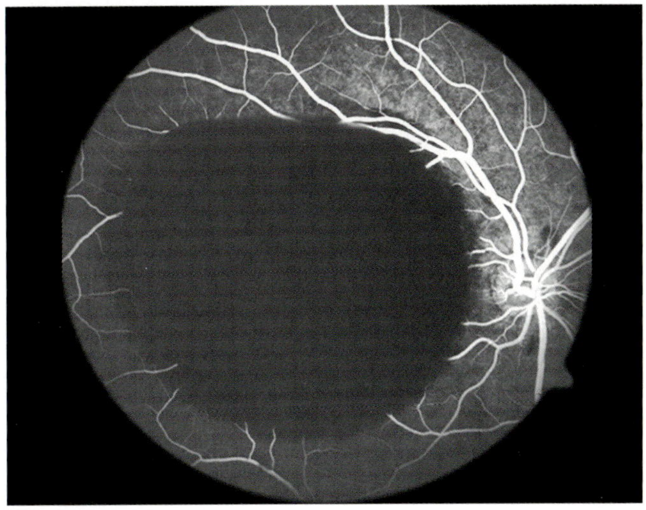

Early arteriovenous phase shows blocked choroidal and retinal fluorescence due to the subhyaloid hemorrhage

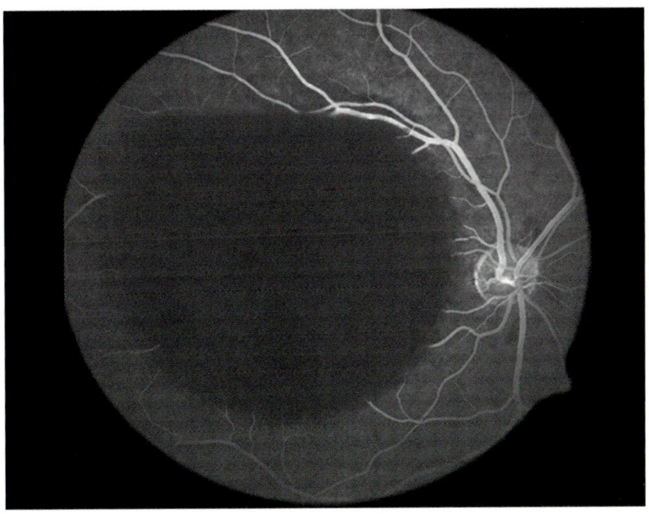

Late arteriovenous phase shows persistence of the blocked fluorescence

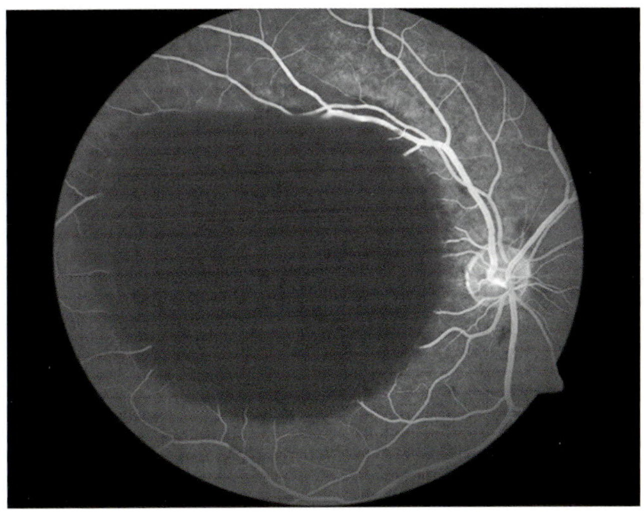

Venous phase also shows persistence of blocked fluorescence with no evidence of any treatable lesion. The patient underwent Nd:YAG hyaloidotomy

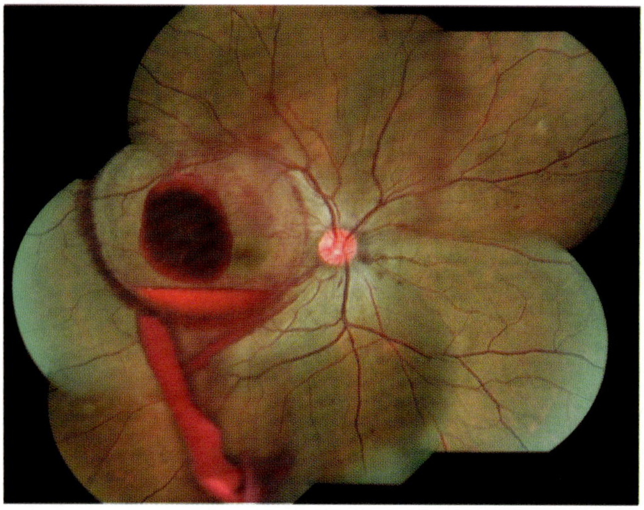

1 hour postlaser hyaloidotomy, fundus examination revealed trickling of the subhyaloid blood inferiorly. Residual sub-ILM and sub-RPE hemorrhage temporal to the fovea is persisting

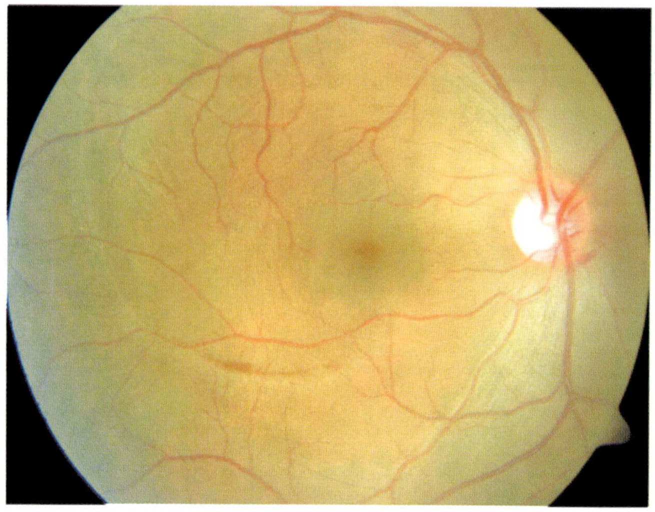

1 month postlaser hyaloidotomy, fundus reveals complete resolution of the blood. Visual acuity recovered to 6/6

CLINICAL NUGGETS

1. YAG laser treatment for Valsalva retinopathy is an effective, noninvasive, and safe procedure for patients with a premacular subhyaloid hemorrhage larger than 3 disc diameter and no longer than 3 weeks of duration.
2. Hyaloidotomy site should be chosen in the inferior edge of the hemorrhage and must be away from the fovea and major vessels.

BIBLIOGRAPHY

1. Durukan AH, Kerimoglu H, Erdurman C, Demirel A, Karagul S. Long-term results of Nd:YAG laser treatment for premacular subhyaloid haemorrhage owing to Valsalva retinopathy. Eye (Lond). 2008;22(2):214-8. Epub 2006 Sep 1.
2. Jones WL. Valsalva maneuver induced vitreous hemorrhage. J Am Optom Assoc 1995;66:301-4.
3. Shukla D, Naresh K, Kim R. Optical coherence tomography findings in Valsalva retinopathy. Am J Ophthalmol 2005;140(1):1346.

38

Chapter

Radiation Retinopathy

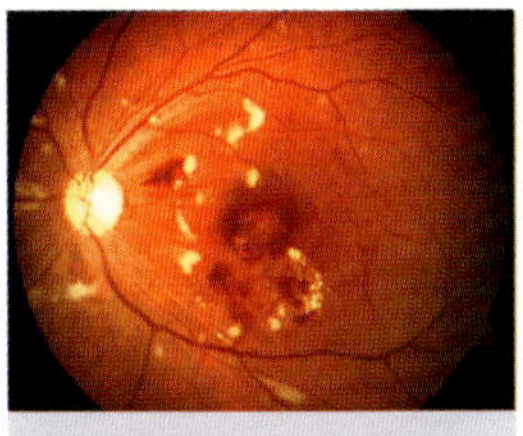

- Radiation retinopathy is a slowly progressive condition with characteristic fundus changes.
- It is predominantly a retinal vascular disorder in which the permeability of the retinal and optic nerve vasculature is affected.
- The changes seen in radiation retinopathy can mimic those seen in diabetic retinopathy.
- Three stages have been described:
  - *Background radiation retinopathy*: This is characterized by microaneurysms, retinal telangiectasia, dot and blot hemorrhages, cotton wool spots, hard exudates and macular edema.
  - *Preproliferative radiation retinopathy*: This is characterized by intraretinal microvascular abnormalities, venous beading and increased number of cotton wool spots.
  - *Proliferative radiation retinopathy*: Neovascularization may occur at the disc or elsewhere in the retina. Vitreous hemorrhage and neovascular glaucoma can result.
- Optic nerve involvement would result in optic disc edema or optic atrophy.

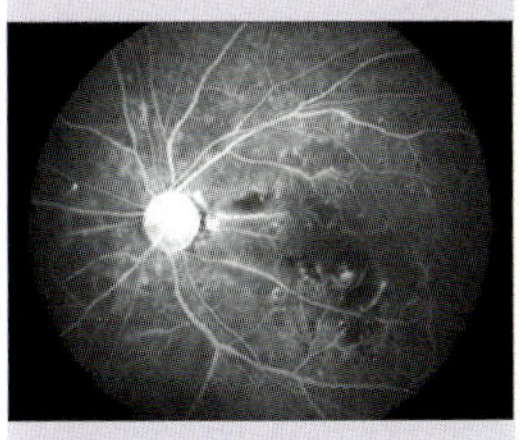

- These changes correlate with the clinical findings and can include areas of capillary non-perfusion, increased capillary permeability and leakage, microaneurysms, IRMA's and neovascularization.
- If optic nerve is affected, then non-perfusion of the optic nerve capillaries is also seen.

CASE 1

A 29-year-old male presented with a history of reduced vision in the left eye of one month duration. He had previously been diagnosed to have an orbital lymphoma and had undergone radiotherapy nine months ago. Visual acuity was 6/6; N6 in the right eye and 6/18; N8 in the left eye. The right eye fundus was normal.

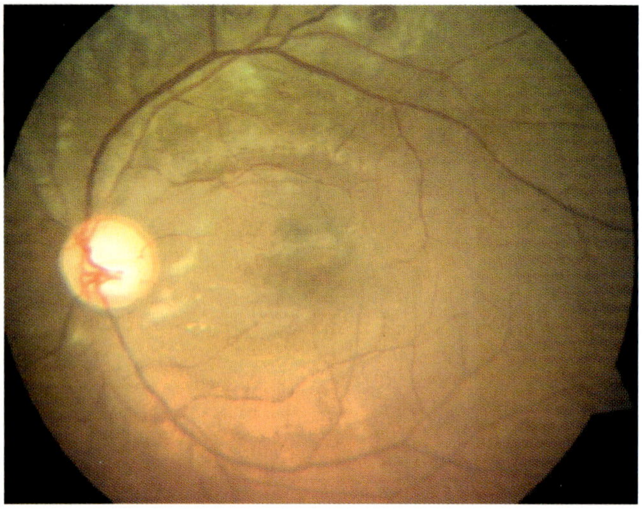

Fundus photograph of the left eye showing cotton wool spots along the superotemporal arcade and temporal to the disc. The macula has a dull appearance

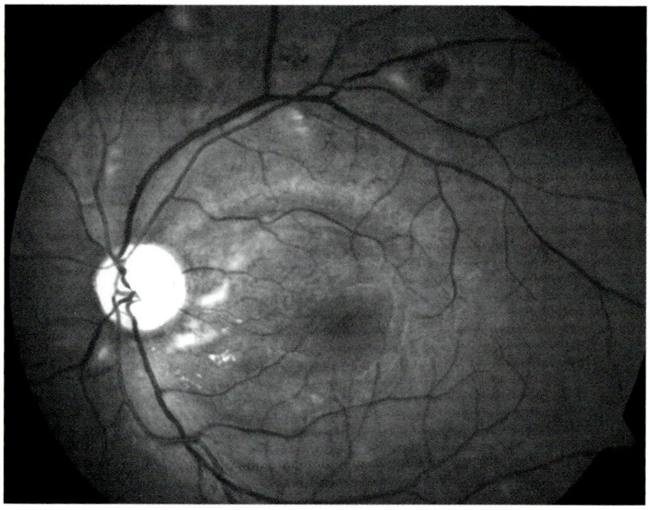

Red free photograph of the left eye. Cotton wool spot and retinal hemorrhages are seen

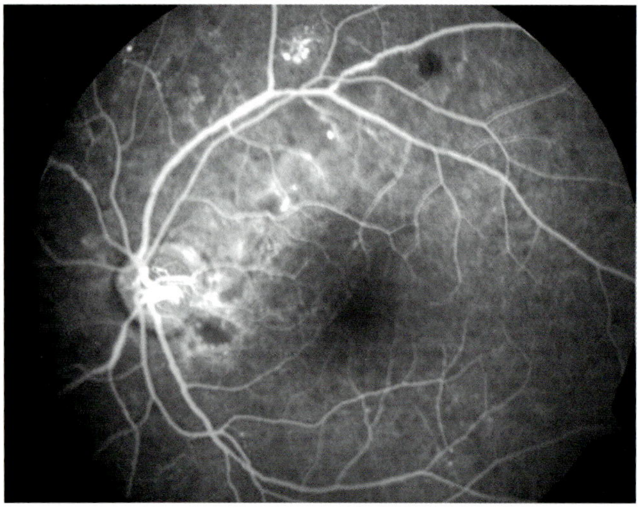

Mid arteriovenous phase showing areas of capillary non-perfusion temporal and superotemporal to the disc. Leakage of the dye from dilated capillaries around the non-perfused areas is seen

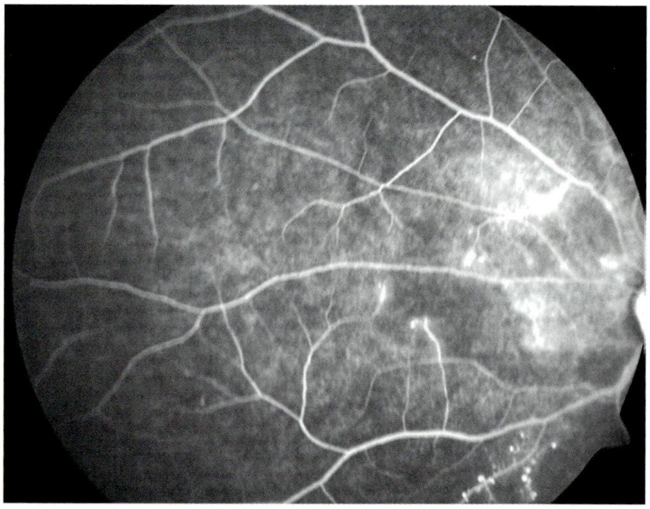

Areas of capillary non-perfusion are seen in the nasal quadrant

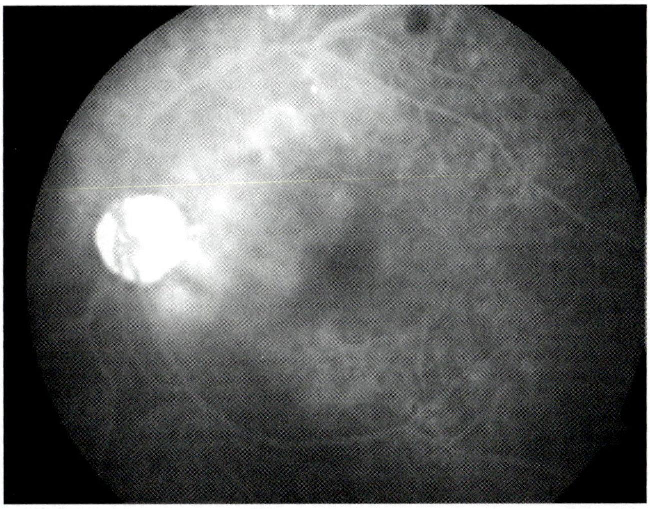

Staining of the retinal tissue from incompetent dilated capillaries is seen in the late phase

COMMENT

This case represents background radiation retinopathy changes. Widespread capillary occlusion is noted.

CASE 2

A 40-year-old male with a history of radiotherapy for nasopharyngeal carcinoma one year back, presented with reduced vision in the left eye. Visual acuity was 6/6; N6 in the right eye and 6/36; N36 in the left eye.

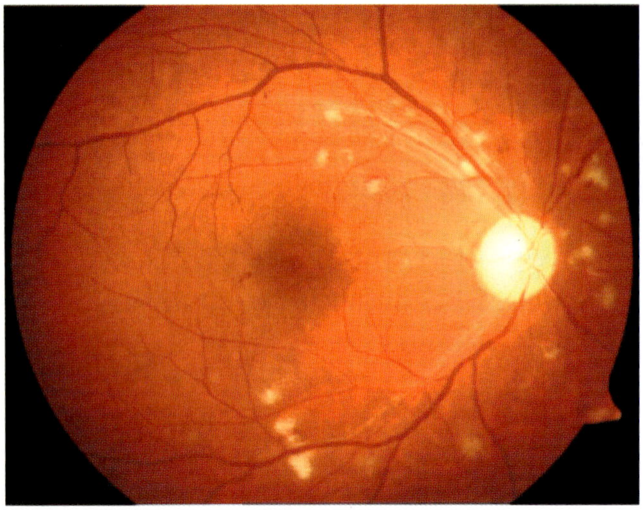

Fundus photograph of the right eye showing multiple cotton wool spots. Fovea has a dull appearance

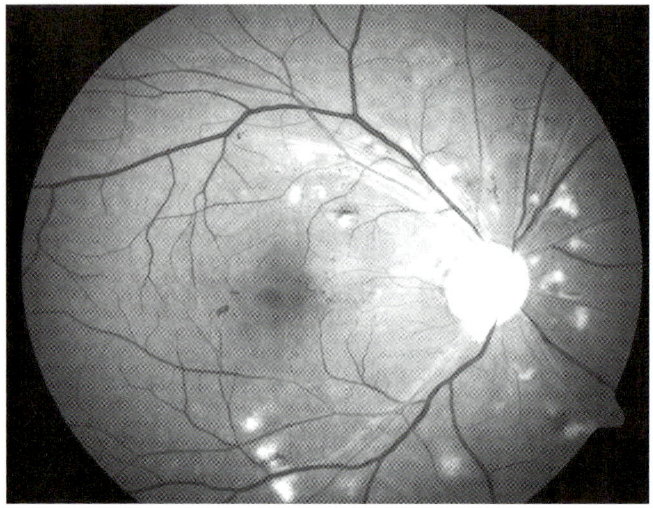

Red free photograph of the right eye

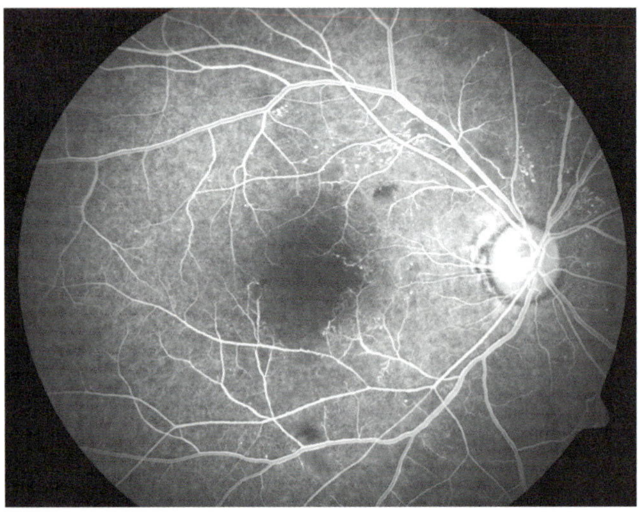

Mid arteriovenous phase showing areas of capillary non-perfusion at the macula. The para- and perifoveal capillaries are affected

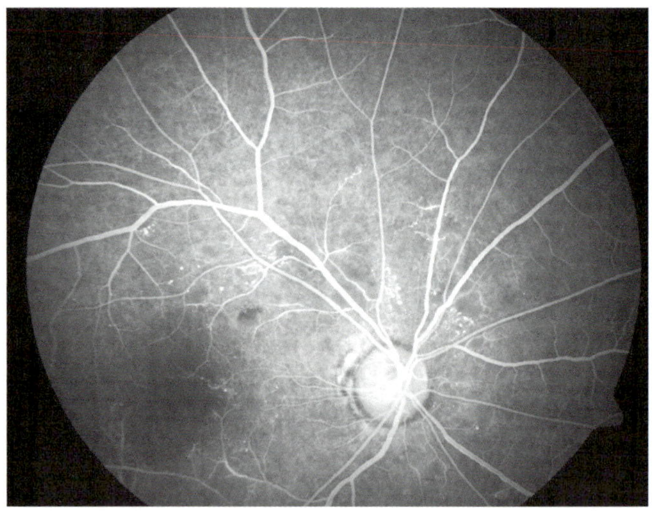

Mid arteriovenous phase shows extensive capillary non-perfusion in the superior and nasal quadrants

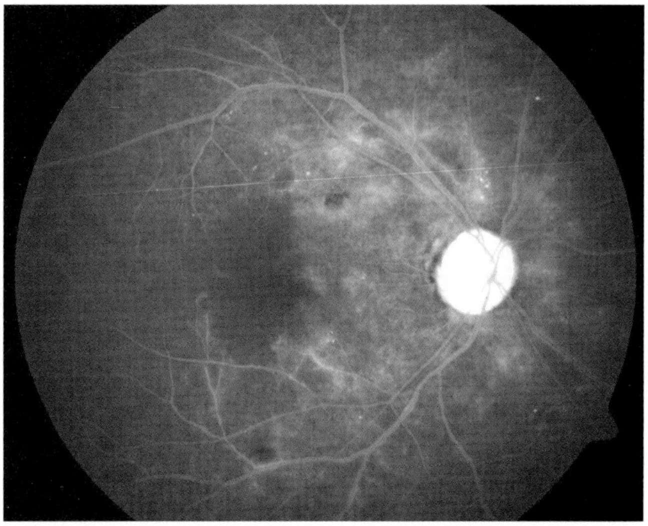

Late phase picture showing staining of the retina around the disc. The fovea remains hypofluorescent

CASE 2 (*Continued*)

Left Eye of the Patient

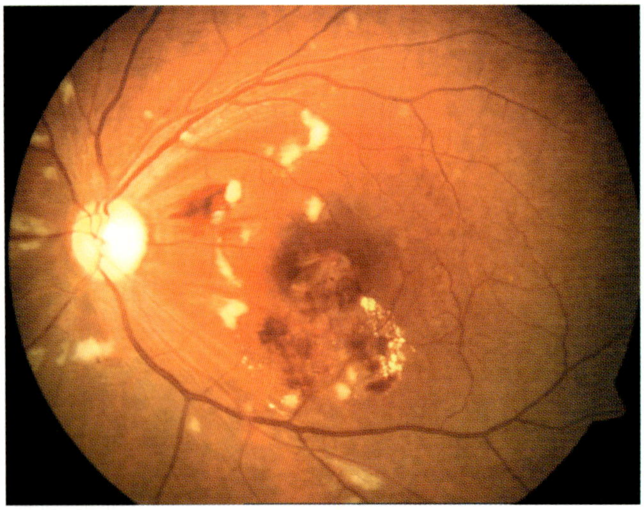

Fundus photograph of the left eye showing cotton wool spots and retinal hemorrhages

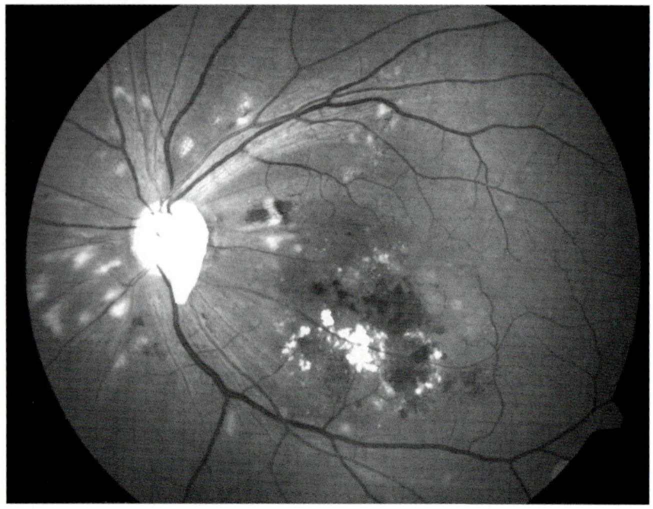

Red free photograph of the left eye

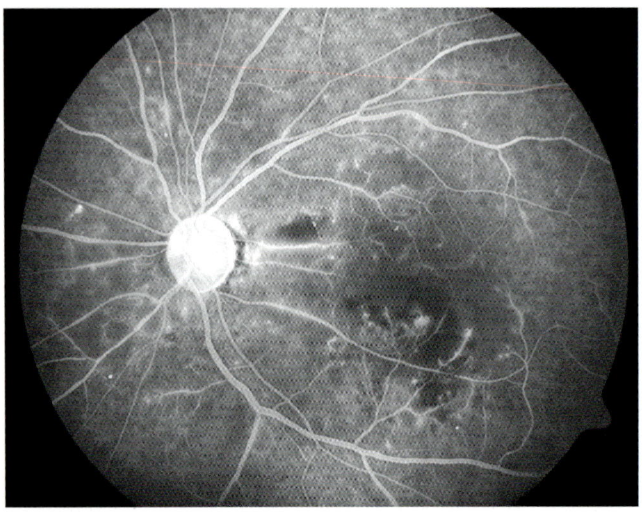

Extensive areas of capillary non-perfusion are seen in all quadrants and at the fovea

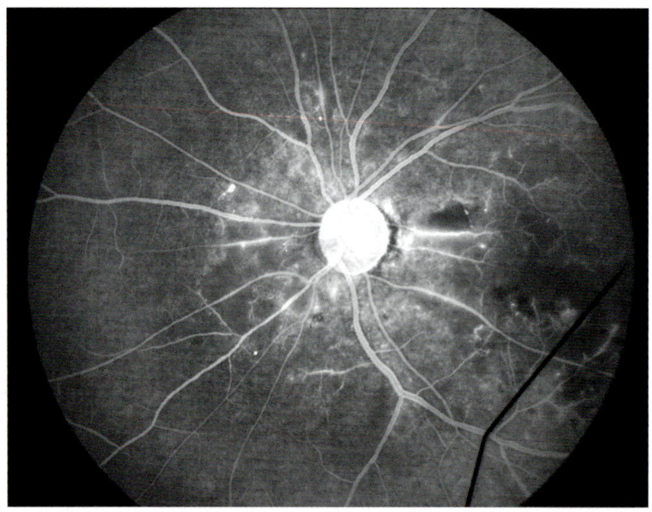

Late phase shows minimal vessel wall staining of the capillaries bordering the areas of non-perfusion. Fovea remains hypofluorescent

COMMENT

Retinal changes seen in radiation retinopathy resembles those seen in diabetic retinopathy.

CASE 3

A 56-year-old lady presented with painless loss of vision in both the eyes for the past 2 months. She was a diagnosed case of ovarian carcinoma treated with 10 cycles of chemotherapy. 8 months back she developed brain metastasis for which radiation was given twice at a gap of 6 months. Her BCVA was 3/60; N36 in the right eye and CF at 50 cm in the left eye.

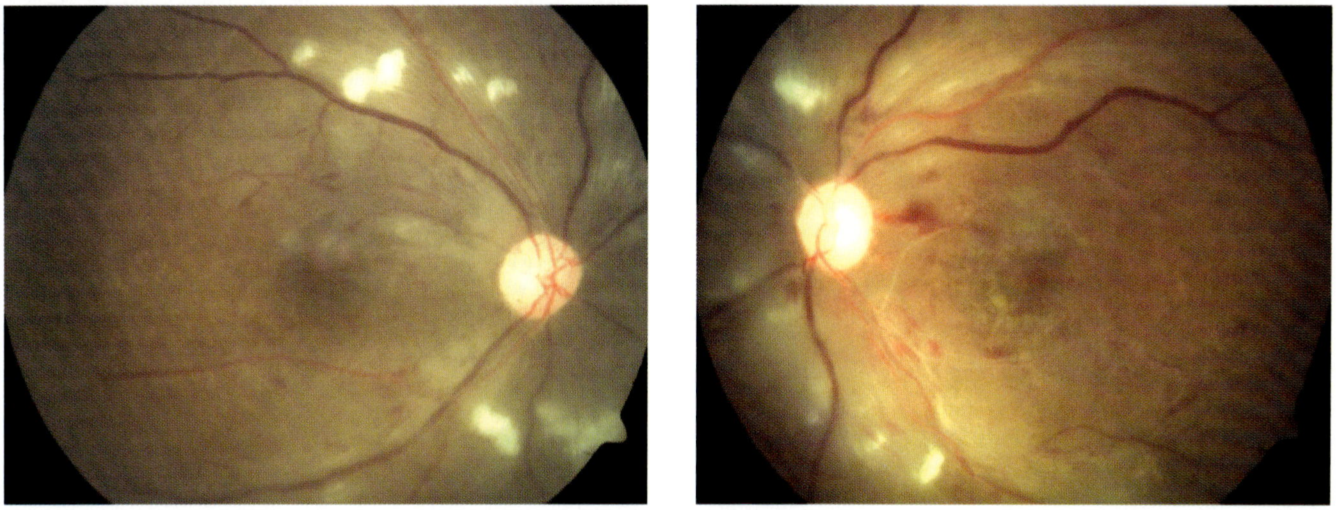

Fundus photograph of both eyes show presence of tortuous vessels, cotton wool spots and few superficial retinal hemorrhages and sclerosed vessels in the left macula with dull, featureless appearance

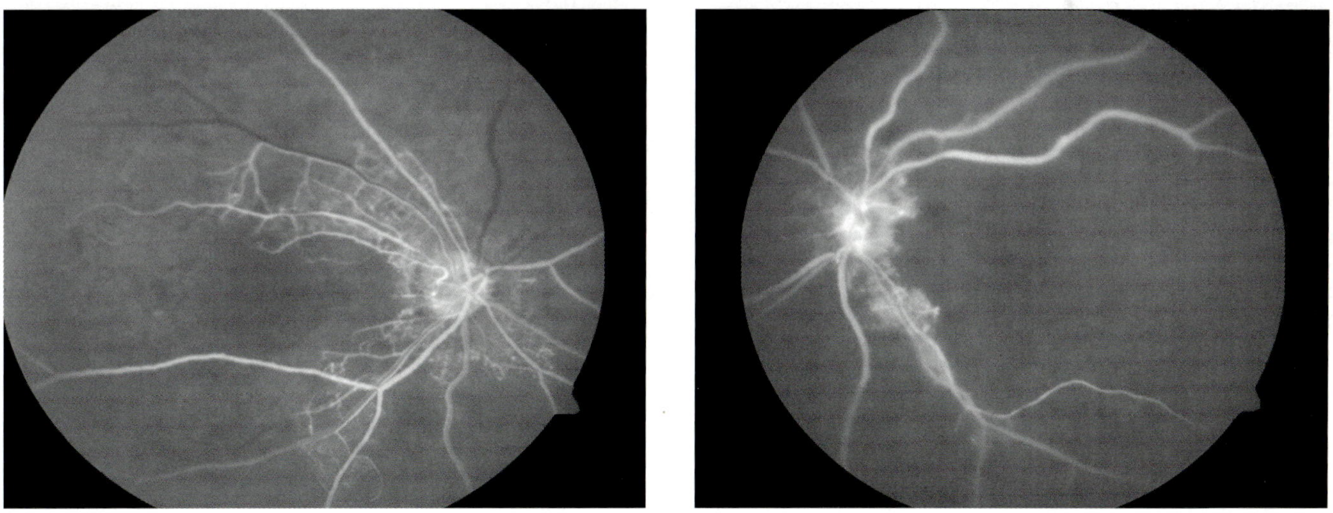

Arterial phase of the angiogram shows non-filling of two prominent vessels in right fundus suggestive of occlusion. Venular tortuosity is seen more in left eye. Multiple microvascular abnormalities are noted along major arcades in both eyes. Macular perfusion is extremely poor especially in the left eye. Hence, other changes which are expected like microaneurysms and cork-screwing of fine vessels are not evident in this case

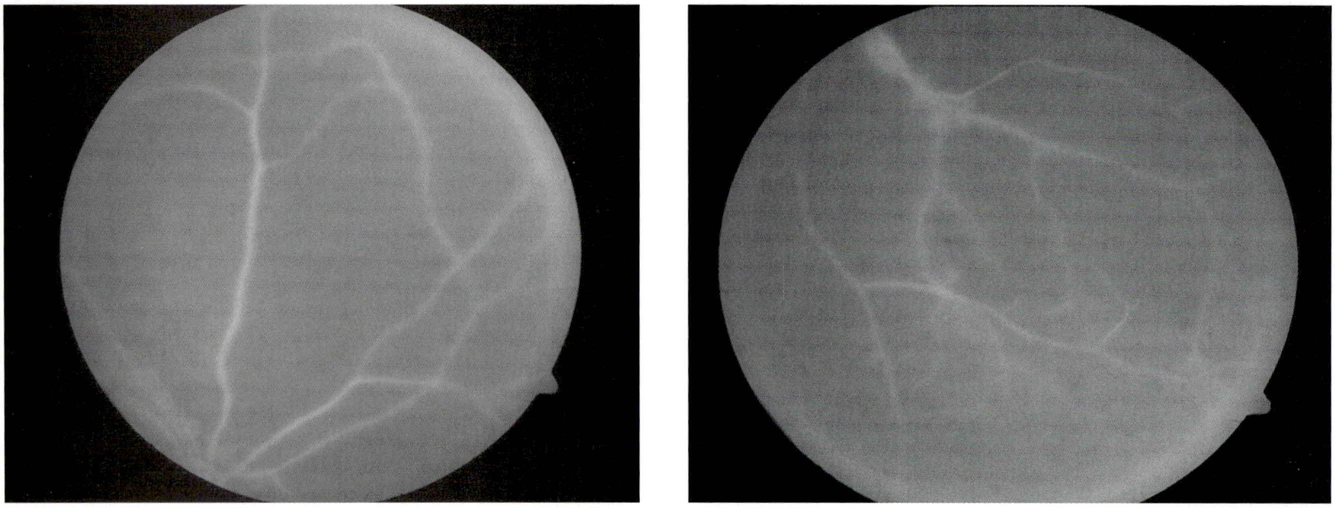

Venous phase of the angiogram showing extensive areas of capillary non-perfusion in all four quadrants. Any neovascularization, if present, shows rapid filling and leakage during this phase. Also, microaneurysms start leaking at the posterior pole

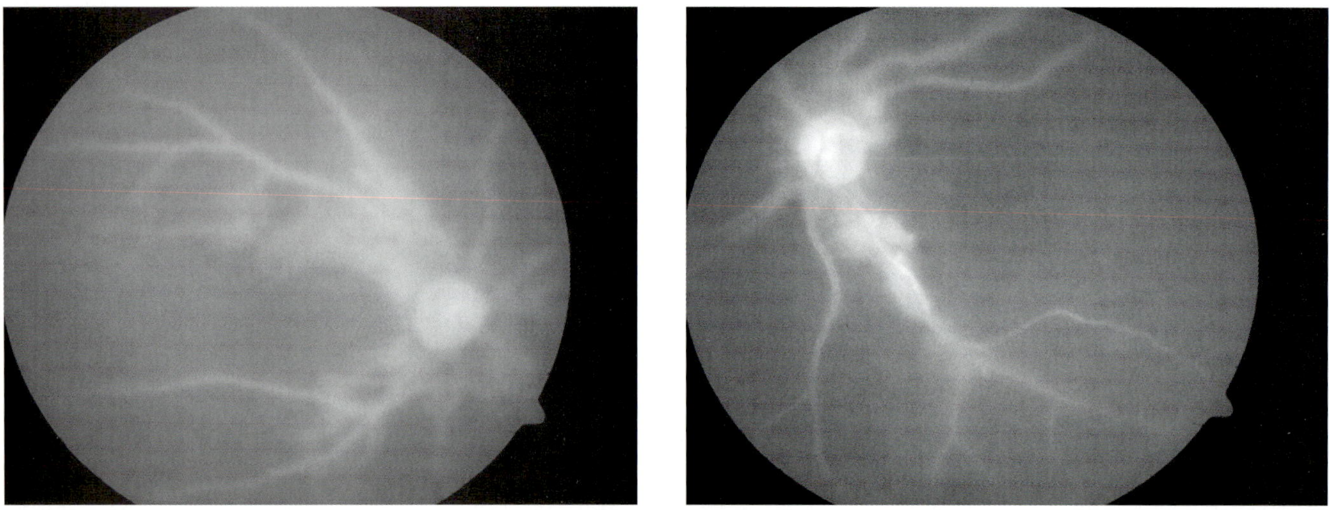

Late phase of the angiogram showing diffuse leakage from abnormal vessels. Usually cystoid macular edema is more common and can be seen as petalloid pooling of dye. Profuse leakage continues from neovascular fronds, if present

CLINICAL NUGGETS

1. Radiation retinopathy can develop 6 months to 8 years following exposure to radiation. Average time is 2-3 years.
2. Radiation retinopathy is rare when the total dose of radiation is less than 3000 rads but has been reported with as little as 1500 rads.

BIBLIOGRAPHY

1. Amoaku WMK, Archer DB. Fluorescein angiographic features, natural course and treatment of radiation retinopathy. Eye 1990;4:657-67.
2. Gass JDM. A fluorescein angiographic study of macular dysfunction secondary to retinal vascular disease. VI. X-ray irradiation, carotid artery and vitritis. Arch Ophthalmol 1968;80:606-17.
3. Hayreh SS. Post radiation retinopathy: A fluorescein fundus angiographic study. Br J Ophthalmol 1970;54: 705-14.

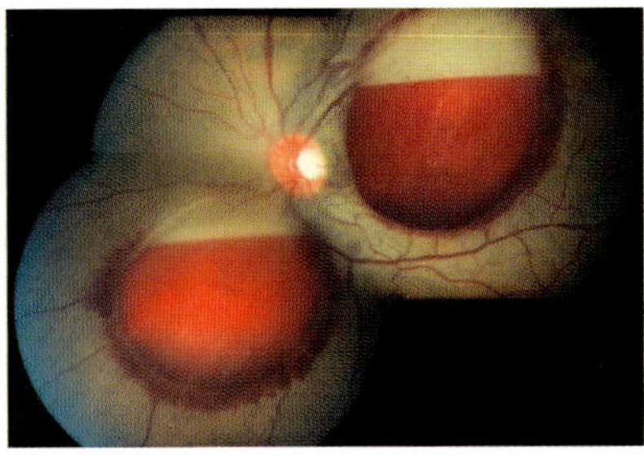

4

Section

Inflammatory Disorders

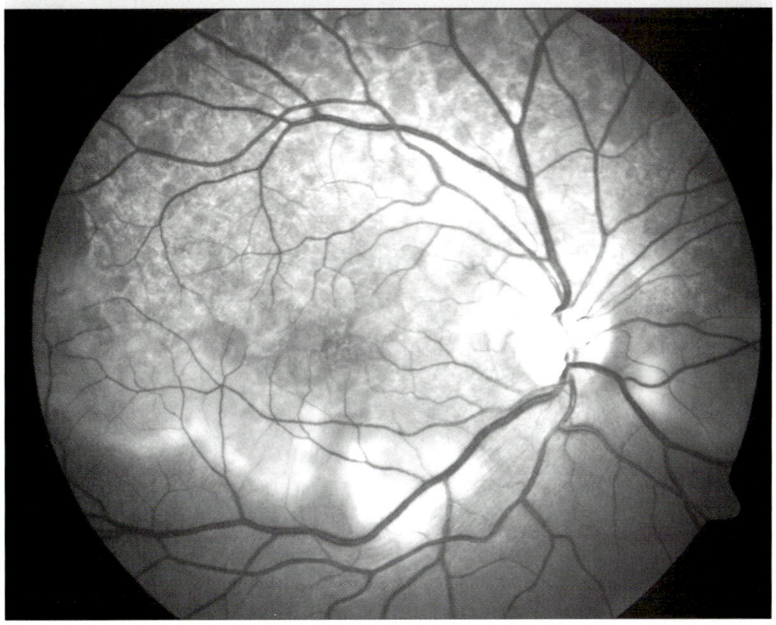

39

Chapter

Acute Retinal Pigment Epitheliitis (Krill's Disease)

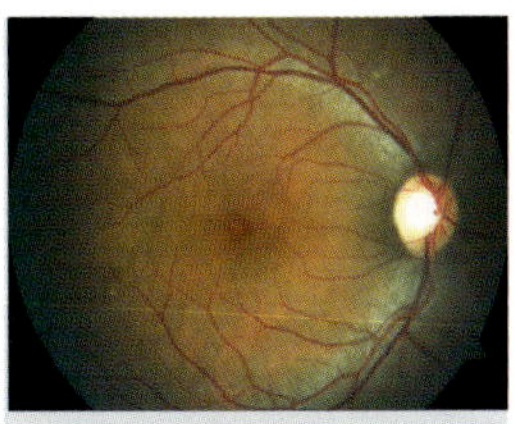

- It is a disease of unknown etiology which affects the pigment epithelium of the posterior pole.
- It predominantly affects young, healthy adults of both genders.
- Patients present with unilateral or bilateral blurred vision and metamorphopsia.
- In certain cases it is associated with viral conditions (Hepatitis C virus).
- Fundus shows yellow to gray lesions located at the pigment epithelium level, surrounded by a yellow halo, usually in the perifoveal area.

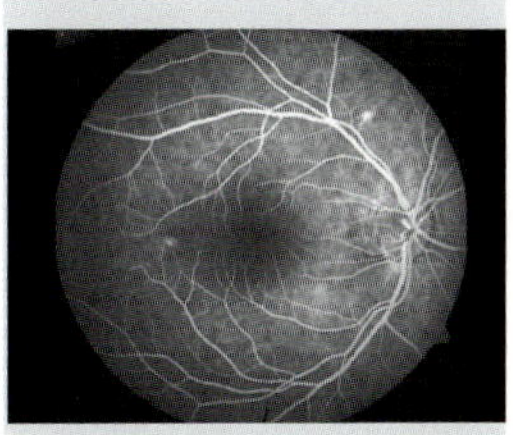

- Fluorescein angiography—shows lesions with a hypofluorescent center surrounded by a hyperfluorescent halo similar to honeycomb appearance.

CASE 1

A 42-year-old man presented with complaints of blurred vision in the right eye of 3 months duration. Visual acuity was 6/12; N10 in the right eye and 6/6; N6 in the left eye.

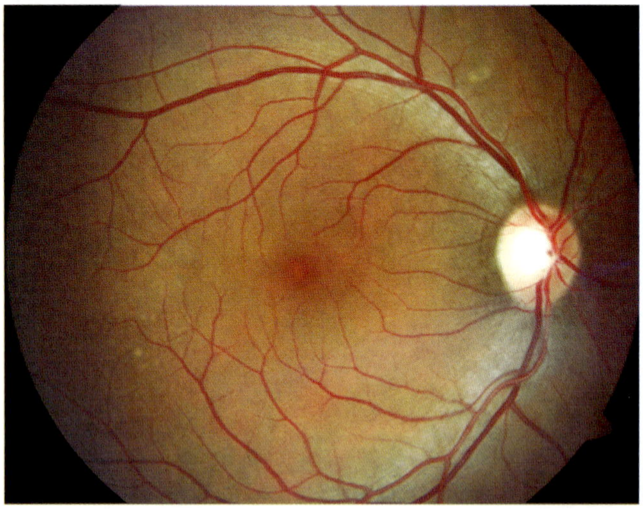

Fundus photo shows small yellow patches temporal to fovea with a hypopigmented spot at the fovea

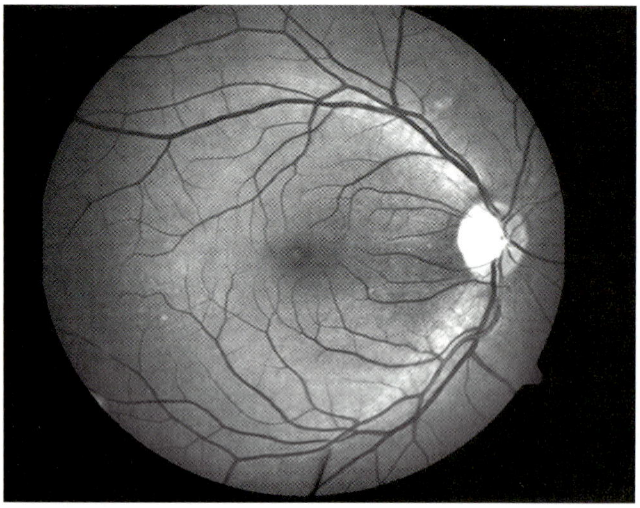

The pale spots are seen better in the red free photo

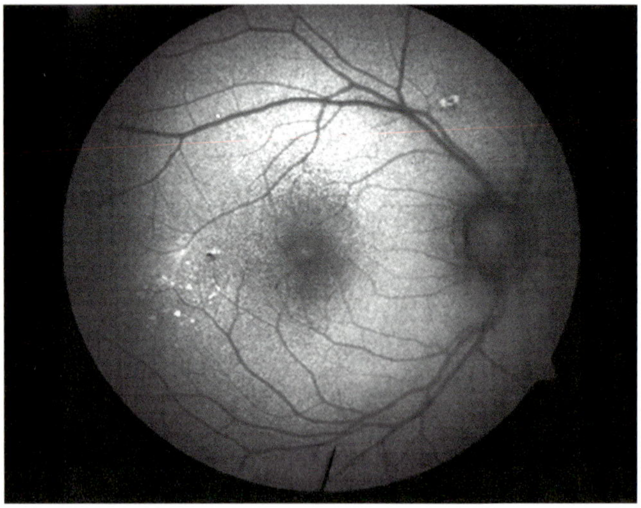

Increased autofluorescence is noted over the lesions

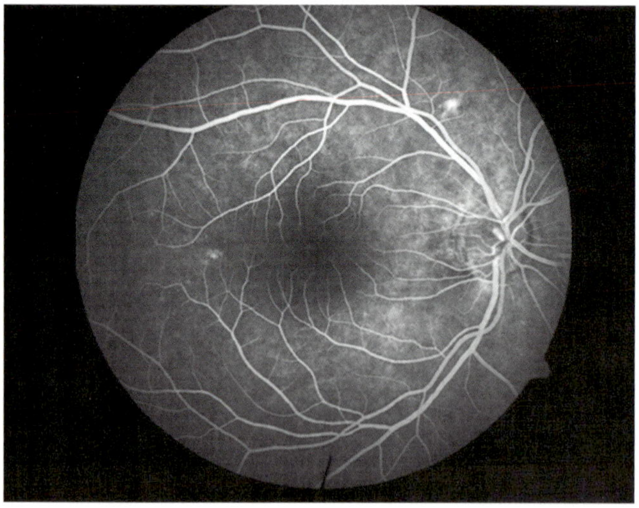

Fluorescein angiography shows hypofluorescent spot surrounded by hyperfluorescence

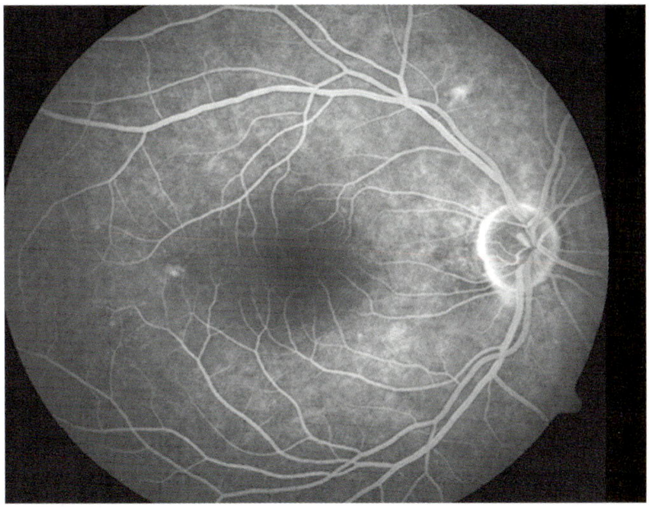

Vitreous cells are typically absent. Late phase photo does not show much change in the fluorescence

COMMENT

It normally resolves spontaneously, but one of the treatments described is the use of NSAIDs.

The differential diagnosis includes APMPPE, acute macular neuroretinopathy, central serous chorioretinopathy and rubella retinopathy.

Spectral-domain optical coherence tomography shows a disruption of the photoreceptor inner segment and outer segment interface associated with a wider disruption of the RPE inner band.

BIBLIOGRAPHY

1. Baillif S, Wolff B, et al. Retinal fluorescein and indocyanine green angiography and spectral-domain optical coherence tomography findings in acute retinal pigment epithelitis. Retina Journal 2011; Vol 31:1-8.
2. Chitum ME, Kallina RE. Acute retinal epithelitis. Ophthalmol 1987;94:1114-9.
3. Deutman AF. Acute retinal pigment epithelitis. Ophthalmologica 1975;171:361-4.
4. Krill AE, Deutman AF. Acute retinal pigment epithelitis. Am J Ophthalmol 1972;74:193-205.
5. Luttrall JK. Acute retinal pigment epithelitis. Am J Ophthalmol 1995;120:389-91.

Chapter 40

Acute Posterior Multifocal Placoid Pigment Epitheliopathy

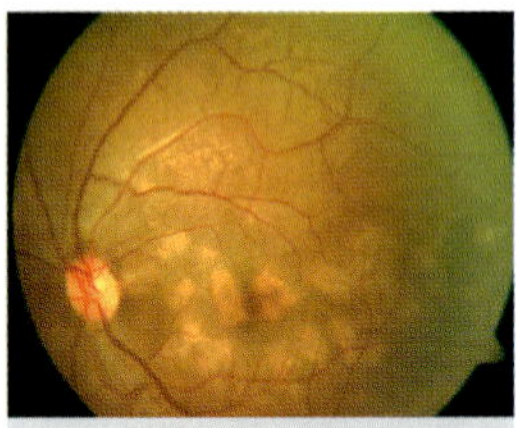

- Acute posterior multifocal placoid pigment epitheliopathy (APMPPE) is characterized by multiple yellow-white placoid lesions in the posterior pole occurring at the RPE/choroid level.
- The lesions are usually discrete and may show considerable variation in size and shape.
- Yellow lesions either represent infiltration of the choroid by inflammatory cells or choroidal hypoperfusion due to obstructive vasculitis or both, leading to opacification of the overlying retinal pigment epithelium.
- Lesions may become confluent.
- The placoid lesions fade and show retinal pigment epithelial changes on resolution. A crop of new active lesions may develop during the healing of the older lesions.

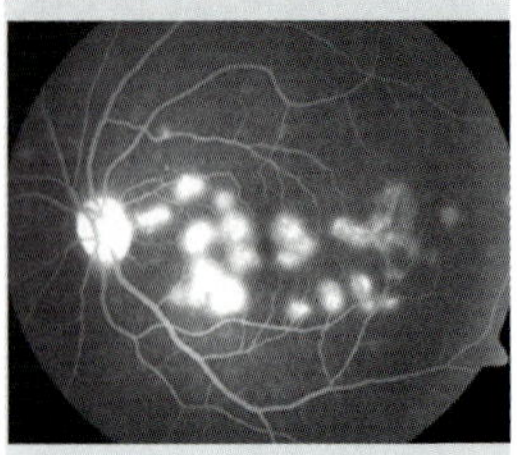

- In the acute stage, the lesions are hypofluorescent due to either blockage of fluorescence by inflammatory cells or due to non-perfusion of choriocapillaris.
- Late hyperfluorescence of the lesions is seen.
- Healed lesions show irregular hyperfluorescence (transmission defects) in the early phase which fades in the later part of the angiogram.

CASE 1

A 40-year-old male presented with history of noticing a central scotoma in the left eye for the past one week. Visual acuity was 6/9; N8 in the left eye.

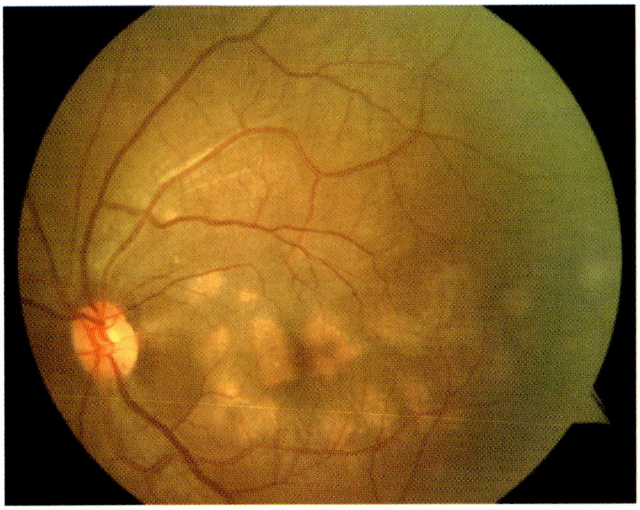

Fundus photograph of the left eye showing multiple dull yellow placoid lesions at the macula

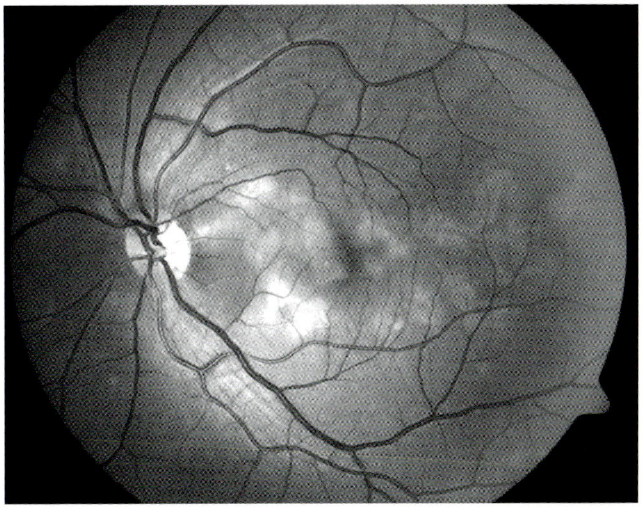

Red free photograph of the left eye

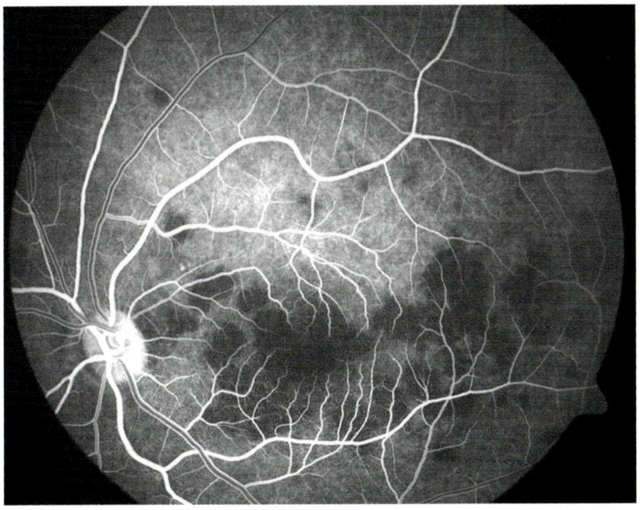

Early arteriovenous phase showing hypofluorescence in the area of the placoid lesions

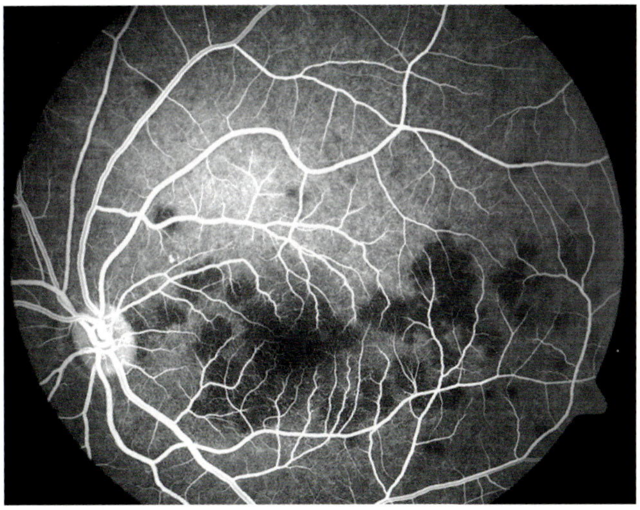

The hypofluorescence is more prominent in the mid-arteriovenous phase due to contrast from the normal surrounding choroidal fluorescence

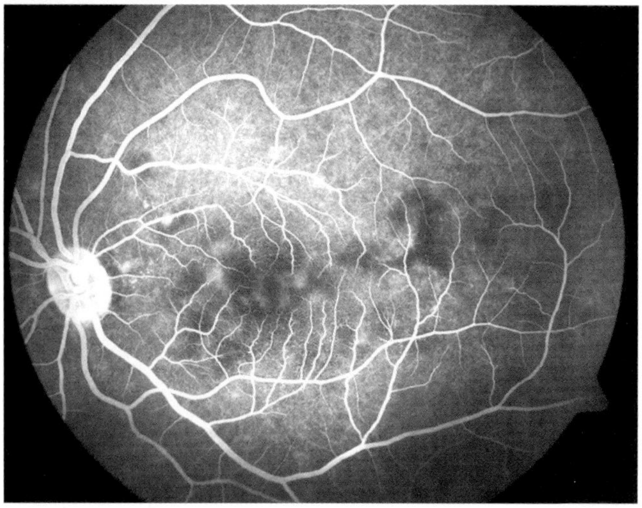

Faint hyperfluorescence is seen within the lesions in the late arteriovenous phase

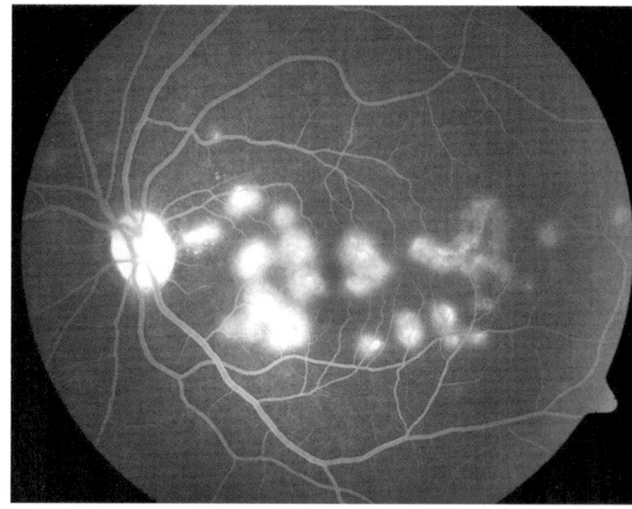

Placoid lesions are hyperfluorescent with fuzzy margins in the late phase

CASE 2

A 49-year-old male presented with history of decreased vision in the right eye for the past ten days. He did not give history of any preceding illness. Visual acuity was 6/60; N36 in the right eye. Left eye was normal.

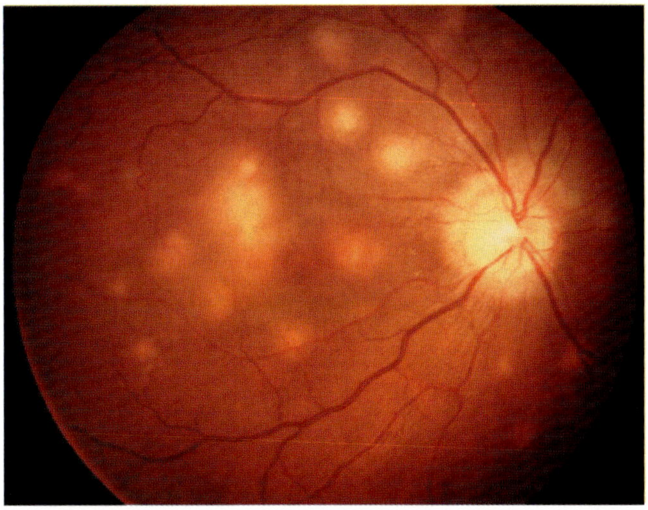

Fundus photograph of the right eye showing multiple placoid lesions at the posterior pole

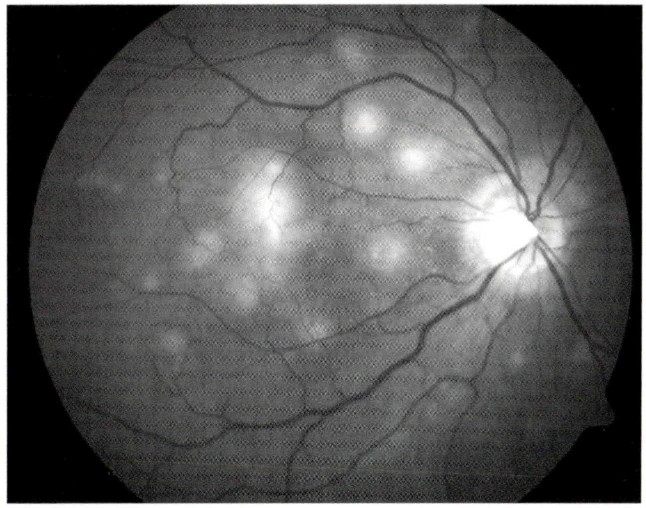

Red free photograph of the right eye

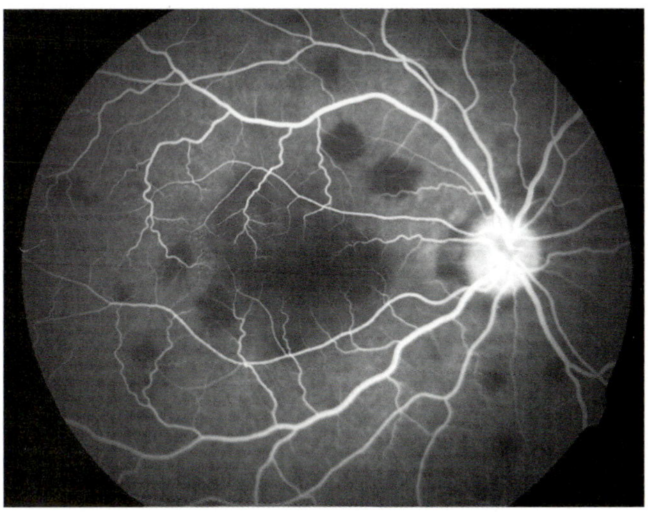

Placoid lesions appear hypofluorescent in the arteriovenous phase. Peripapillary hypofluorescence is seen corresponding to the lesions seen in the fundus photograph

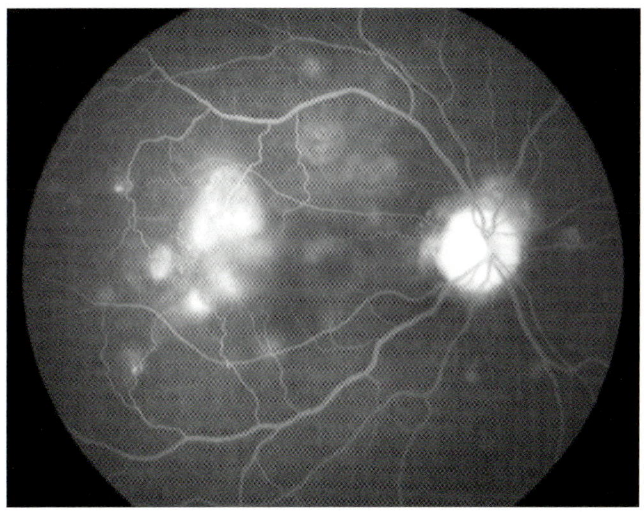

Placoid lesions appear hyperfluorescent in the late phase. Hyperfluorescence is also noted in the peripapillary region

COMMENT

Active placoid lesions of APMPPE appear hypofluorescent in the early phase and hyperfluorescent with fuzzy margins in the late phase.

CASE 2 (*Continued*)

The patient was observed without treatment. Six weeks later vision had improved to 6/18; N12. Fundus examination showed a combination of healed and active lesions.

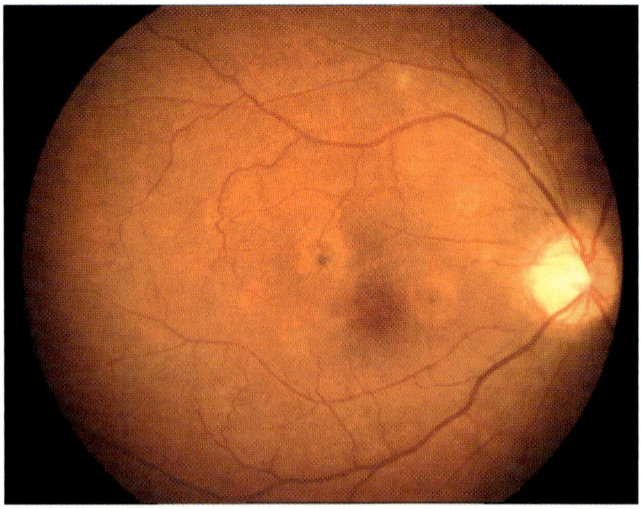

Lesions just nasal and temporal to the fovea appear healed with pigmentary changes seen in the center. Faint dull yellow placoid lesions are still made out in the temporal and superior part of the macula

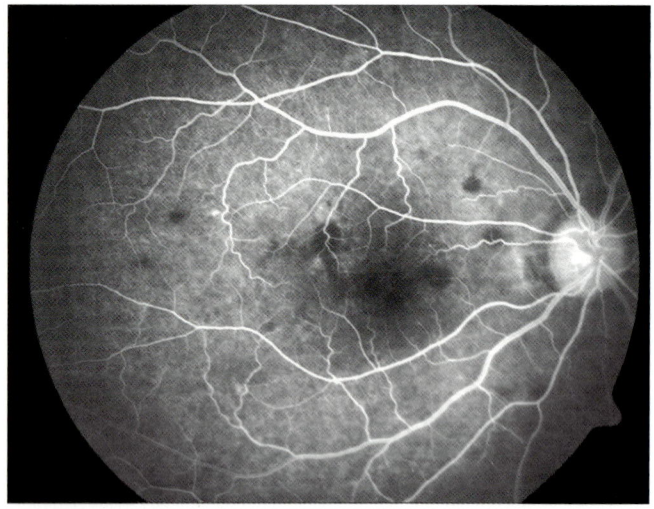

All the lesions appear hypofluorescent. Faint hyperfluorescence due to transmission defect is seen around the healed lesion just temporal to the fovea. The hypofluorescence around the disc seen in the active stage has reduced

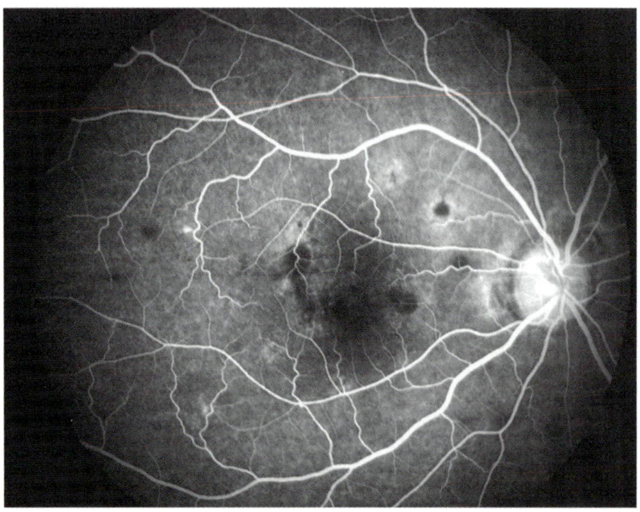

Arteriovenous phase shows the healed lesions to have a central hypofluoresence with a rim of hyperfluorescence due to transmission defect. The active lesions are still clearly visualized

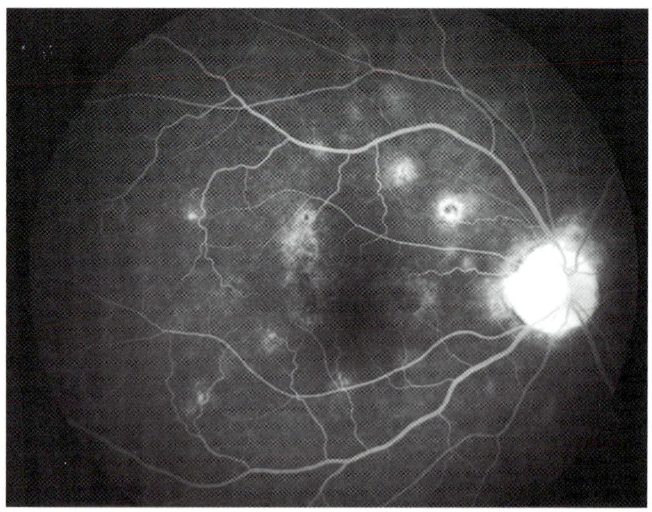

Late staining of the active placoid lesion in the temporal and superior part of the macula is seen. Peripapillary staining is less than that in the active stage

COMMENT

Healed APMPPE lesions show some hyperfluorescence due to transmission defect in the early phase. They are hyperfluorescent in the late phase with well defined margins.

CASE 3

A 49-year-old male presented with floaters in the right eye since 4 days. His visual acuity in the right eye was 6/6; N6. Left eye was normal.

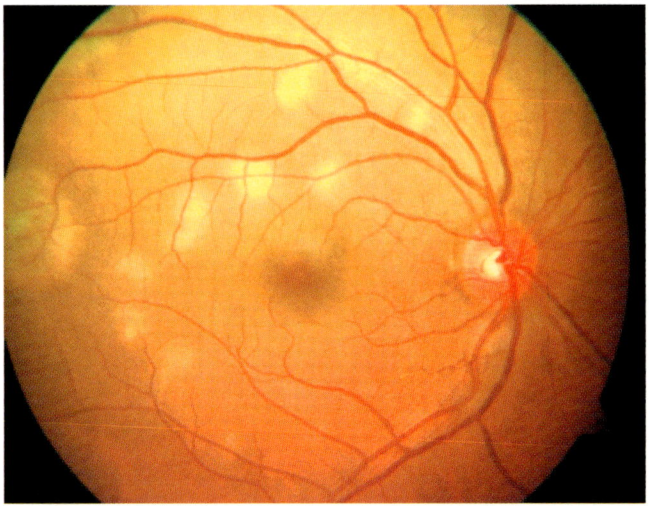

Color fundus photo of right eye showing yellow placoid lesions at macula

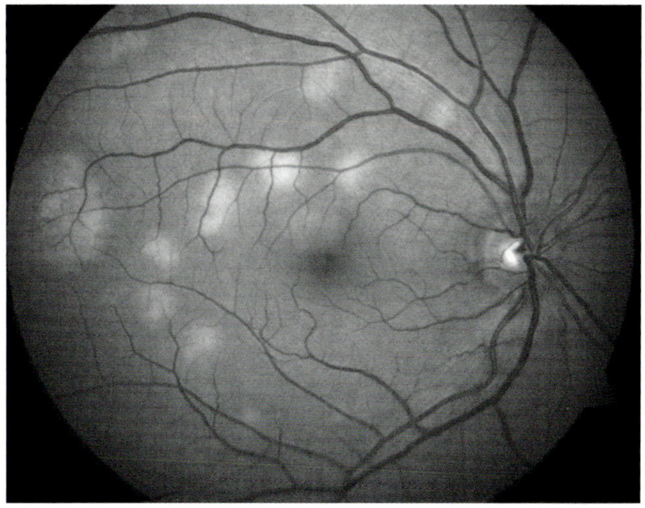

Red free photograph of right eye

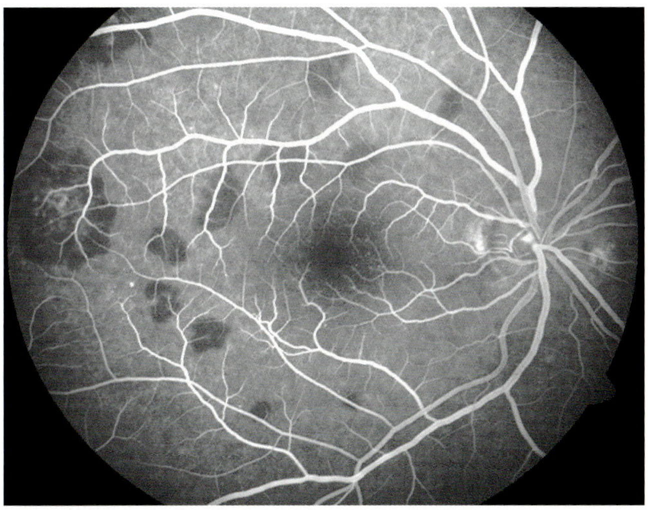

Early arteriovenous phase showing hypofluorescent lesions

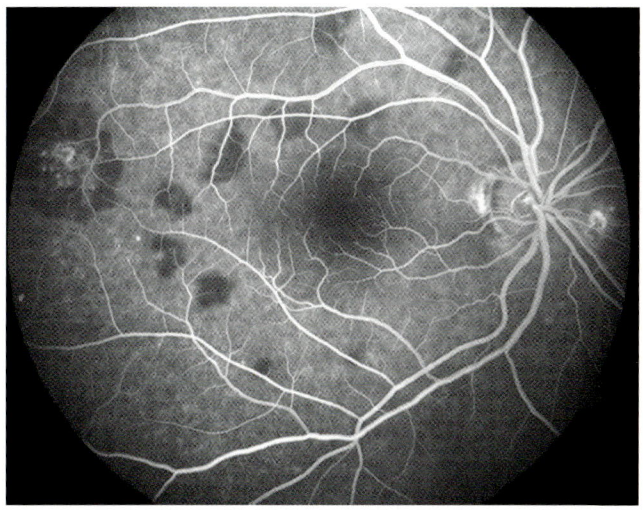

Midarteriovenous phase showing prominent hypofluorescent lesions due to contrast from normal surrounding choroidal fluorescence

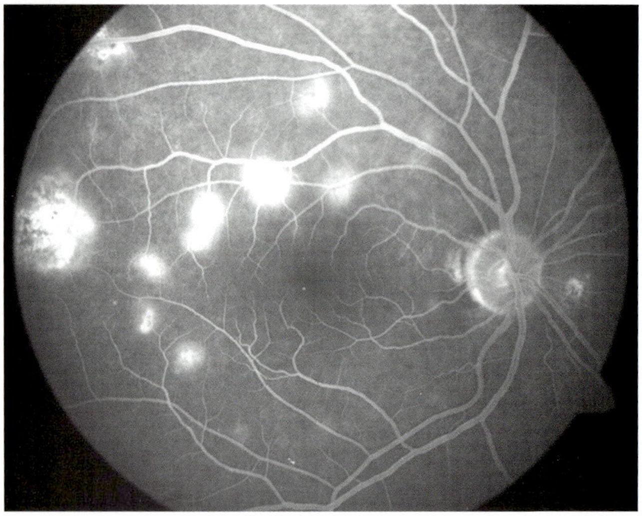

Placoid lesions are hyperfluorescent in late phase with fuzzy margins

CLINICAL NUGGETS

1. Early serpiginous choroidopathy may be confused with APMPPE but it affects an older age group, runs a recurrent course and has a poor prognosis.
2. MEWDS presents with acute visual loss in healthy young adults. The lesions are smaller, unilateral and at the level of outer retina and RPE. FFA shows more numerous lesions than seen clinically.
3. APMPPE is associated with systemic conditions like tuberculosis, hepatitis B vaccination, mumps, Wegener's granulomatosis, polyarteritis nodosa, ulcerative colitis, sarcoidosis and Lyme disease.

BIBLIOGRAPHY

1. Burés-Jelstrup A, Adán A, Casaroli-Marano R. Acute posterior multifocal placoid pigment epitheliopathy. Study of 16 cases. Arch Soc Esp Ophthalmol. 2007;82(5): 291-7.
2. Fiore T, Iaccheri B, Androudi S, Papadaki TG, Anzaar F, Brazitikos P, D'Amico DJ, Foster CS. Acute posterior multifocal placoid pigment epitheliopathy: outcome and visual prognosis. Retina. 2009; 29(7):994-1001.

Chapter 41

Geographic Helicoid Peripapillary Choroidopathy

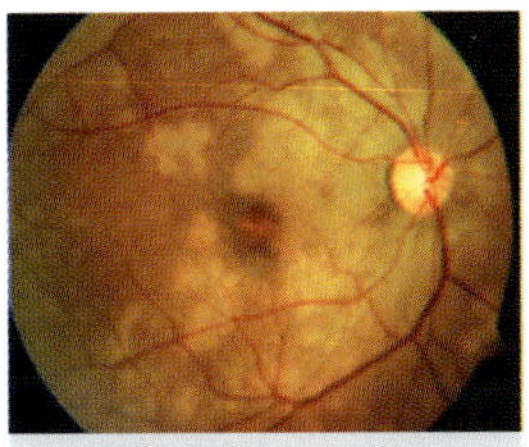

- Serpiginous choroiditis or geographic helicoid peripapillary choroidopathy (GHPC) is a bilateral, chronic progressive inflammatory condition affecting the retinal pigment epithelium and the inner choroid at the posterior pole.
- It is typically seen in young and middle-aged patients with no sex predilection.
- In its active stage, cream or yellow colored lesions are seen at the level of the retinal pigment epithelium extending in a helicoid manner from the optic disc. Typical pseudopod like extensions are seen around the edge of the lesions.
- Healing starts centrally and results in pigmentary alteration within the lesion.
- Skip or satellite lesions can occur.

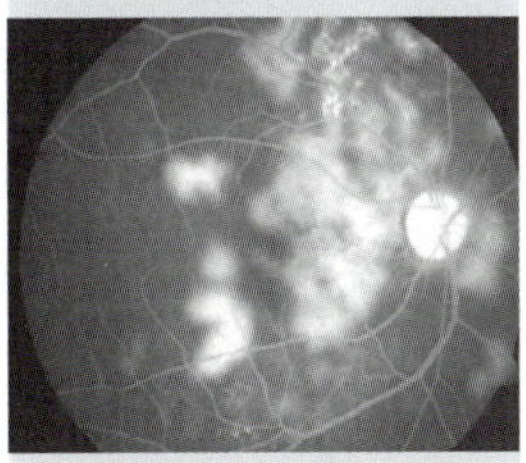

- Active lesions are hypofluorescent in the early phases and show staining with fuzzy borders in the later part of the angiogram.
- Angiographic appearance of healed lesions depends on the extent of atrophy of the retinal pigment epithelium and choriocapillaris. When retinal pigment epithelium is predominantly affected with relative preservation of the choriocapillaris, the angiogram will show mottled hyperfluorescent defects within the lesion in the early phase. If the choriocapillaris are also significantly atrophied, the angiogram will remain hypofluorescent in the early phases with the scleral staining seen through in the late phase. Pigment clumps associated with the lesion will block the choroidal fluorescence.

CASE 1

A 31-year-old female presented with history of episodes of pain and redness in both eyes for the past one year. She was diagnosed to have episcleritis in both eyes. Visual acuity was 6/6; N6 in both eyes. Fundus examination in both eyes showed active GHPC.

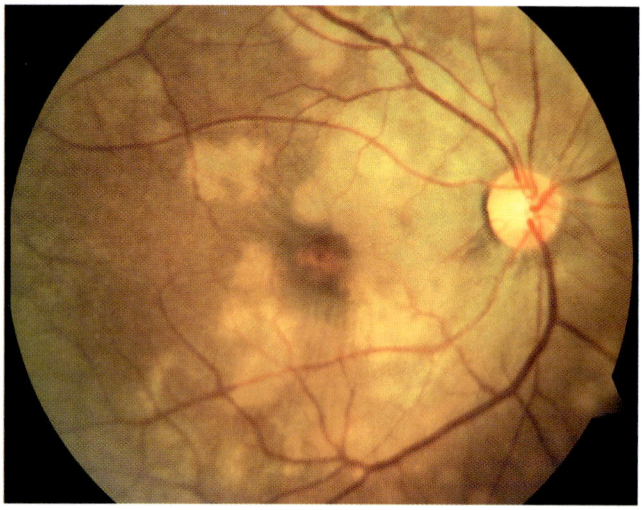

Fundus photograph of the right eye showing active GHPC. Few skip lesions are seen temporally

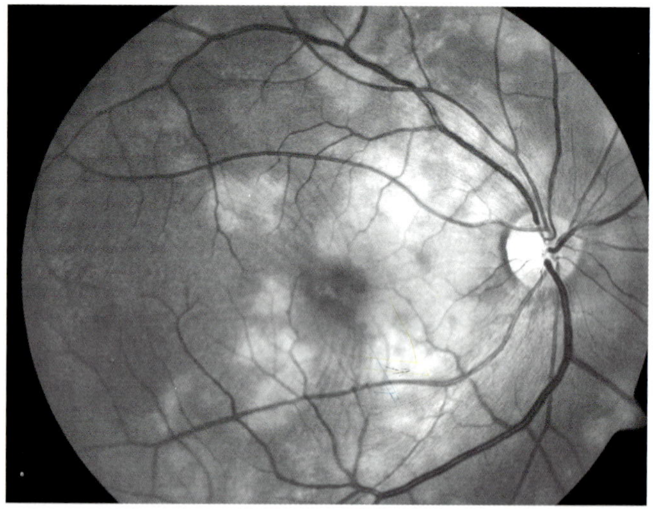

Red free photograph of the right eye

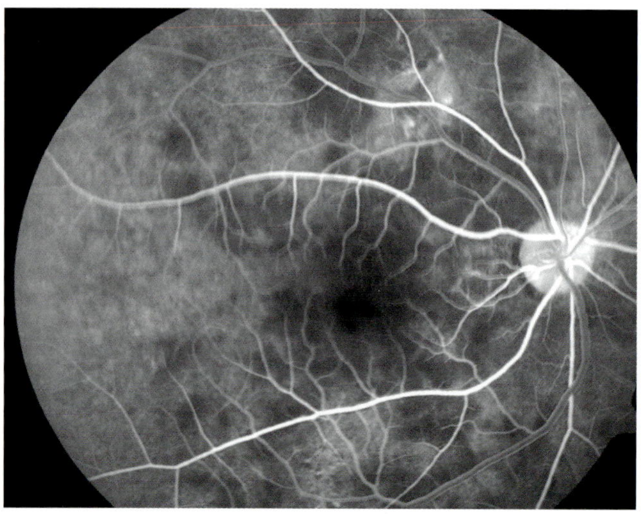

The lesions appear hypofluorescent in the early arteriovenous phase. Few specks of transmitted hyperfluorescence are seen superiorly

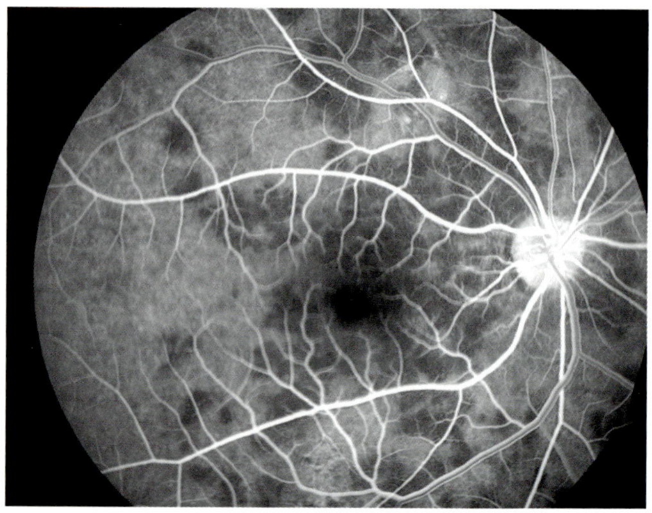

The lesions remain hypofluorescent in the mid arteriovenous phase

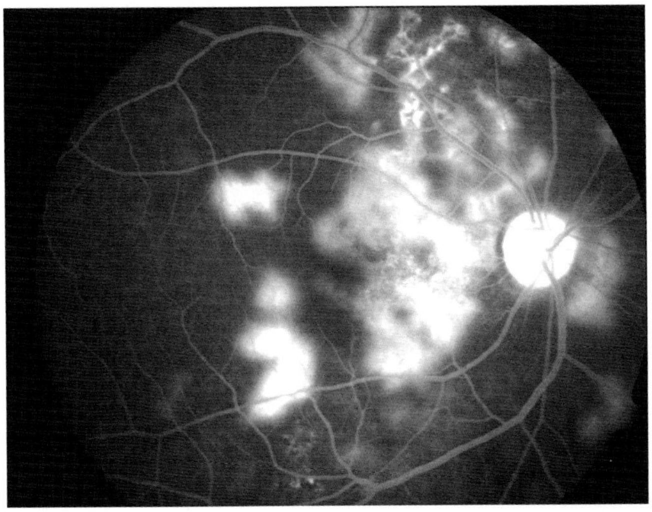

Late phase shows hyperfluorescence with fuzzy margins

COMMENT

Active GHPC lesions are hypofluorescent in the early phase and hyperfluorescent with fuzzy margins in the late film.

CASE 2

A 26-year-old male presented with decreased vision in the right eye of one month duration. Visual acuity was 6/12; N10. Left eye was normal.

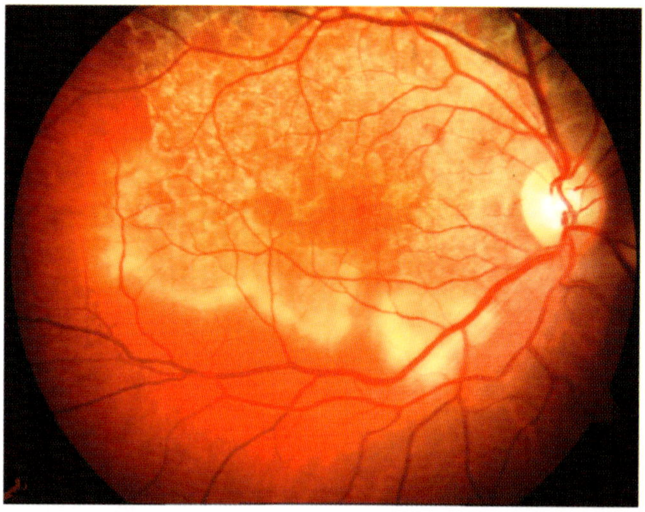

Fundus photograph of the right eye showing GHPC. The inferior edge of the lesion appears active while the rest of the lesion is healed

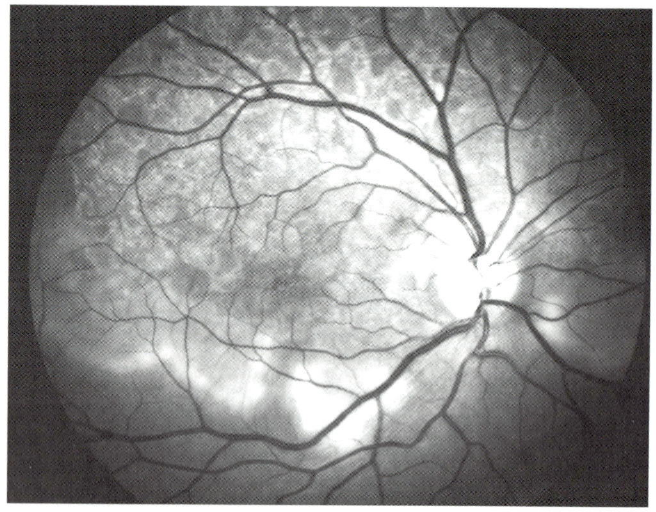

Red free photograph of the right eye

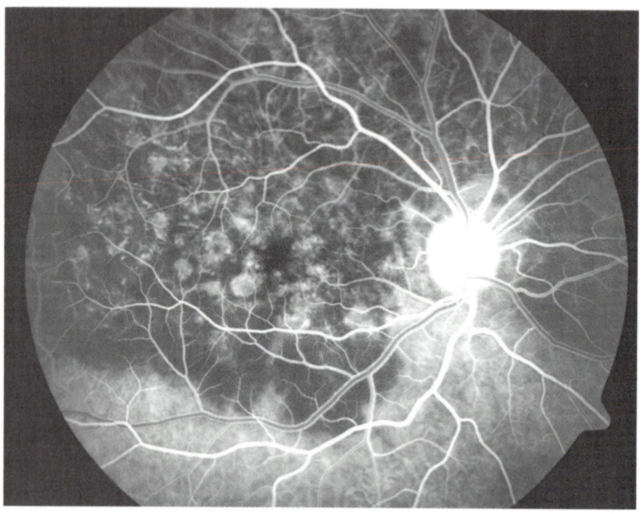

The inferior active part appears hypofluorescent. Irregular hyperfluorescence is seen in the healed area

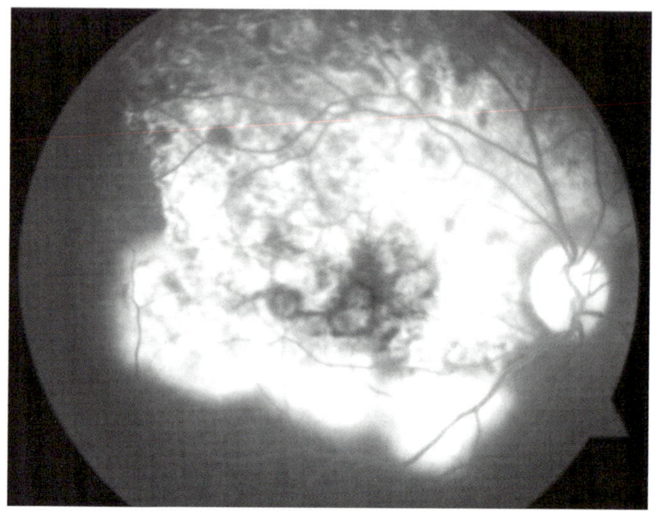

Marked fuzzy hyperfluorescence is seen in the area of the active disease. Hyperfluorescence due to staining is also noted in the healed part. However, its edges remain well defined in contrast to the fuzzy margins of the inferior active part

COMMENT

This case illustrates the difference between active and healed GHPC. Healed lesions have well defined borders even in the late phase while the active lesion shows increased hyperfluorescence with fuzzy margins in the late phase.

CASE 2 (*Continued*)

Patient was treated with systemic steroids. Four months later, visual acuity had improved to 6/9; N6. Fundus examination showed healed lesions.

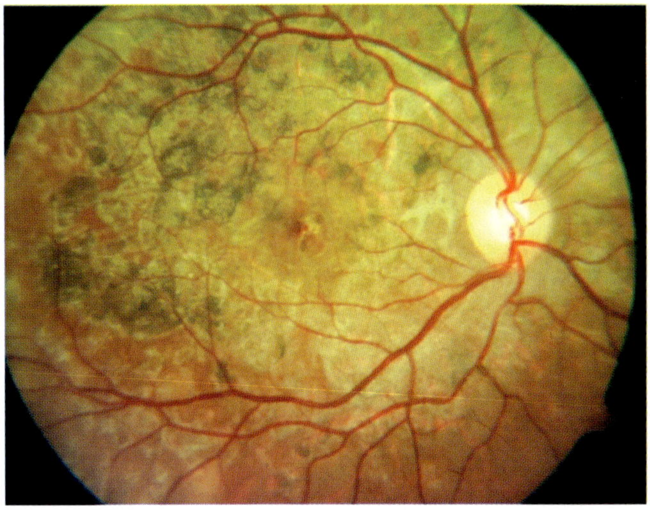

Fundus photograph of the right eye showing healed GHPC

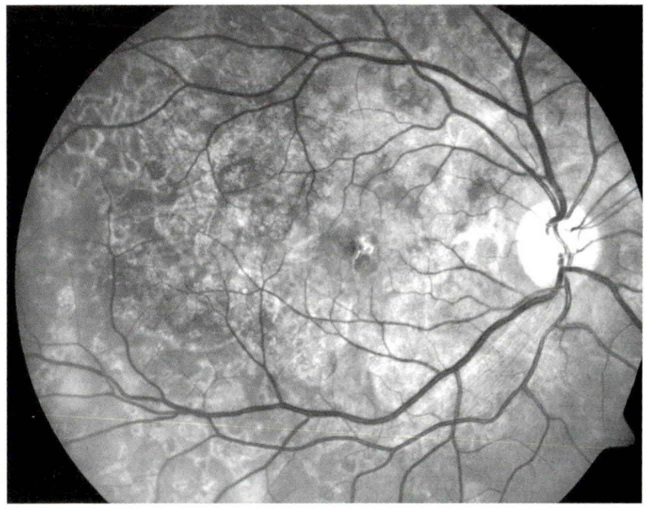

Late phase shows hyperfluorescence with fuzzy margins

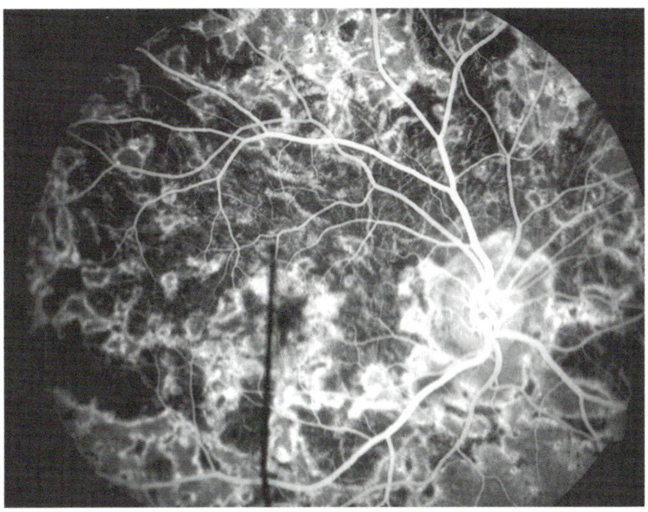

Central hypofluorescence with a rim of hyperfluorescence is seen in the healed lesions

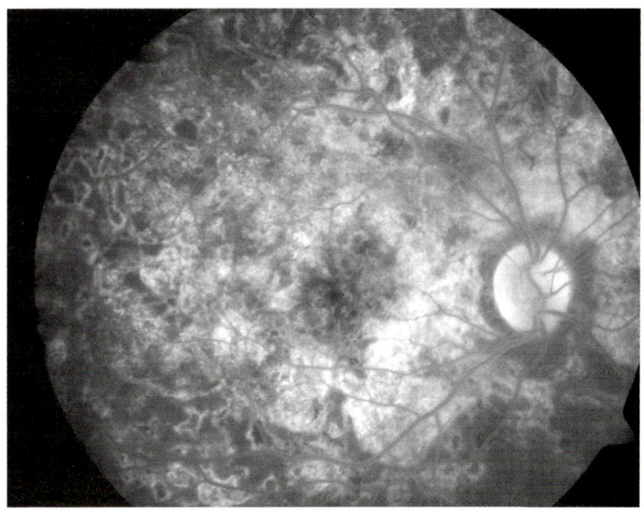

Late hyperfluorescence of the healed lesion occurs due to increased visibility of the scleral staining and due to staining of the scar tissue. Note that the edges of the lesions remain discrete

COMMENT

Geographic helicoid peripapillary choroidopathy (GHPC) lesions progressively increase in size. Fluorescein angiography is extremely useful to monitor this progression.

CASE 3

A 29-year-old male presented with history of reduced vision of two weeks duration. Visual acuity was 6/36; N36.

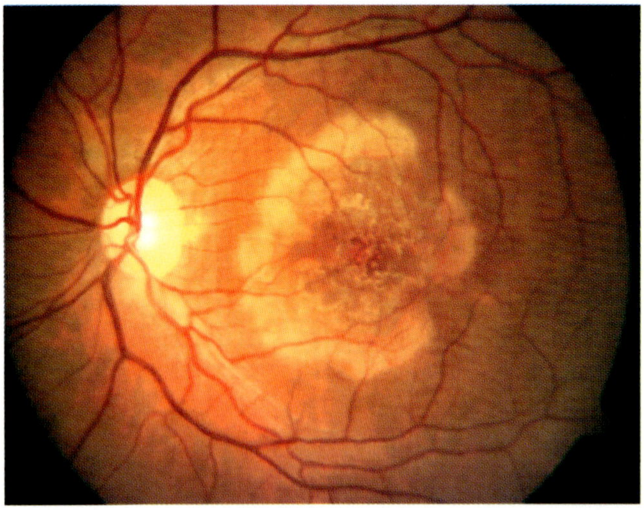

Fundus photograph of the left eye showing macular GHPC. The edges of the lesion appears active while the center of the lesion appears healed

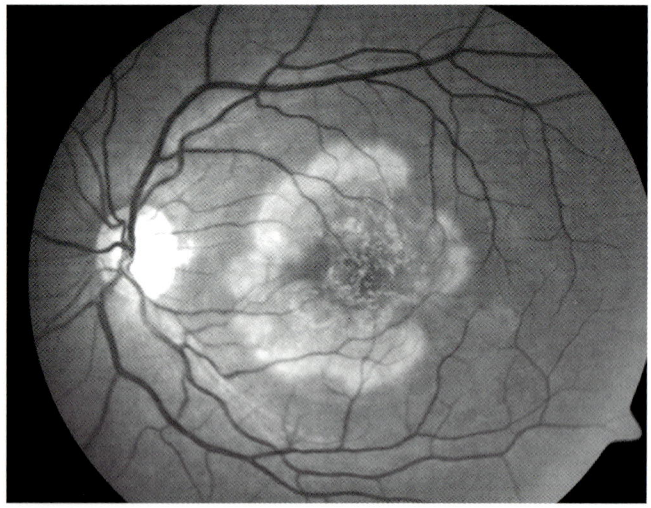

Red free photograph of the left eye

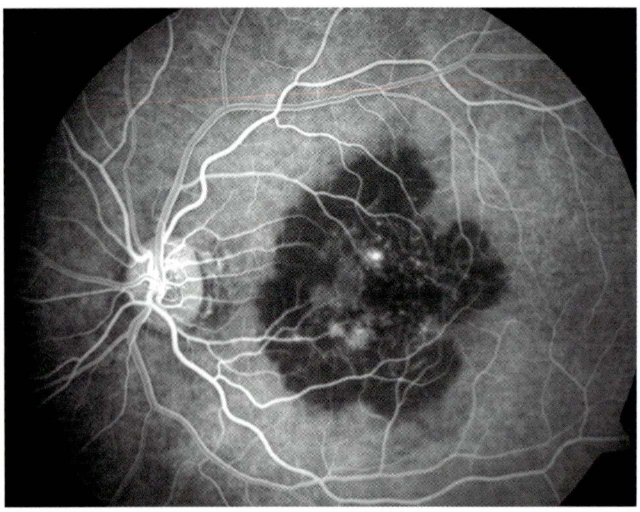

Early arteriovenous phase showing hypofluorescence along the active edge of the lesion. Irregular central hyperfluorescence is seen

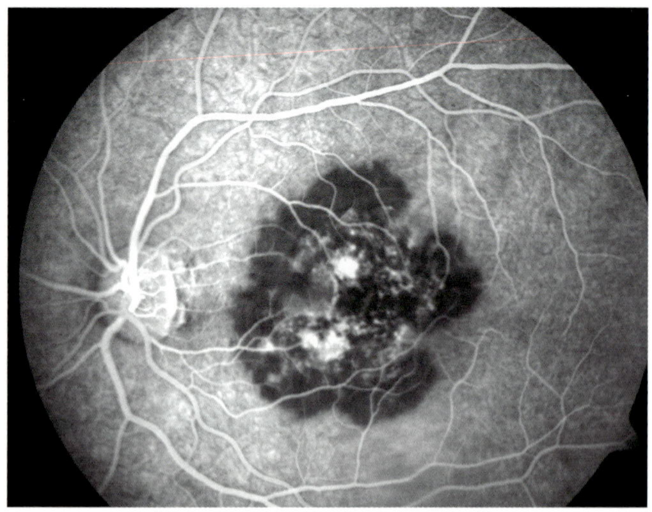

Mid arteriovenous phase show hypofluorescence of the active edge

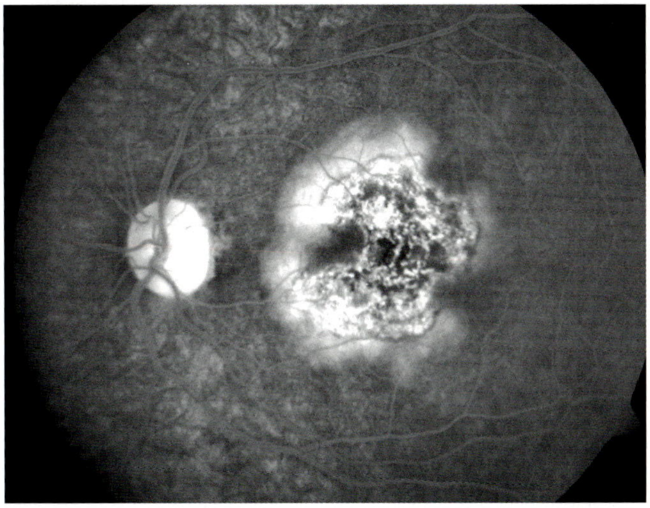

Late fuzzy hyperfluorescence is seen in the active part of the lesion. Irregular hyperfluorescence is noted in the central healed part

COMMENT

GHPC need not always be peripapillary, as seen in this case of macular GHPC.

CLINICAL NUGGETS

1. Geographic helicoid peripapillary choroidopathy (GHPC) is a chronic, typically bilateral, episodic disease with a poor visual prognosis.
2. Geographic helicoid peripapillary choroidopathy (GHPC) typically affects the young to middle-aged patient with no sex predilection.
3. Geographic helicoid peripapillary choroidopathy (GHPC) lesions are typically peripapillary, but macular lesions can also occur.
4. Skip or non-contiguous lesions can occur and probably represent new foci of involvement.
5. Systemic steroids, antiviral and immunosuppressive drugs have been tried in the treatment of GHPC.
6. APMPPE lesions usually resolve spontaneously and visual prognosis is excellent in contrast to GHPC.
7. Active lesion of toxoplasmosis is characterized by prominent vitreal inflammation and unlike serpiginous choroiditis, they can occur anywhere in the fundus. These patients have a positive toxoplasmosis serology.
8. Multifocal choroiditis is clinically distinct from serpiginous choroiditis by the smaller lesions and the prominent vitritis.

BIBLIOGRAPHY

1. Abrez H, Biswas J, Sudharshan S. Clinical Profile, Treatment, and Visual Outcome of Serpiginous Choroiditis. Ocular Immunology and Inflammation, 2007;15:325-5.
2. Lim WK, Buggage RR, Nussenblatt, RB. Serpiginous Choroiditis: Major review. Survey of Ophthalmology 2005;50:3.

42

Chapter

Vogt-Koyanagi-Harada Syndrome

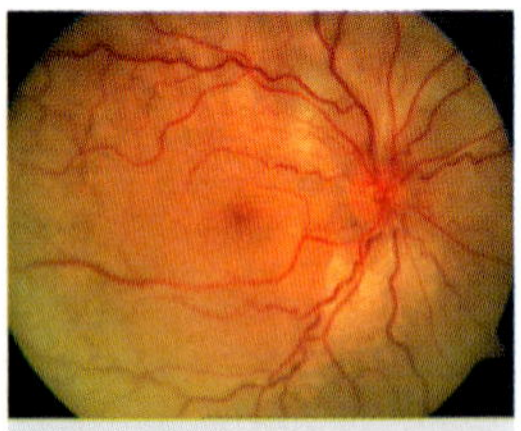

- Vogt-Koyanagi-Harada (VKH) syndrome is a bilateral disorder, commonly seen in the second to fourth decade of life.
- It is a panuveitis associated with exudative retinal detachment and is more common in darkly pigmented individuals and in patients with oriental ancestry.
- Acute stage is characterized by massive infiltration of the choroid with inflammatory cells.
- Localized or extensive exudative retinal detachment is the most common finding and is associated with cells in the vitreous and anterior chamber. The detachment usually begins in the posterior pole and may be multifocal. Focal yellow-white lesions may be seen at the retinal pigment epithelial layer. The optic nerve head is hyperemic.
- The resolved stage is characterized by a 'sunset glow' fundus.

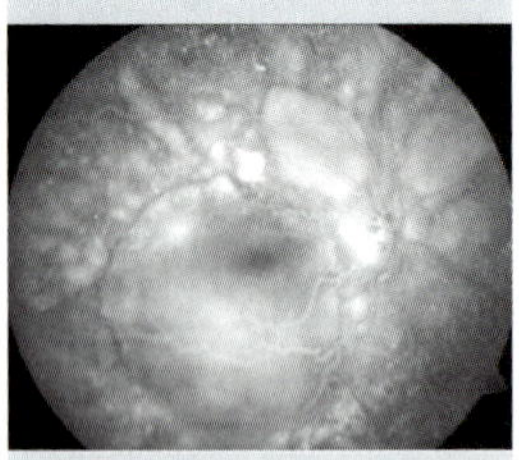

- Typically, innumerable tiny leaks at the level of the retinal pigment epithelium are seen in the early phase of the angiogram.
- In the late phase, characteristic pooling of the dye occurs in the areas of exudative retinal detachments.
- Late staining of the optic nerve head is seen.
- In the resolved stage, transmission window defects are noted in the areas of retinal pigment epithelium atrophy. Areas of hyperpigmentation cause blocked fluorescence.

CASE 1

A 55-year-old female presented with sudden loss of vision in the right eye for the past 4 days. Visual acuity was counting fingers close to face in the right eye and 6/6; N6 in the left eye. Vitreous cells were seen in the right eye.

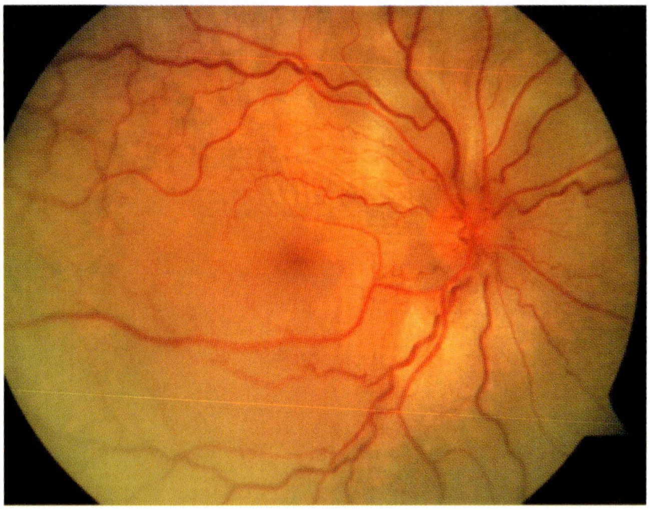

Fundus photograph of the right eye showing pockets of subretinal fluid at the posterior pole. The disc is hyperemic

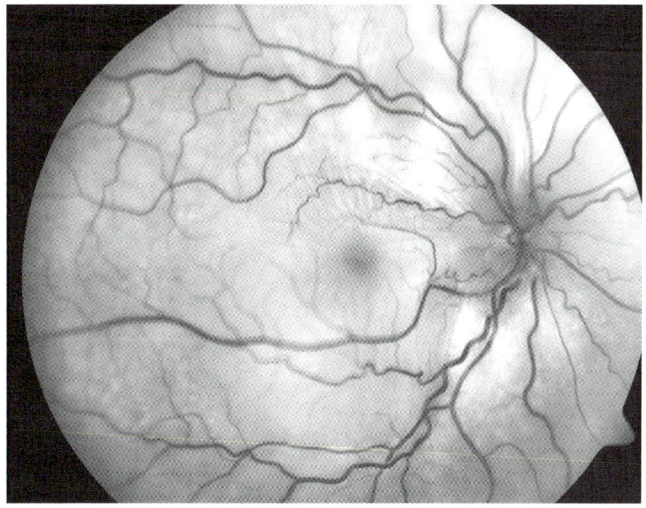

Red free photograph of the right eye

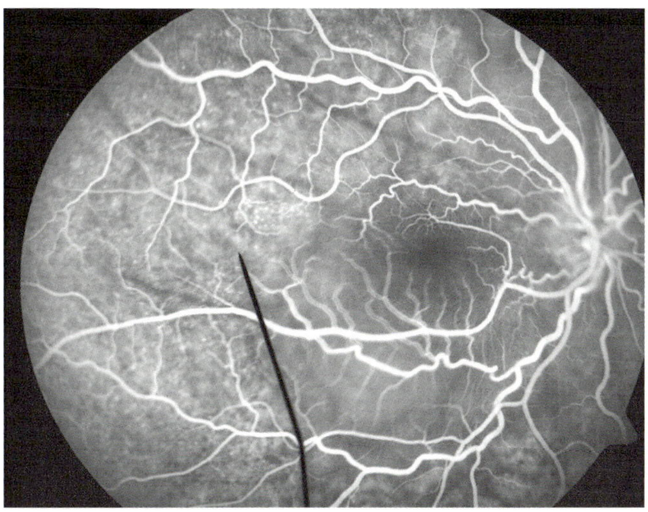

Midarteriovenous phase showing blurring of the choroidal fluorescence in the region of the subretinal fluid. A cluster of pinpoint hyperfluorescence is seen temporal to the fovea

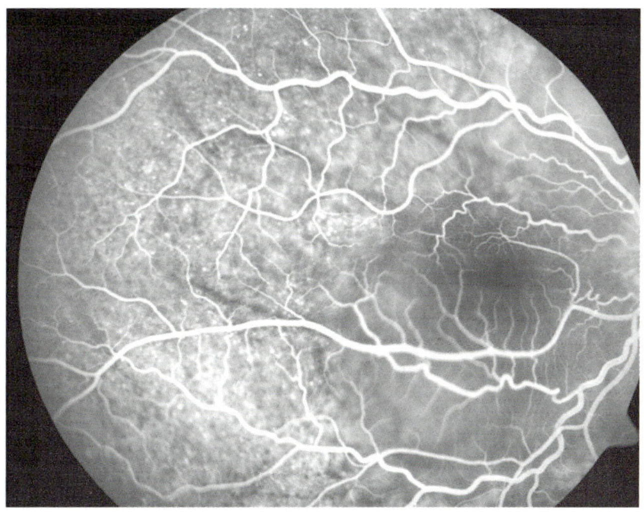

The areas of pinpoint hyperfluorescence are better seen in the late arteriovenous phase

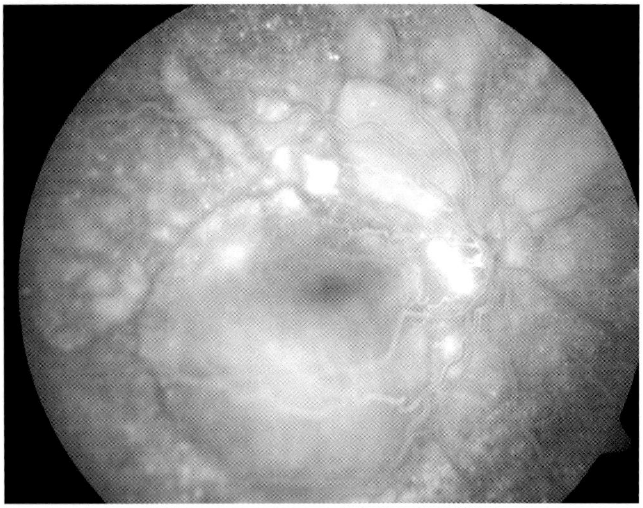

Characteristic extensive pooling of the dye in the subretinal space is seen in the late phase

COMMENT

Multiple pinpoint hyperfluorescent spots in the arteriovenous phase with extensive late pooling of the dye in the subretinal space is typical of VKH.

CASE 2

A 15-year-old girl presented with decreased vision in the left eye of one day duration. Visual acuity was 1/60 in the left eye and 6/9; N12 in the right eye. She was found to have an exudative retinal detachment at the maculae in both eyes.

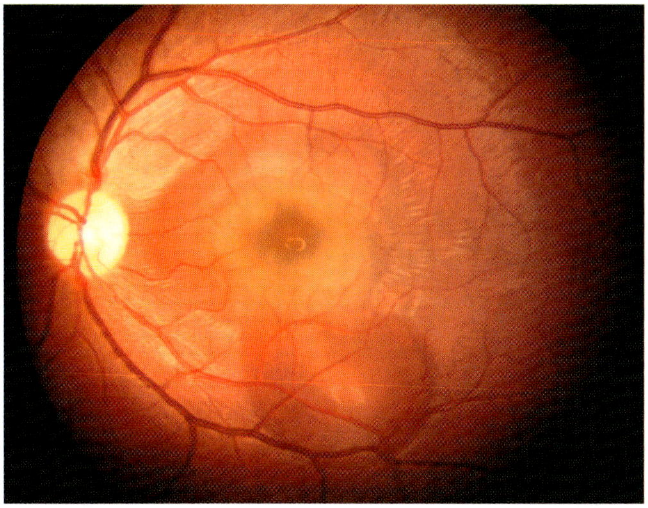

Fundus photograph of the left eye showing pockets of subretinal fluid at the macula

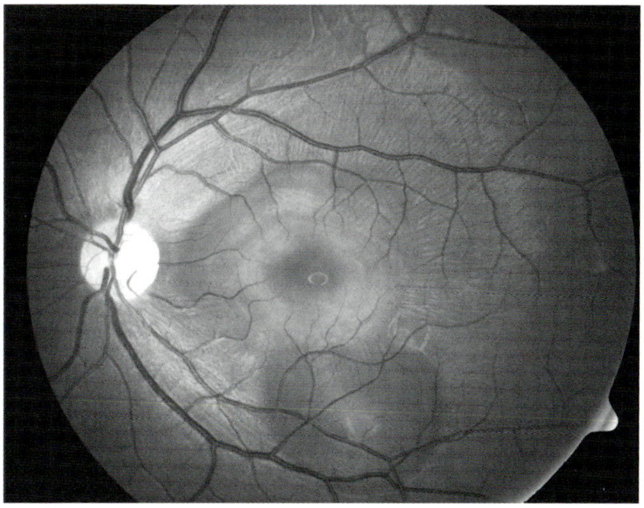

Red free photograph of the left eye

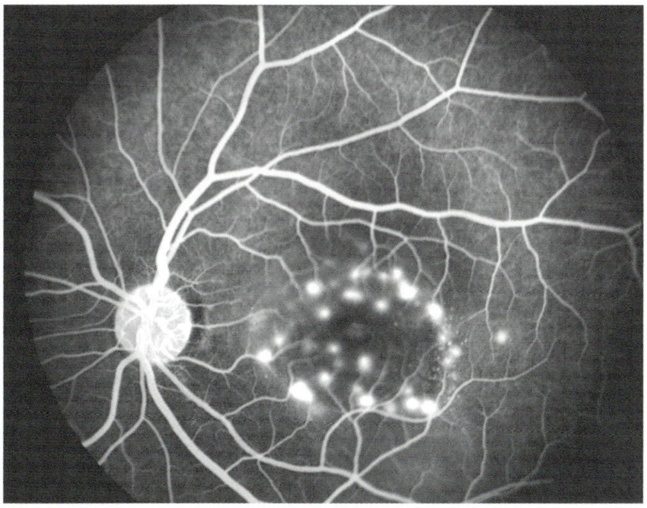

Multiple hyperfluorescent points are seen in the mid-arteriovenous phase

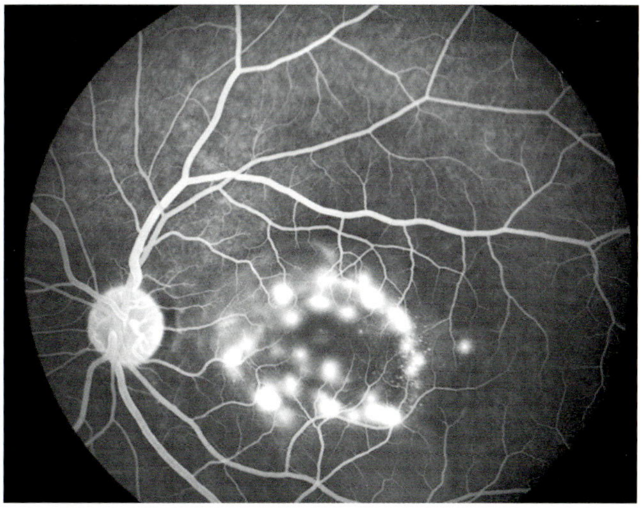

The leakage is seen to increase as the angiogram progresses

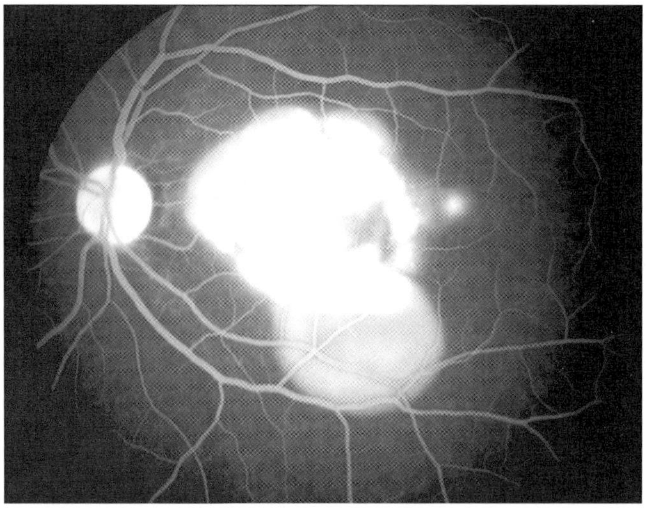

Late phase shows significant pooling of the dye in the subretinal space

CASE 2 (*Continued*)

Right Eye of the Patient

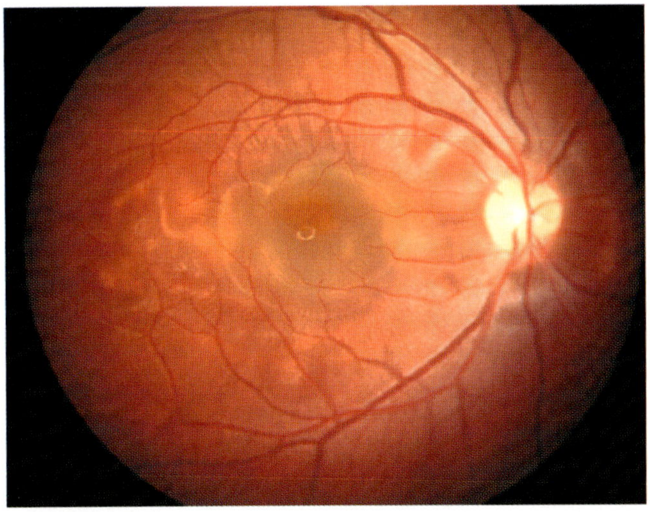

Fundus photograph of the right eye showing exudative detachment at the macula

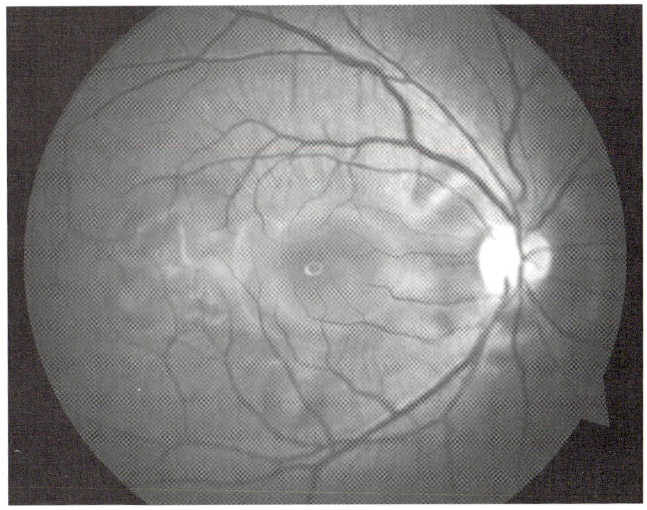

Red free photograph of the right eye

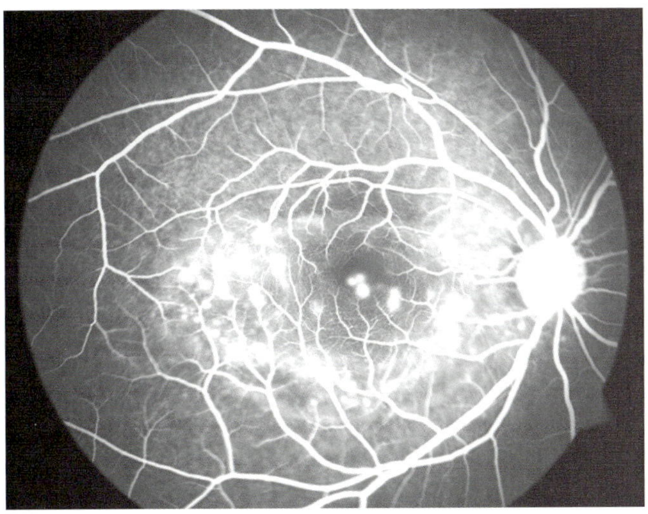

Midarteriovenous phase showing multiple points of dye leakage at the RPE level

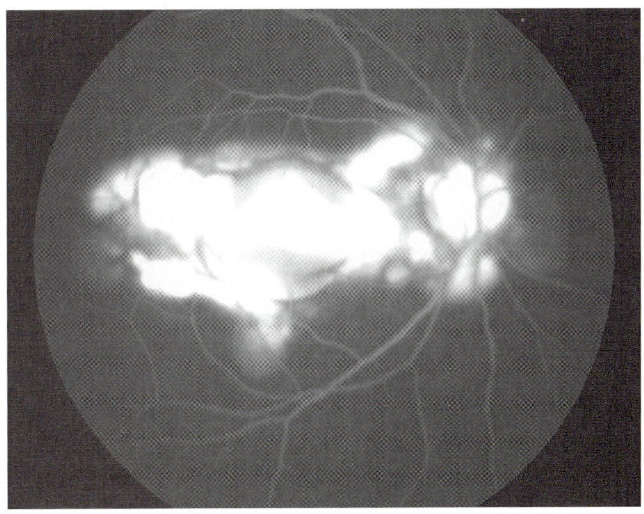

Late phase showing extensive pooling of the dye in the subretinal space

COMMENT

Unlike in CSC, the leaks in VKH are innumerable.

Late pooling of the dye that occurs in CSC is never so extensive as in VKH. In CSC, the entire extent of neurosensory elevation is never filled up with dye even in the very late phase.

Late staining of the disc is a common finding in VKH.

CASE 3

A 17-year-old girl presented with history of decreased vision in the right eye of one month duration. Visual acuity was 1/60 in the right eye and 6/6; N6 in the left eye.

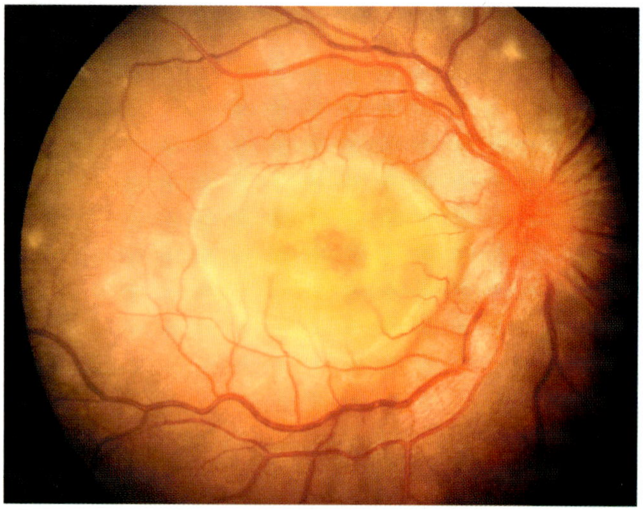

Fundus photograph of the right eye showing an exudative detachment at the macula. The disc is hyperemic

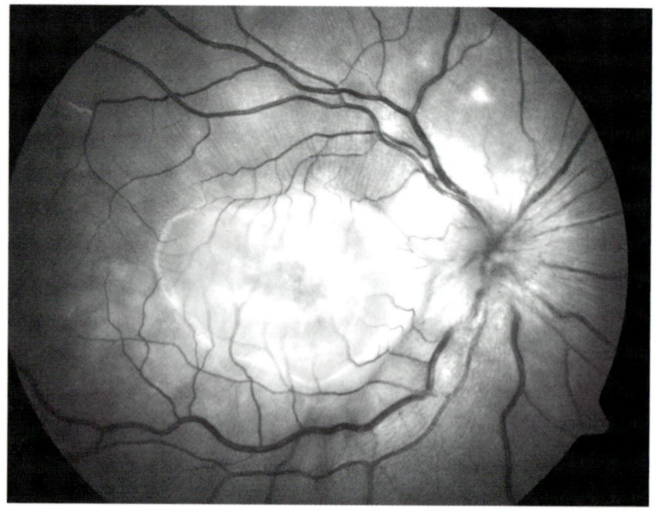

Red free photograph of the right eye

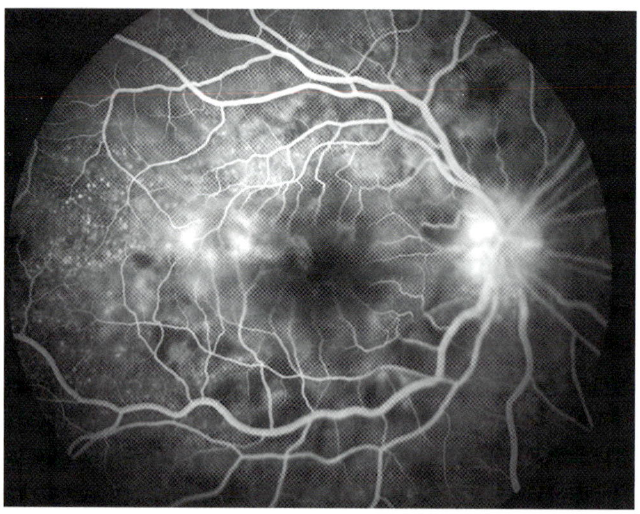

Mid arteriovenous phase showing pinpoint hyperfluorescence temporally. The disc capillaries are dilated and the margins are blurred

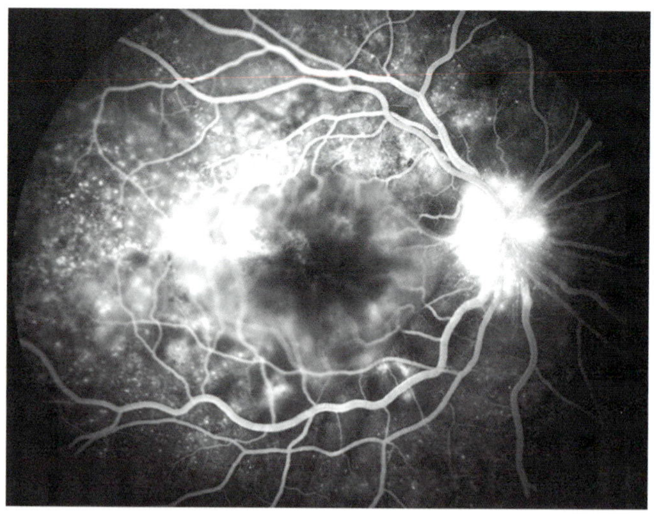

The pinpoint hyperfluorescence is well seen in the late arteriovenous phase

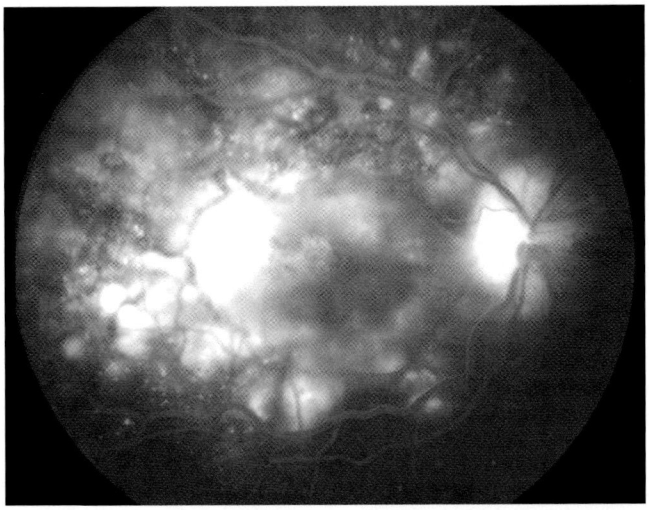

Pooling of the dye in the subretinal space is seen in the late film. Increased disc staining is evident

CASE 3 (*Continued*)

Left Eye of the Patient

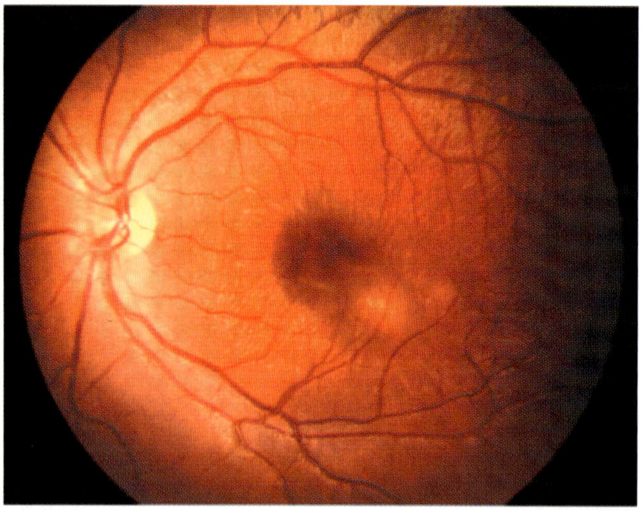

Fundus photograph of the left eye showing a pocket of turbid subretinal fluid inferotemporal to the foveal center

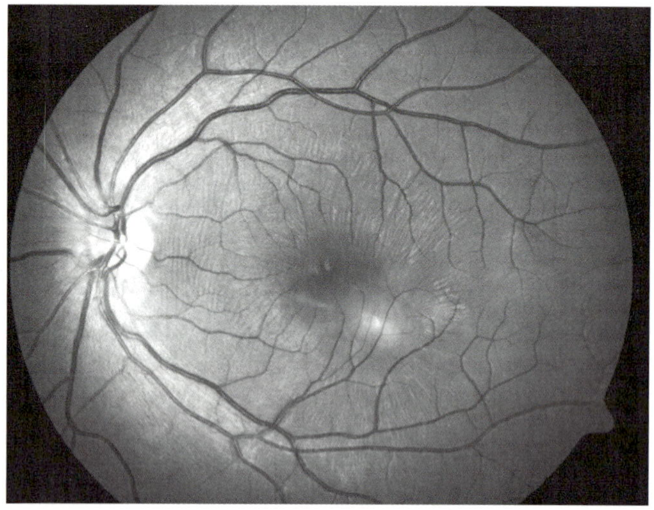

Red free photograph of the left eye

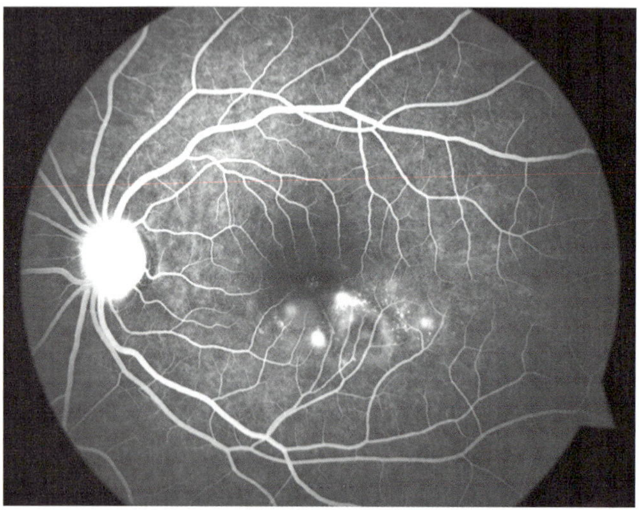

Arteriovenous phase showing hyperfluorescent points inferotemporal to the fovea

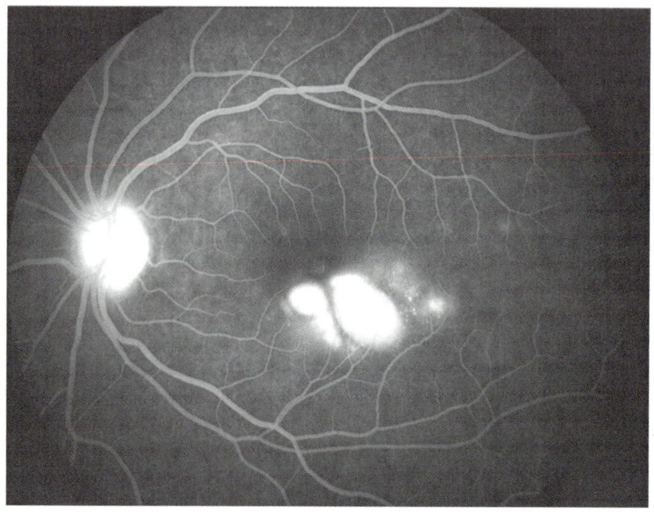

Late pooling of the dye is seen. The dye fills the entire area of neurosensory detachment. Increased staining of the disc is seen

COMMENT

It is important to differentiate VKH from central serous chorioretinopathy as the treatment of the two conditions is different.

Age, visual acuity, presence of vitreous cells, disc involvement, ultrasound and the angiographic findings help to differentiate the two.

CASE 4

A 40-year-male patient presented with blurring of vision in the left eye since 2 days. His visual acuity was 6/6; N6 in both eyes. After being diagnosed of VKH syndrome, the patient was treated with a course of IVMP and systemic steroids.

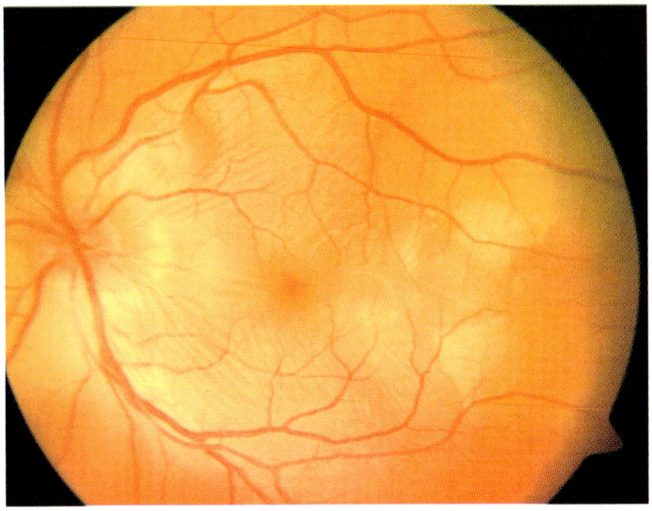

Color fundus photo of left eye showing disc hyperemia and edema along with pockets of subretinal fluid at the posterior pole

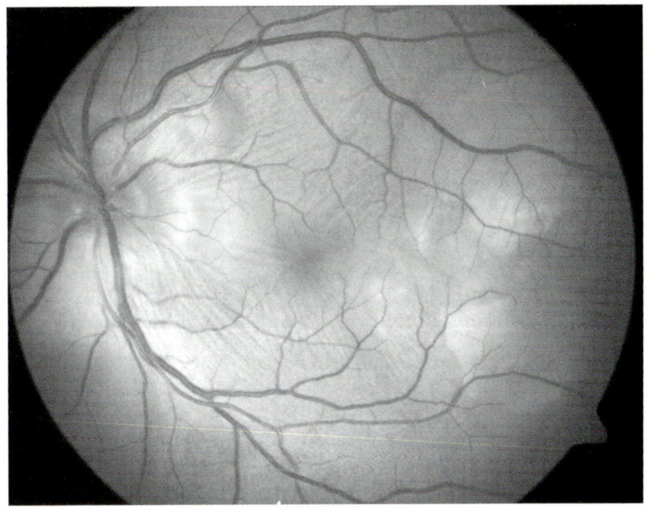

Red free photo of left eye

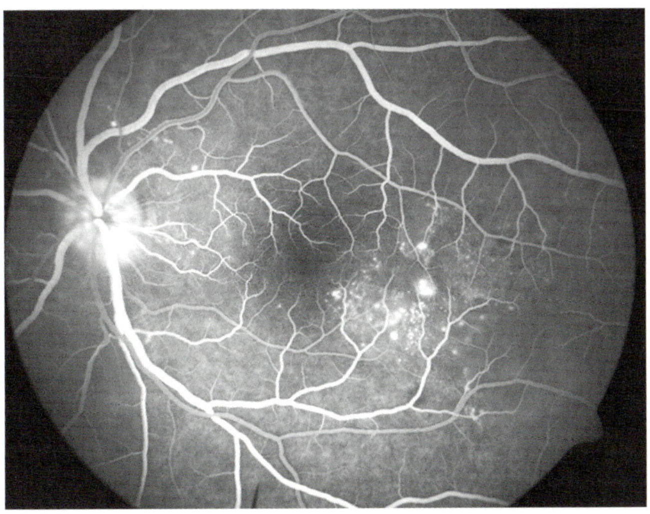

Early arteriovenous phase showing 'pin head leaks' which is characteristic of VKH

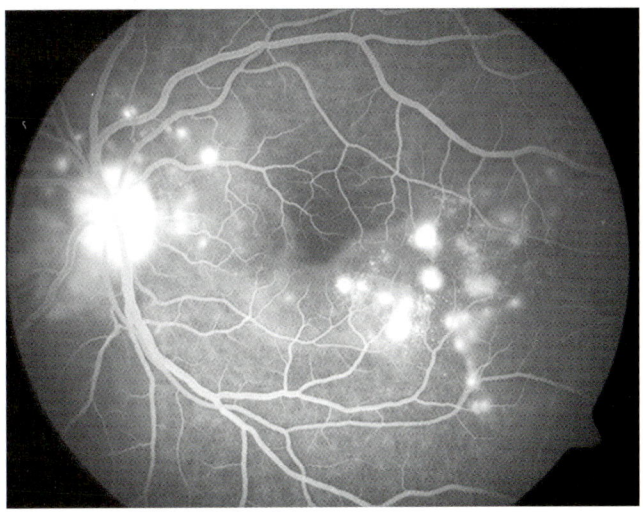

Midarteriovenous phase showing increase in size of leaks

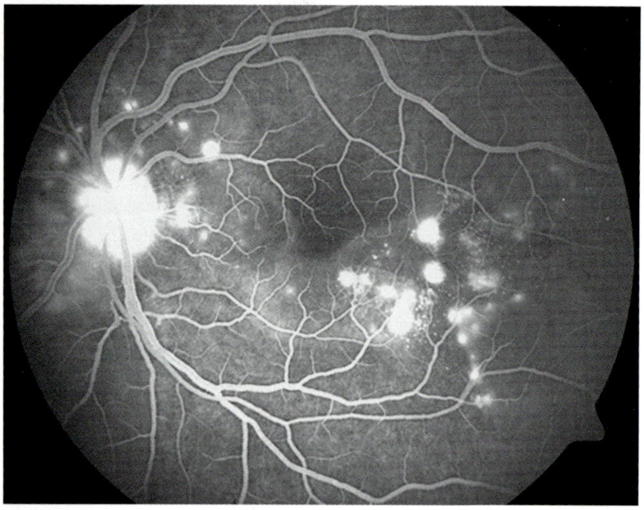

Late arteriovenous phase showing further increase in the size of leaks along with disc staining

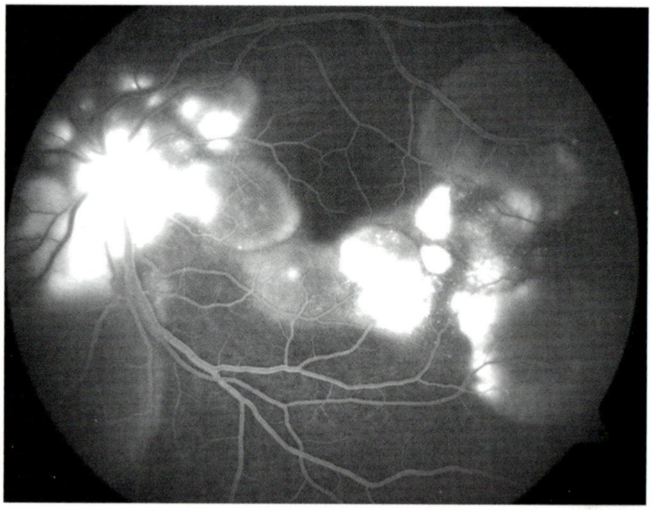

Late phase showing pooling of dye in subretinal space along with disc staining and leakage

CLINICAL NUGGETS

1. The condition has to be differentiated from sympathetic ophthalmia which has a similar angiographic finding, but is unilateral and has history of penetrating injury or ocular surgery in the fellow eye.
2. Posterior scleritis also has a similar angiographic picture, but is usually unilateral and has classical T-sign on ultrasonography in majority of cases along with pain on ocular movements.

BIBLIOGRAPHY

1. Bordaberry MF. Vogt-Koyanagi-Harada disease: diagnosis and treatments update. Curr Opin Ophthalmol. 2010;21(6):430-5.
2. Chee SP, Jap A, Cheung CM. The prognostic value of angiography in Vogt-Koyanagi-Harada disease. Am J Ophthalmol. 2010 Dec;150(6):888-93. Epub 2010 Oct 8.
3. Yamaguchi Y, Otani T, Kishi S. Tomographic Features of Serous Retinal Detachment with Multilobular Dye Pooling in Acute Vogt-Koyanagi-Harada Disease. Am J Ophthalmol 2007;144:260-65.

43

Chapter

Sympathetic Ophthalmitis

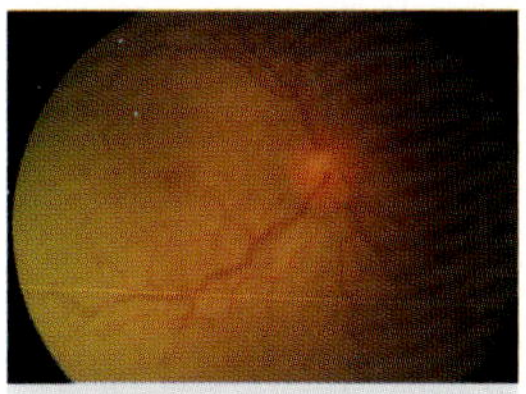

Sympathetic ophthalmitis (SO) is a bilateral, granulomatous panuveitis that occurs after penetrating injury to one eye. The traumatized eye is called the *exciting eye* and the noninjured eye is called the *sympathizing eye*.

Sympathetic ophthalmitis has been reported after various surgical procedures such as cataract surgery, cyclodestructive procedures, enucleation/evisceration and even after proton beam radiation to choroidal melanomas.

The latent period from injury is usually between 2 weeks and 3 months with more than 90 percent cases occurring within 1 year. The exciting eye is usually traumatized, hyperemic and irritable while symptoms in the sympathizing eye vary from mild photophobia to excruciating pain.

Ultrasound examination shows a thickened choroid.

Optical coherence tomography (OCT) is a useful noninvasive tool to quantify the extent of serous retinal detachment and follow the response to corticosteroid therapy. Gupta et al reported reversible elongation of the photoreceptor layer in eyes with acute SO using spectral domain OCT.

The main differential diagnosis of SO is Vogt-Koyangi-Harada (VKH) syndrome. The critical factor is the history of penetrating ocular trauma or intraocular surgery in the recent past. Systemic features such as vitiligo, poliosis, dysacusis and cerebrospinal fluid (CSF) pleocytosis are uncommon in SO and favor VKH.

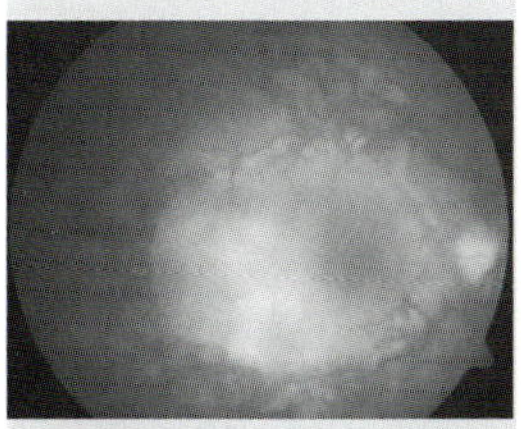

In acute phase of SO, the fluorescein angiography typically demonstrates multiple hyperfluorescent points of leakage at the level of the RPE in the venous phase (starry sky appearance). In severe cases, these may coalesce with pooling of dye beneath exudative neurosensory detachment. The optic disc may demonstrate leakage in the later phases.

Indocyanine green angiography (ICGA) may reveal dark spots or hypofluorescent foci in the choroid due to the inflammatory foci which act as space occupying lesions. Hyperfluorescent pinpoint spots corresponding to Dalen-Fuch nodules may also be seen corresponding to those seen on fundus photograph when angiography is performed relatively early in the disease course. Diffuse late hyperfluorescence alternating with hypofluorescence may also be seen due to leakage from large choroidal vessels. Disc hyperfluorescence in ICGA indicates severe disease.

CASE 1

A 40-year-old man presented with pain and redness with gradually progressive visual blurring in the left eye since the past 2 weeks. He had sustained penetrating injury to the right eye 6 months back following road traffic accident. He underwent surgery in his right eye elsewhere and was referred to our center for further management. On examination, right eye was prephthisical with silicone oil in AC. Left eye had BCVA of 6/24; N18.

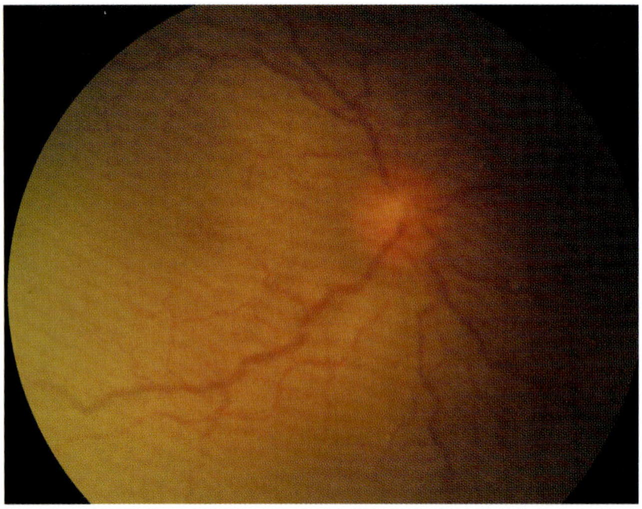

Fundus photograph of the right eye reveals the presence of pockets of subretinal fluid over the posterior pole

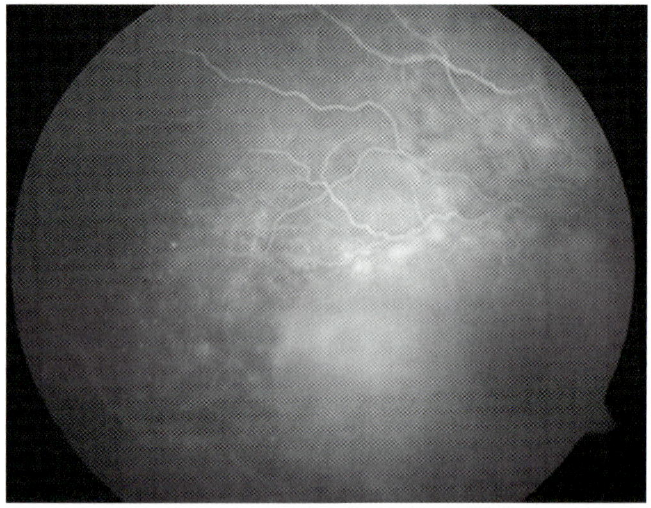

A-V phase reveals multiple pin-point leakages giving a starry-sky appearance, suggestive of sympathetic ophthalmitis

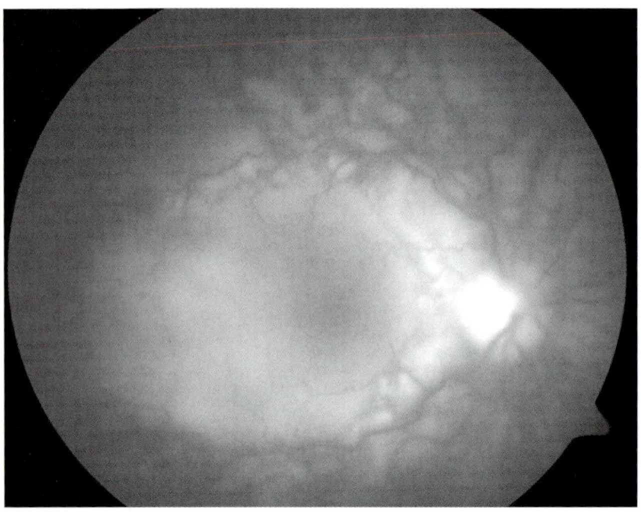

Late phase angiogram reveals coalescence of leakage points resulting in a large area of pooling of the dye under the macula. Note the disc staining and leakage

COMMENT

This patient was treated with high dose oral prednisolone and azathioprine. His vision improved to 6/12; N10 within 1 week of treatment. He was on a tapering dose of oral steroids and immunosuppressives at the last visit.

CLINICAL NUGGETS

1. The critical factor in clinical suspicion of SO is the history of penetrating ocular trauma or intraocular surgery.
2. The initial approach in most cases is to suppress the immune response with intensive corticosteroid therapy using high dose pulse intravenous methylprednisolone followed by a slow taper of oral steroids.

BIBLIOGRAPHY

1. Galor A, Davis JL, Flynn HW Jr, Feuer WJ, Dubovy SR, Setlur V, et al. Sympathetic ophthalmitis: incidence of ocular complications and vision loss in the sympathizing eye. Am J Ophthalmol 2009;148:704-10.
2. Gass JD. Sympathetic ophthalmitis following vitrectomy. Am J Ophthalmol 1982;93:552-8.
3. Gupta V, Gupta A, Dogra MR, Singh I. Reversible retinal changes in the acute stage of sympathetic ophthalmitis seen on spectral domain optical coherence tomography. Int Ophthalmol, 2011. [Epub ahead of print], PMID: 21331811.
4. Holland G. About the indications and time for surgical removal of an injured eye. Klin Monatsbl Augenheilkd 1964;145:732-40.
5. Liddy L, Stuart J. Sympathetic ophthalmitis in Canada. Can J Ophthalmol. 1972;7:157-9.
6. Makley TA Jr, Azar A. Sympathetic ophthalmitis. A long-term follow-up. Arch Ophthalmol 1978;96:257-62.
7. Marak GE Jr. Recent advances in sympathetic ophthalmitis. Surv Ophthalmol 1979;24:141-56.
8. Saatci AO, Paşa E, Söylev MF, Koçak N, Durak I, Kaynak S. Sympathetic ophthalmitis and indocyanine green angiography. Arch Ophthalmol 2004;122:1568-9.
9. Sampangi R, Venkatesh P, Mandal S, Garg SP. Recurrent neovascularization of the disc in sympathetic ophthalmitis. Indian J Ophthalmol 2008;56:237-9.
10. Sharp DC, Bell RA, Patterson E, Pinkerton RM. Sympathetic ophthalmitis. Histopathologic and fluorescein angiographic correlation. Arch Ophthalmol 1984;102:232-5.
11. Vianna RN, Ozdal P, Souza Filho JP, Deschênes J. Choroidal neovascularization associated with sympathetic ophthalmitis: case report. Arq Bras Ophthalmol 2005;68:397-400.

44 Chapter

Behçet's Syndrome

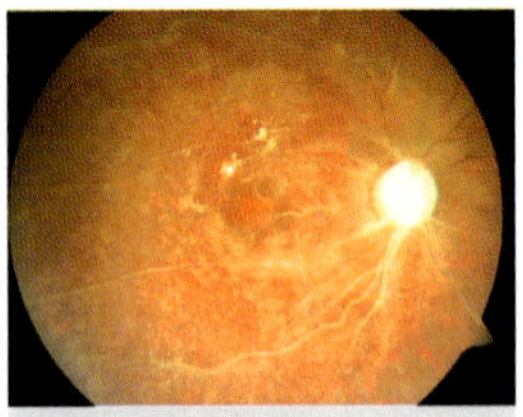

- Behçet's syndrome is an idiopathic, multisystem disease characterized by recurrent episodes of orogenital ulceration and vasculitis which may involve small, medium and large veins and arteries.
- Ocular disease is usually bilateral.
- It can present as recurrent, acute anterior uveitis with hypopyon, retinal infiltrates, retinal vasculitis, macular edema, ischemic optic neuropathy and vitritis.
- Retinal vasculitis in Behçet's disease involves both arteries and veins, is diffuse and occlusive, with significant vitritis.
- It is associated with HLA B51.
- Treatment is with oral steroids, immunosuppressives and biologicals.
- Prognosis is guarded due to the development of optic atrophy in end stage disease with 20 percent of eyes becoming blind despite treatment.

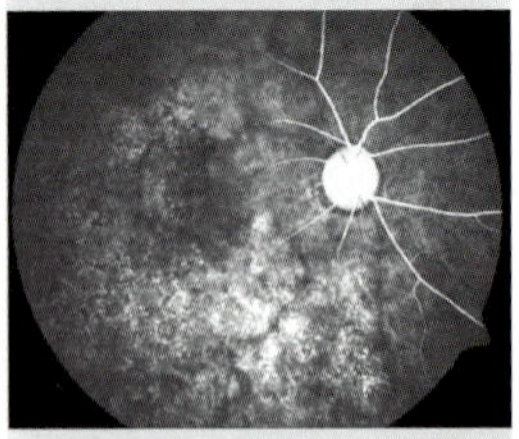

Fundus fluorescein angiography shows diffuse retinal vascular leakage and occlusion of retinal vessels.

- Fluorescein leakage from retinal vessels may be seen before any clinical signs of vasculitis.
- During acute inflammation, retinal vascular leakage is prominent, especially in the radial peripapillary area.
- Affected retinal and optic nerve vessels leak fluorescein profusely during early transit phase and their walls stain in late transit phase.
- Fluorescein angiography may also reveal macular ischemia and cystoid macular edema.

CASE 1

A 19-year-old male presented with decreased vision in the right eye since one month and sudden loss of vision in the left eye since one day. He had a history of genital ulcers. BCVA in the right eye was 6/18; N6 and NPL in the left eye. The patient was diagnosed of Behçet's disease and treatment initiated with immunosuppressive agents (cyclosporine) and oral steroids.

At Presentation

Right Eye

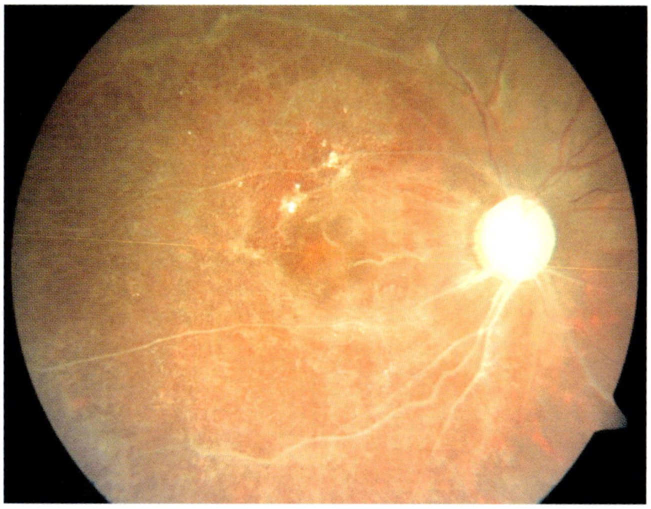

Color fundus photo of the right eye shows marked disc pallor, sclerosed vessels with very few perfused vessels along the superior arcades. Diffuse RPE atrophy and patches of subretinal scarring can be noted in the macula

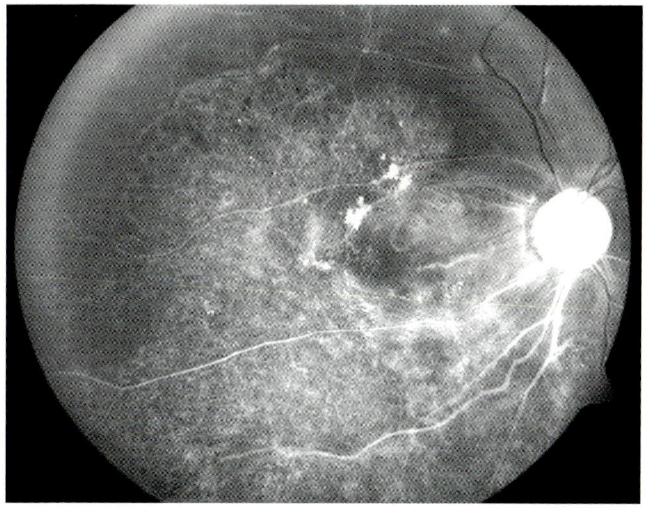

Red free photograph highlights the extent of RPE degeneration

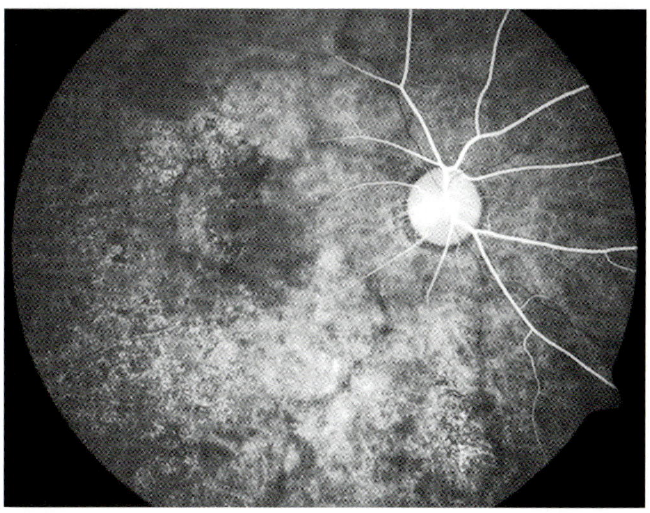

Arterial phase angiogram shows thin caliber of vessels and gross RPE window defects along with nonperfusion areas in the macula

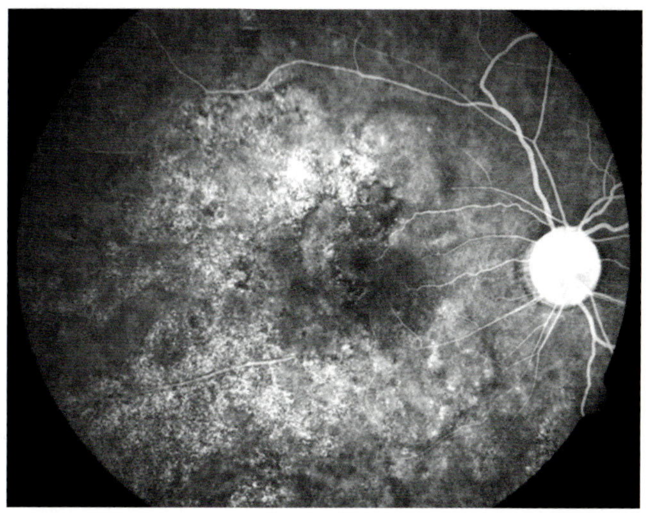

Late phase shows disc staining with late filling of sclerosed vessels

Left Eye

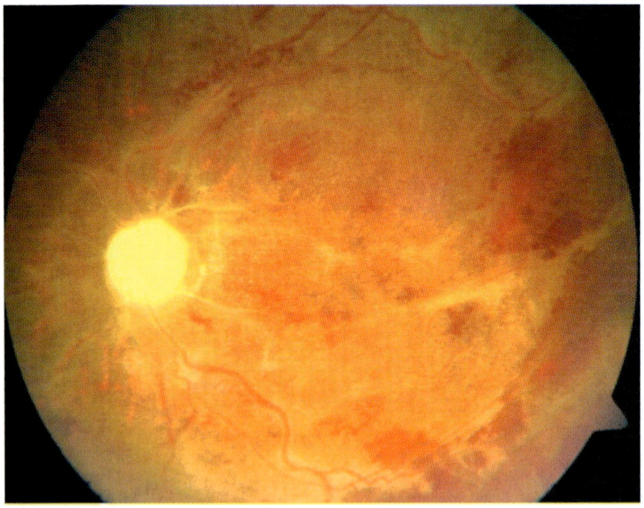

Color fundus photo of the Left eye shows optic atrophy, sheathed vessels emerging from the disc, subretinal hemorrhage and gross RPE atrophy seen over the posterior pole

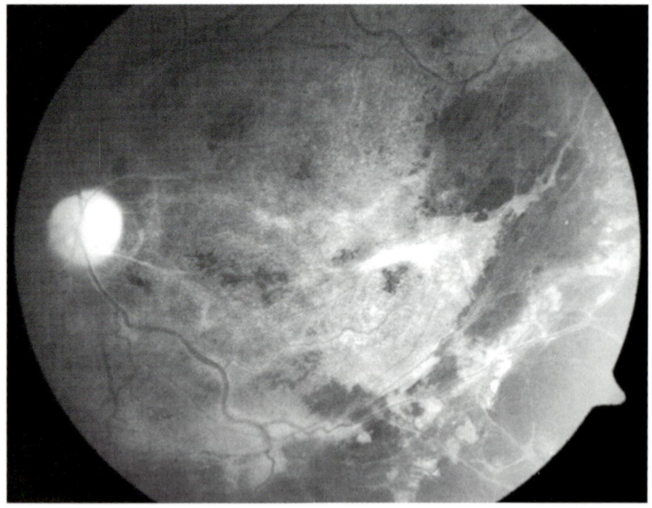

Red free photo of the left eye highlights the extent of subretinal hemorrhage

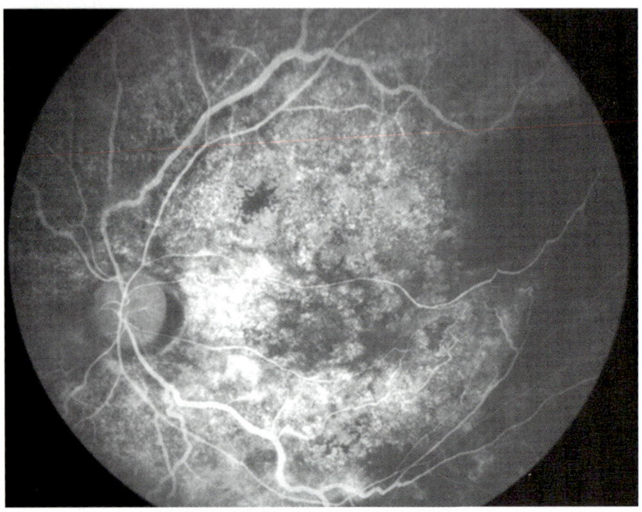

Early arteriovenous phase shows RPE window defects with macular nonperfusion

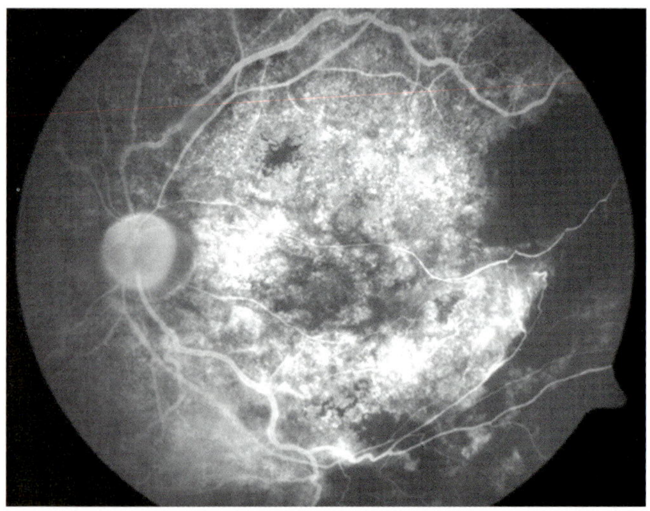

Late phase shows blocked fluorescence corresponding to subretinal blood temporal to macula

At Last Visit

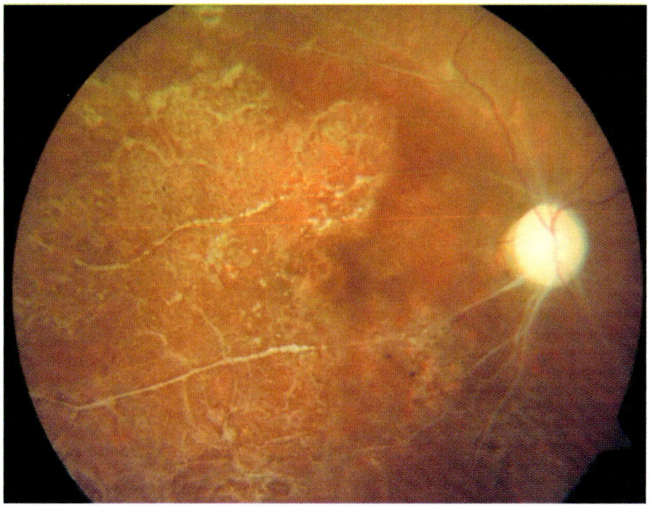

Color fundus photo of the right eye shows advanced disc pallor with more prominent RPE atrophy and subretinal scars at the macula

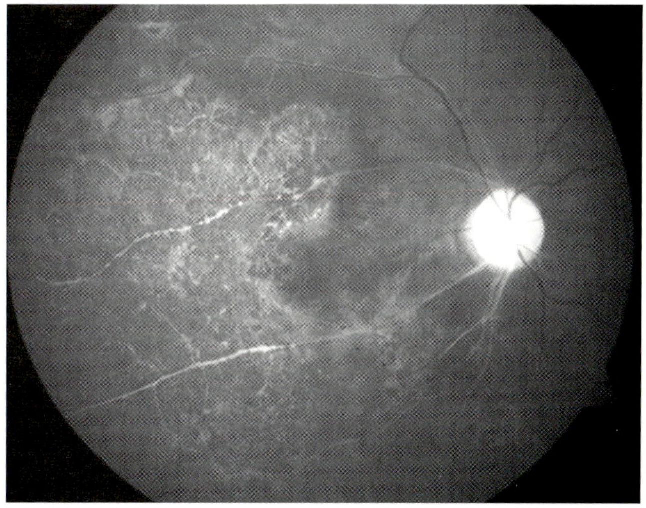

Red free photo highlights the extent of RPE degeneration

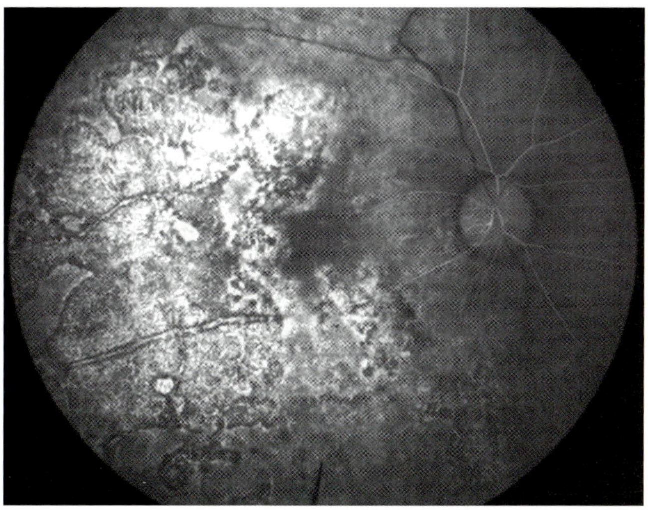

Arterial phase shows filling of the arcade vessels with RPE window defects at the macula

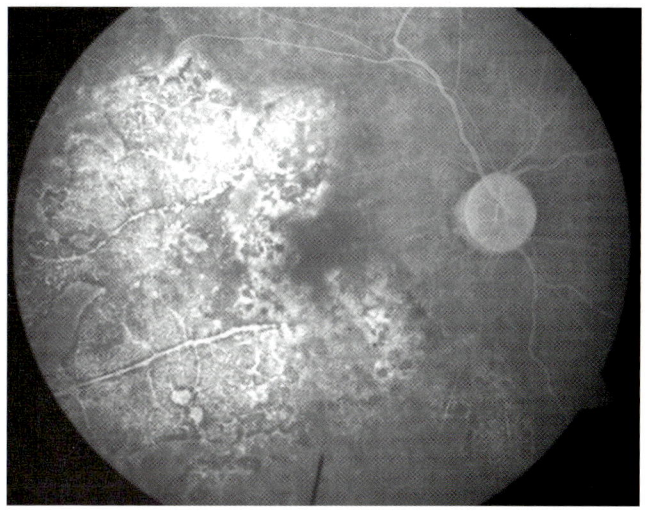

Late phase shows prominent staining due to the scar along with window defects and surrounding pseudo-blocked fluorescence due to normal RPE

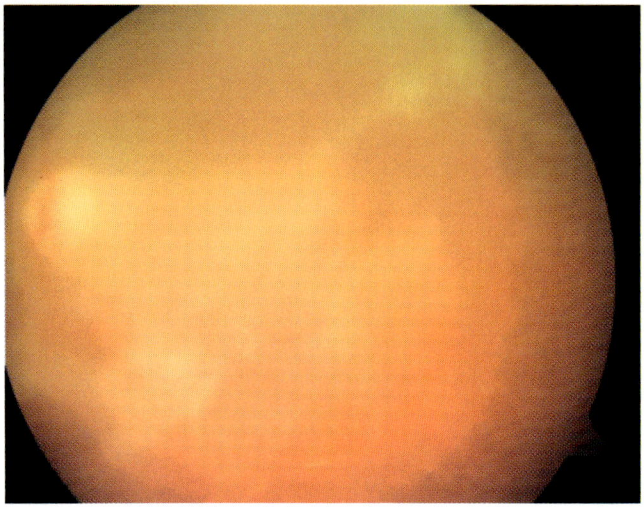

Color fundus photo of the left eye shows media haze increased due to vitritis and moderate cataractous changes. Note the deep retinal hemorrhage along the arcade

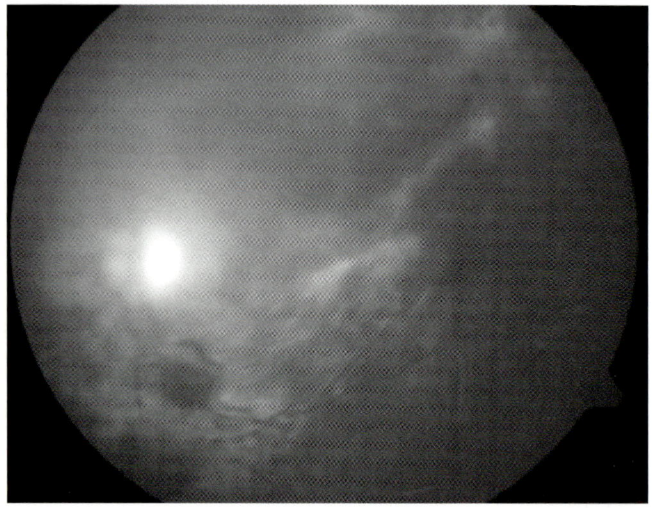

Red free photo of the left eye

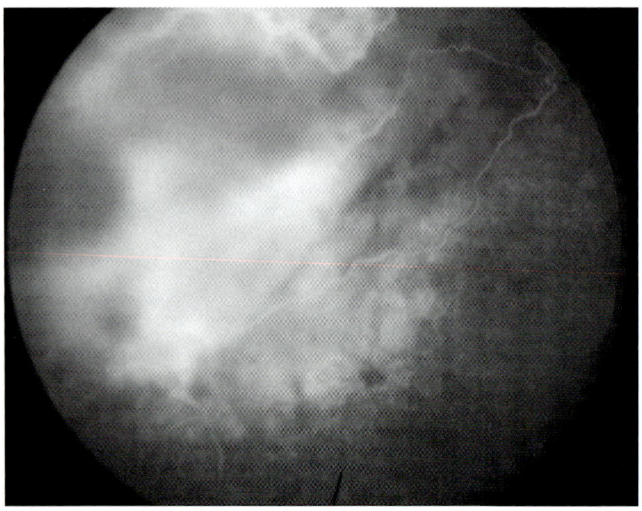

Midarteriovenous phase shows diffuse dye leakage in vitreous and dye leak from the retinal vessels

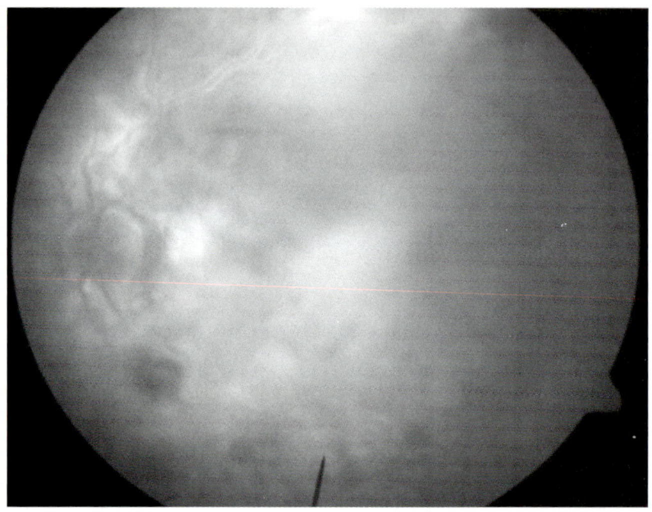

Late phase shows staining of the vessels and blocked fluorescence corresponding to the retinal hemorrhages

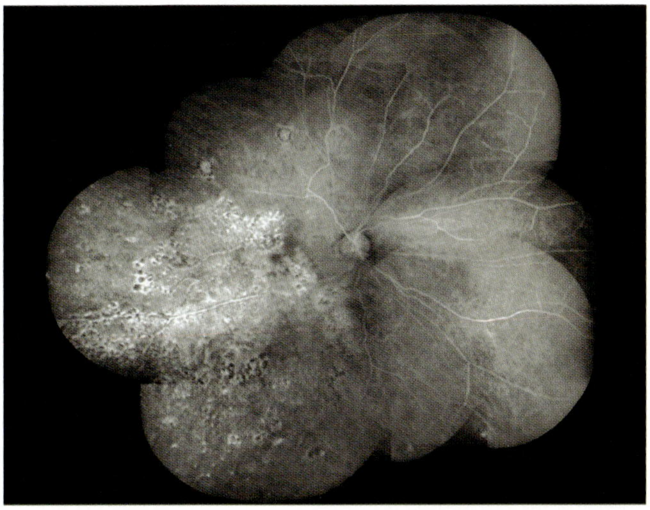

Montage angiogram image reveals the extensive retinal involvement

CLINICAL NUGGETS

1. Vasculitis in Behçet involves both arteries and veins, is diffuse, occlusive and associated with vitritis.
2. Hypopyon in Behçet is mobile and shifts with gravity in contrast to immobile fibrinous hypopyon in spondyloarthropathies.

BIBLIOGRAPHY

Sachdev N, Kapali N, Singh R, Gupta V, Gupta A. Spectrum of Behçet's disease in the Indian population. Int Ophthalmol. DOI 10.1007/s10792-008-9273-8.

45 Chapter

Intermediate Uveitis

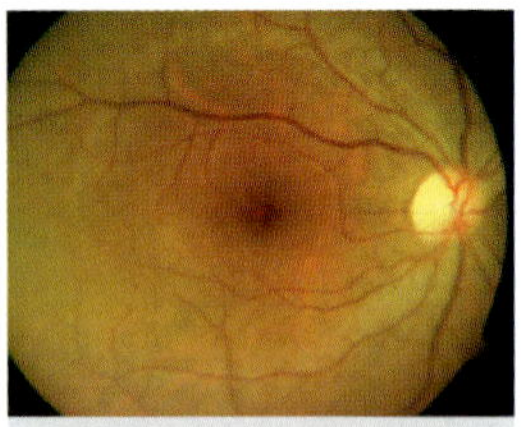

- Intermediate uveitis or pars planitis is a common chronic inflammatory disorder causing marked inflammatory exudative response in the peripheral retina.
- Vitreous cells are invariably present and may range from mild to severe.
- Yellow-white exudates may collect over the inferior vitreous base overlying the pars plana and the peripheral retina—when this is significant it is called 'snowbanking'.
- Cystoid macular edema is very common and important cause of visual loss in this condition.
- Disc edema can also be present.

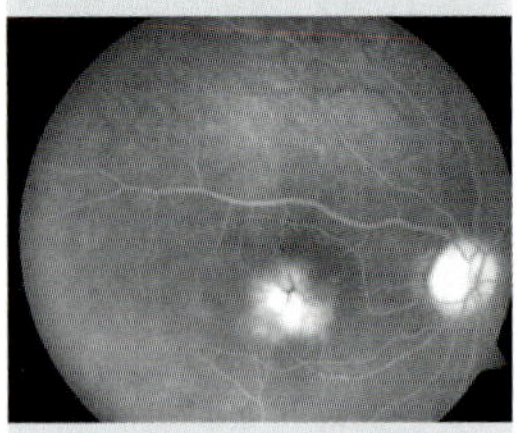

- Fluorescein angiography is useful in evaluating cystoid macular edema in intermediate uveitis. This is especially true in cases in which the vitritis does not allow a very clear visualization of the posterior pole.
- Leakage from the perifoveal capillaries is seen in the arteriovenous phase of the angiogram. This is generally more extensive than that seen in aphakic cystoid macular edema. Cystoid changes are very well noted in the late phase of the angiogram.
- Leakage of the dye and staining of the vessel wall may occur in larger vessels. Increased disc staining is common and well seen in the late phase.

CASE 1

A 42-year-old female presented with blurring of vision in the right eye for the past two months. Visual acuity was 6/24; N18. Exudates were noted over the pars plana.

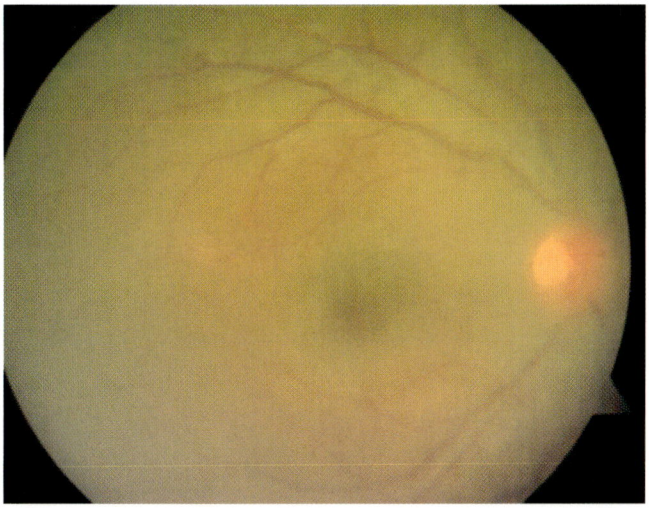

Fundus photograph of the right eye. Vitreous haze precludes evaluation of the finer retinal details

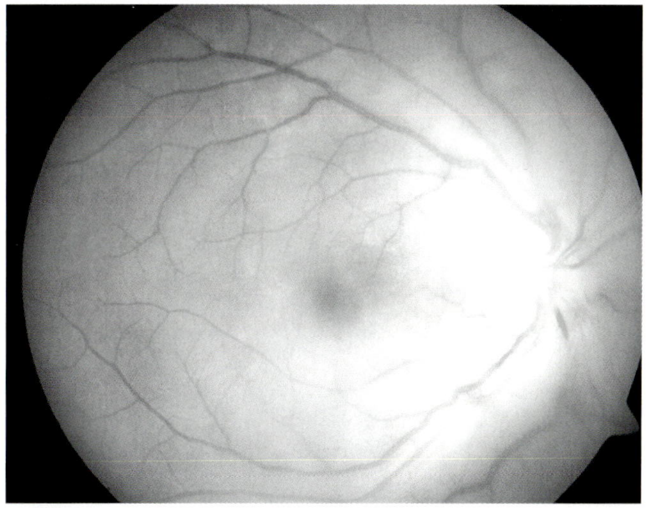

Red free photograph of the right eye

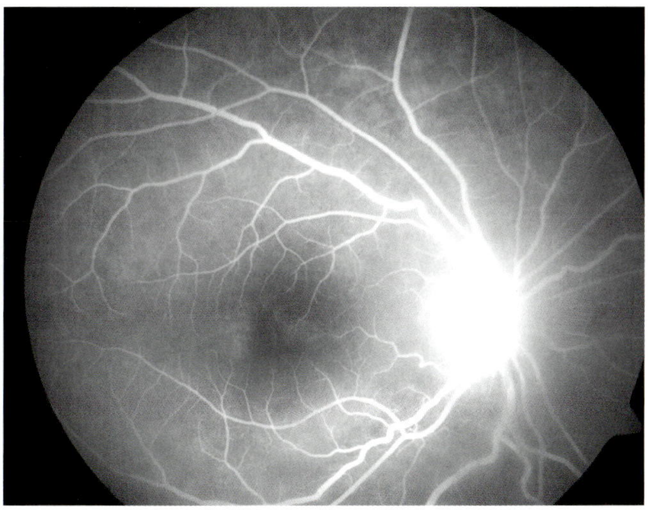

Increased hyperfluorescence of the disc is seen. Faint hyperfluorescence is seen in the perifoveal region

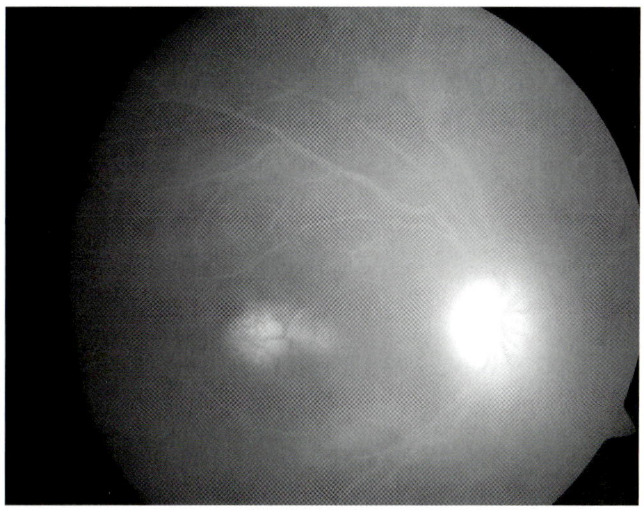

Late phase shows the accumulation of the dye in cystoid spaces at the fovea

COMMENT

Due to presence of vitreous haze, biomicroscopic evaluation of the macula is sometimes difficult in case of intermediate uveitis. Fluorescein angiography helps to detect macular edema in such situations.

CASE 2

A 34-year-old female presented with episodes of blurring of vision and floaters in both eyes for the past three years. She had received periocular steroids in both eyes in the past. Visual acuity was 6/18; N6 in the right eye and 6/12; N6 in the left eye. Vitreous cells were noted in both eyes.

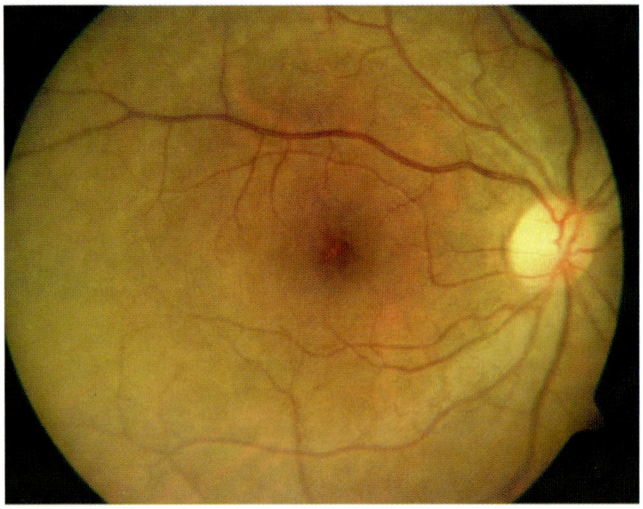

Fundus photograph of the right eye. Biomicroscopic examination had shown retinal thickening at the fovea

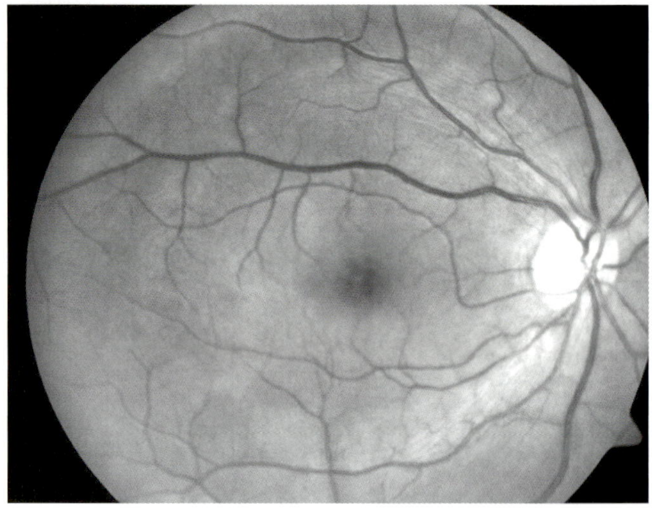

Red free photograph of the right eye

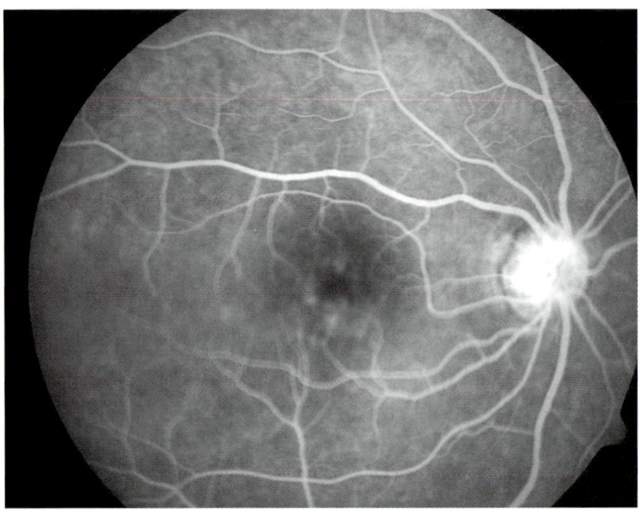

Mid arteriovenous phase shows dilation of the parafoveal capillaries with early leakage of the dye

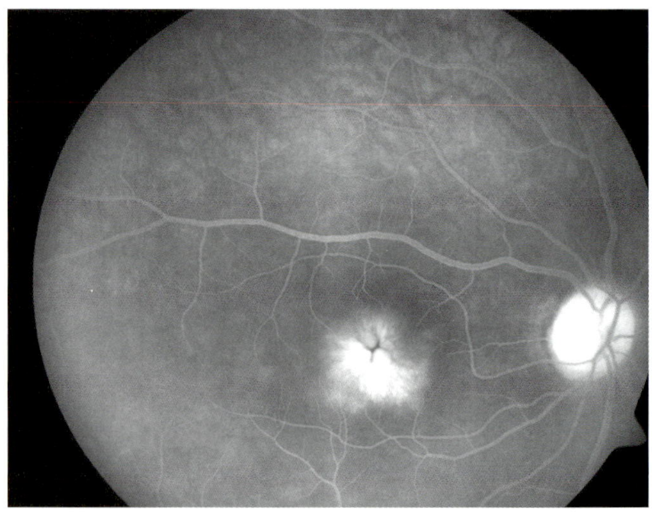

Cystoid macular edema is well seen in the late phase

CASE 2 (*Continued*)

Left Eye of the Patient

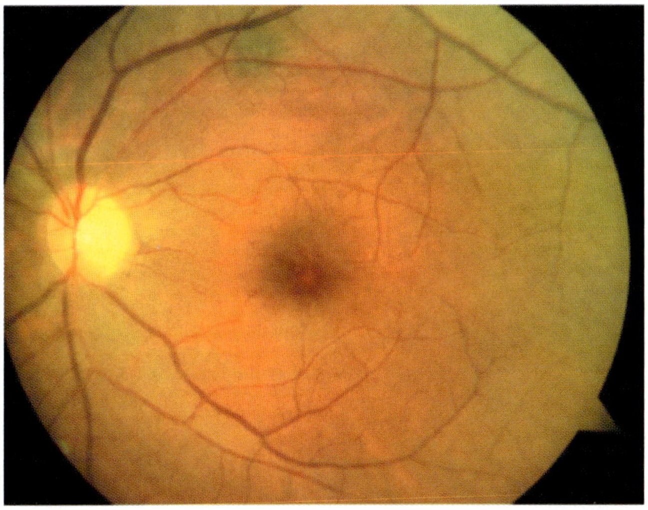

Fundus photograph of the left eye

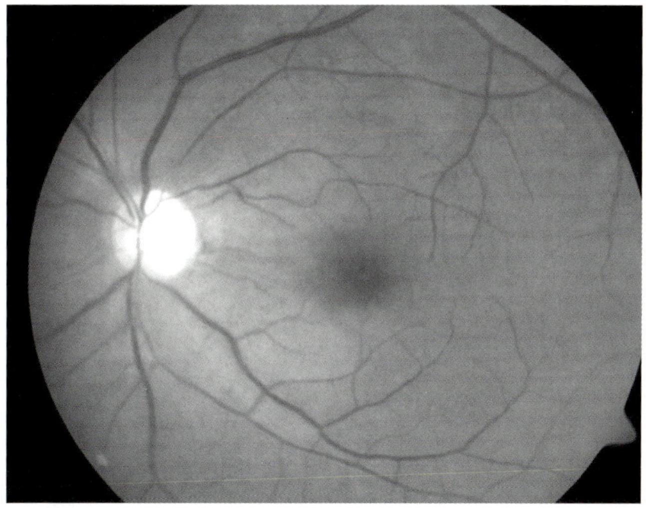

Red free photograph of the left eye

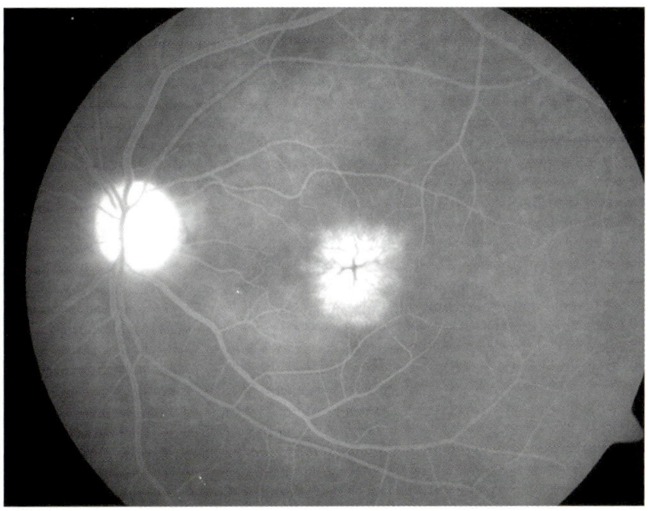

Late phase showing cystoid macular edema

COMMENT

Cystoid macular edema and increased disc staining are typical angiographic findings in intermediate uveitis.

CLINICAL NUGGET

Optical coherence tomography (OCT) is useful in monitoring the macular edema and the response to treatment.

46

Chapter

Birdshot Retinochoroidopathy

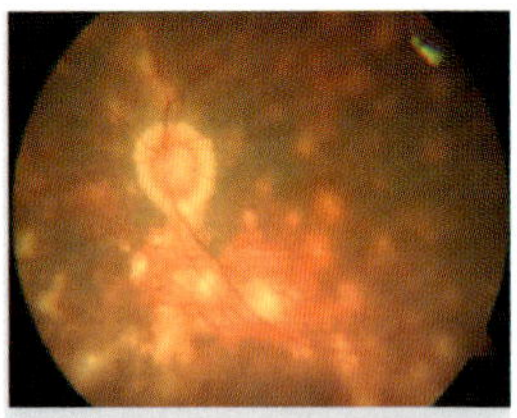

- Birdshot retinochoroidopathy is a rare, bilateral disorder occurring more commonly in females in the fifth to seventh decade of life.
- The lesions are typically flat, creamy yellow in color and distributed throughout the fundus.
- They appear to radiate linearly from the optic disc.
- These lesions are choroidal infiltrates.
- Some degree of vitritis is common in this disorder.
- Cystoid macular edema and disc edema are frequently present.

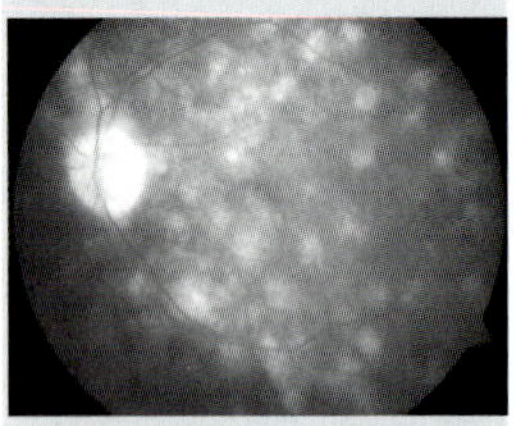

- The lesions of birdshot retinochoroidopathy usually do not show hypo- or hyperfluorescence in the early phase. Mild hyperfluorescence is seen in the late phase of the angiogram.
- Arterial filling may be delayed.
- Leakage from the perifoveal capillaries and from larger vessels may be seen in the late phase.
- Cystoid macular edema is commonly seen.

CASE 1

A 60-year-old male patient presented with history of reduced vision in the left eye for the past several years. He had been diagnosed to have panuveitis in both eyes and had lost vision in the right due to secondary glaucoma. Visual acuity in the left eye was 6/36; N36.

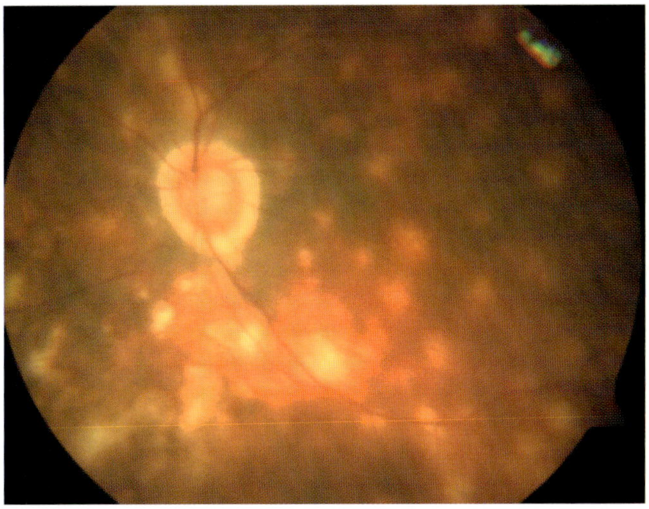

Fundus photograph of the left eye showing multiple flat creamy yellow lesions

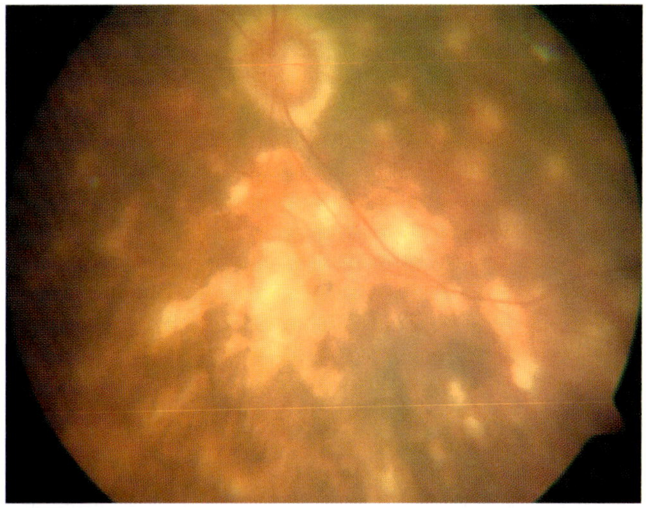

Fundus photograph showing the inferior midperiphery

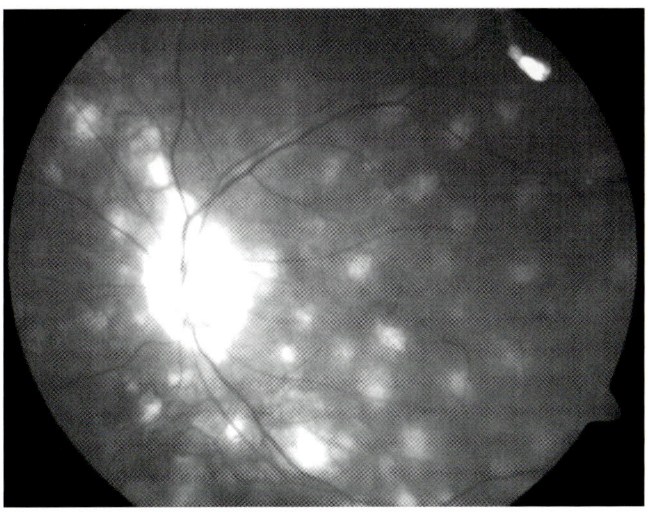

Red free photograph of the left eye

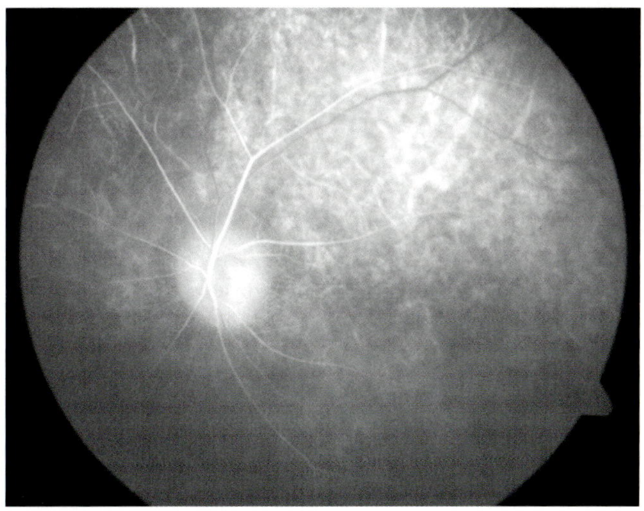

The lesions are not seen in the early arteriovenous phase

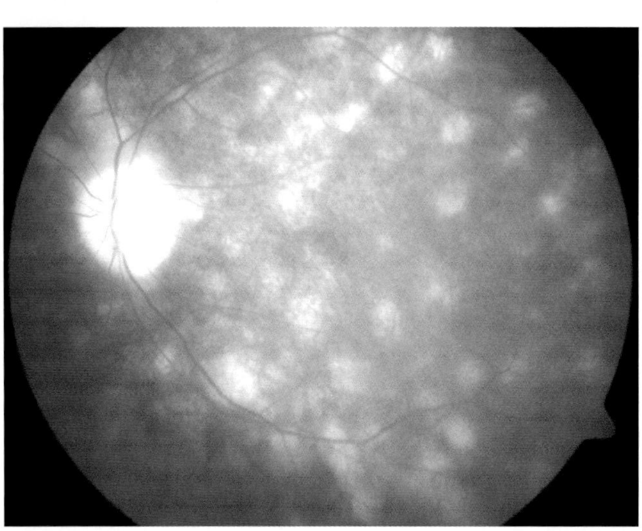

Late phase showing hyperfluorescence of the lesions

COMMENT

In contrast to APMPPE and GHPC, the lesions in birdshot retinochoroidopathy do not show hypofluorescence in the early phase.

CASE 2

A 41-year-old lady presented with decreased vision along with flashes in both eyes. Visual acuity was 6/24 in right eye and and 6/6 in the left eye.

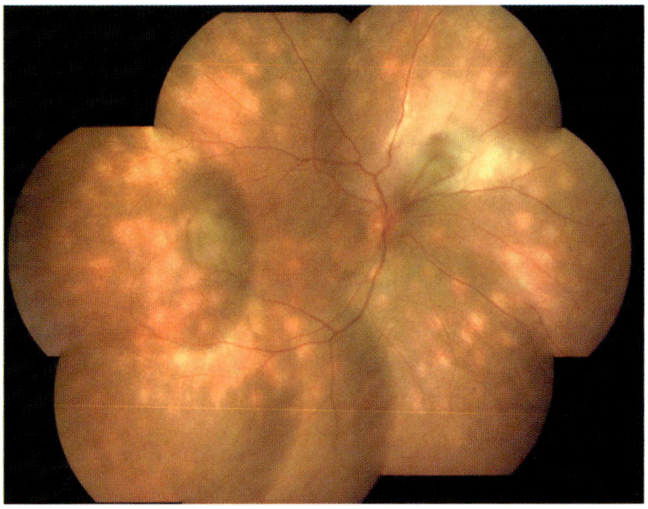

Color montage fundus picture of right eye

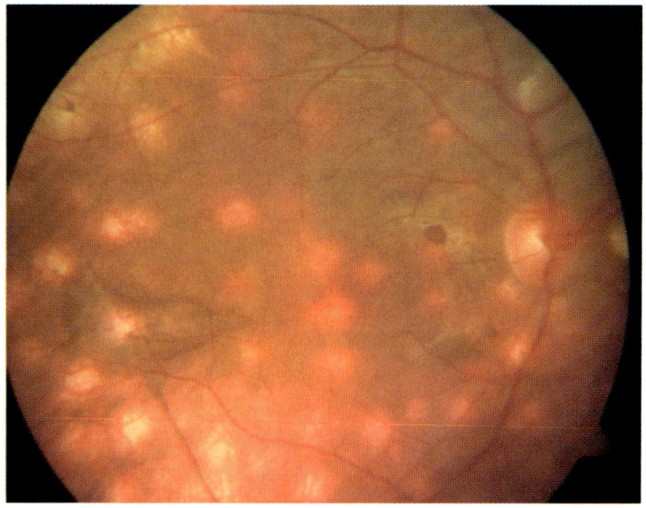

Color fundus photo of right eye showing multiple, creamy yellow, flat lesions throughout the fundus

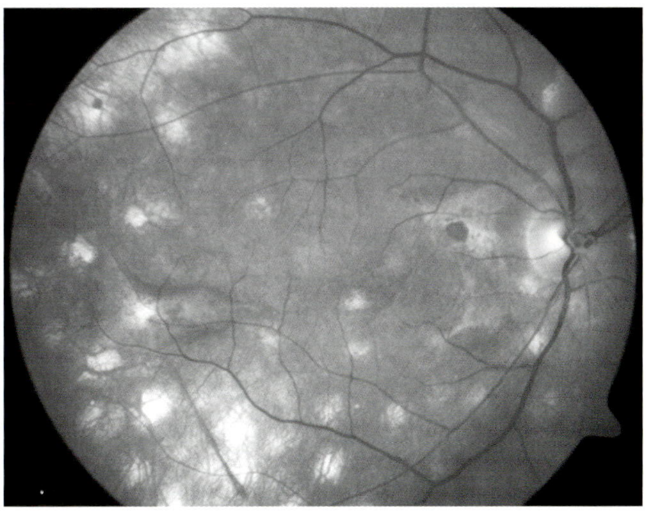

Red free photograph of right eye

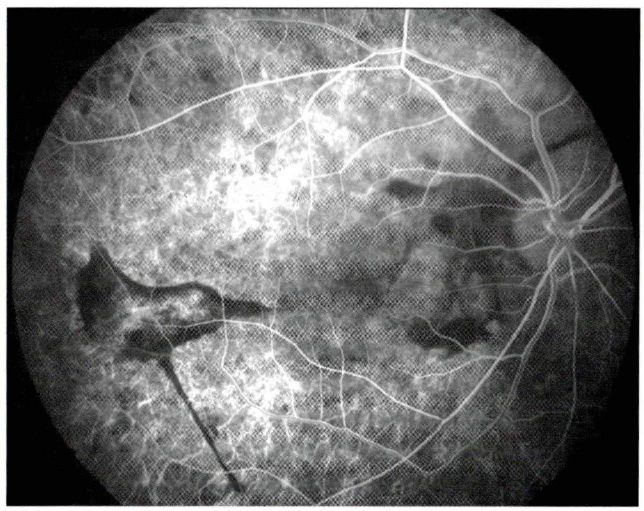

Lesions not seen in early arteriovenous phase

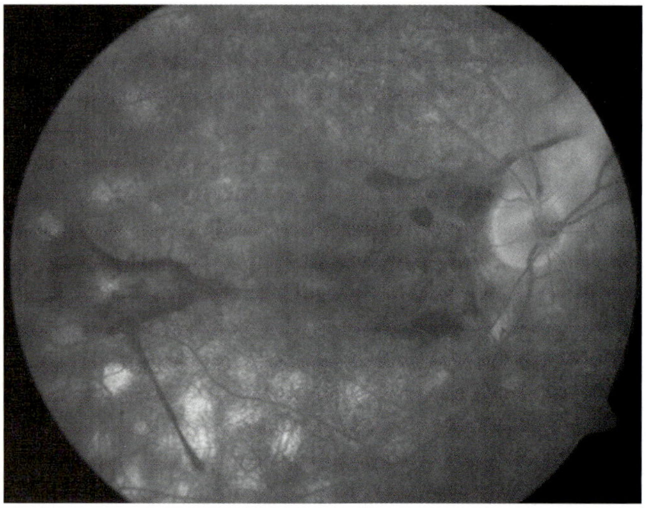

Hyperfluorescent lesions seen in the late phase of angiogram

CLINICAL NUGGETS

1. The fundus spots appear several years after the onset of vitritis, vasculitis, and CME, resulting in misdiagnosis.
2. The introduction of early therapy based on ERG findings may have a significant impact on the prognosis.

BIBLIOGRAPHY

1. Levinson RD, Gonzales CR. Birdshot retinochoroidopathy: immunopathogenesis, evaluation, and treatment. Ophthalmol Clin North Am. 2002;15(3):343-50, vii.
2. Thorne JE, Jabs DA, Peters GB, Hair D, Dunn JP, Kempen JH. Birdshot retinochoroidopathy: ocular complications and visual impairment. Am J Ophthalmol. 2005;140(1):45-51.

47

Chapter

Multiple Evanescent White Dot Syndrome

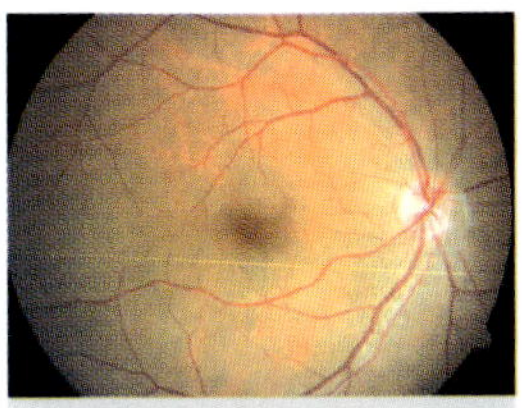

- Clinical examination reveals multiple, gray-white, flat, subretinal lesions over the posterior pole.
- Lesions are subtle and require careful examination for accurate diagnosis.
- Foveal granularity is characteristic. However, other features may include optic disc edema, vitritis and RAPD.
- Visual field testing reveals an enlarged blind spot. Visual field defect persists even after the disappearance of the lesions.
- The differential diagnosis includes APMPPE, birdshot retinochoroidopathy, acute retinal pigment epitheliitis, and diffuse unilateral subacute neuroretinitis.

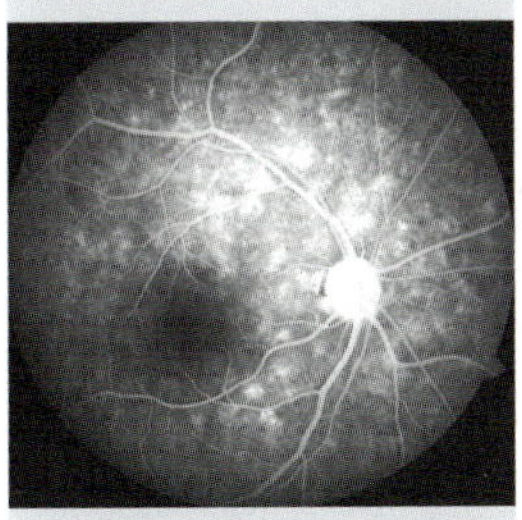

Fundus fluorescein angiography demonstrates hyperfluorescence corresponding to white spots. Other features may include mild macular edema, retinal vascular sheathing and disc leakage.

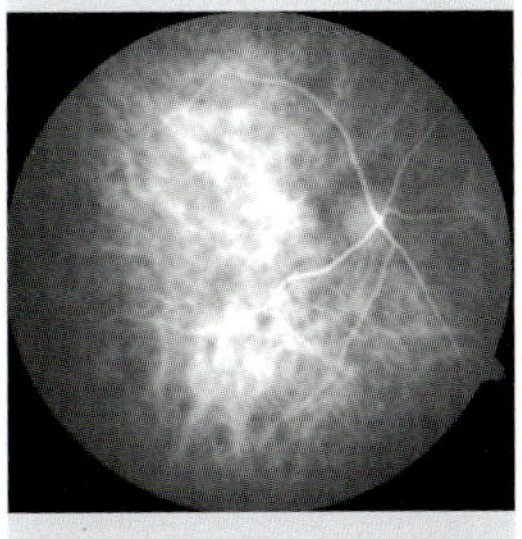

Indocyanine green angiography demonstrates multiple hypofluorescent spots in the posterior pole and hypofluorescence around the optic nerve head. The hypofluorescent spots persist until the patient recovers.

CASE 1

A 35-year-old lady presented with pain in both eyes, which was occasional and associated with redness for the past 4 months. On examination, best corrected visual acuity was 6/5; N6 in both eyes. She had been diagnosed earlier as 'resolving choroiditis'. Slit-lamp examination revealed no evidence of active or healed anterior uveitis. Intraocular pressure in both eyes was within normal limits.

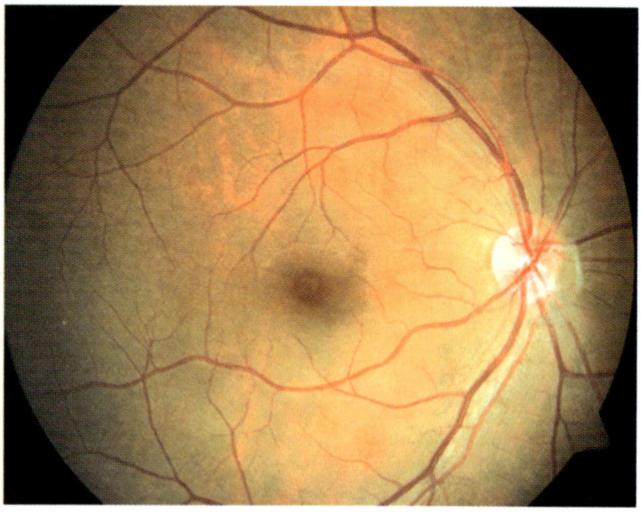

Fundus examination revealed a few subtle white spots over the posterior pole

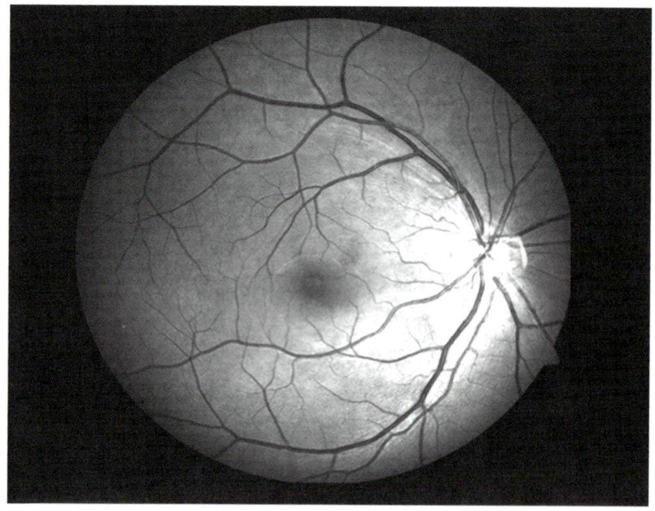

Red free photograph of the right eye

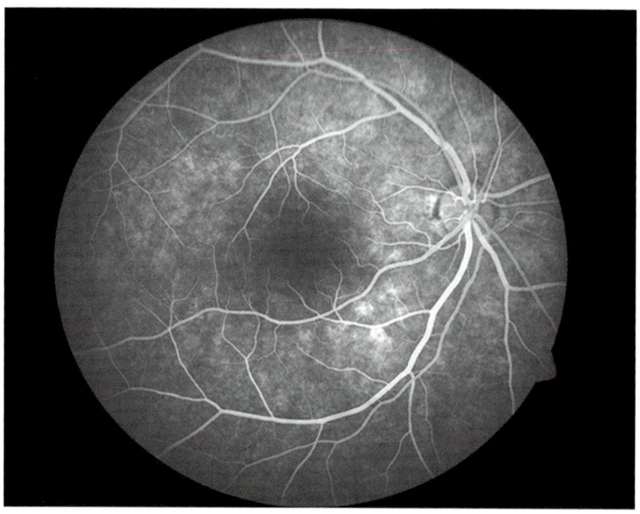

A-V phase fundus fluorescein angiography shows multiple hyperfluorescent spots over the posterior pole

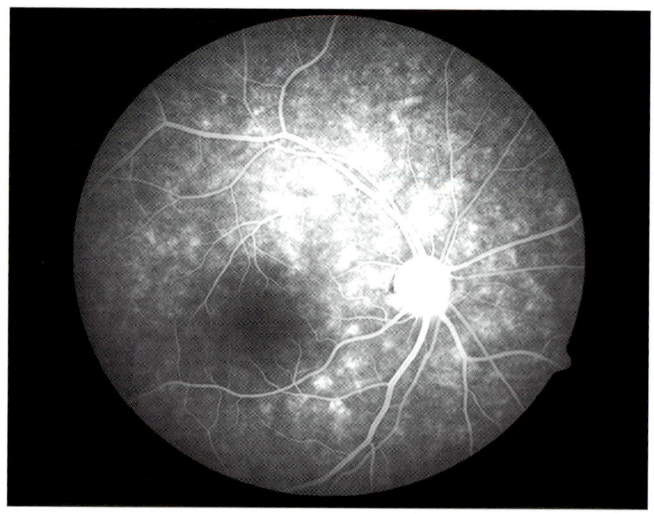

Venous phase fundus fluorescein angiography showed an increase in intensity of the hyperfluorescent lesions

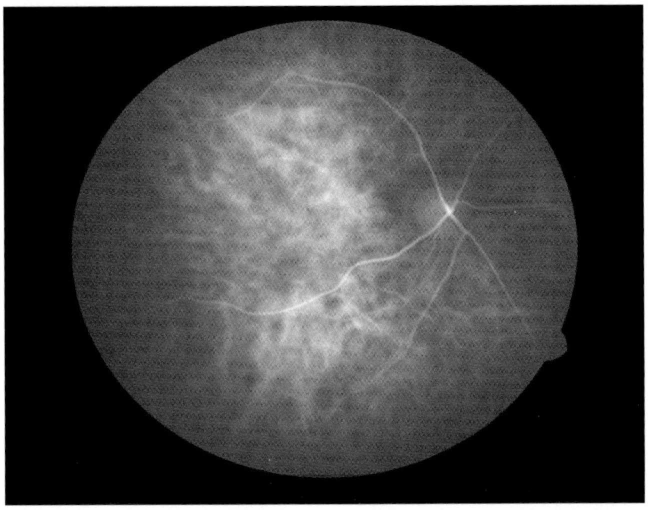

ICG angiography demonstrates multiple hypofluorescent spots in the posterior pole and hypofluorescence around the optic nerve head

48 Chapter

Punctate Inner Choroidopathy

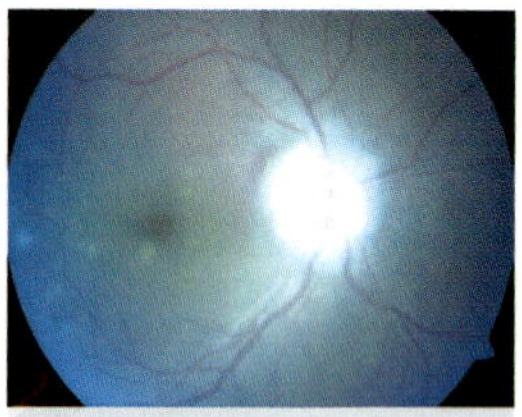

Punctate inner choroidopathy (PIC) was first described by Watzke and associates in 1984. This rare condition is also one of the entities grouped under AZOOR. Other terms used to describe this condition include multifocal inner choroiditis and pseudohistoplasmosis. It typically affects young, moderately myopic women with bilateral ocular involvement. Patients usually presents with blurring of vision, central and peripheral scotoma and photopsia.

Signs

1. Absence of vitreous inflammation and anterior segment inflammation.
2. Yellowish-white lesions at the level of inner choroid or retinal pigment epithelium usually at the posterior pole and occasionally midperiphery and nasal to optic disc.
3. Active lesions frequently have overlying serous detachment and heal to form atrophic scars with variable pigmentation.

Diagnosis

FFA: Active lesions—Early hyperfluorescence and late leak.
Chronic scar—Staining in late phase of angiogram.
CNVM—Hyperfluorescence with late leakage.
OCT: Useful in documenting subretinal serous collections overlying the active lesions.

CASE 1

A 32-year-old female patient with history of recurrent uveitis presented with OU—blurring and floaters since 8 months. BCVA OD—6/9; OS—6/12.

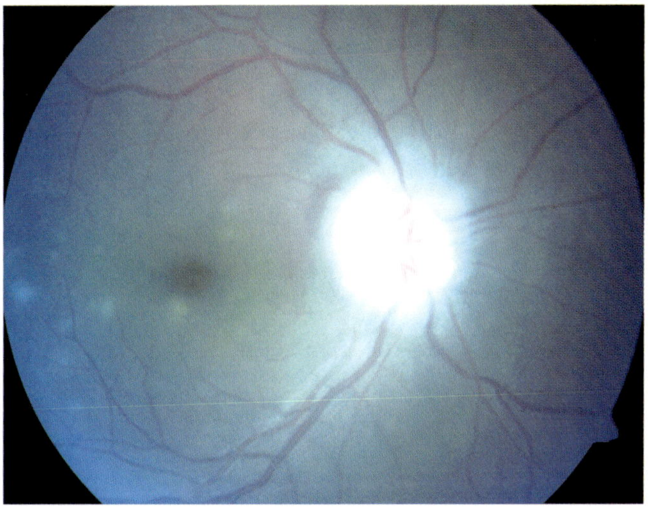

Color fundus photo of the right eye reveals hyperaemic disc with poorly defined margins and well-defined yellowish-grey subretinal lesions over the posterior pole

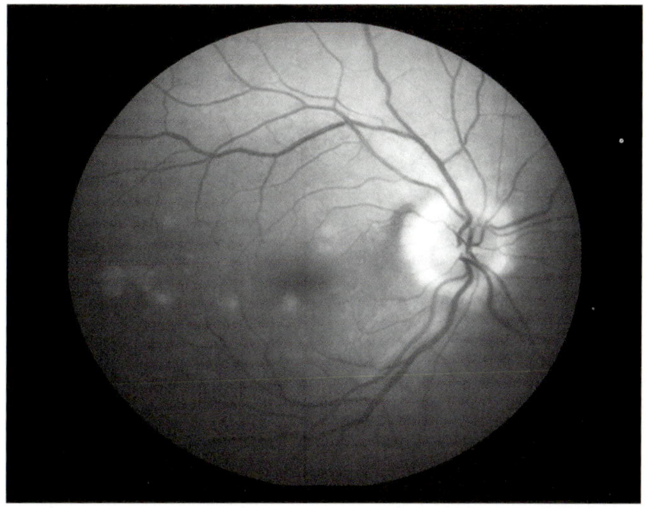

Red free image highlights the posterior pole tesions with a cresentic peripapillary shadow. Retinal vessels can be seen passing above the posterior pole lesions confirming its subretinal location

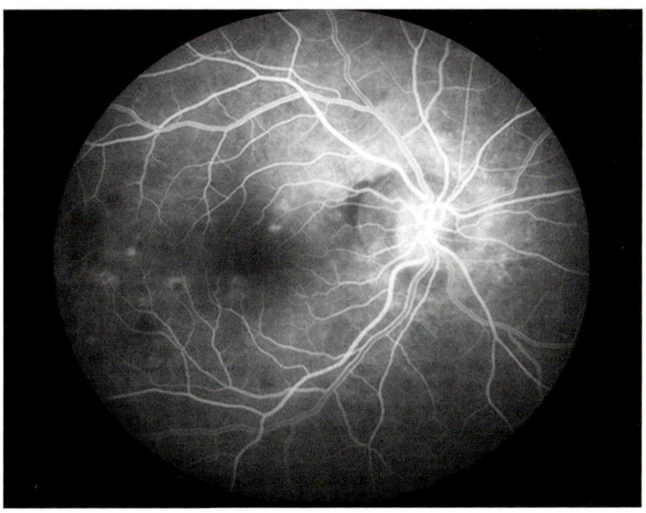

Early phase of FFA shows multiple early hyperfluorescent lesions over the post pole and area of blocked fluorescence in the peripapillary area

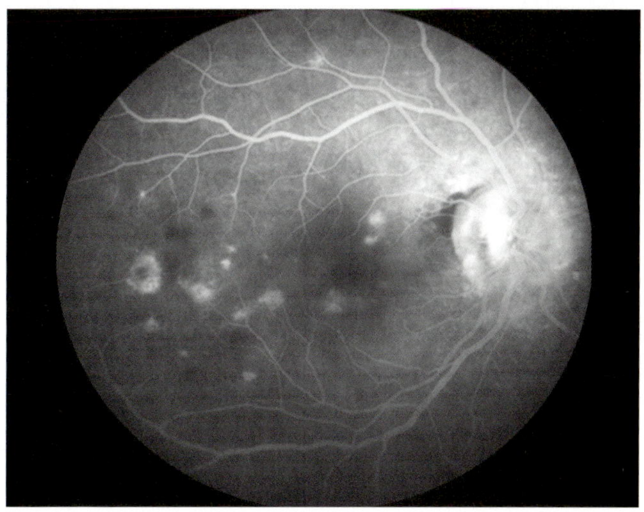

Late phase of FFA shows active leakage from the corresponding areas and area of blocked fluorescence surrounded by hyperfluorescence in peripapillary area

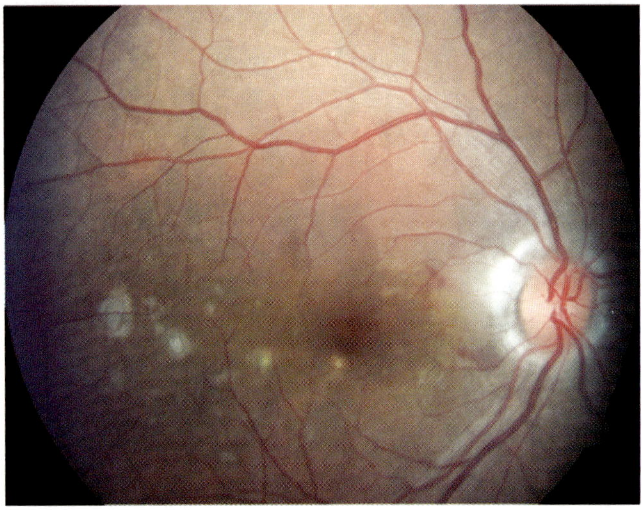

Following oral steroid therapy fundus photo shows healed well-defined atrophic choroidal lesions with resolving peripapillary CNVM inferotemporal to disc with subretinal hemorrhage

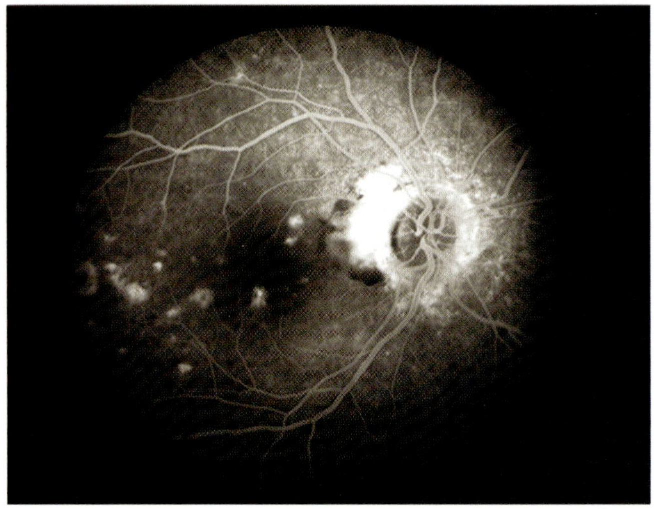

Late phase of FFA showing staining of the CNVM with blocked fluorescence in peripapillary area and multiple well-defined lesions over posterior pole with no leakage

CLINICAL NUGGETS

1. Differential diagnosis include myopic fundus, POHS, multifocal choroiditis and panuveitis, APMPPE.
2. Treatment:
   - Most cases are self-resolving, so warrant just careful close observation.
   - When vision is decreased due to serous RD systemic and periocular steroids may be given.
3. Key Features:
   - Many patients are even asymptomatic and detected on routine examination.
   - CNVM may develop from active lesions or more commonly from edges of atrophic scars which need treatment according to its location.

BIBLIOGRAPHY

1. Branzas D, et al. Choroidal neovascularization due to PIC: long-term follow-up and review of literature. Cli Ophthalmol 2010;4:871-6.
2. Gass JD. Stereoscopic Atlas of Macular Diseases Diagnosis and Treatment. St Louis: Mosby-Year Book Inc;1987.
3. Morgan CM, Schatz H. Recurrent multifocal choroiditis. Ophthalmol, 1986;93(9):1138-47.
4. Taira K, Nakazawa M, Takano Y, Ota T. Acute zonal occult outer retinopathy in the fellow eye 5 years after presentation of punctate inner choroidopathy. Graefes Arch Clin Exp Ophthalmol. 2005;29:1-3.

Chapter 49 Acute Retinal Necrosis

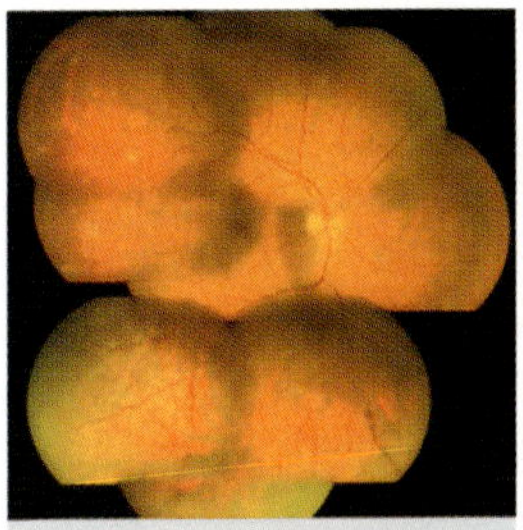

- It is a type of necrotizing herpetic retinitis characterized by a triad of peripheral foci of retinal necrosis, occlusive arteriolitis and vitritis.
- The peripheral lesions are initially discrete and progressively coalesce to form 360 degrees creamy white retinitis with scalloped posterior border.
- In 36 percent of the patients the other eye is involved within 6 weeks if no antiviral treatment is given.
- Retinal hemorrhages are rare and the posterior pole is spared.
- Disc edema and macular edema can be seen.
- Exudative retinal detachment can be seen in severe inflammation.
- Seventy-five percent of patients develop multiple posterior breaks and rhegmatogenous retinal detachment.

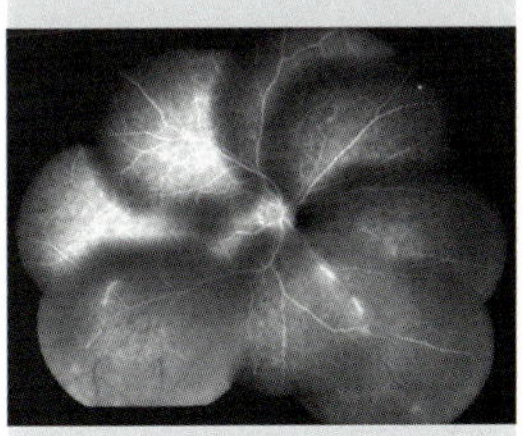

- In active disease, the areas of retinal necrosis appear hypofluorescent throughout the angiogram with no filling of arterioles suggestive of occlusive arteriolitis.
- Dye leakage from the retinal capillaries is seen at the junction of involved and uninvolved retina.
- Disc leakage and cystoid macular edema can be seen in late phases.
- In healed retinitis, the areas of scarring show sheathing of vessels with no retinal perfusion and hyperfluorescent staining in late phases.

CASE 1

A 49-year-old male presented with visual loss since 3 weeks in the left eye and since 3 days in the right eye. He had been treated with intravenous acyclovir (elsewhere) for 3 days before presentation. Aqueous tap PCR was positive for varicella zoster virus.

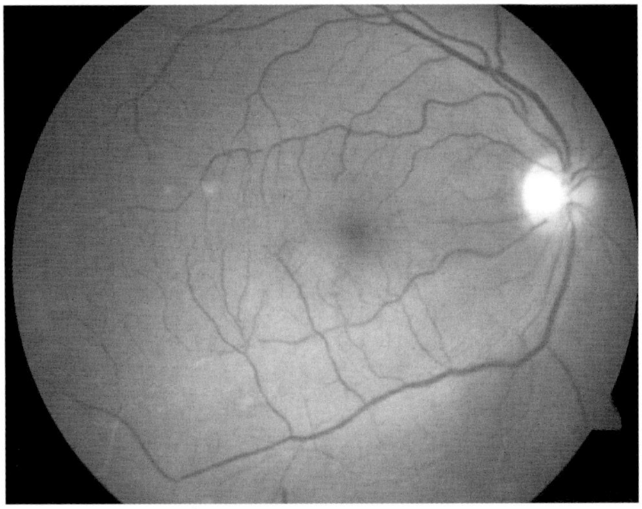

Red free photo of right eye showing occluded temporal branch arterioles

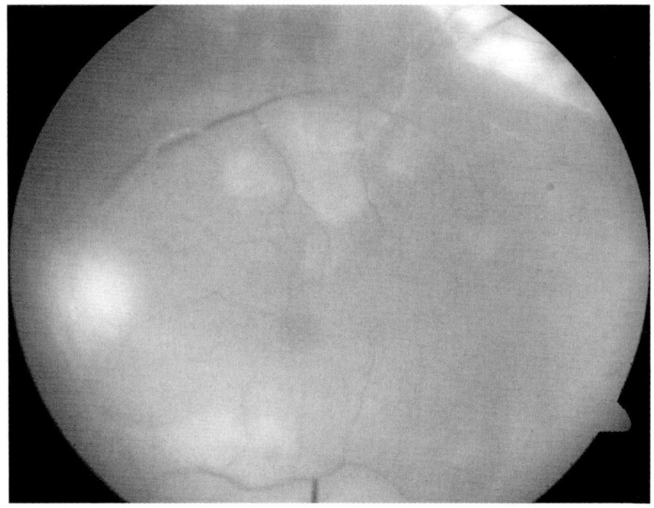

Red free photo of left eye shows hazy media due to vitritis with occluded temporal arterioles with retinal necrosis in the superotemporal quadrant

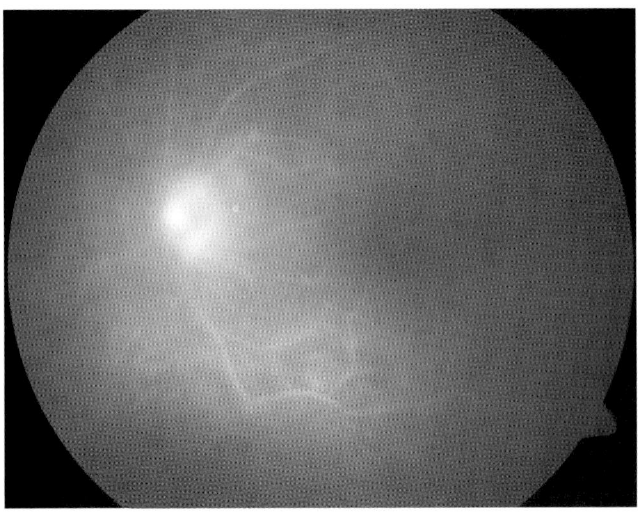

Recirculation phase reveals optic disc staining, generalized retinal vessel staining and nonperfused retinal arterioles, nasally

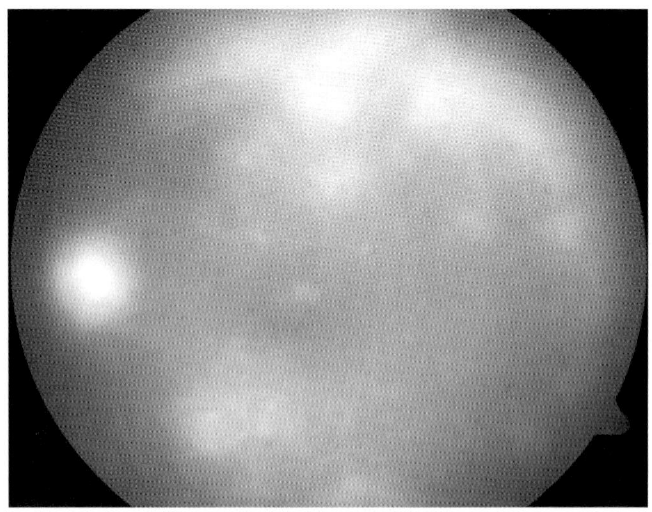

Late phase shows disc staining and intense retinal leakage at the posterior edge of the necrosed retina in the superotemporal quadrant

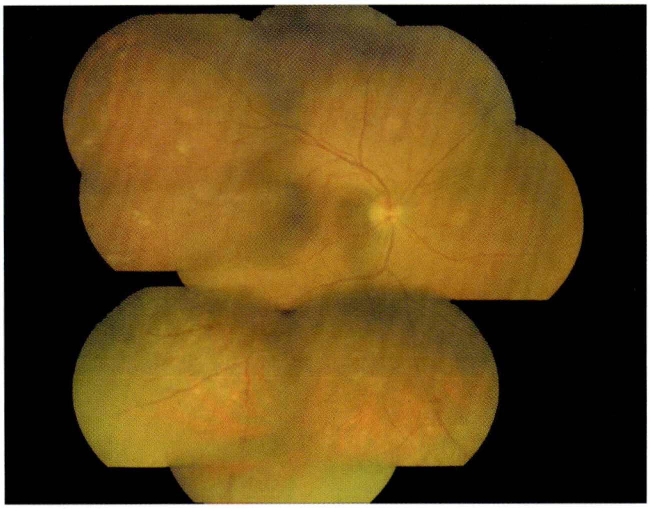

A color photo montage of the right eye showing occluded arterioles in the temporal and inferior mid-periphery with a large area of retinal whitening inferotemporally suggestive of active retinal necrosis

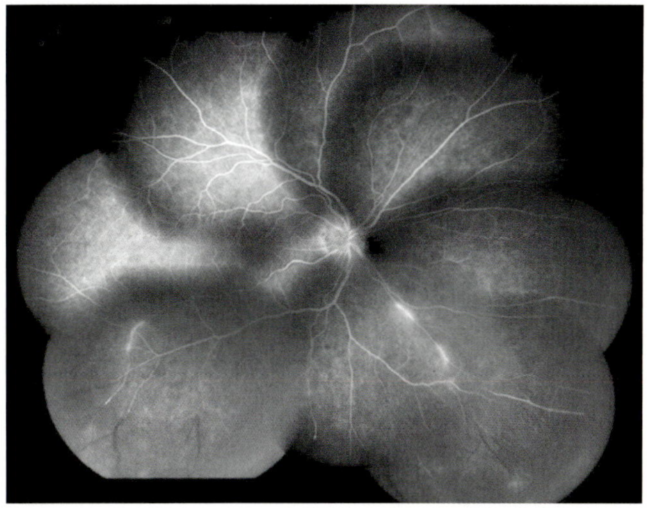

A composite photo of the angiogram of the right eye shows the non-filling arterioles in the inferior and temporal periphery with staining of vessels at the border of involved and uninvolved retina

COMMENT

ARN is usually characterized by severe vitritis therefore fluorescein angiography is done only in cases of a dilemma in diagnosis.

Cystoid macular edema and disc edema can be seen in late phases despite hazy media due to vitritis.

Posterior Scleritis

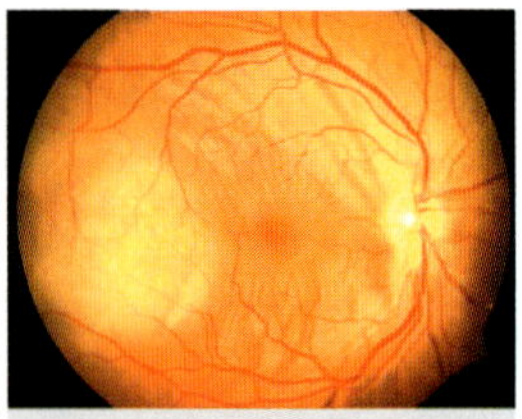

Posterior scleritis constitutes two percent of all cases of scleritis.

It occurs more commonly in females (65%) and usually manifests before the age of 40 years.

Mostly, it occurs unilaterally. However, bilateral affection has been reported in 10-35 percent cases.

Patients present with mild to excruciating periocular pain, headache, diminution of vision, proptosis and diplopia in extreme cases. Nearly 60 percent cases develop anterior scleritis during sometime of their disease course.

The various ocular signs associated with posterior scleritis include:
- Associated anterior scleritis
- Serous retinal detachments
- Optic disc swelling
- No abnormalities (9%)
- Visible subretinal mass
- Elevated intraocular pressure
- Choroidal folds
- Annular choroidal detachments
- Transient induced myopia or hyperopia.

Posterior scleritis can be associated with a systemic disease in 30 percent cases. This is more often noted in patients with combined anterior and posterior scleritis and age more than 40 years at presentation. Commonly associated systemic diseases include:

- Rheumatoid arthritis
- Wegener's granulomatosis
- Systemic vasculitis
- Vogt-Koyanagi-Harada (VKH) syndrome
- Relapsing polychondritis
- Systemic lymphoma and leukemia.

The common causes of visual loss include:
- Macular changes
  - Retinal pigment epithelium (RPE) changes
  - Epiretinal membrane (ERM) formation
  - Macular hole/cyst
- Optic atrophy.

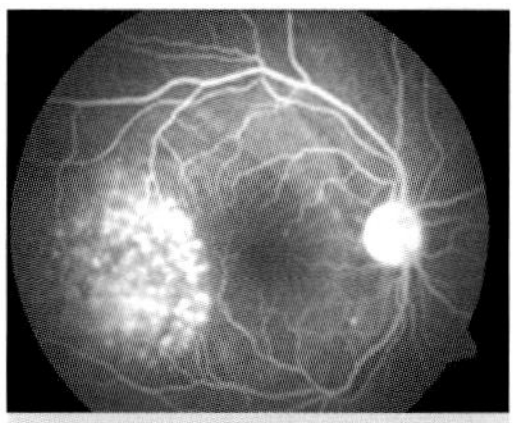

Fundus fluorescein angiography (FFA) reveals multiple pinpoint hyperfluorescent spots overlying the subretinal lesion suggestive of leakage. It may also show a mottled aspect of the choroidal fluorescence, disc hyperfluorescence and late pooling suggestive of serous retinal detachments. Late phase angiogram usually reveals intense, diffuse hyperfluorescence overlying the lesion with confluence of the pinpoint hyperfluorescent points noted in earlier phases.

CASE 1

A 53-year-old healthy lady presented with complaints of blurring of vision in the right eye since one week. Her BCVA at presentation was 6/6; N12 in the right eye and 6/6; N6 in the left.

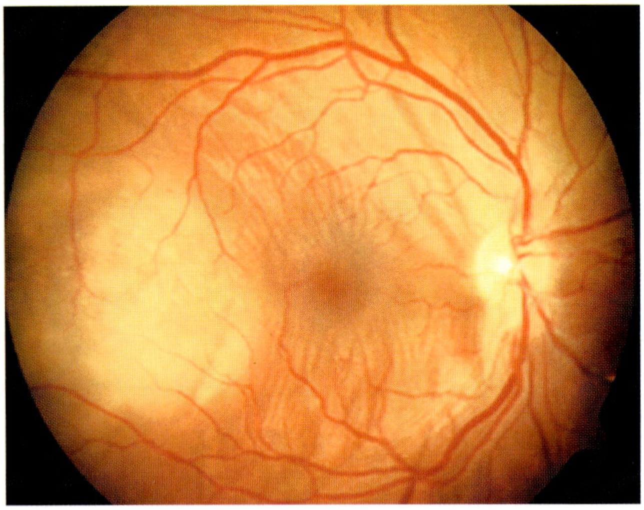

Color fundus photograph of the right eye reveals a large, yellowish subretinal mass lesion temporal to the fovea. Prominent choroidal folds are noted at the macula

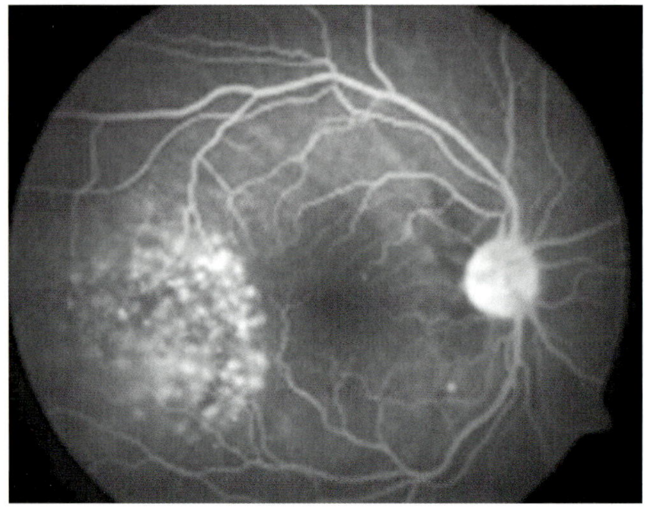

Late A-V phase angiogram reveals multiple pinpoint hyperfluorescent spots overlying the subretinal lesion suggestive of leakage. Alternate hypo- and hyperfluorescent bands in the macula correspond to the choroidal folds

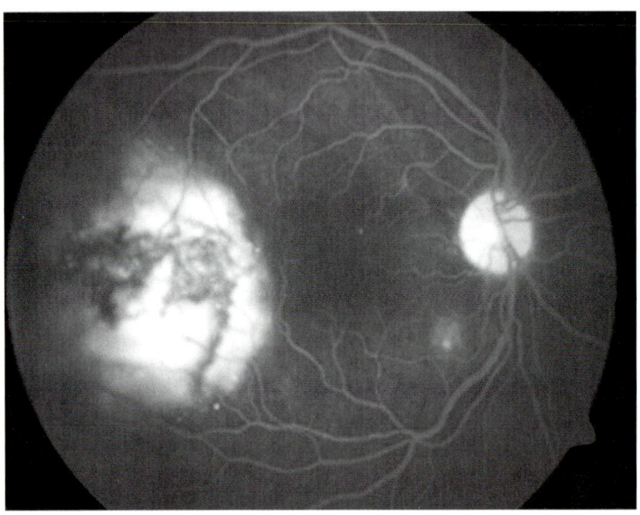

Late phase angiogram reveals intense, diffuse hyperfluorescence overlying the lesion with confluence of the pinpoint hyperfluorescent points noted in earlier phases

COMMENT

This patient was treated with tapering dose of oral steroids. There was complete resolution of the lesion with restoration of normal vision after 6 weeks.

CLINICAL NUGGETS

Differential diagnosis for posterior scleritis includes:

A. Fundus mass
   - Malignant melanoma
   - Metastatic carcinoma
   - Choroidal hemangioma
   - Benign reactive lymphoid hyperplasia.

B. Choroidal folds, disc edema
   - Orbital neoplasms
   - Hypotony
   - Graves' disease.

C. Choroidal detachment
   - Uveal effusion syndrome
   - Angle closure glaucoma.

D. Exudative macular detachment
   - CSR
   - VKH
   - PIC
   - APMPPE.

- Posterior scleritis is often an under-diagnosed condition.
  Careful clinical assessment and high quality ultrasound are required for proper management.
  Ultrasound B scan reveals;
  - Thickened posterior coats
  - Fluid in Tenon's capsule
  - Optic disc swelling
  - Distended optic nerve sheath
  - Scleral nodules.
- Goals of therapy
  - Block inflammatory process and prevent trigger of destructive cascade
  - Prevent visual loss
  - Prevent progression of underlying disease.
- Every patient of posterior scleritis, whatever type or severity, must be treated as if they have a potentially blinding condition.
- Patients more than 50 years of age have more systemic disease association, more chances of visual loss and need far more aggressive immunosuppressive treatment.

BIBLIOGRAPHY

1. Biswas J, Mittal S, Ganesh SK, Shetty NS, Gopal L. Posterior scleritis: Clinical profile and imaging characteristics. Indian J Ophthalmol 1998;46:195-202.
2. McCluskey PJ, Watson PG, Lightman S, Haybittle J, Restori M, Branley M. Posterior scleritis: clinical features, systemic associations, and outcome in a large series of patients. Ophthalmol 1999 Dec; 106(12):2380-6.

51 Chapter

Choroidal Granuloma

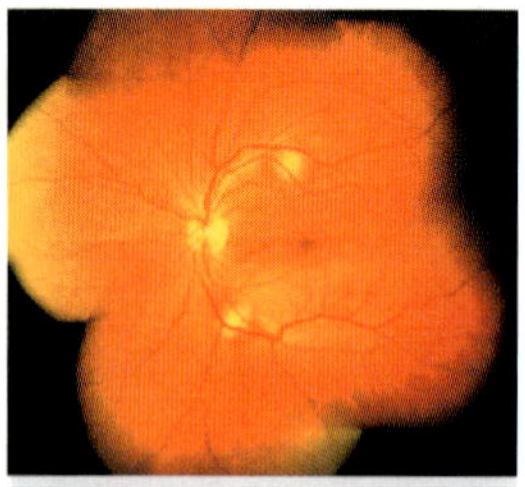

Choroidal granuloma is characterized by a subretinal mass lesion which has yellowish-white creamy color with retinal edema over it and surrounding exudative fluid.

Differential diagnosis of choroidal granuloma includes:[1]

- Tubercular granuloma
- Sarcoid granuloma
- Amelanotic melanoma
- Choroidal hemangioma
- Metastatic lesion

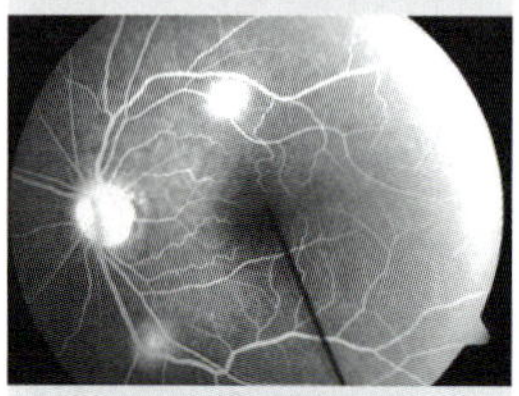

- Fluorescein angiography in active lesions shows early choroidal hypofluorescence due to blockage from the mass.
- Fluorescein angiography in inactive lesions displays retinal pigment epithelium window defects.

CASE 1

A 32-year-old female presented with blurring of vision in the left eye since last 6 months. At presentation, BCVA was 6/18; N10 in that eye. Anterior segment examination was normal. 2+ vitreous cells were noted. Systemic evaluation revealed raised serum levels of angiotensin converting enzyme and hilar lymphadenopathy on CT chest. Other investigations were unremarkable.

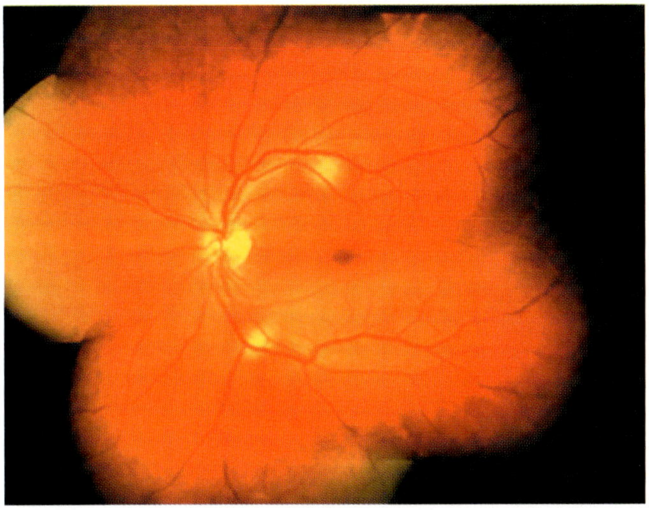

Fundus examination of left eye showed two discrete, elevated, choroidal granulomas, superotemporal and inferior to the disc

FFA

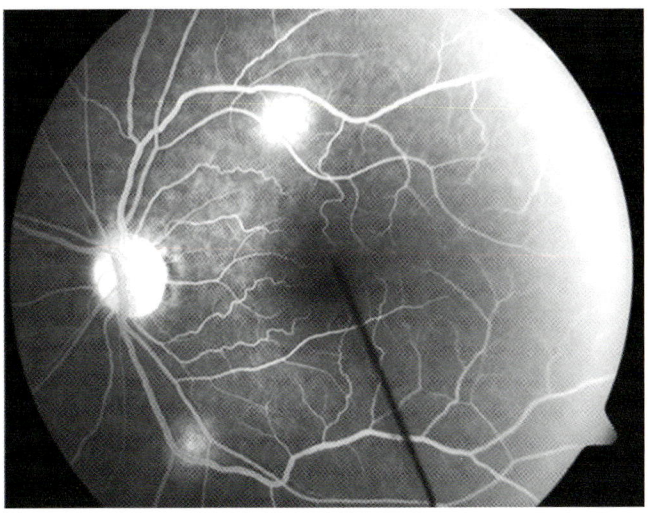

Arteriovenous phase shows two spots of hyperfluorescence from the lesions, which continued to leak throughout the remainder of the angiogram. This leakage would pool in the subretinal space in areas of neurosensory retinal detachment

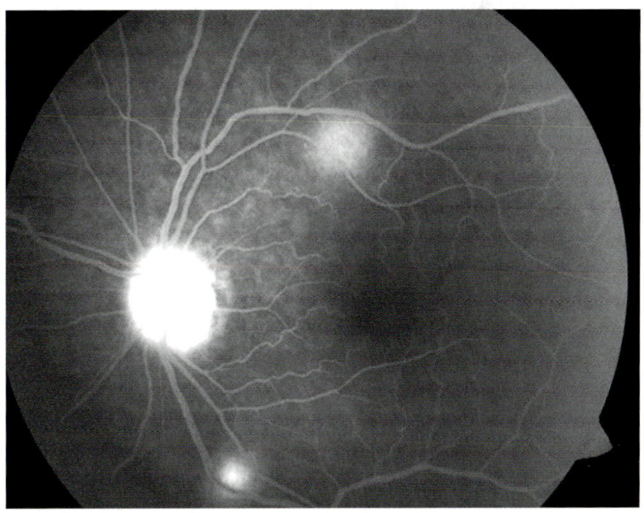

Late phase showing staining of the choroidal mass

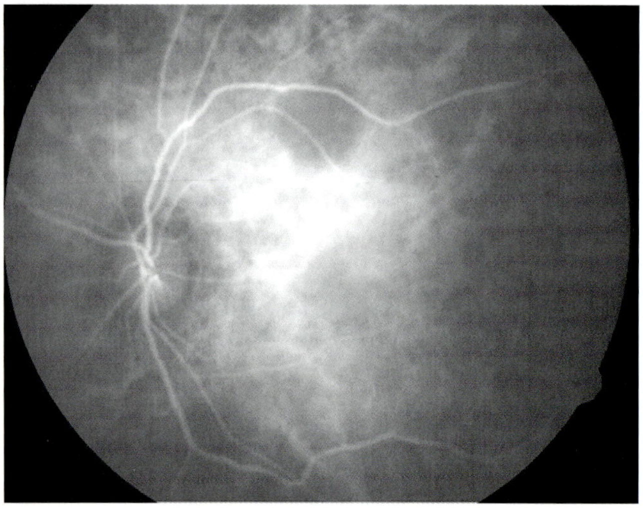

Early phase ICG angiography reveals blockage of fluorescence because of the choroidal granuloma. Choroidal granuloma lesions on ICG angiography remain hypofluorescent in early and mid phases

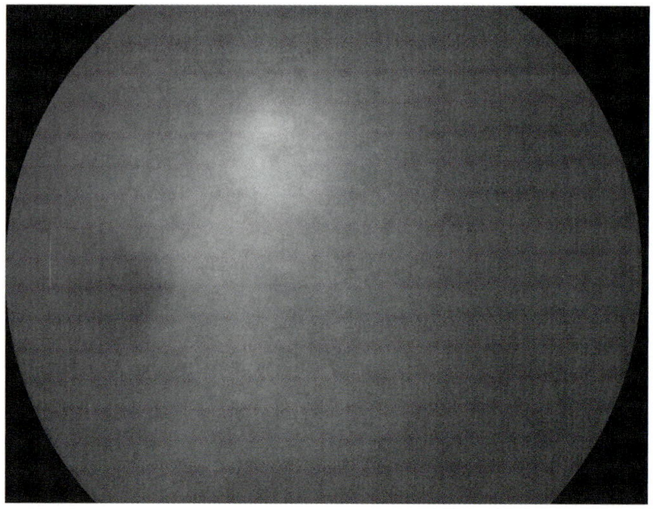

Late phase ICG angiography reveals hyperfluorescence due to staining of the choroidal granuloma superotemporal to the disc

CLINICAL NUGGETS

1. Fluorescein angiography in active lesions shows early choroidal hypofluorescence due to blockage from the mass.
2. Fluorescein angiography in inactive lesions displays retinal pigment epithelium window defects.
3. Solitary tubercular choroidal granuloma can be misdiagnosed as choroidal melanoma due to multiplicity of clinical findings, which can cause diagnostic delay.[2,3]
4. *Tubercular granuloma:* Most common presentation is a solitary granuloma which can occur at the posterior pole, although multiple choroidal granulomas can be seen in cases of miliary tubercles and in immunosuppressed patients.[4]
5. Sarcoid choroidal granuloma may be single or multiple and can present in the optic nerve, peripheral retina, pars plana and anterior choroid.

REFERENCES

1. Desia UR, Tawansy KA, Joondeph BC, Schiffman RM. Retina 2001;21:40-7.
2. Marback EF, Mendes E Jr, Oliveira C, Parikh JG, Rao NA. J Ophthal Inflamm Infect. DOI: 10.1007/s12348-010-0010.
3. Karim A, Laghmari M, Boutimzine N, Lamarti A, Ibrahimy W, Issakali N. Choroidal granuloma revealing tuberculosis. A case report. J Fr Ophthalmol 2003; 26:614-7.
4. Cangemi FE, Friedman AH, Josephberg R. Tuberculoma of choroid. Ophthalmol 1980;87:252-8.

52 Chapter

Other Inflammatory Disorders

PARASITIC TRACTS

CASE 1

A 49-year-old female presented with decreased vision in the right eye for the past one month. Visual acuity was 6/12; N8 in the right eye.

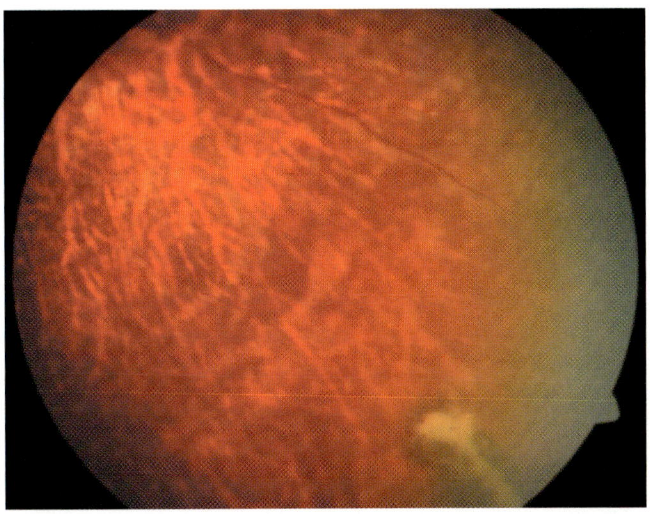

Fundus photograph showing the dead parasite in the inferonasal periphery. The parasitic tracts are seen

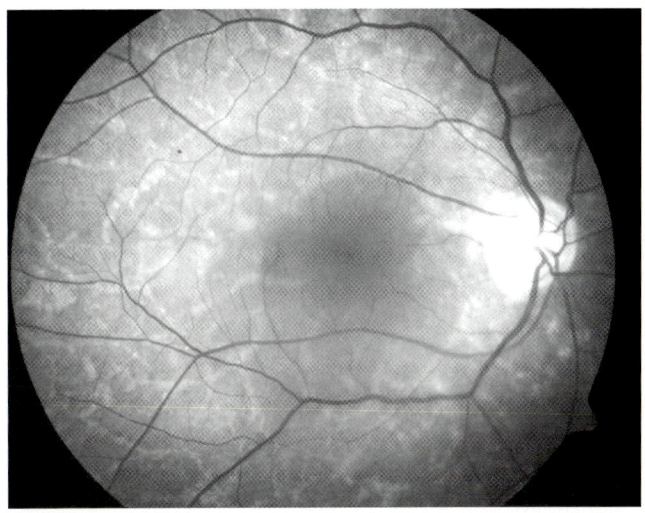

Red free photograph showing the posterior pole. The linear tracts are well seen

CASE 1 (*Continued*)

Right Eye of the Patient

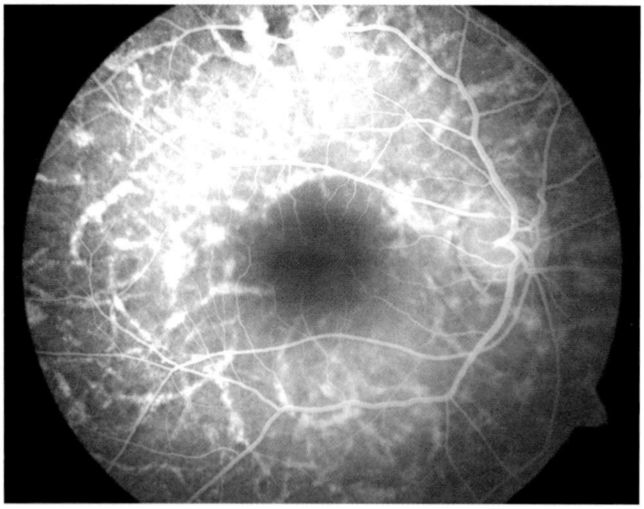

The parasitic tracts appear hyperfluorescent due to transmission window defects

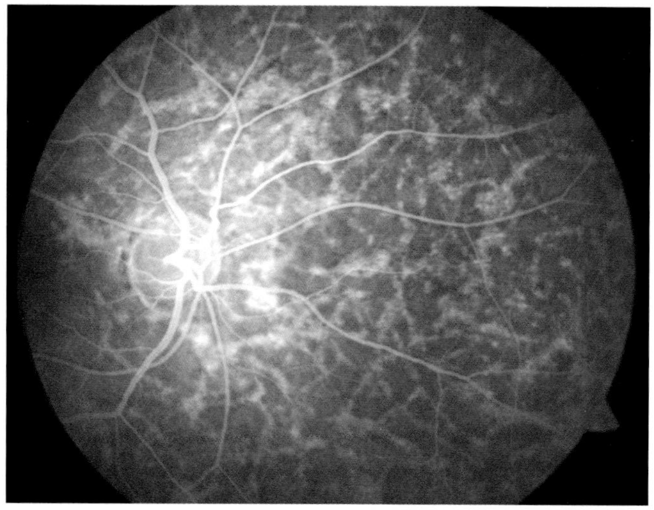

Tracts seen nasally

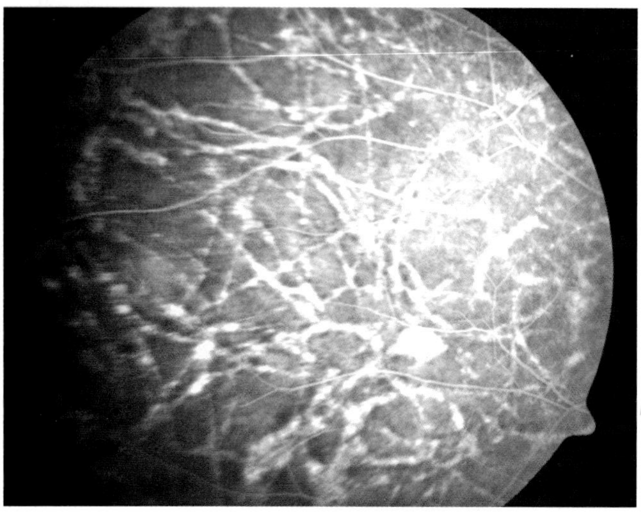

The criss-crossing tracts seen in the temporal periphery

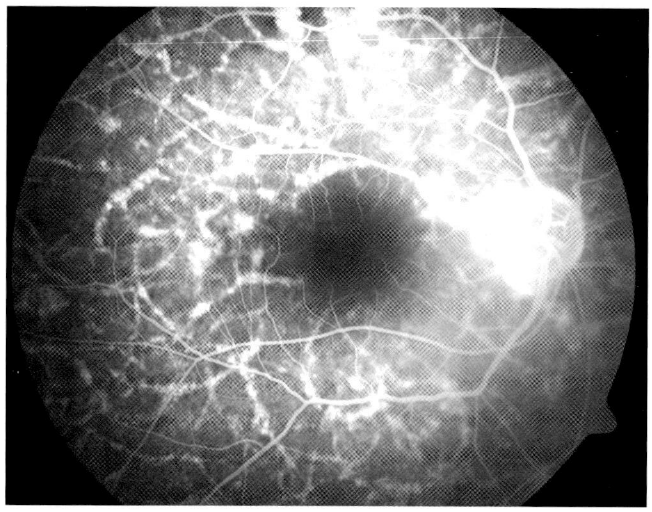

Late phase angiogram showing some fading of the hyperfluorescence along the tracts

PARASITIC TRACTS

CASE 2

A 42-year-old lady presented with metamorphopsia in the right eye followed by diminution of vision since 2 months and redness and watering since 15 days. Best corrected visual acuity was 6/18; N18 in right eye and 3/60; N6 in left eye. Left eye was amblyopic. Right fundus showed multiple retinal pigment epithelial tracts in the mid-peripheral retina and choroidal neovascularization with subretinal hemorrhage at the macula. Clinical findings were confirmed on FFA and OCT.

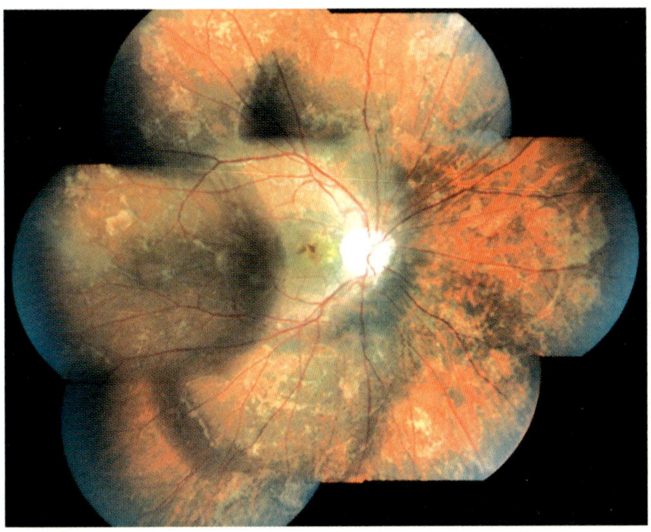

Color fundus montage of the right eye reveals several irregular, curvilinear depigmented subretinal lesions spread over the entire fundus. Subfoveal hemorrhage with yellow-gray CNV nasal to fovea can be made out

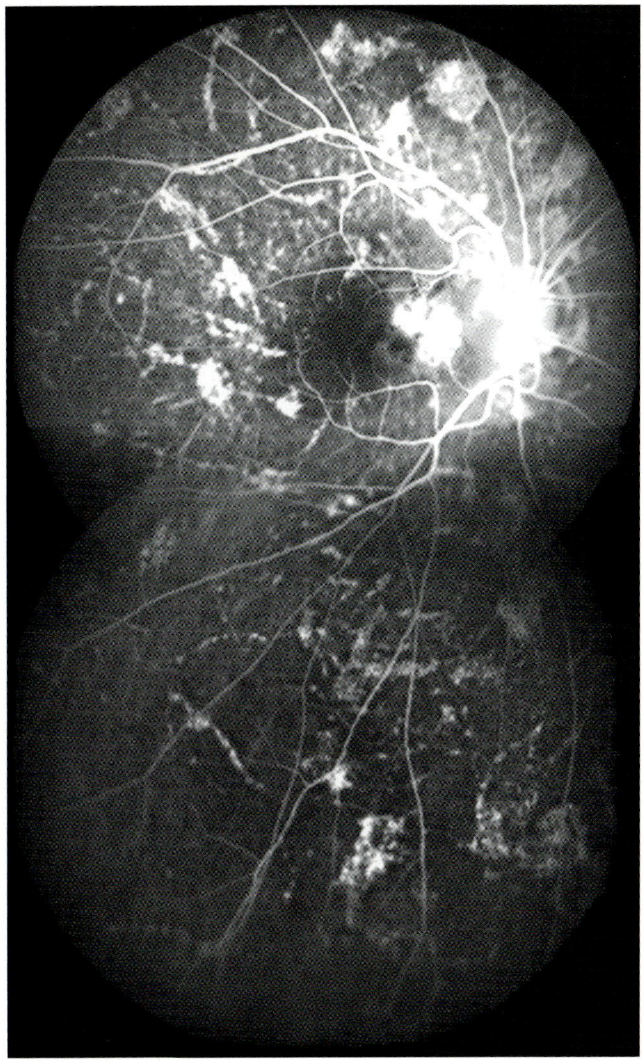

FFA montage of the same eye reveals several window defects corresponding to the atrophic RPE tracts. Hyperfluorescence due to intense leakage from the CNV nasally abutting the fovea can be seen. Blocked fluorescence is due to subretinal hemorrhages

DISSEMINATED CHOROIDITIS

CASE 3

A 22-year-old male was examined for decreased vision in the right eye for the past six months. He had been treated with systemic steroids for his ocular problem. Visual acuity was 6/24; N6 in the right eye and 6/6; N6 in the left eye.

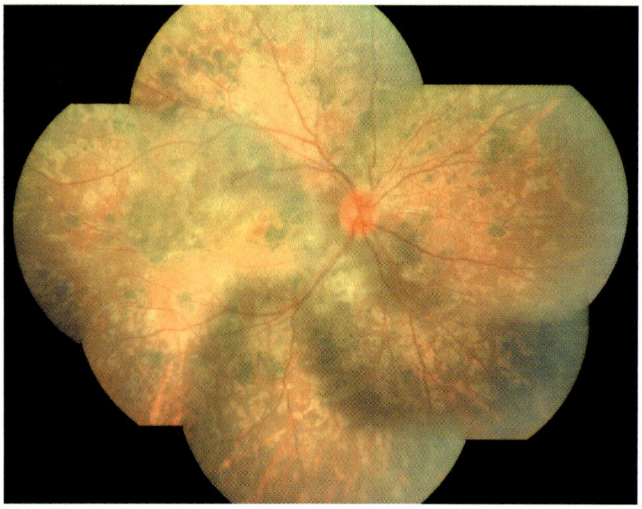

Montage picture of the right eye fundus showing disseminated healed choroiditis

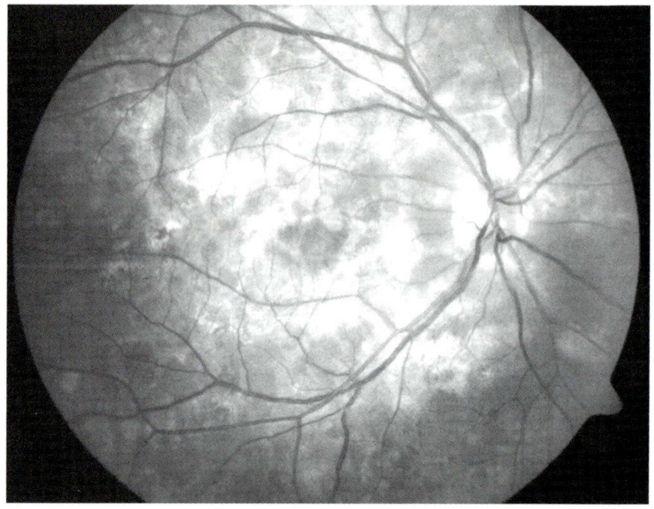

Red free photograph of the right eye

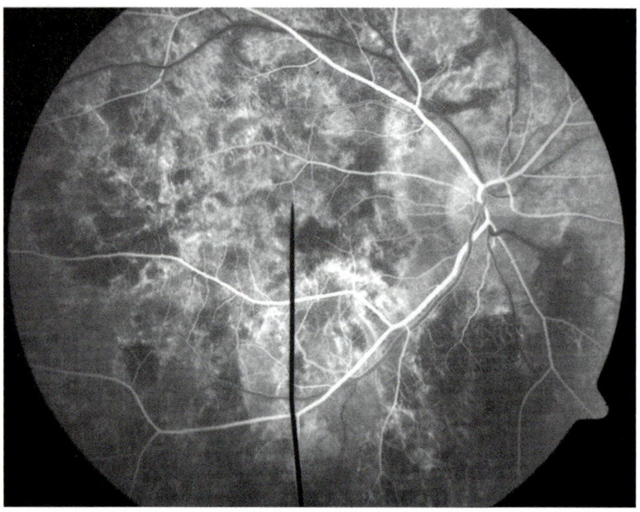

Arterial phase of the angiogram showing the lesion to be hypofluorescent

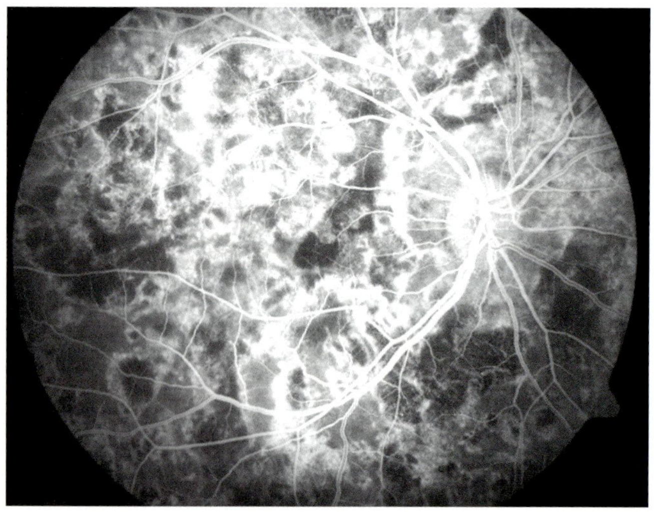

Arteriovenous phase shows the healed lesion to be hypofluorescent in the center with a rim of hyperfluorescence

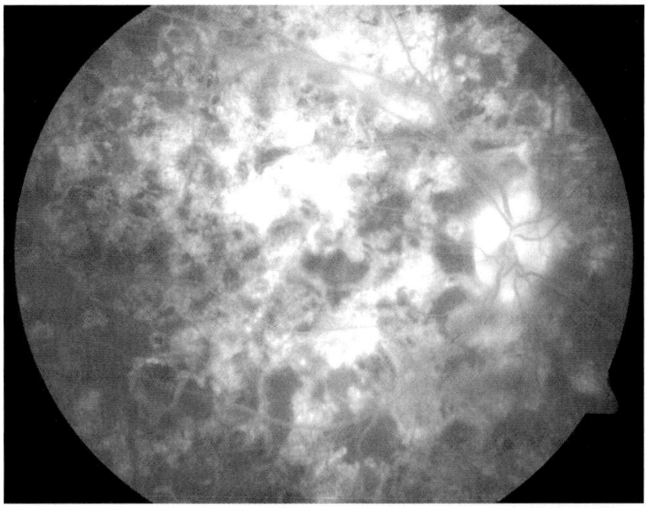

Late phase angiogram showing staining of the scar tissue. The central blocked fluorescence due to pigment hypertrophy still persists

TOXOPLASMIC RETINOCHOROIDITIS

CASE 4

A 24-year-old male presented with reduced vision in the right eye of one week duration. Visual acuity was 6/9; N6. He had been previously diagnosed to have healed toxoplasmic retinochoroiditis.

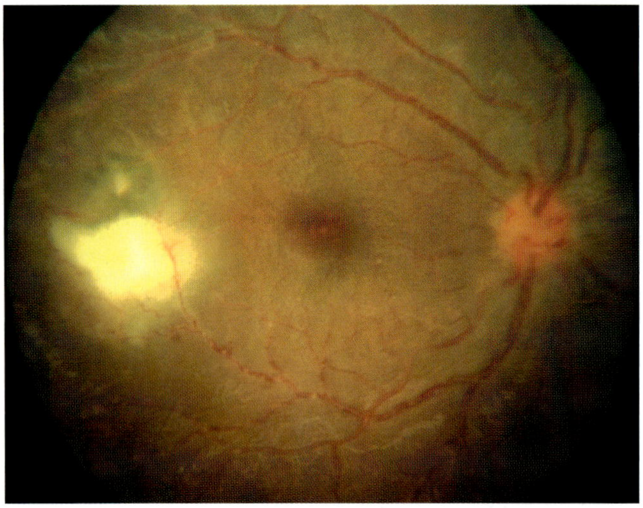

Fundus photograph of the right eye showing an active retinochoroiditis patch adjacent to a healed lesion. Overlying vitreous haze is seen

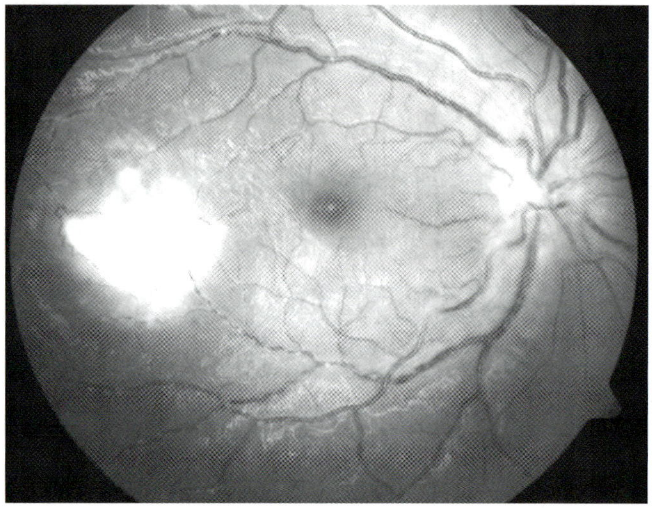

Red free photograph of the right eye

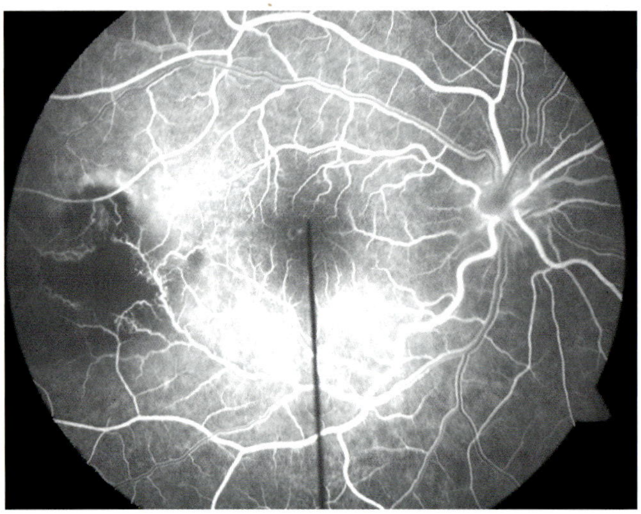

Early arteriovenous phase showing hypofluorescence in the region of the active and healed lesion

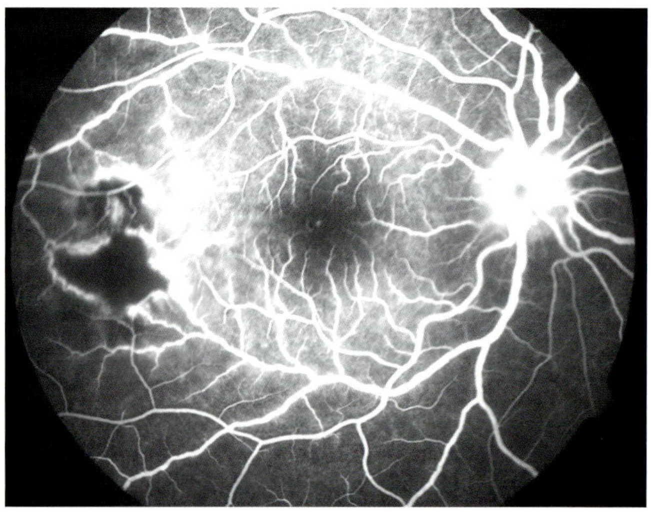

Hypofluorescence is persisting in the late part of the arteriovenous phase. Minimal leakage of the dye from the walls of the adjacent retinal vessels is seen

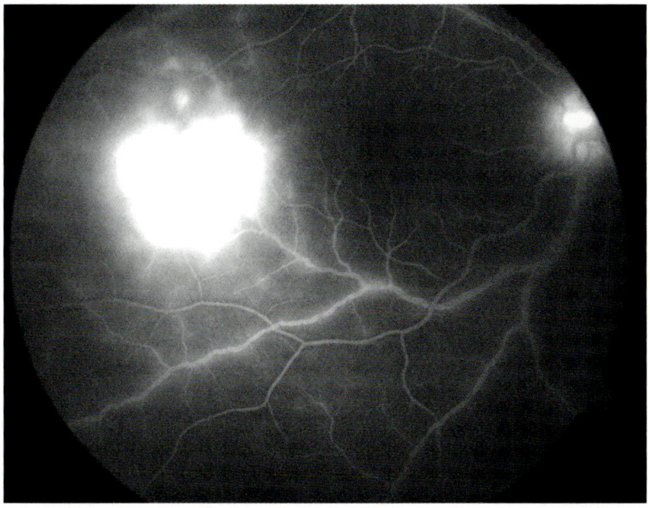

Late phase shows hyperfluorescence of the active lesion. Staining of the vessel walls and the disc are also seen

COMMENT

Early hypofluorescence with late intense hyperfluorescence with fuzzy margins are typical findings in active toxoplasmic retinochoroiditis. Recurrent lesions usually occur at the edge of the old healed lesion.

CLINICAL NUGGETS

1. APMPPE is usually a self-limiting disease; rarely it recurs.
2. Vogt-Koyanagi-Harada syndrome is a systemic disorder involving the eye, ear, skin and the meninges.
3. Dalen-Fuchs nodules can occur in VKH syndrome.
4. Ultrasonography shows a characteristic low reflective thickening of the choroid in VKH.
5. Birdshot chorioretinopathy is closely linked to HLA-A29.

BIBLIOGRAPHY

1. De Laey JJ. Fluorescein angiography in posterior uveitis. Int Ophthalmol Clin 1995;35:33-58.
2. Gass JD. Acute posterior multifocal placoid pigment epitheliopathy. Arch Ophthalmol 1968;80:177-85.
3. Gass JD. Vitiliginous chorioretinitis. Arch Ophthalmol 1981;99:1778-87.
4. Hyvarinen L, Maumenee AE, George T, Weinstein GW. Fluorescein angiography of the choriocapillaris. Am J Ophthalmol 1969;67:653-66.
5. Schatz H, Maumenee AE, Patz A. Geographic helicoids peripapillary choroidopathy. Trans Am Acad Ophthalmol Otolaryngol 1974;78:OP747-761.

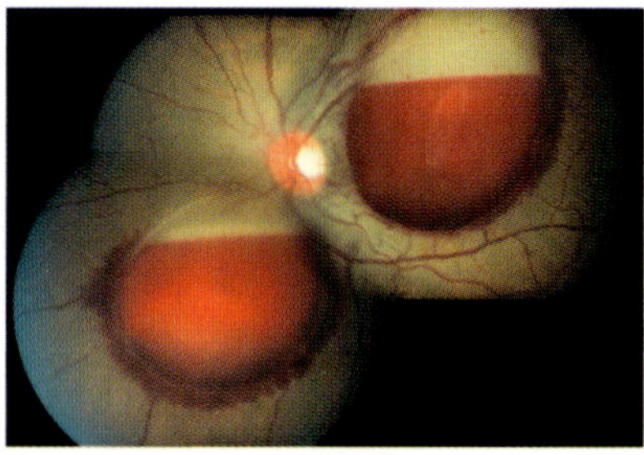

5

Section

Heredomacular Dystrophy

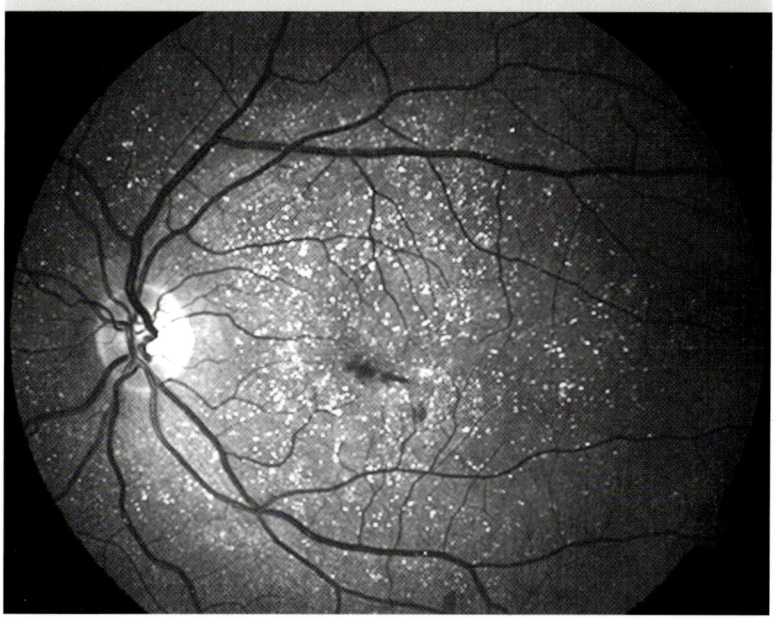

Chapter 53

Bietti's Crystalline Dystrophy

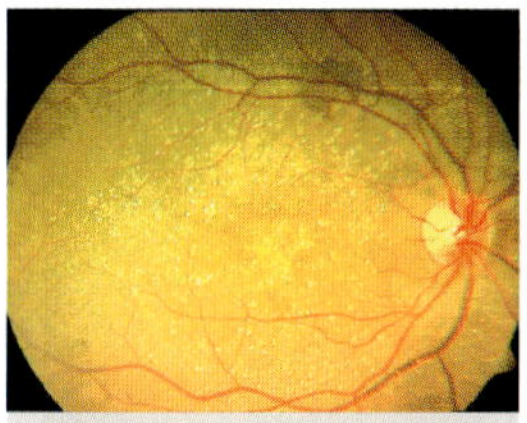

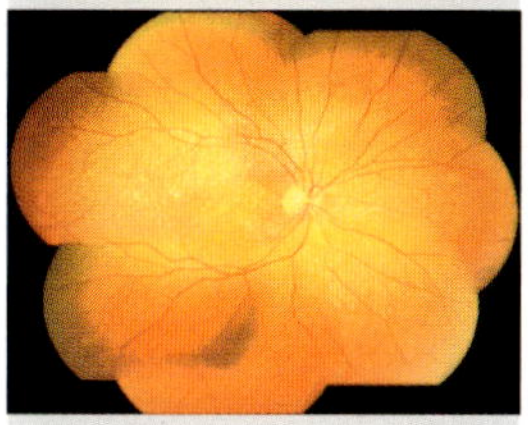

Bietti's crystalline dystrophy (BCD) is a condition comprising of tapetoretinal degeneration with small glittering crystals in the posterior pole of the fundus, atrophy of the retinal pigment epithelium (RPE) and choroidal sclerosis associated with sparkling yellow crystals in the superficial paralimbal cornea.

- It is associated with derangement of lipid metabolism.
- It's onset is in the third decade.
- Inheritance is autosomal recessive.
- Mutation in CYP4V2 gene has been reported.
- Late stages can be associated with nyctalopia.
- Long-term follow-up of cases of BCD have demonstrated a progression of patient's symptoms, visual field defects and electrophysiologic results.
- Causes of visual loss could be due to foveal atrophy or CNVM.

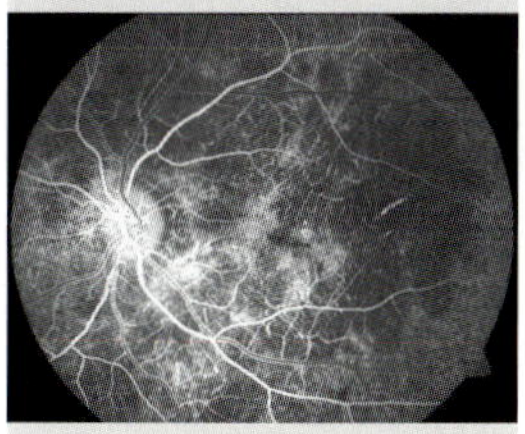

Fundus fluorescence angiography (FFA) shows early intense hyperfluorescence and late washout because of RPE atrophy.

Prominent choroidal vessels are also seen. Can be associated with hyperfluorescence secondary to CNVM.

CASE 1

A 31-year-old gentleman presented with metamorphopsia in left eye of one week duration with night vision problems. He reported no family history of similar problems. In this case the patient had CNVM in left eye (arrow).

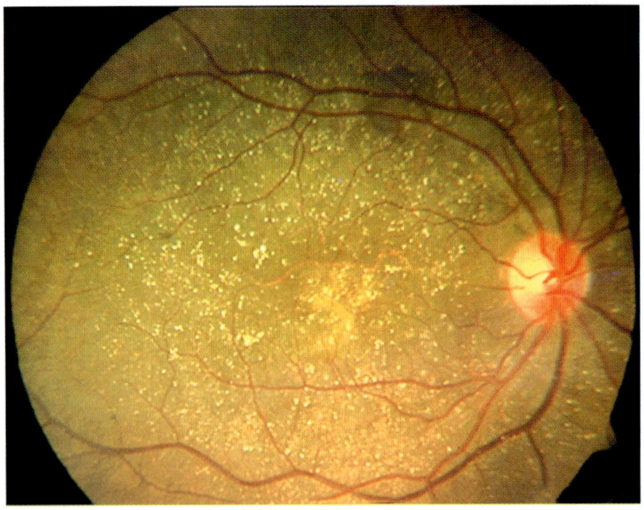

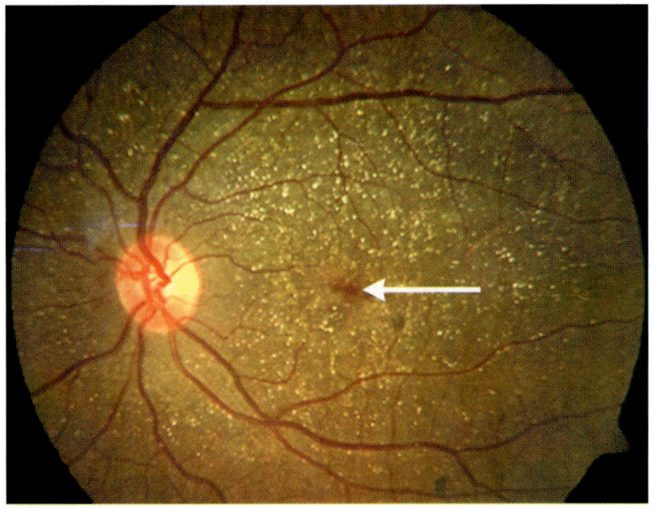

Color fundus photographs of both the eyes reveal multiple, crystalline, refractile, subretinal deposits over the posterior pole with RPE alterations. Left eye also reveals fresh subfoveal hemorrhage (arrow) signifying the possibility of an underlying CNVM

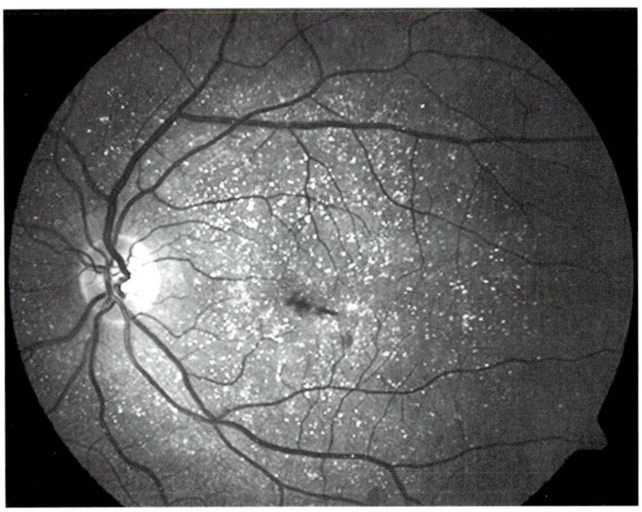

Red free photograph of the left eye highlights the subfoveal hemorrhage and the scattered crystalline deposits

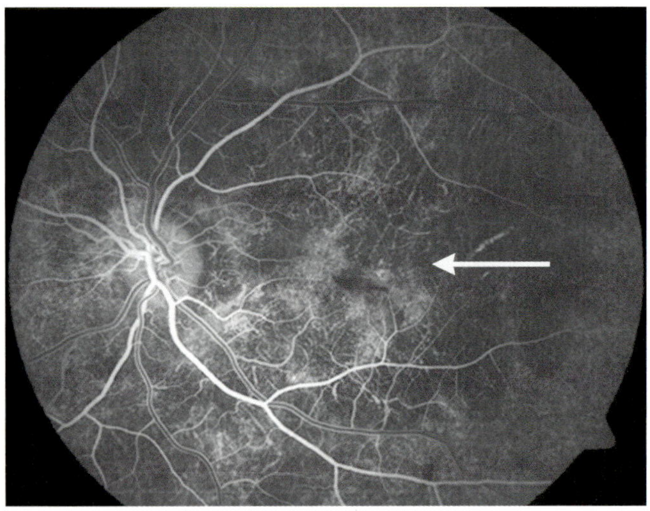

Early arteriovenous phase fluorescein angiography reveals the lacy pattern hyperfluorescence suggestive of classic subfoveal CNVM (arrow)

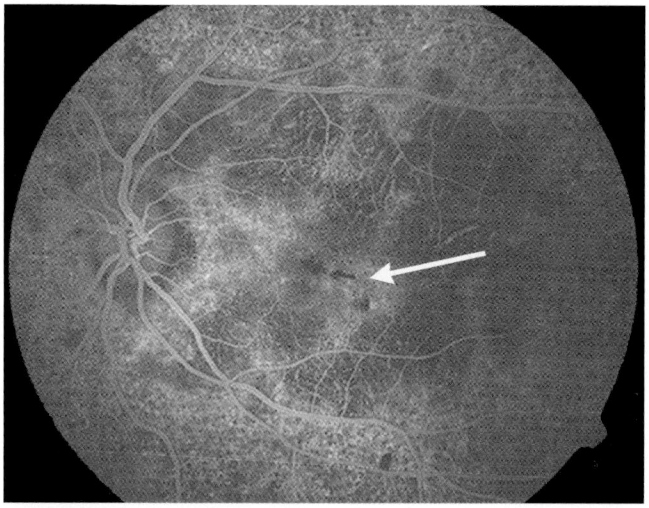

Late phase fluorescein angiography reveals staining of the subfoveal CNVM (arrow)

CASE 1 (*Continued*)

The patient underwent treatment with intravitreal injection of anti-VEGF agent.

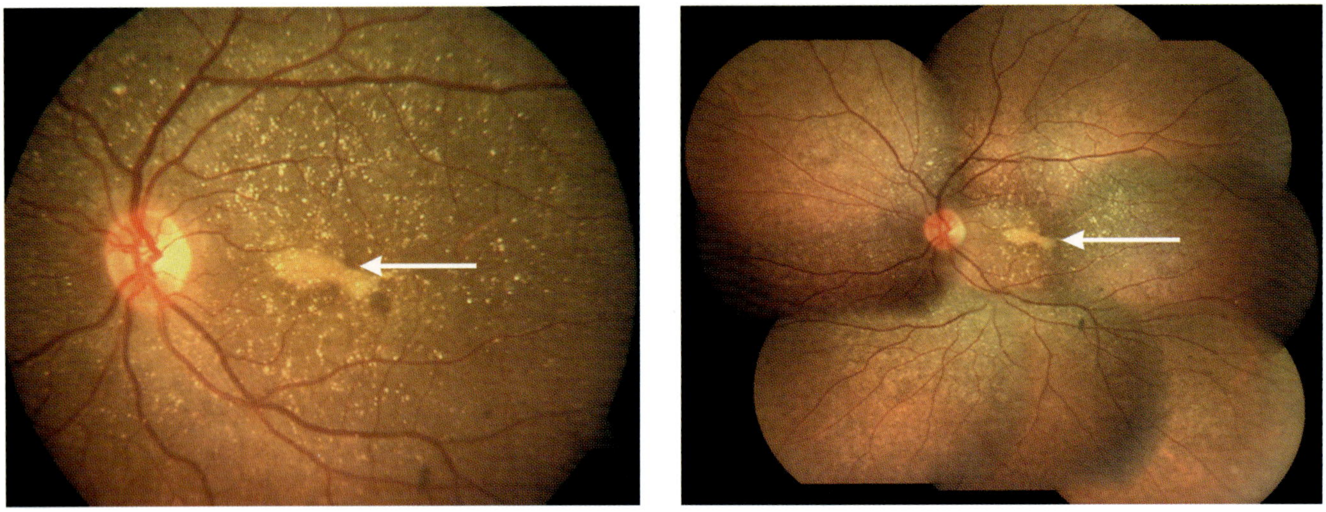

On follow-up, six weeks after the injection, fundus examination revealed scarred CNVM (arrow). Clinical findings were confirmed on OCT

CLINICAL NUGGETS

1. Bilateral crystalline dystrophy.
2. History of drug intake to rule out other causes of crystalline dystrophy.
3. Derangement in lipid metabolism.
4. HVF and mf-ERG correlate with fundus findings.
5. Classification is based on ERG.

BIBLIOGRAPHY

1. Wilson DJ, Weleber RG, Klein ML, et al. Bietti's crystalline dystrophy— A clinicopathologic correlative study. Arch Ophthalmol. 1989;107(2):213-21.
2. Mansour AM, Uwaydat SH, Chan CC. Long-term follow-up in Bietti crystalline dystrophy. Eur J Ophthalmol. 2007;17(4):680-2.

54

Chapter

Best's Disease

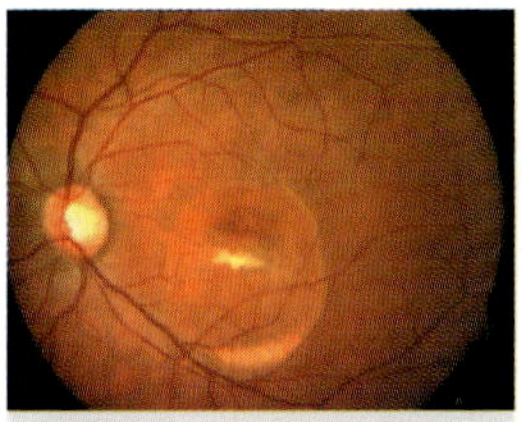

- Best's disease or vitelliform macular dystrophy is an autosomal dominant disorder with variable penetrance and expressivity.
- It primarily affects the RPE layer.
- The Arden's index in the electro-oculogram is markedly reduced in this condition.
- The various stages described include:
  - Previtelliform stage
  - Vitelliform stage
  - Pseudohypopyon stage
  - Vitelliruptive stage
  - Atrophic stage.

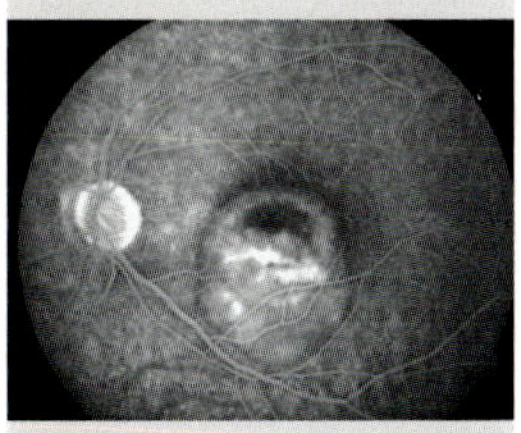

- Depends on the stage of the disease.
- In the vitelliform stage, the early phases of angiogram shows some blocked choroidal fluorescence in the region of the lesion. In the later phase of the angiogram, the vitelliform lesion may appear nonfluorescent or may appear to fluoresce slightly.
- In the subsequent stages when the yellow material disrupts, the angiogram shows areas of hyperfluorescence within the lesion and late staining.
- In the atrophic stage, the large choroidal vessels may be visualized within the atrophic lesion.
- Angiography in Best's disease permits the detection of choroidal neovascularization.

CASE 1

A 36-year-old female presented with history of decreased vision in both eyes for the last ten years. Visual acuity was 6/60; N36 in both eyes. Electroretinogram was normal in both eyes while the electro-oculogram showed markedly subnormal Arden's index. Both eyes had similar fundus findings.

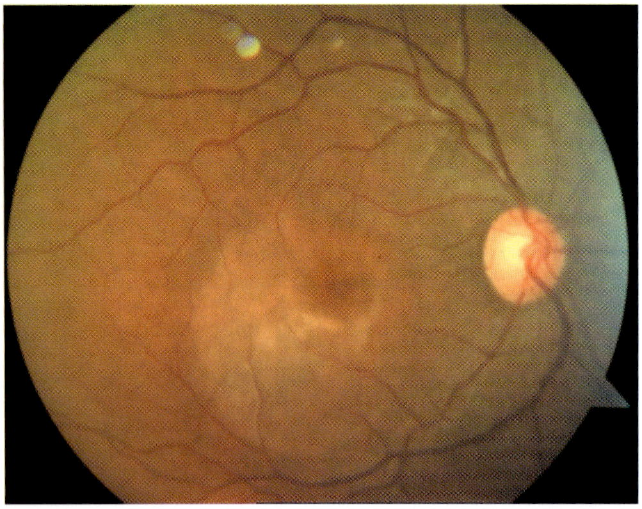

Fundus photograph of the right eye showing a well-demarcated round lesion in the macula with dull yellow organized subretinal deposits in the center. RPE alteration is seen within the lesion

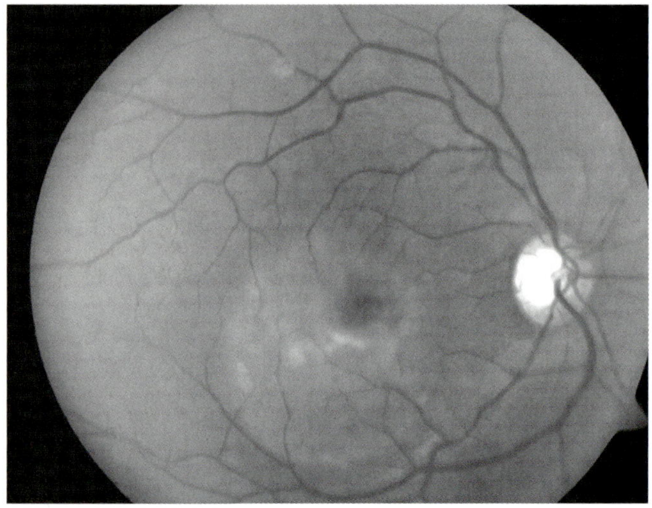

Red free photograph of the right eye

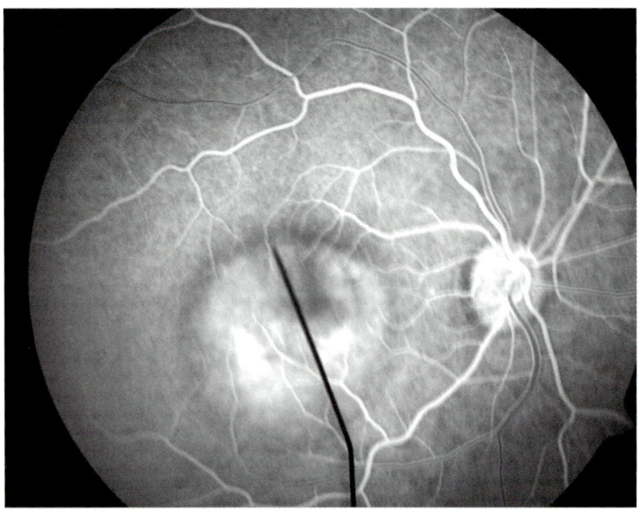

Early arteriovenous phase shows hyperfluorescence within the lesion. A rim of hypofluorescence is seen surrounding the lesion

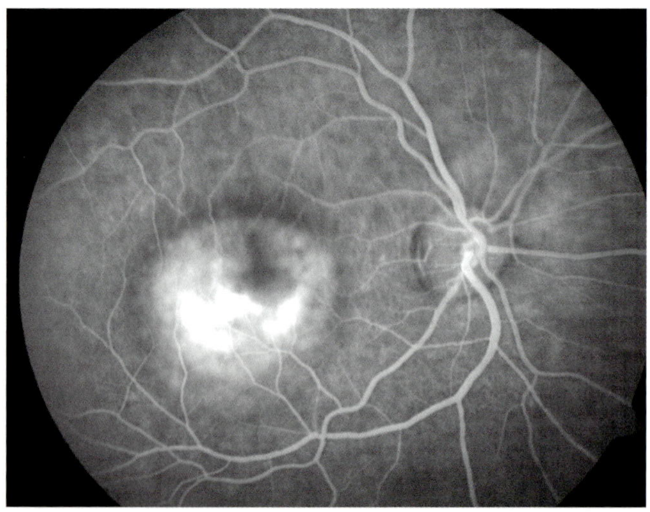

The hyperfluorescence has increased in the arteriovenous phase with one area of more intense hyperfluorescence

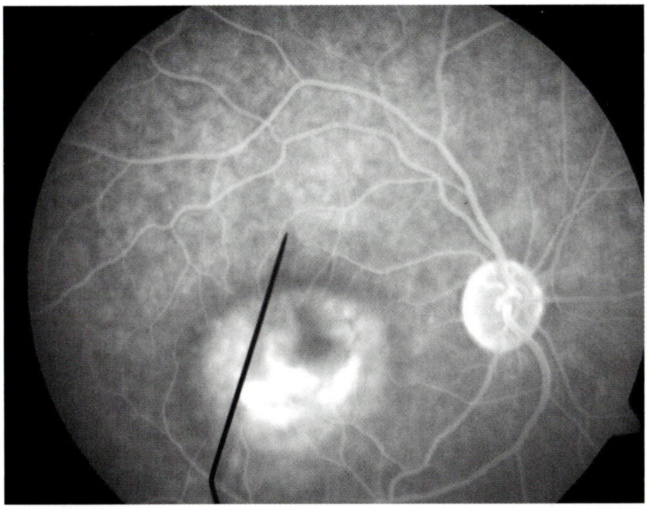

Late phase angiogram showing fading of the hyperfluorescence. Staining of the subretinal organized deposits is seen

COMMENT

Irregular hyperfluorescence is commonly seen within the lesion and occurs due to RPE alterations. Some fuzziness within the lesion is usually seen in the late phase.

CASE 2

A 41-year-old male presented with history of difficulty in reading small print. Visual acuity was 6/18; N10 in the right eye and 6/9; N8 in the left eye. Electro-oculogram showed markedly subnormal Arden's index.

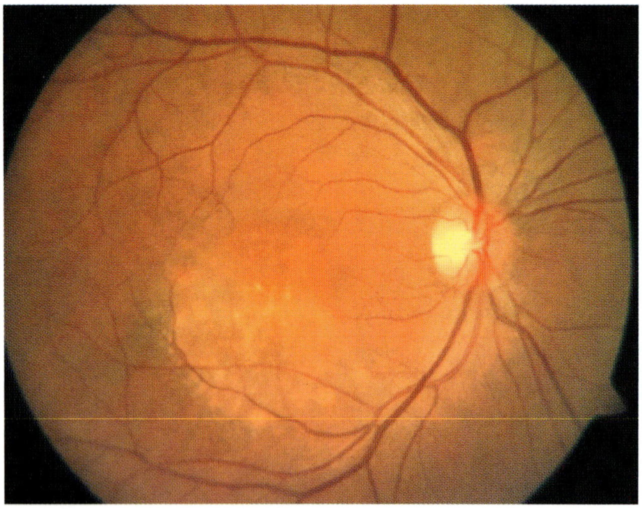

Fundus photograph of the right eye showing scattered dull yellow subretinal deposits in the macula. RPE alterations are seen

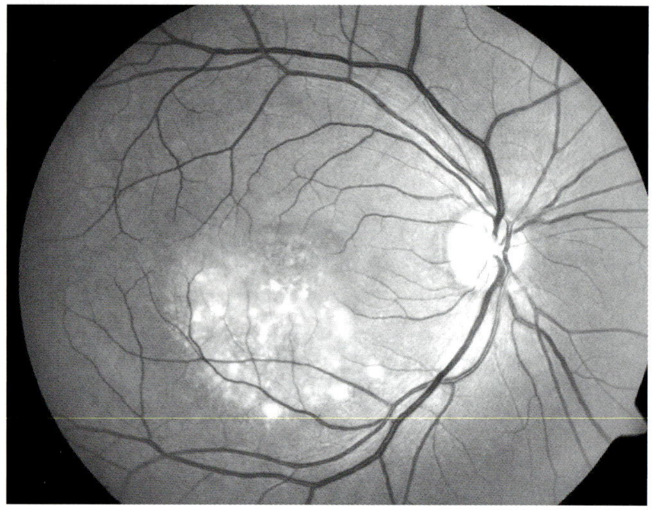

Red free photograph highlights these changes

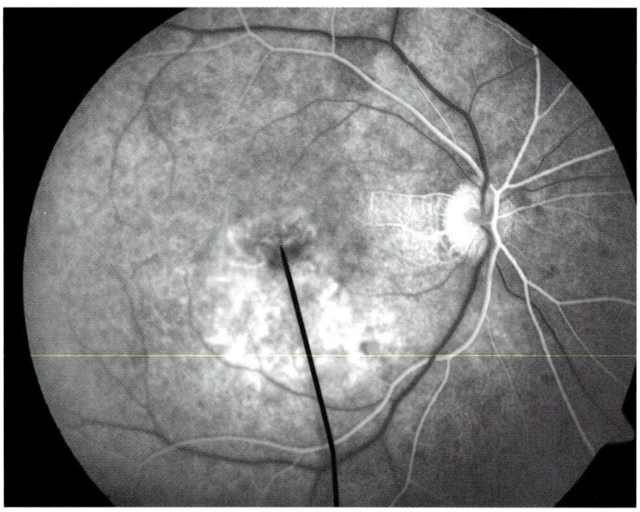

Arterial phase shows irregular hyperfluorescence in the area of the lesion

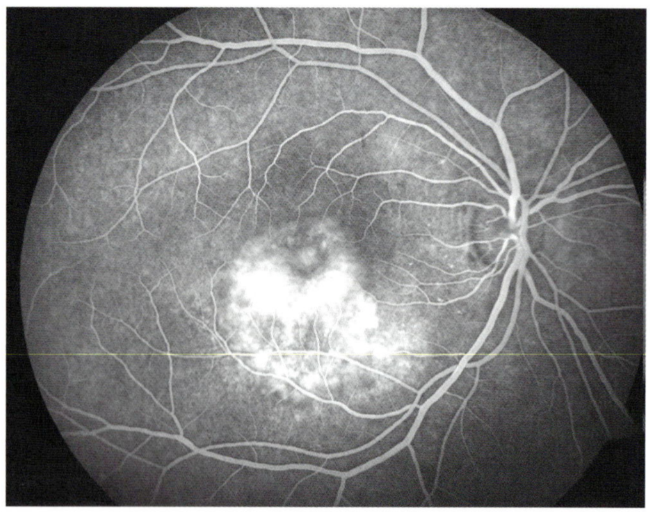

The hyperfluorescence has increased in the arteriovenous phase with some fuzziness of the fluorescence

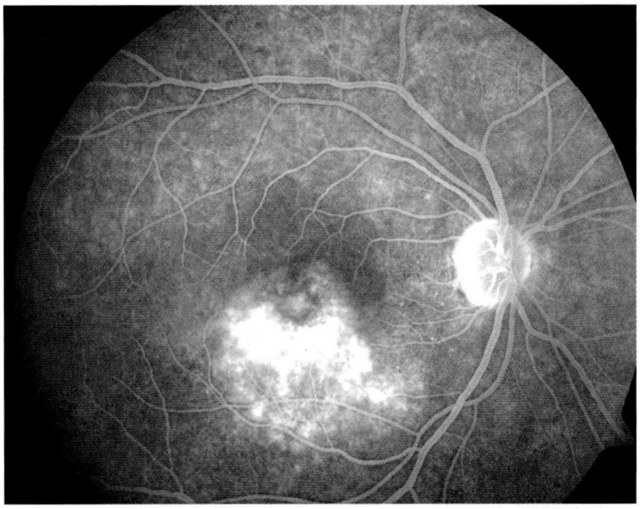

Late phase angiogram shows fading of the fluorescence indicating transmission defect

CASE 2 (*Continued*)

Left Eye of the Patient

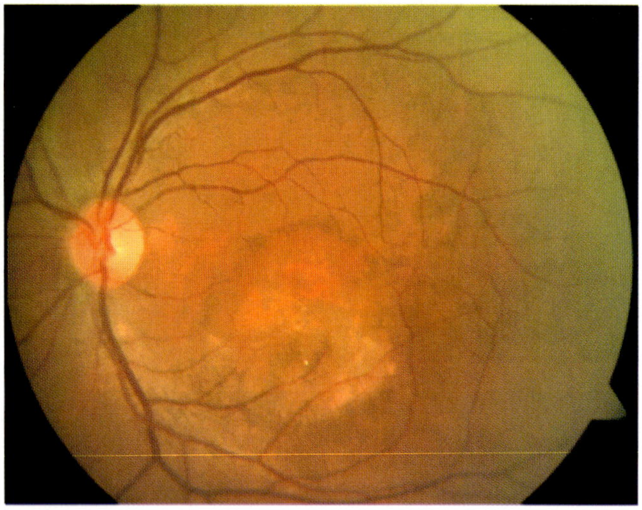

Fundus photograph of the left eye showing RPE alterations with scattered subretinal yellow deposits in the macula

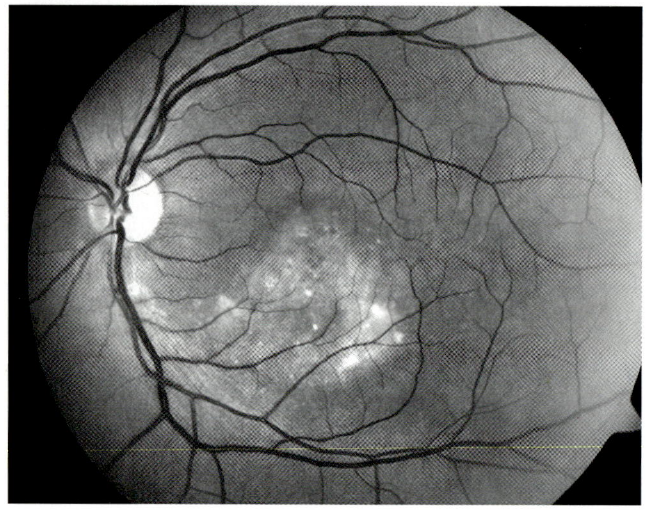

Red free photograph of the left eye

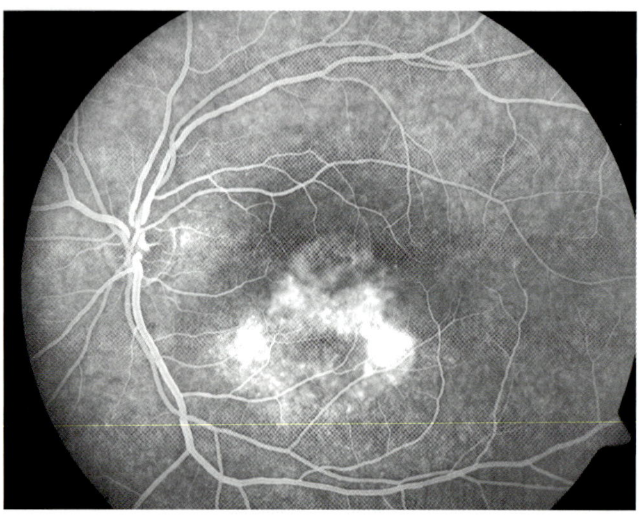

Early hyperfluorescence is seen within the lesion due to transmission defect

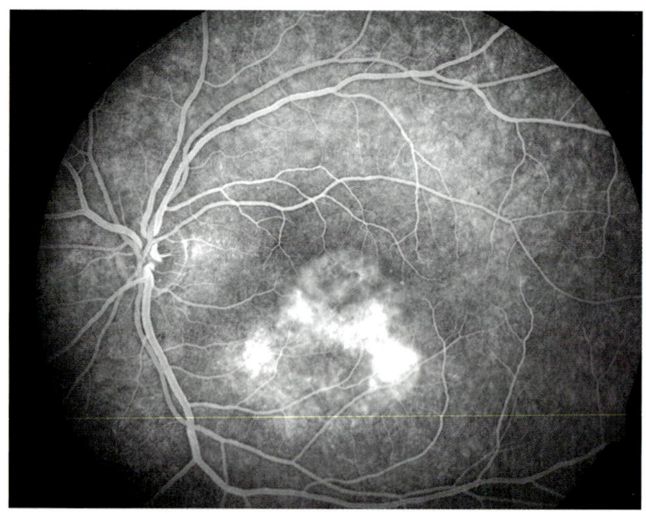

Increase in the hyperfluorescence is seen in the mid-arteriovenous phase

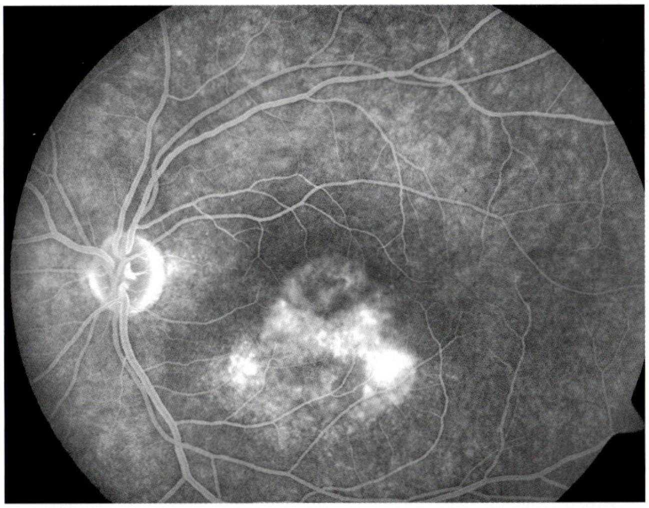

The hyperfluorescence fades in the late films

COMMENT

In cases with bilateral, symmetrical, round lesions at the fovea with some evidence of subretinal deposits, Best dystrophy should be considered. Fluorescein angiogram will show transmission defects at the site of the lesion. Electro-oculogram is diagnostic.

CASE 3

A 29-year-old male presented with history of decreased vision in the right eye noticed for the last one year. Visual acuity was 6/9; N6 in the right eye and 6/6; N6 in the left eye. The Arden's index was reduced.

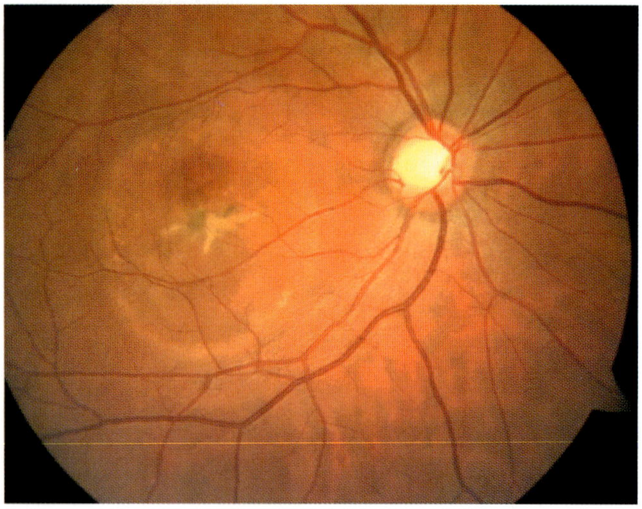

Fundus photograph of the right eye showing the vitelliruptive stage of Best disease. Subretinal deposits are seen as a rim inferiorly. A scar is noted at the fovea

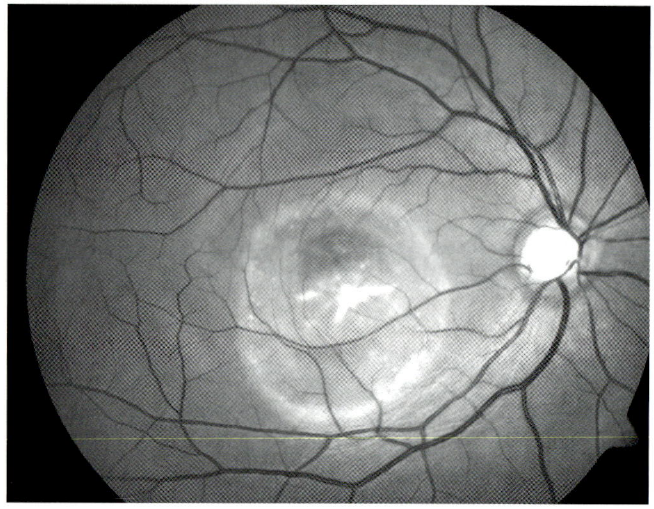

Red free photograph of the right eye

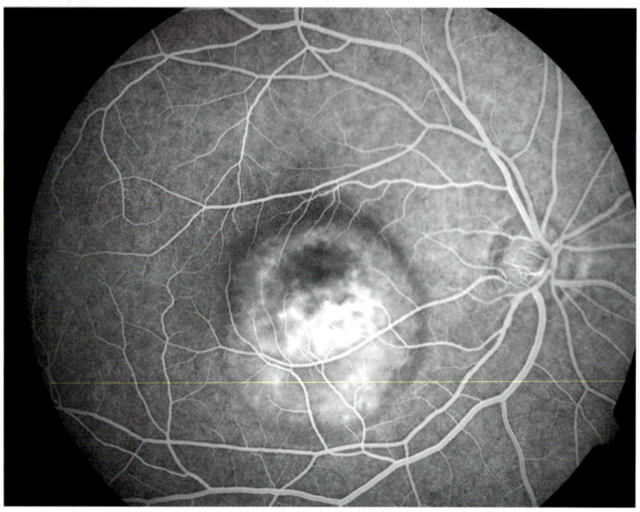

Hyperfluorescence is seen in the area of the lesion in the arteriovenous phase. Increased hyperfluorescence is seen in the center and a rim of hypofluorescence is seen surrounding the lesion

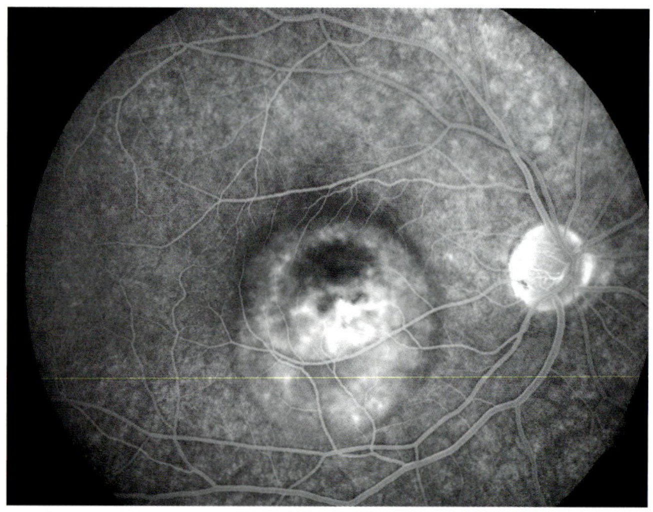

Fading of the hyperfluorescence is seen. Staining of the central scar is seen in the late film

CASE 3 (*Continued*)

Left Eye of the Patient

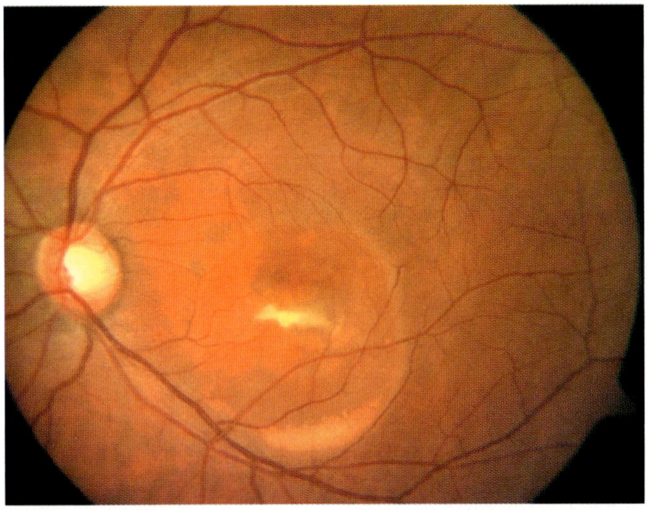

Fundus photograph of the left eye showing a pseudohypopyon. A subretinal scar is seen centrally

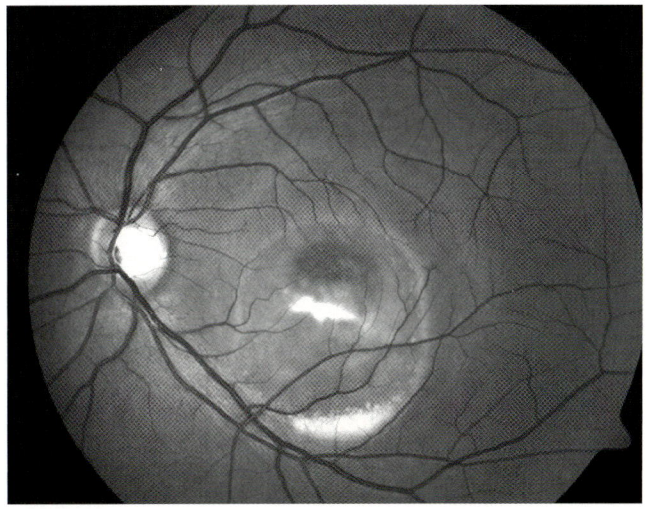

Red free photograph of the left eye

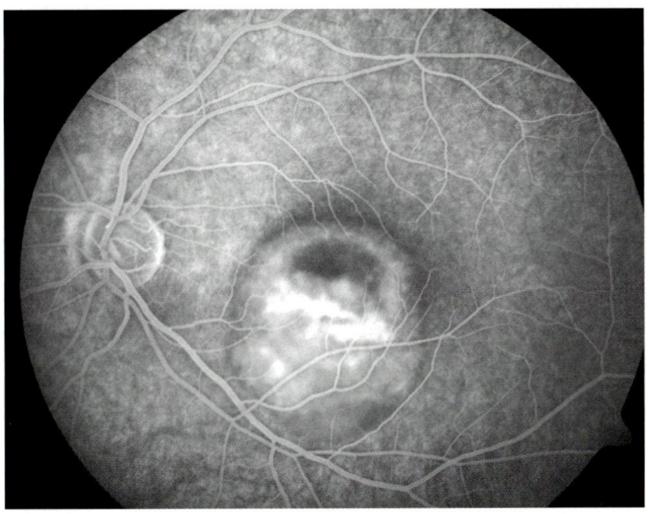

Arteriovenous phase showing transmitted hyperfluorescence within the lesion. The scar shows intense hyperfluorescence

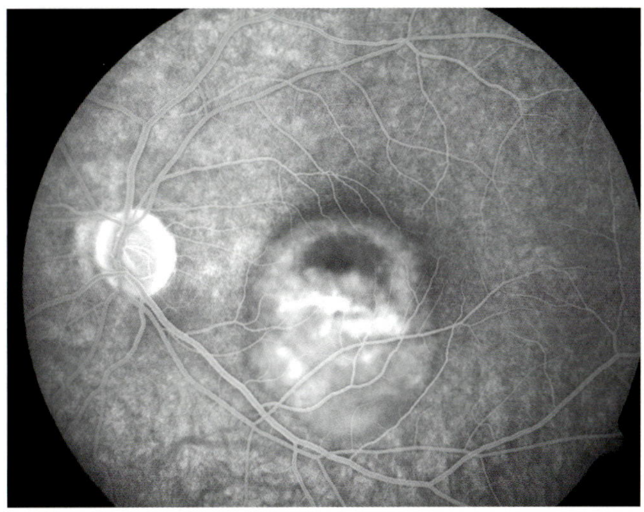

Late phase shows staining of the central scar

COMMENT

Development of CNVM is known to occur in patients with Best dystrophy. The CNVM tends to remain small and results in a scar formation.

CASE 4

A 23-year-old healthy gentleman, presented with distortion of central visual field, gradual and progressive for the past one year. He had a BCVA of 3/60; N36 in right eye and 6/9; N6 in the left eye. Clinical evaluation and FFA/OCT revealed Best's vitelliform dystrophy in both eyes with active CNVM in the right eye. EOG showed unreliable responses due to poor fixation. ERG was normal. Patient underwent intravitreal injection bevacizumab in the right eye.

At Presentation

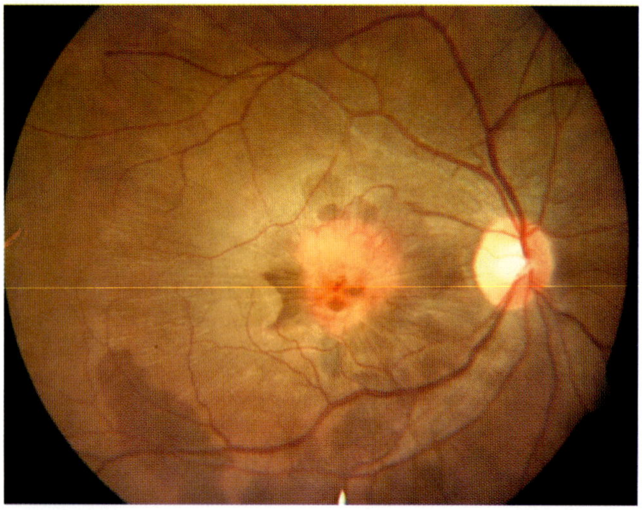

Color fundus photo of the right eye reveals a subfoveal vitelliform lesion associated with a yellowish-gray CNV, subretinal and subretinal pigment epithelium hemorrhages extending up to the inferotemporal vascular arcade. Subretinal fluid and ILM striae are also noted

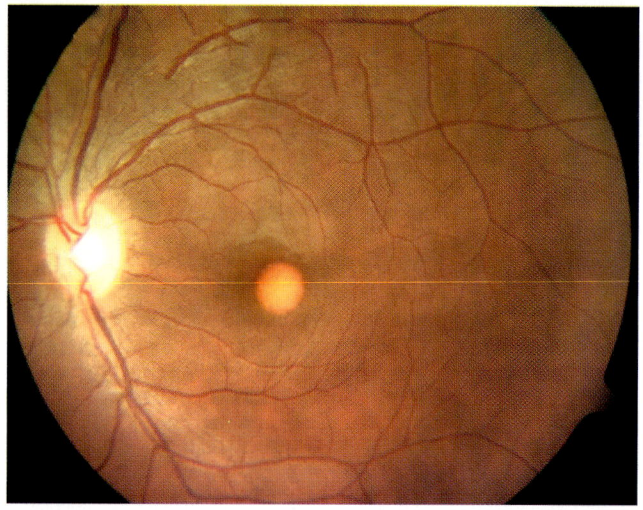

Color fundus photo of the left eye shows an egg yolk appearance at the fovea characteristic of Best's disease

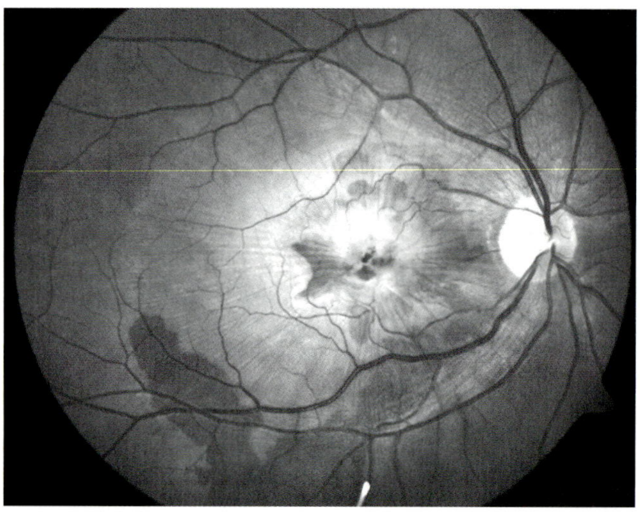

Red free photograph of the right eye highlights the extent of subretinal hemorrhage

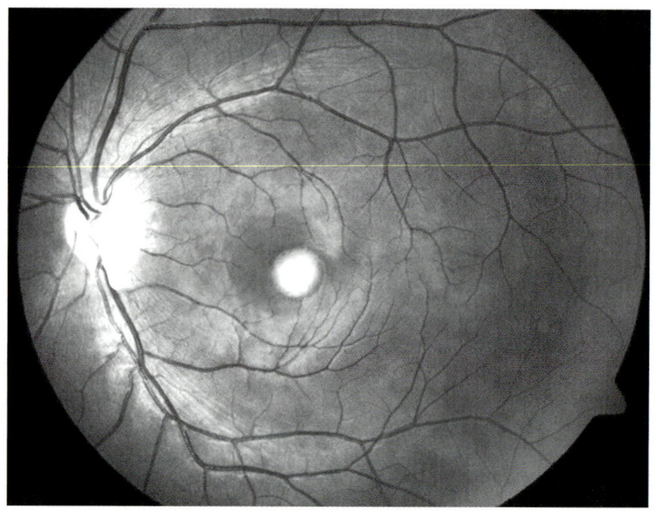

Red free photograph of the left eye highlights the vitelliform lesion at the fovea

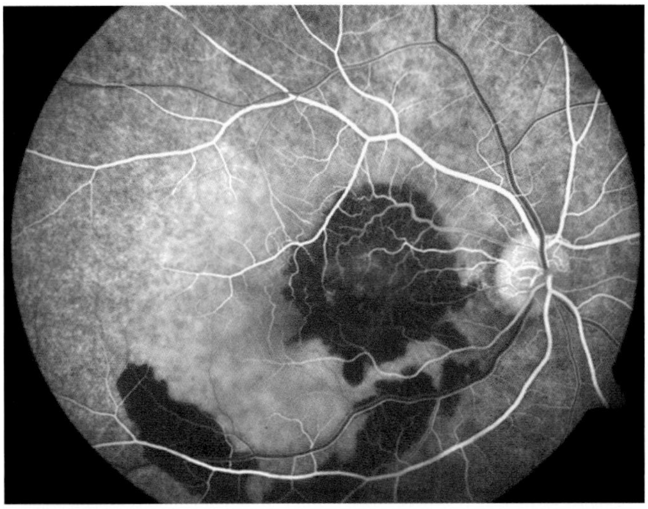

Early A-V phase angiography reveals lacy pattern of hyperfluorescence from the choroidal neovascular membrane. Blocked fluorescence corresponds to the subretinal and sub-RPE hemorrhages

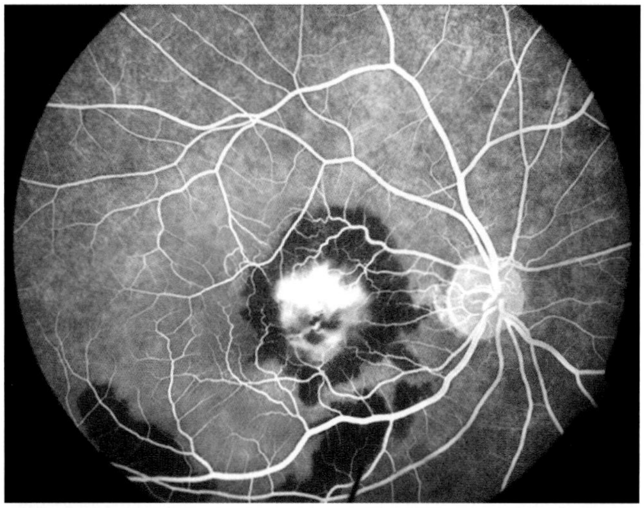

Late A-V phase angiography reveals intense hyperfluorescence from the choroidal neovascular membrane

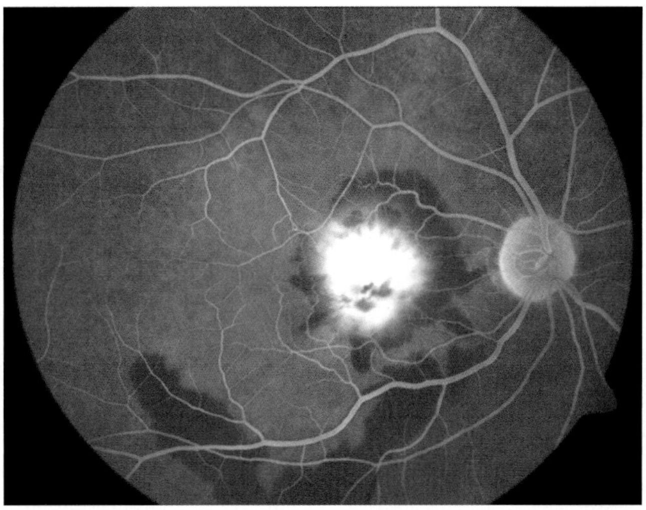

Late phase angiography reveals intense leakage from the choroidal neovascular membrane

Visit 2

Five weeks later, BCVA in the right was 3/36; N36 in the right eye. Repeat FFA and OCT revealed reduced size of CNVM but persistence of SRF for which he underwent a 2nd injection of bevacizumab.

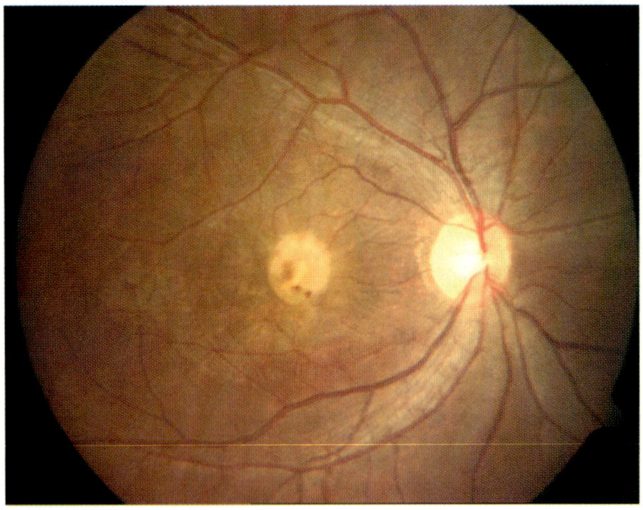

Color fundus photo of the right eye shows regressing choroidal neovascular membrane with marked resolution of subretinal hemorrhage and reduction of subretinal fluid at fovea

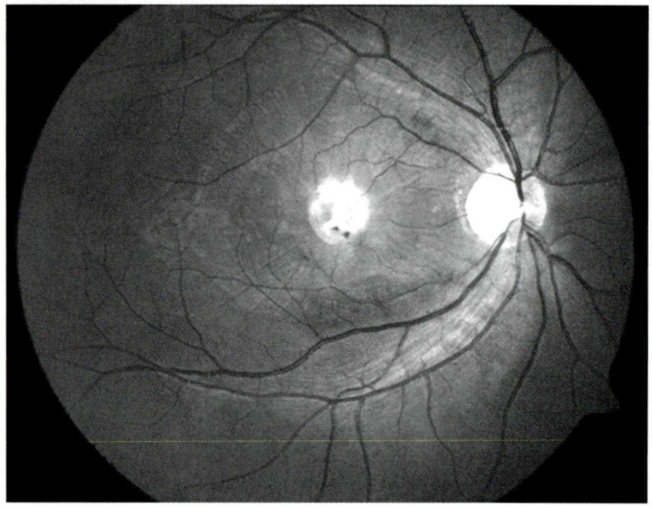

Red free photograph of the right eye highlights the significant reduction of subretinal hemorrhage

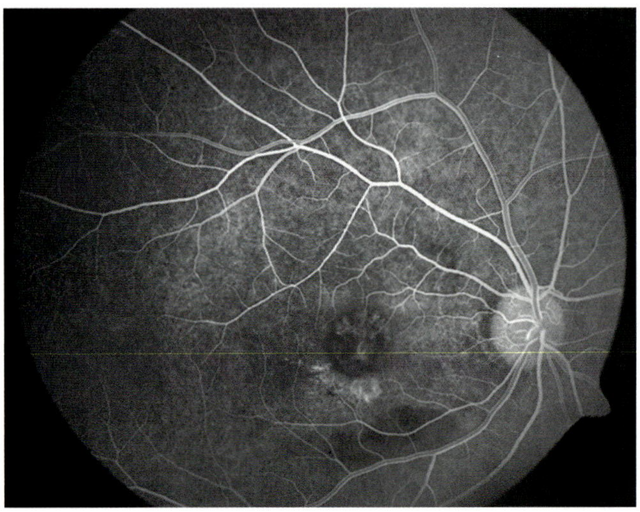

Early A-V phase angiography reveals reduced leakage from choroidal neovascular membrane in right eye

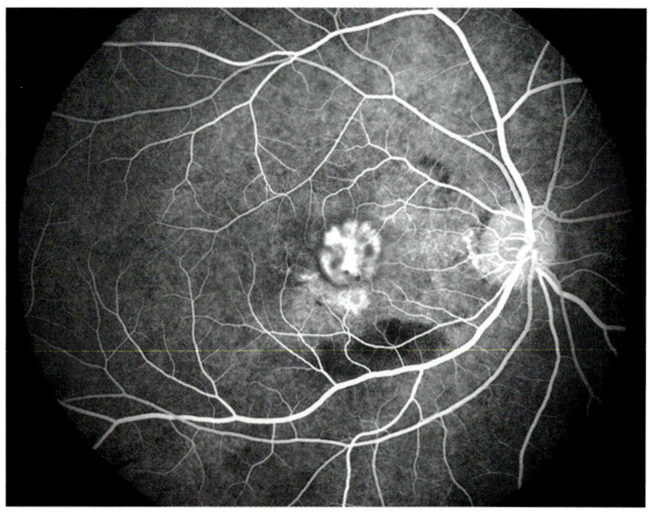

Late A-V phase angiography reveals comparatively reduced leakage from choroidal neovascular membrane

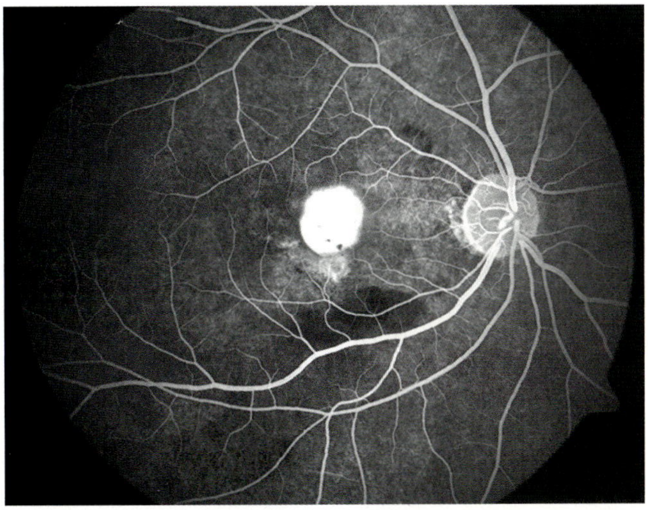

Late phase angiography shows intense hyperfluorescence due to leakage from choroidal neovascular membrane

Visit 3

The patient reported eight weeks after third injection of bevacizumab. BCVA was maintained (3/36; N36). Repeat FFA (not shown here) revealed persistence of lacy hyperfluorescence in the right eye for which a 3rd injection of bevacizumab was administered.

Visit 4

One month later, BCVA had improved to 6/45; N12 in the right eye. This was maintained till last follow-up, 2 years after initial presentation.

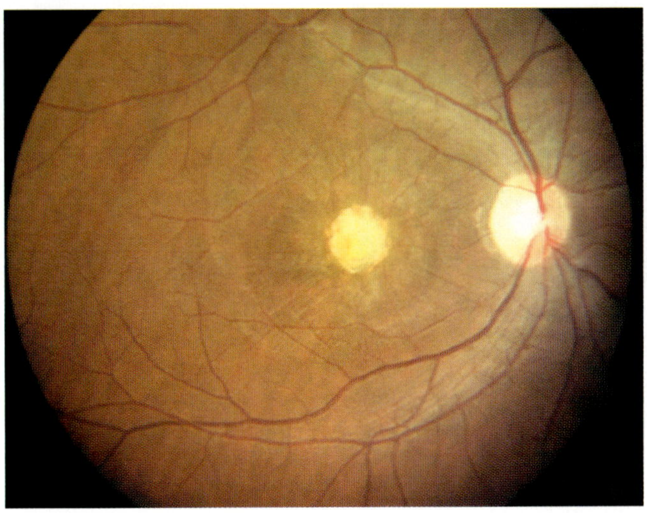

Fundus examination of right eye shows a completely regressed CNV with internal limiting membrane striae

CASE 5

A 10-year-old boy from abroad, presented with sudden diminution of vision in both eyes since the last ten days. His visual acuity was 6/18; N6 in right eye and 6/45; N8 in left eye. The patient underwent PDT for CNVM in the right eye.

Visit 1

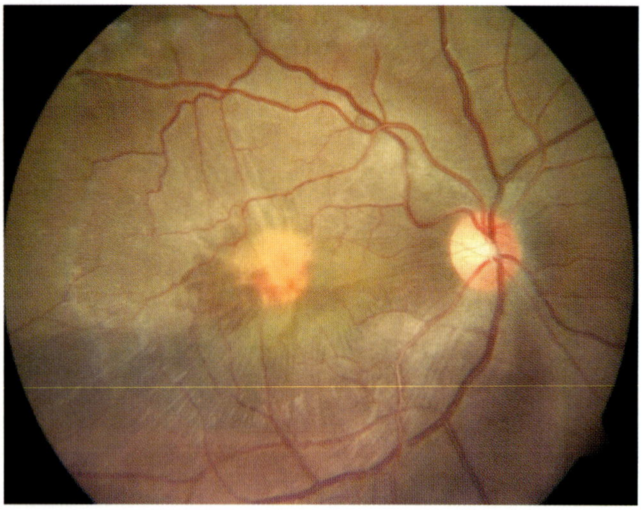

Color fundus photo of the right eye reveals a subfoveal vitelliform lesion associated with a yellowish-gray CNV, subretinal and subretinal pigment epithelium hemorrhages extending up to the inferotemporal vascular arcade

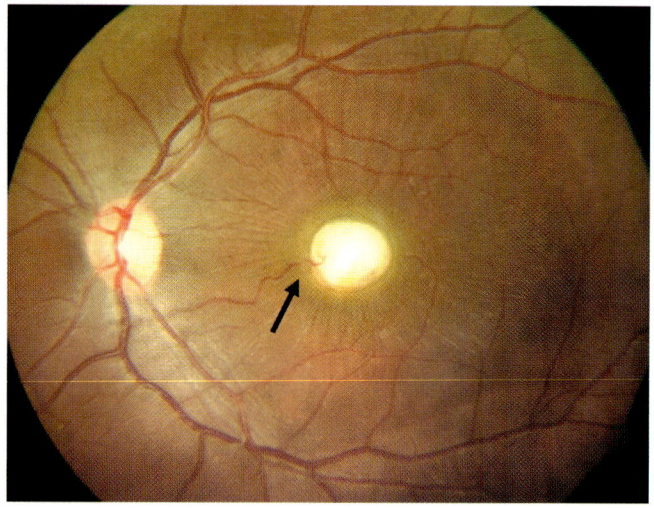

Color fundus photo of the left eye shows an egg yolk appearance at the fovea characteristic of Best's disease. A retinochoroidal anastomosis is prominently seen (arrow)

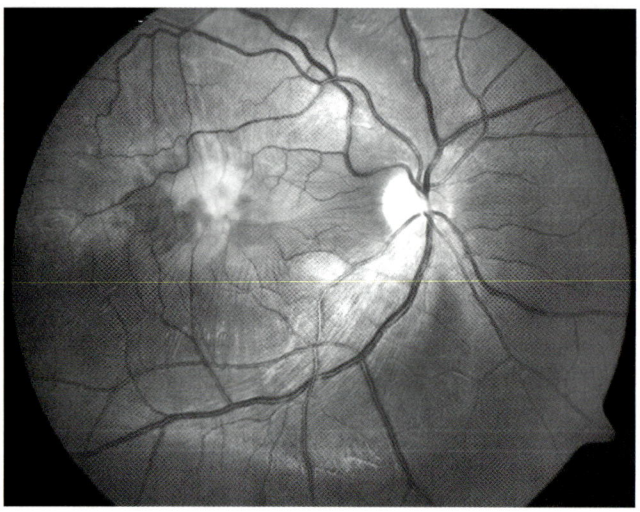

Red free photograph of the right eye highlights the extent of subretinal hemorrhage

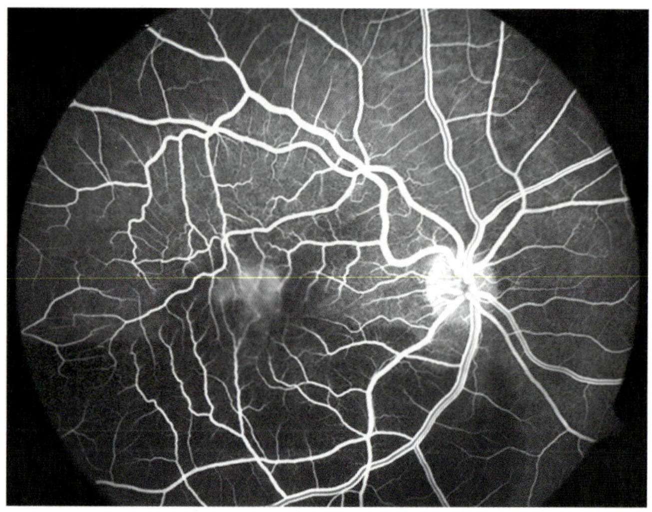

Early A-V phase angiography reveals lacy pattern of hyperfluorescence from the choroidal neovascular membrane. Blocked fluorescence corresponds to the subretinal and sub-RPE hemorrhages

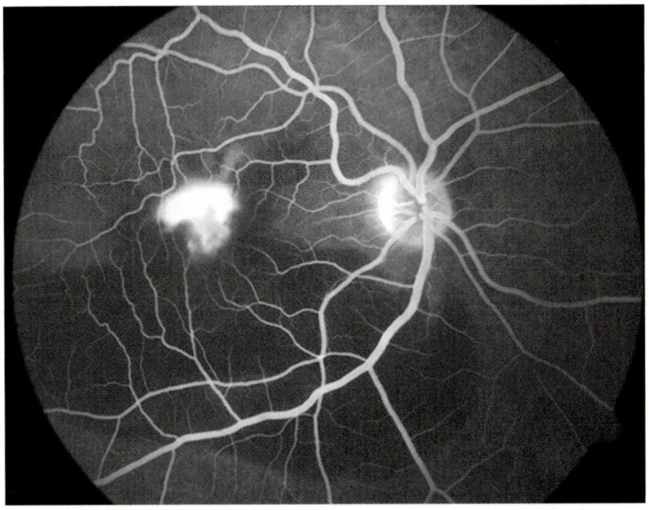

Late A-V phase angiography reveals intense hyperfluorescence from the choroidal neovascular membrane

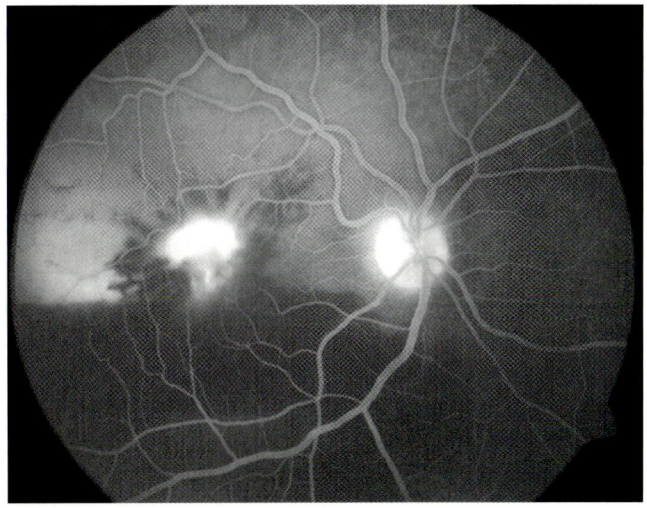

Late phase angiography reveals intense leakage from the choroidal neovascular membrane

Visit 2

One month post-PDT, BCVA was 6/36; N8 in the right eye. FFA was repeated which showed reduced activity of CNVM but SRF persisted. The patient was watched and no further treatment was undertaken.

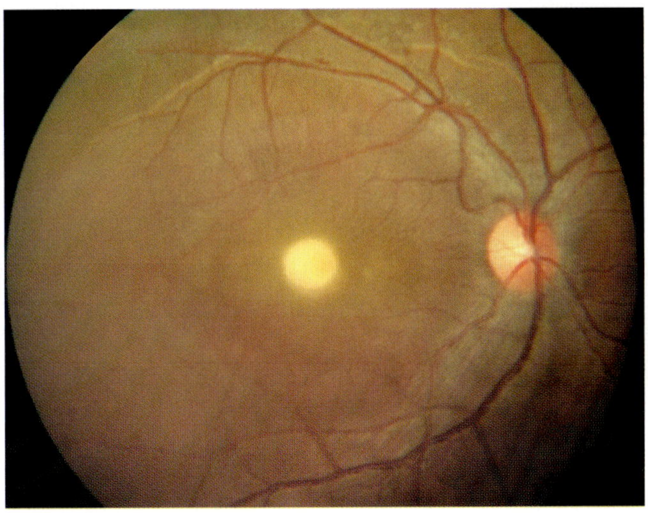

Color fundus photo of the right eye shows regressing choroidal neovascular membrane with marked resolution of subretinal hemorrhage and reduction of subretinal fluid at fovea

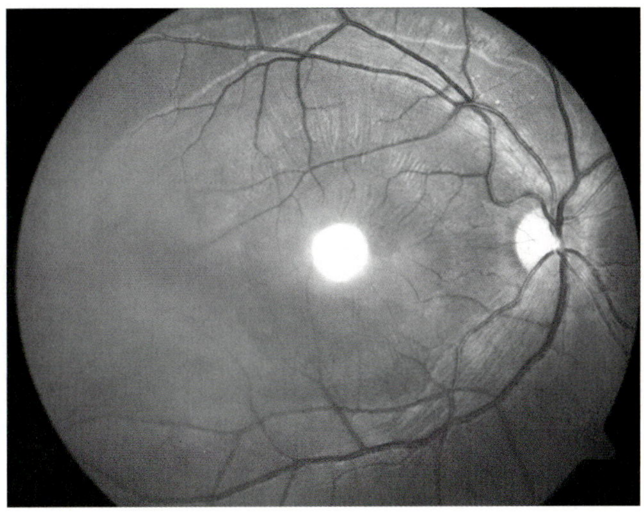

Red free photograph of the right eye highlights the significant reduction of subretinal hemorrhage

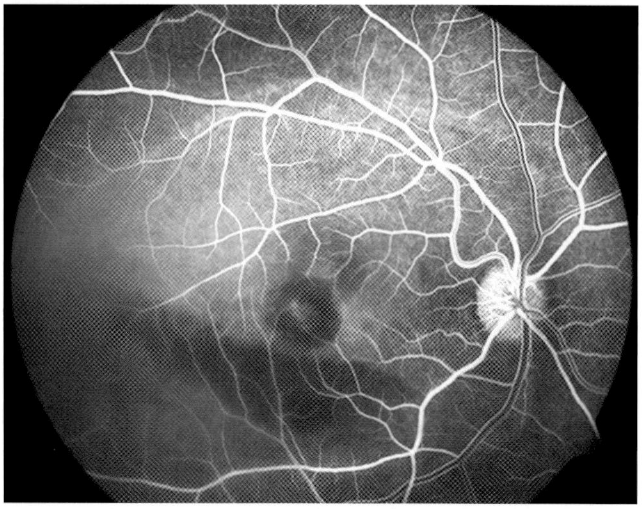

Early A-V phase angiography reveals reduced leakage from choroidal neovascular membrane in right eye

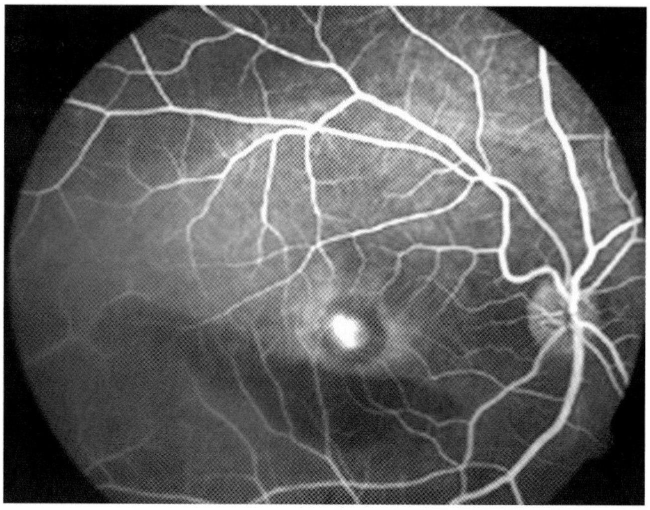

Late A-V phase angiography reveals comparatively reduced leakage from choroidal neovascular membrane

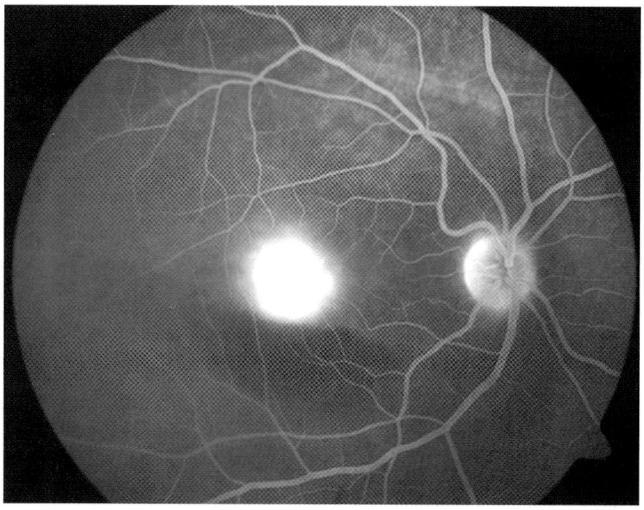

Late phase angiography shows intense hyperfluorescence due to leakage from choroidal neovascular membrane

Visit 3

The patient next presented 5 years later. BCVA was 6/24; N6 in the right eye and 6/9; N6 in the left. Fundus examination revealed scarred CNVM in the right eye which was confirmed on FFA and OCT.

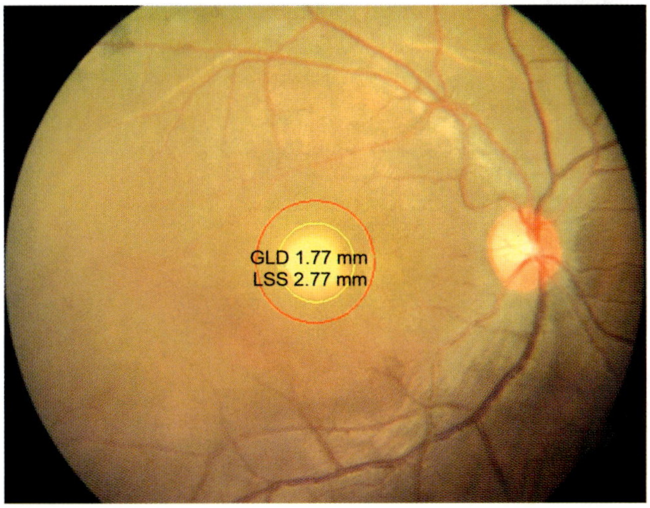

Fundus examination of right eye shows a completely regressed CNV

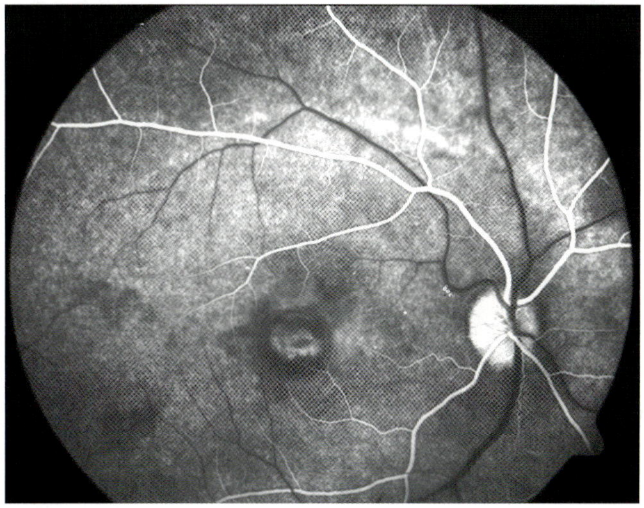

Arterial phase angiogram reveals lacy pattern within the regressed CNV and surrounding window defects

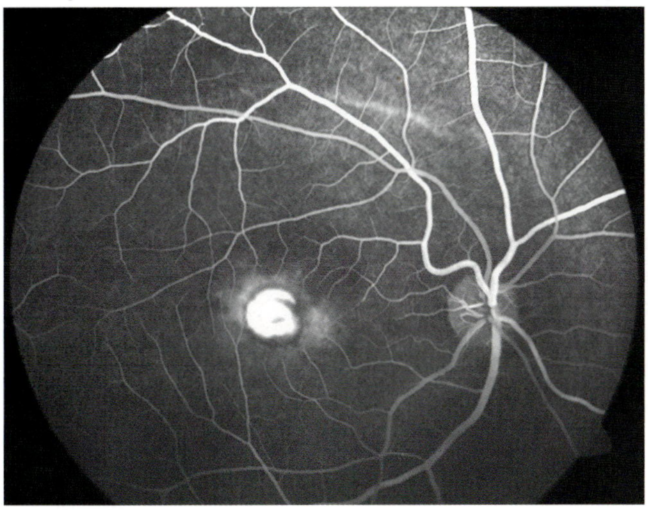

Early A-V phase angiogram reveals hyperfluorescence restricted within the confines of the CNV

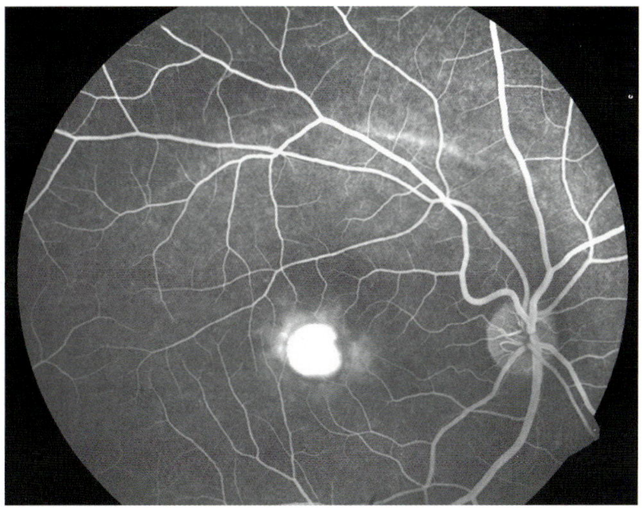

Late A-V phase angiogram reveals hyperfluorescence suggestive of staining of the CNV

BIBLIOGRAPHY

1. Rishi P, Sharma T, Lingam G. Photodynamic Therapy for Childhood Choroidal Neovascular Membrane Associated with Best's Vitelliform Dystrophy. RETINAL Cases & Brief Reports. 2009;3(3):288-92, Summer.
2. Rishi E, Rishi P, Mahajan S. Intravitreal bevacizumab for choroidal neovascular membrane associated with Best's vitelliform dystrophy. Indian J Ophthalmol. 2010; 58(2):160-2.

55
Chapter

Stargardt's Disease (Fundus Flavimaculatus)

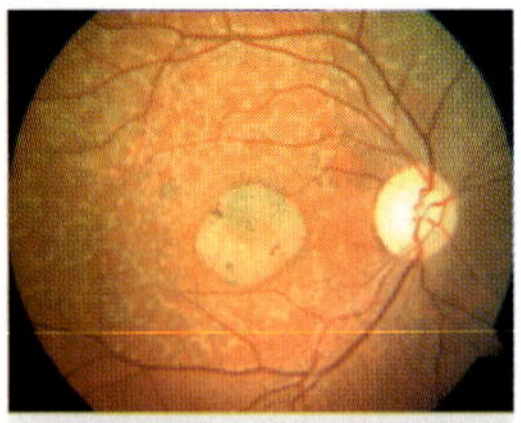

- Stargardt's disease and fundus flavimaculatus can be considered to represent different stages of the same disease.
- It is predominantly an autosomal recessive disorder.
- Visual loss starts early, usually in childhood or early adulthood.
- Fundus may be normal in the early stages. However with time, atrophic macular changes and associated retinal flecks develop.

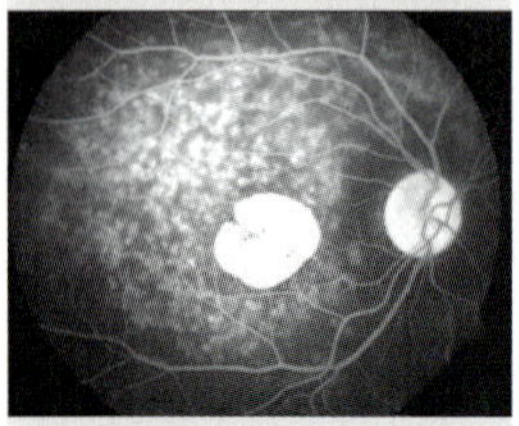

- The characteristic feature of Stargardt's disease on fluorescein angiogram is the absence of choroidal fluorescence or the 'silent choroid'. This is considered almost pathognomonic of Stargardt's disease.
- Lipofuscin-like material deposition in the retinal pigment epithelium is probably responsible for blockage of the underlying choroidal fluorescence.
- The retinal vessels especially the retinal capillary network are seen more prominently against the dark background.
- The atrophic macular lesion shows up as a hyperfluorescent area due to window defect.
- Multiple irregular hyperfluorescent spots that do not precisely correspond to the flecks are seen in the midperipheral retina.

CASE 1

A 14-year-old male presented with inability to see the blackboard at school for the last six months. Visual acuity was 6/24; N12 in both eyes.

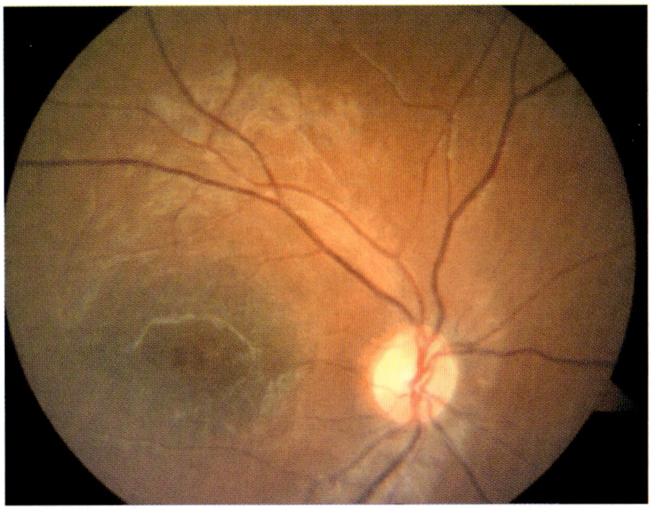

Fundus photograph of the right eye showing RPE alterations at the fovea

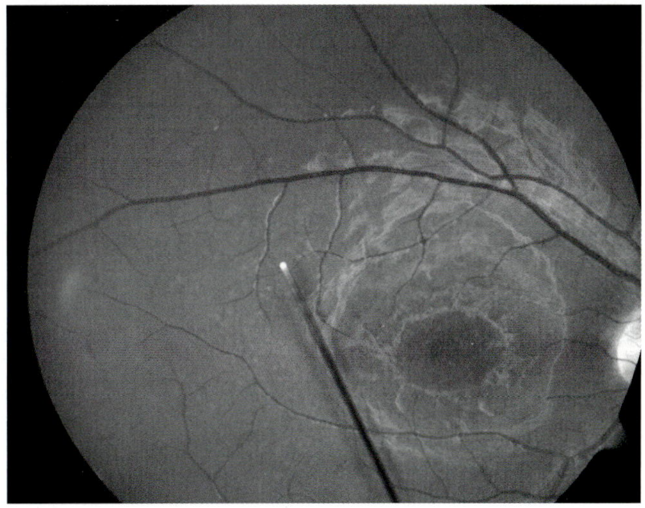

Red free photograph of the right eye

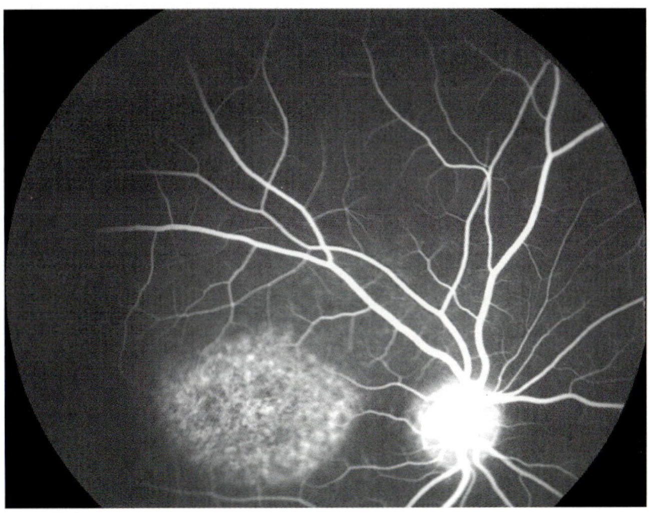

Arteriovenous phase of the angiogram showing stippled hyperfluorescence in foveal region due to transmission defects. Choroidal fluorescence is not seen in the rest of the areas

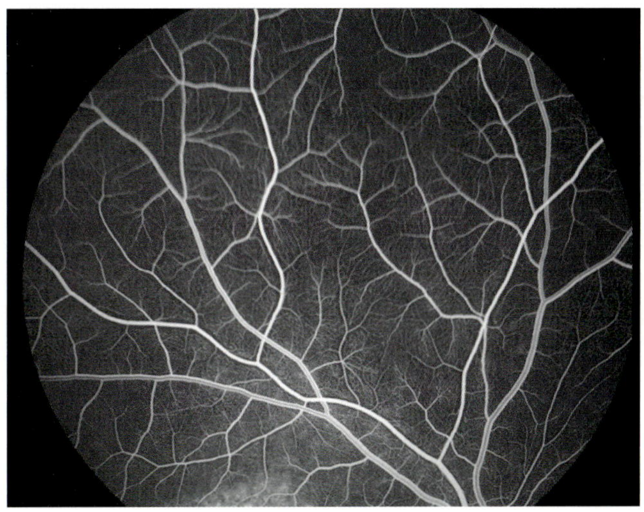

No choroidal fluorescence is seen even in the mid-periphery of the fundus

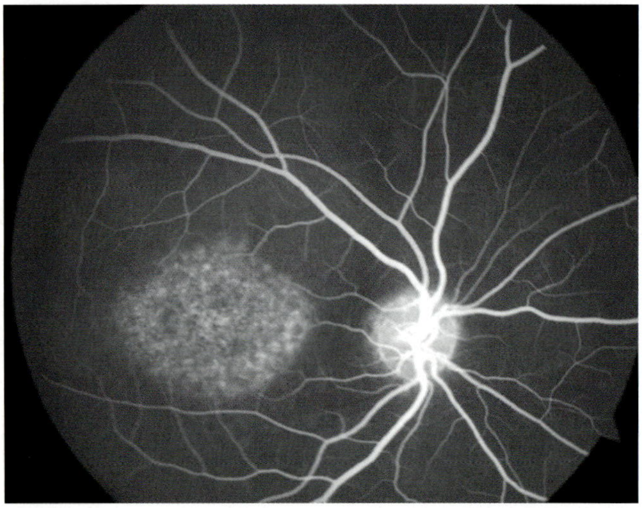

Fading of the hyperfluorescence is seen in the foveal region in the late phase, indicating a window defect. Silent choroid can still be appreciated

COMMENT

Presence of lipofuscin like material in the RPE blocks the background choroidal fluorescence giving rise to the 'silent choroid' picture in the angiogram.

The retinal vessels stand out against the dark background.

CASE 2

A 16-year-old male presented with a history of decreased vision in both eyes for the past four years. Visual acuity was 6/36; N12 in both eyes.

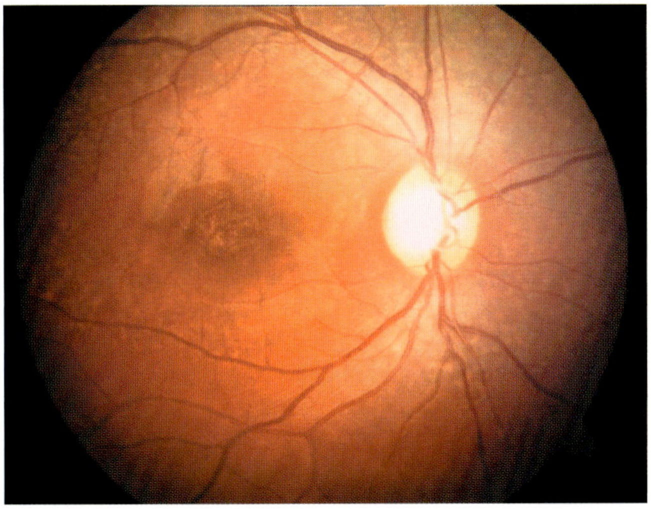

Fundus photograph of the right eye showing an atrophic lesion at the fovea with multiple irregular flecks at the posterior pole

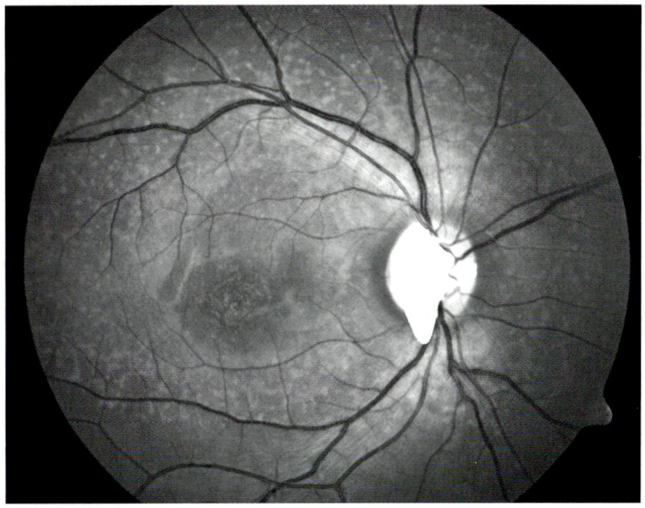

Red free photograph of the right eye

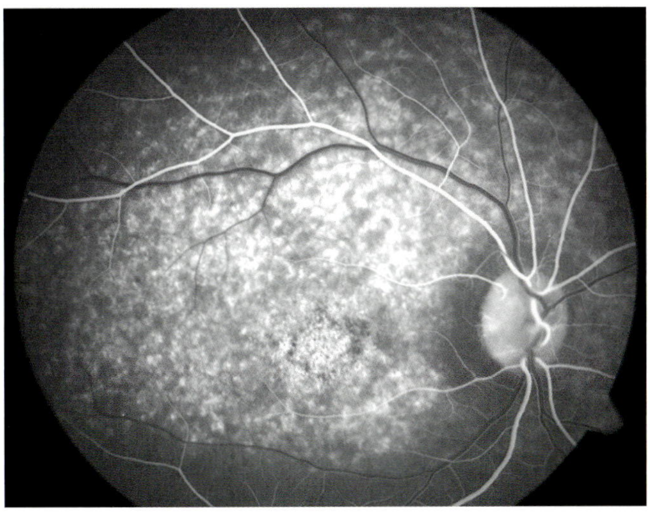

Arterial phase showing irregular transmitted hyperfluorescence. The choroidal fluorescence is absent in the peripapillary region

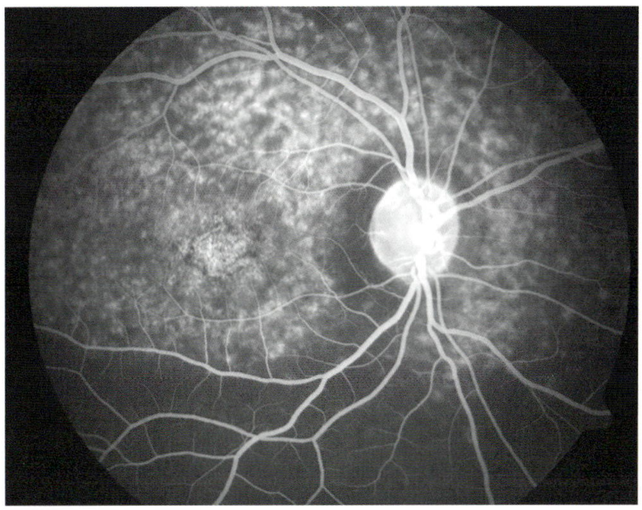

Marked increase in the hyperfluorescence is seen in the transit phase. No choroidal fluorescence is seen in the peripapillary region and in the midperiphery

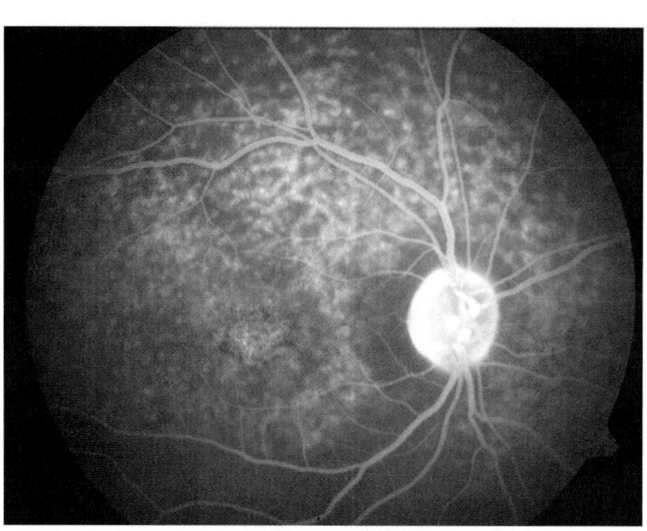

Fading of the transmitted hyperfluorescence is seen in the late phase

CASE 2 (*Continued*)

Left Eye of the Patient

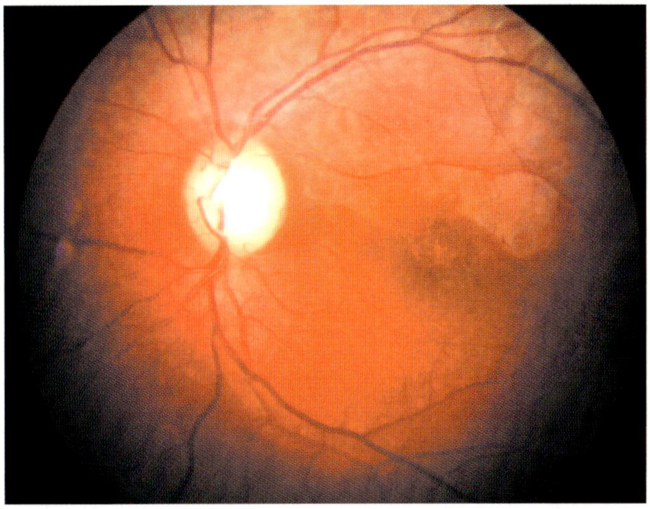

Fundus photograph of the left eye showing RPE alterations at the fovea. Retinal flecks were noted throughout the posterior pole

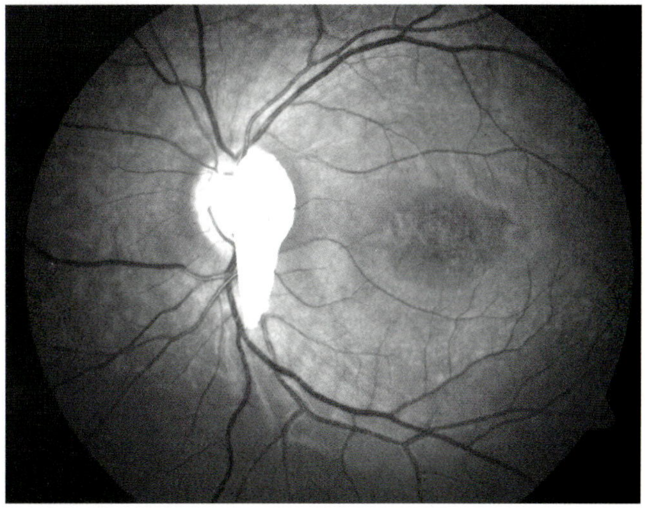

Red free photograph of the left eye

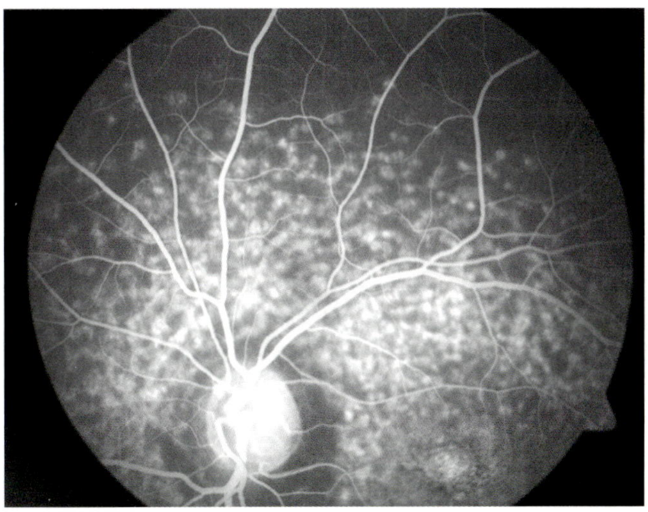

Transmitted hyperfluorescence is seen in the region of the flecks and the atrophic macular lesion. No choroidal fluorescence is seen in the peripapillary region and in the midperiphery

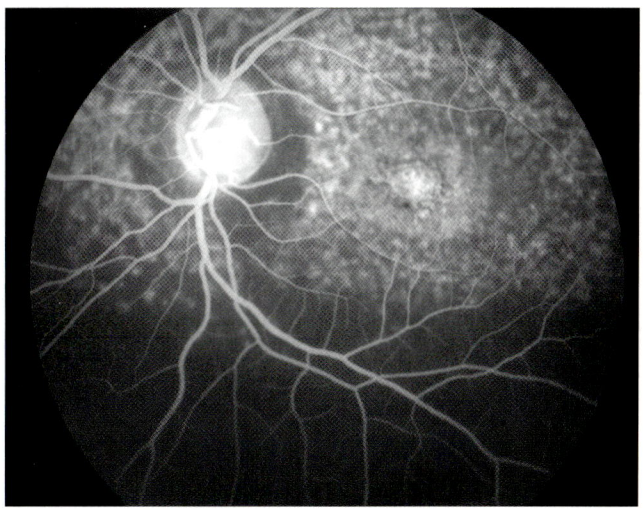

Some fading of the hyperfluorescence is seen in the later phase of the angiogram

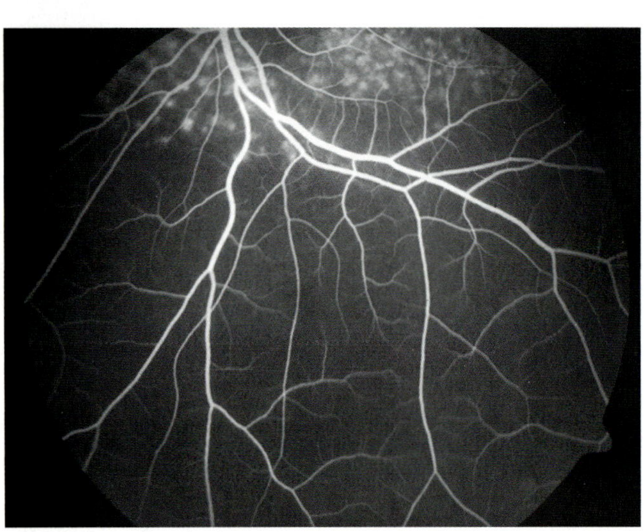

Absence of the choroidal fluorescence is seen in the inferior midperiphery

COMMENT

Even in patients with extensive flecks, the silent choroid is still evident in the peripapillary region, in between flecks and in the midperiphery.

CASE 3

A 13-year-old child was brought for examination with history of defective vision for the past six months. Visual acuity was 6/18; N6 in the right eye and 6/36; N10 in the left eye.

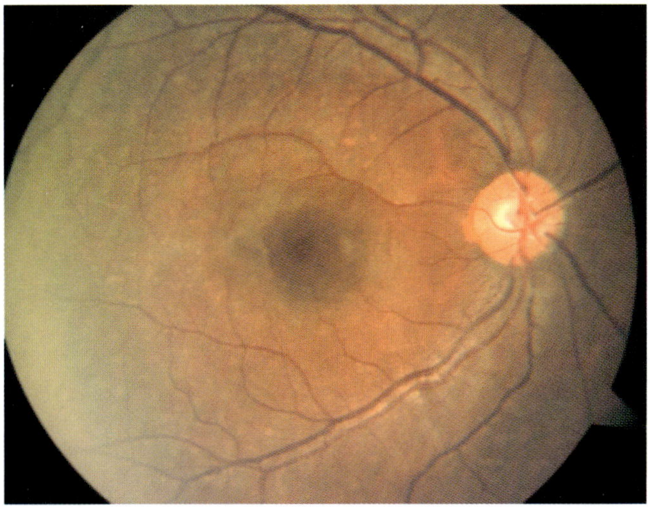

Fundus photograph of right eye with retinal flecks. No atrophic lesion is seen at the fovea

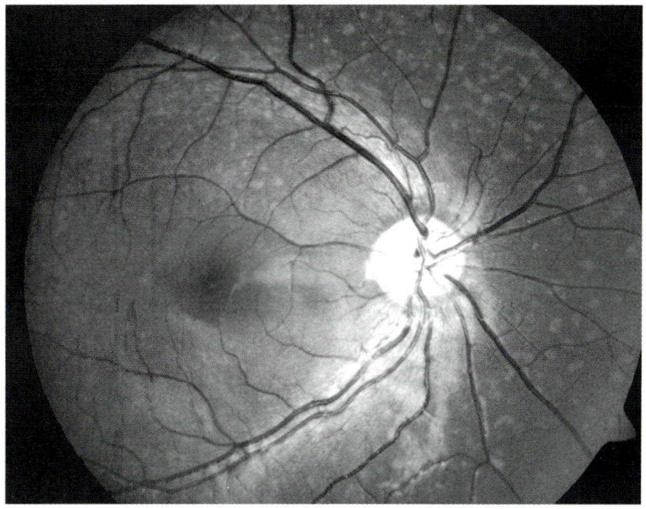

Red free photograph showing the retinal flecks

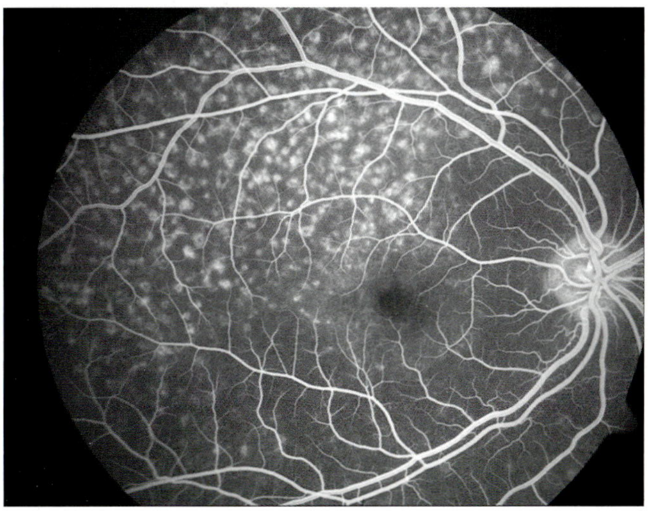

Hyperfluorescence is seen in the region of the retinal flecks. No choroidal fluorescence is seen elsewhere

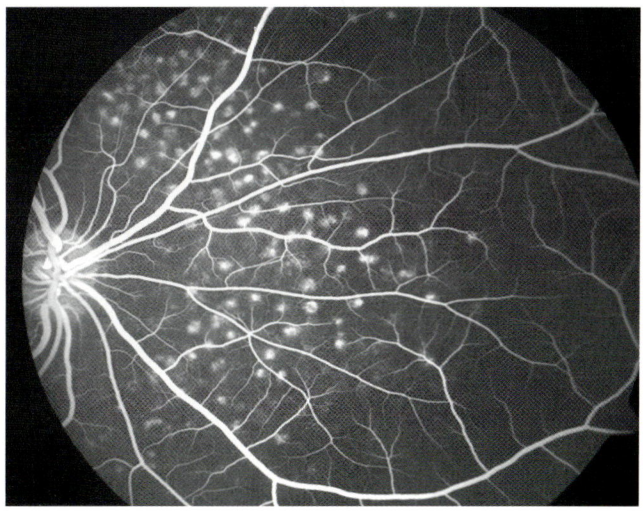

Increased hyperfluorescence at the flecks with a silent choroid is seen in the nasal retina

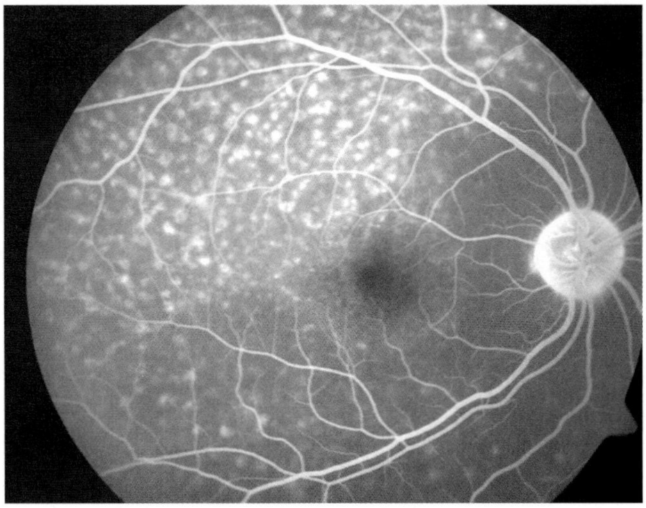

Fading of the hyperfluorescence is seen suggesting a transmission window defect

CASE 3 (*Continued*)

Left Eye of the Patient

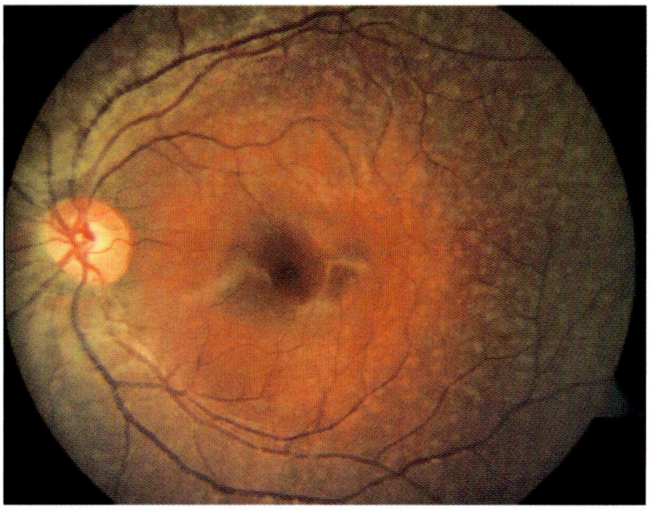

Fundus photograph of the left eye. No atrophic lesion is seen at the fovea

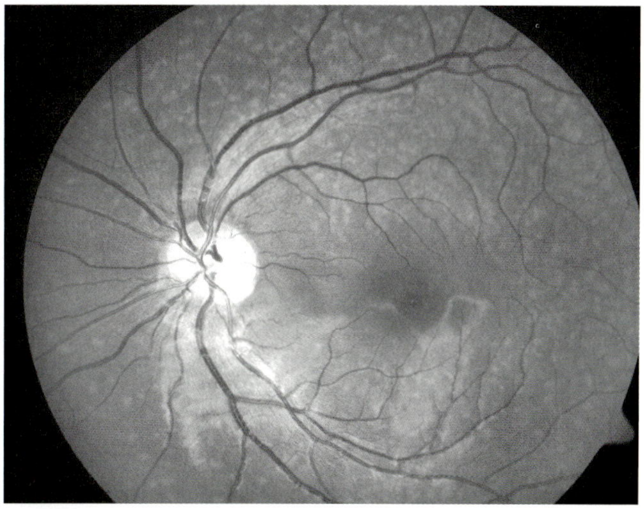

Red free photograph showing the retinal flecks in the superior part of the macula and in the superior mid periphery

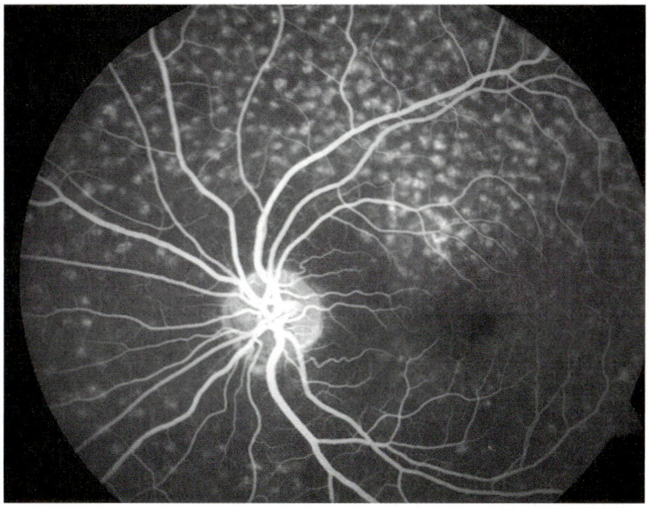

Increased hyperfluorescence is seen in the region of the retinal flecks in the transit phase of the angiogram. No choroidal fluorescence is seen elsewhere

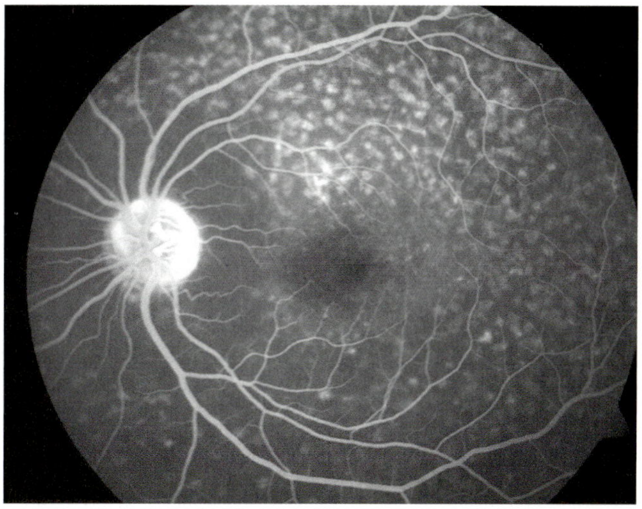

Late phase of the angiogram showing fading of the hyperfluorescence

COMMENT

Fluorescein angiogram is able to detect more flecks than is clinically visible.

CASE 4

A 33-year-old male presented with history of decreased vision in both eyes for the past five years. Visual acuity was 6/60; N12 in both eyes.

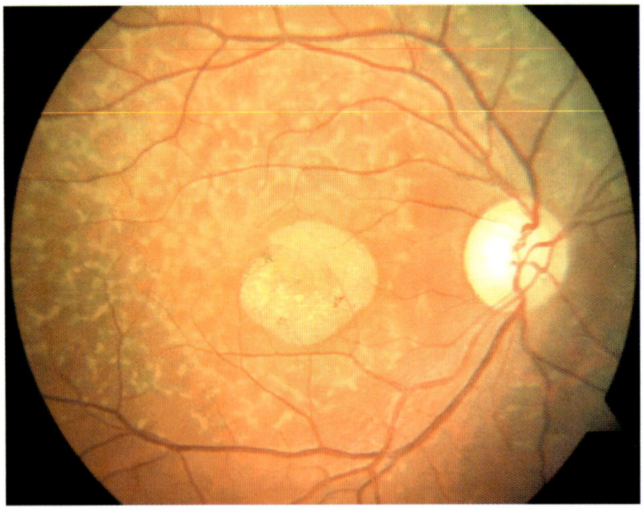

Fundus photograph of the right eye showing a large atrophic patch at the fovea. Numerous atrophic flecks are seen throughout the posterior pole

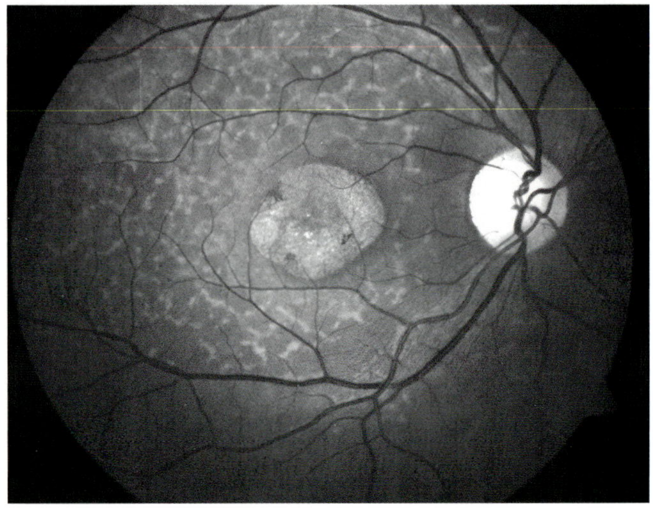

Red free photograph of the right eye

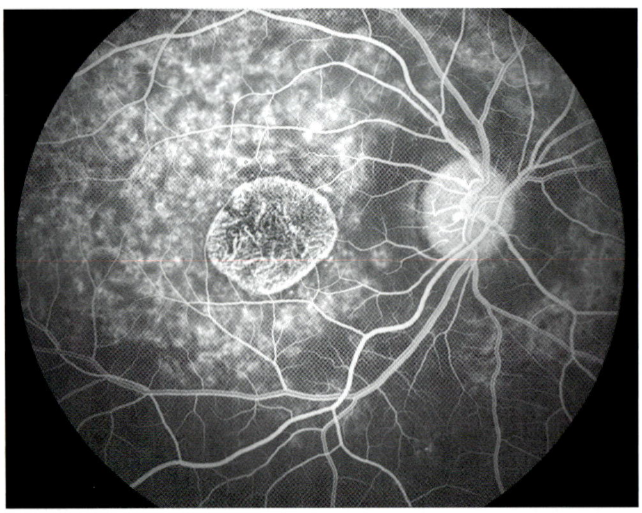

Mid arteriovenous phase shows hypofluorescence in the region of the foveal atrophic lesion. Large choroidal vessels are seen within. Irregular hyperfluorescence is seen elsewhere in the macula. No choroidal fluorescence is seen in the peripapillary region and in the midperiphery

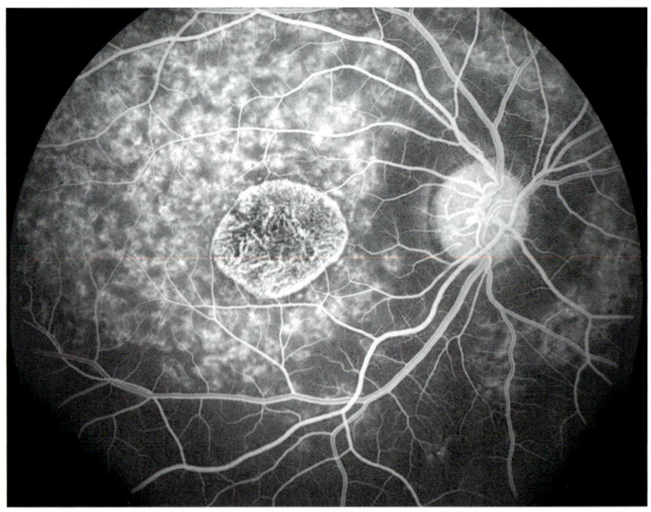

Irregular hyperfluorescence has increased in the arteriovenous phase of the angiogram

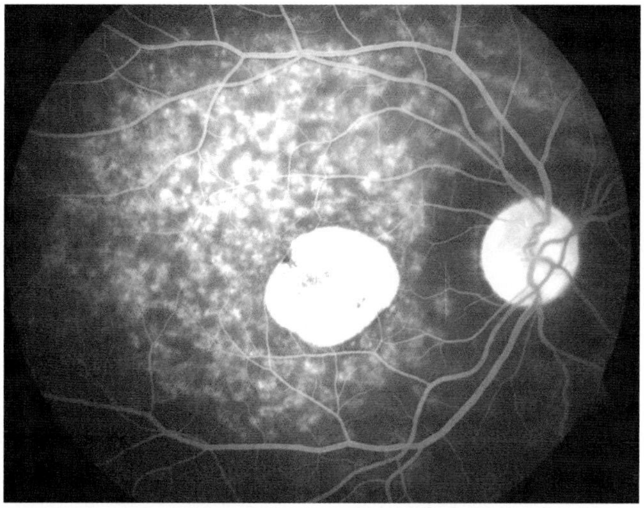

Fading of the hyperfluorescence is seen in the area of the flecks. The central atrophic area is hyperfluorescent due to the scleral staining being seen through

CASE 4 (*Continued*)

Left Eye of the Patient

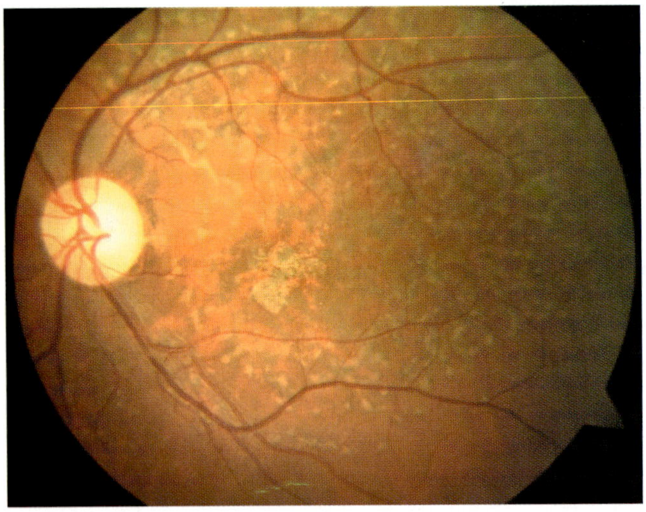

Fundus photograph of the left eye showing similar changes as the right eye

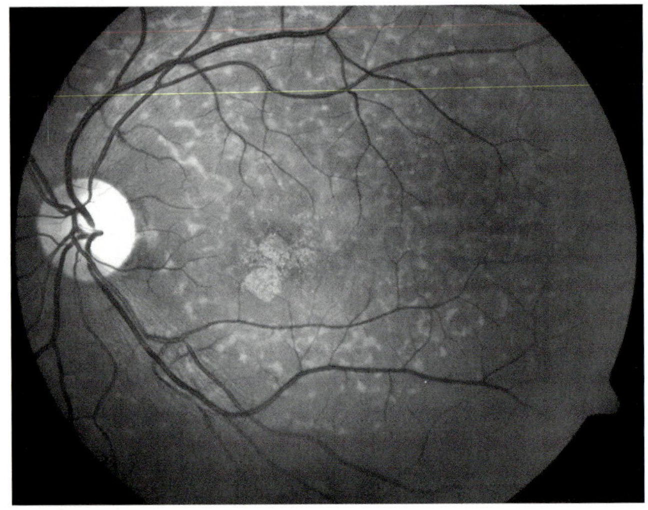

Red free photograph of the left eye

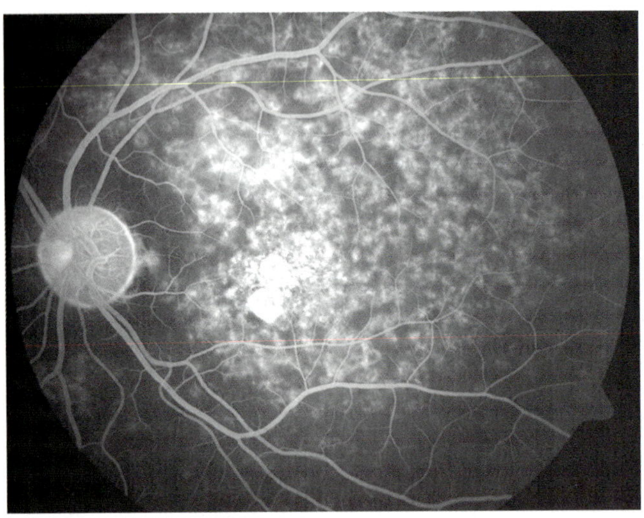

Increased hyperfluorescence is seen in the area of the flecks. Choroidal silence is seen in the peripapillary region and in the mid periphery

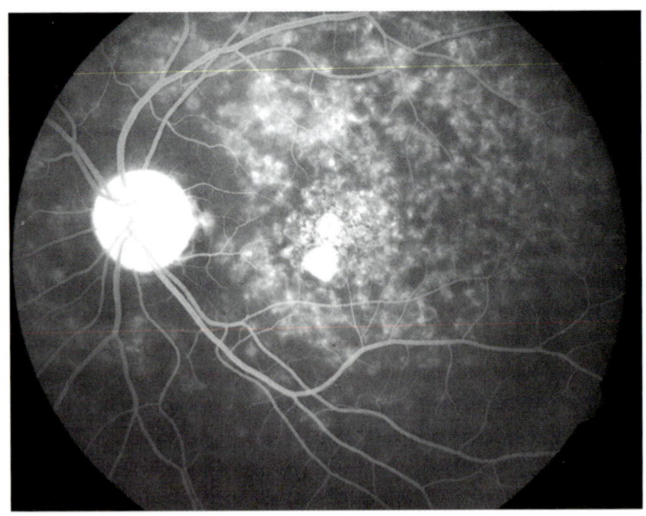

Late phase showing fading of the irregular hyperfluorescence. The atrophic central lesion shows hyperfluorescence due to scleral staining

COMMENT

Angiogram showing the absence of the choroidal fluorescence in the peripapillary region and in the midperiphery.

The atrophic changes occurring at the fovea is well seen in the angiogram.

CASE 5

A 31-year-old male presented with diminution of vision in the right eye with limited spontaneous improvement. Vision was 6/9; N6 in the right eye and 6/6; N6 in the left eye.

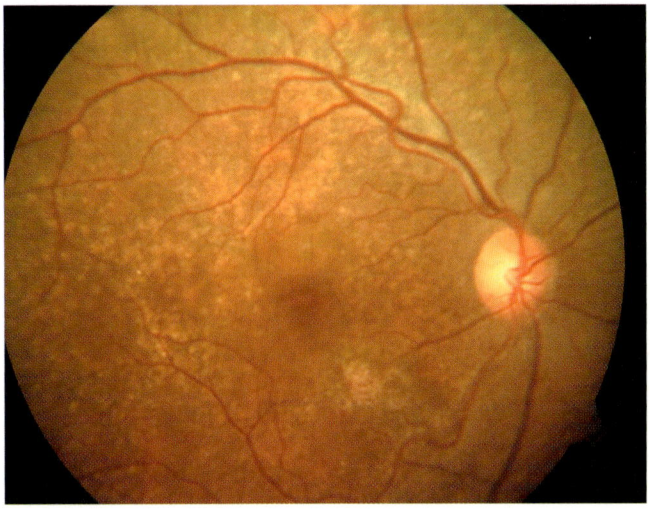

Fundus photograph of the right eye shows numerous yellowish white flecks all over the posterior pole. A well defind grayish-white lesion is seen inferonasal to the fovea with surrounding subretinal hemorrhage

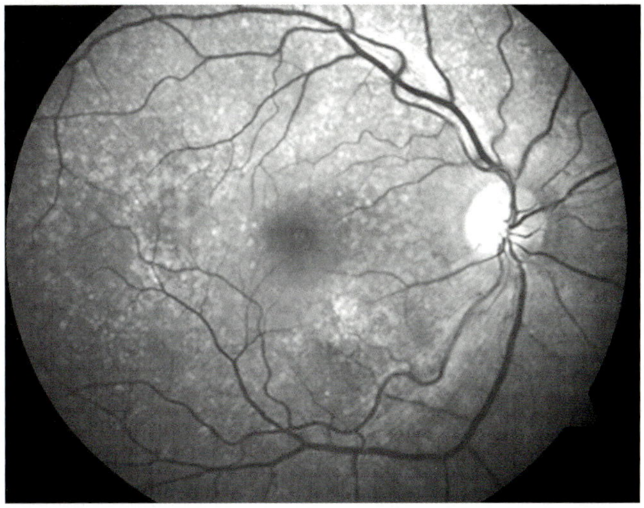

Red free photograph showing retinal flecks and classic CNVM

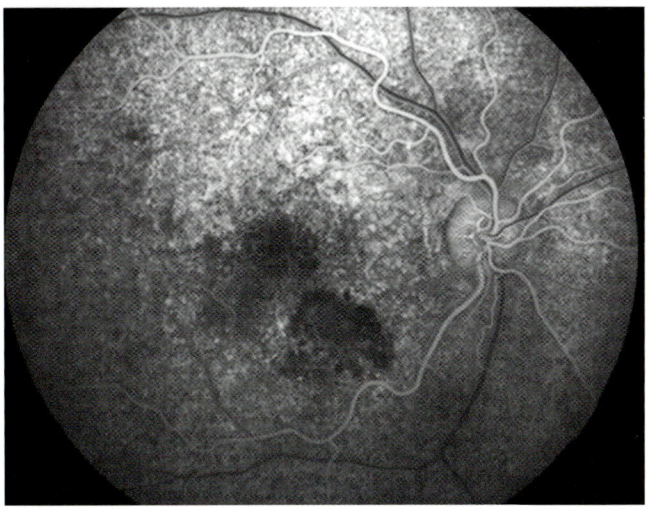

Early arteriovenous phase showing blocked fluorescence because of subretinal hemorrhage with lacy network of vessels suggestive of a classic CNVM

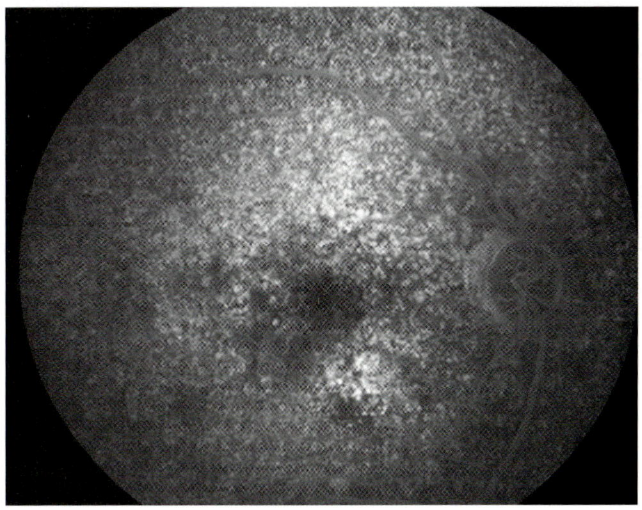

Hyperfluorescence due to the CNVM increases in intensity in the late phase

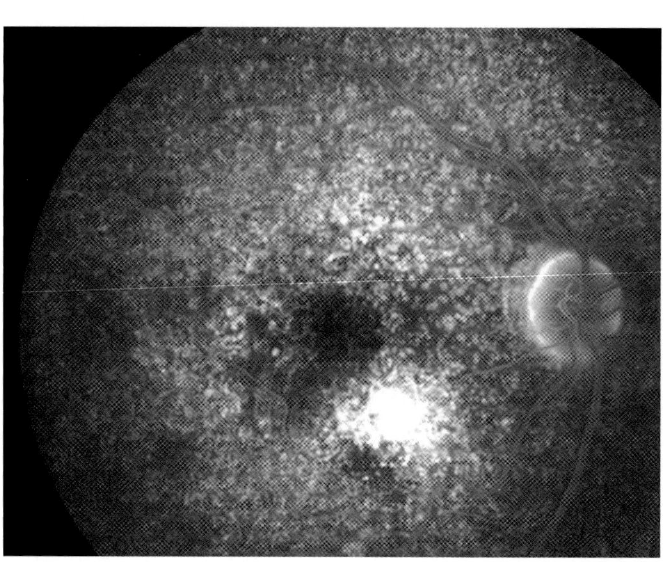

Late phase of the angiogram with intense hyperfluorescence suggestive of leakage from CNVM with its staining

56

Chapter

Progressive Cone Dystrophy

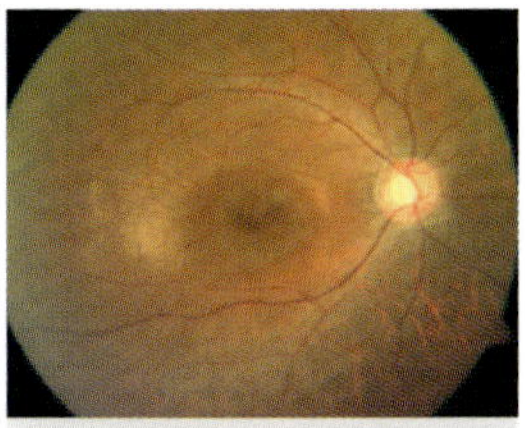

- The mode of inheritance is usually autosomal dominant
- The onset of symptoms is usually in early childhood. However, a subgroup of patients may have onset of symptoms in the third or fourth decade of life
- Common symptoms include reduced vision, photoaversion, nystagmus and color vision defect. Though photophobia and nystagmus can be early signs of the disease; they are seen to diminish with increasing age.
- The fundus appearance in this condition can vary. It could be normal in early stages. A classical bull's eye lesion may develop in the macular region. Alternately, pigment stippling or a large atrophic area may develop in the macular region. Late features may include mild temporal disc pallor as well as arteriolar attenuation.

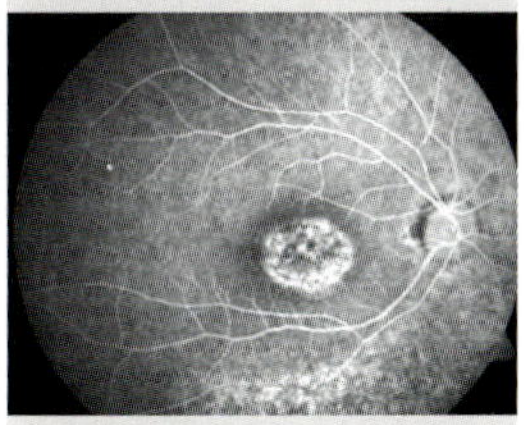

- Fluorescein angiography depends on the type of lesion seen in the fundus.
- In cases with a bull's eye maculopathy, a horizontally ovoid zone of hyperfluorescence is seen surrounding a hypofluorescent center at the macula.
- In patients with pigment stippling, the fluorescein angiogram show diffuse stippled hyperfluorescence.
- In patient with a large atrophic lesion, a hyperfluorescent window defect is seen in the area of the lesion.

CASE 1

A 39-year-old male presented with reduced vision in both eyes for the past five years. Visual acuity was 6/12; N6 in both eyes. A bull's eye like lesion was seen in both eyes. Color vision was severely affected. The cone responses in the electroretinogram were markedly reduced.

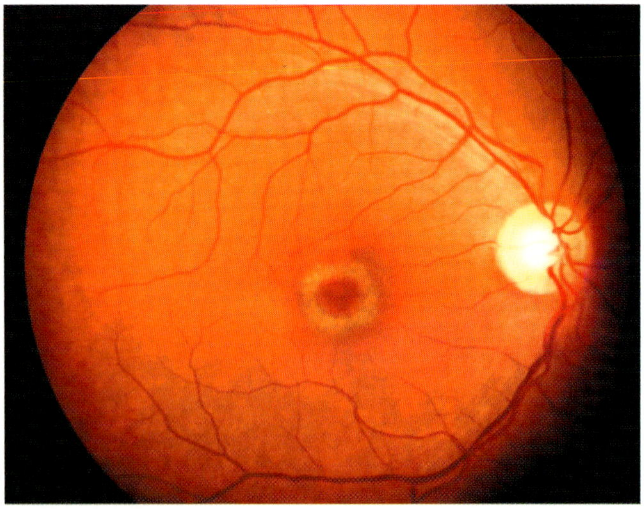

Fundus photograph of the right eye showing a bull's eye like lesion at the fovea

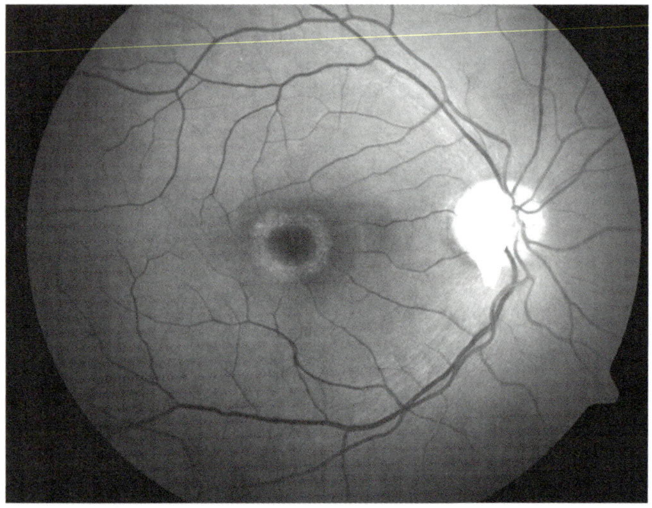

Red free photograph showing the foveal lesion

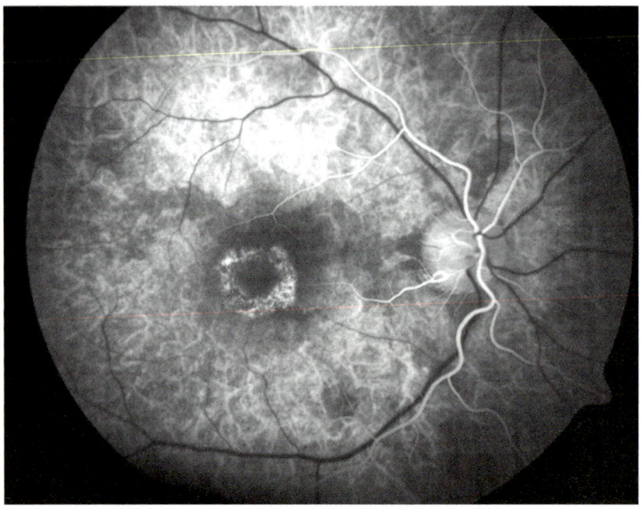

Arterial phase of the angiogram showing the hyperfluorescence due to transmission defect at the fovea

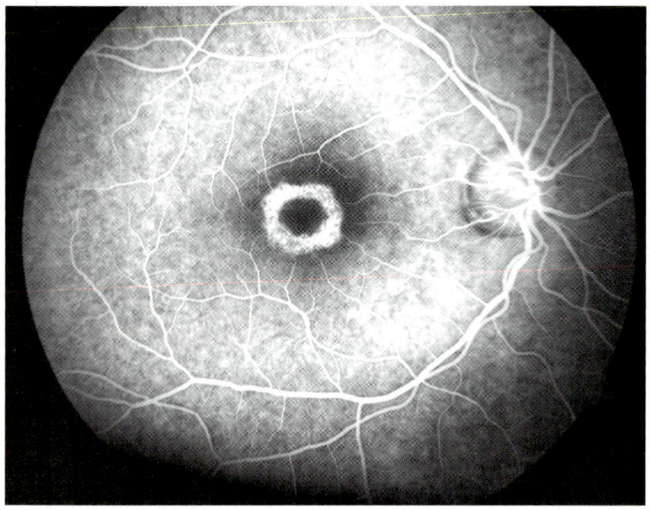

Arteriovenous phase showing increased transmission defect seen through the annular atrophy at the fovea

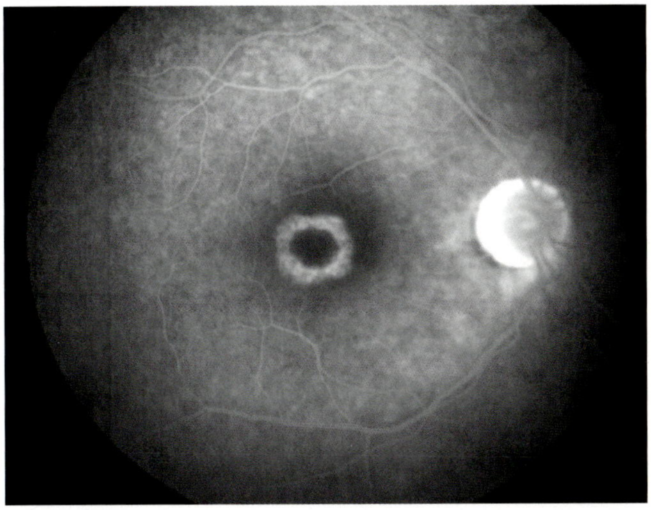

Late phase shows fading of the hyperfluorescence indicating it to be a transmission window defect

COMMENT

The bull's eye lesion is very well seen in the angiogram. The central normal hypofluorescence is surrounded by a ring of hyperfluorescence due to transmission defects.

CASE 2

A 34-year-old male presented with history of photoaversion and reduced vision in both eyes. Visual acuity was 6/24; N12 in the right eye and 6/60; N12 in the left eye. The cone response was significantly reduced in the electroretinogram.

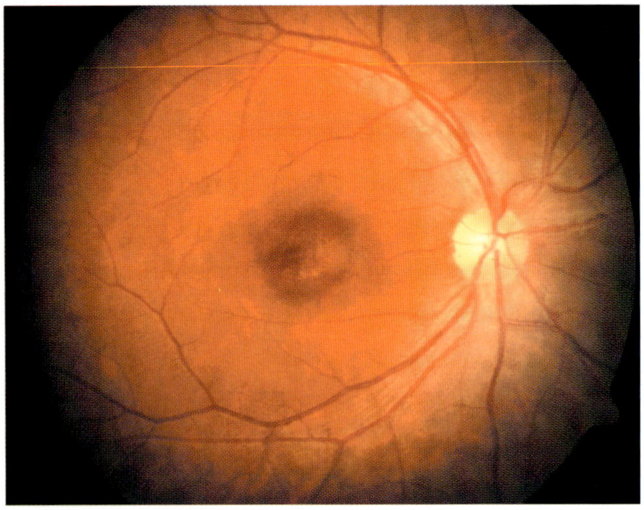

Fundus photograph of the right eye showing an atrophic lesion at the fovea

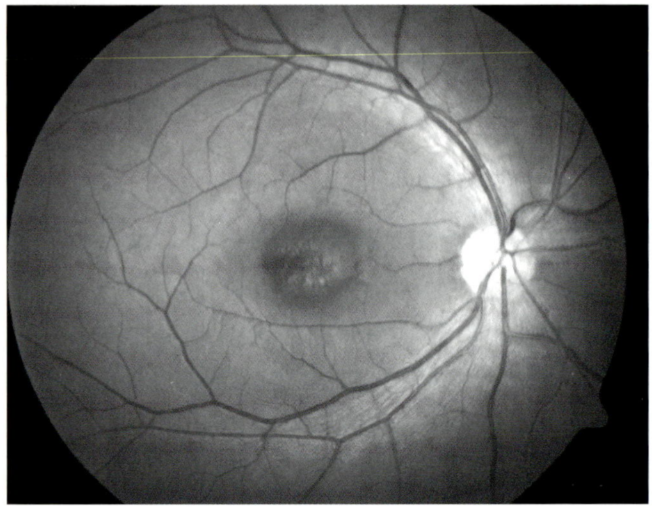

Red free photograph of the right eye

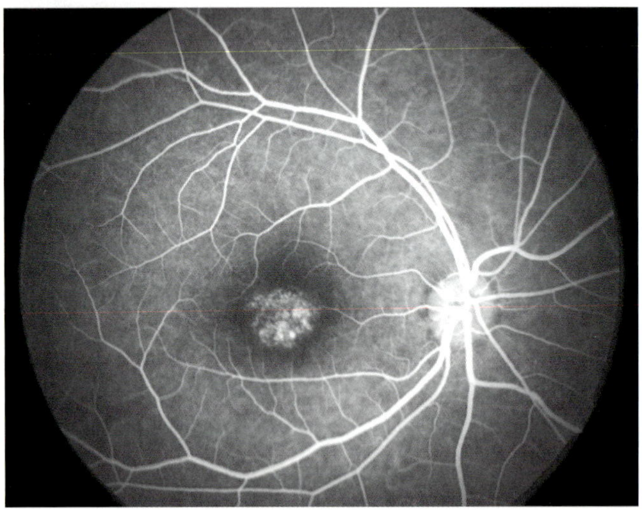

Arteriovenous phase of the angiogram showing transmitted irregular hyperfluorescence within the atrophic lesion

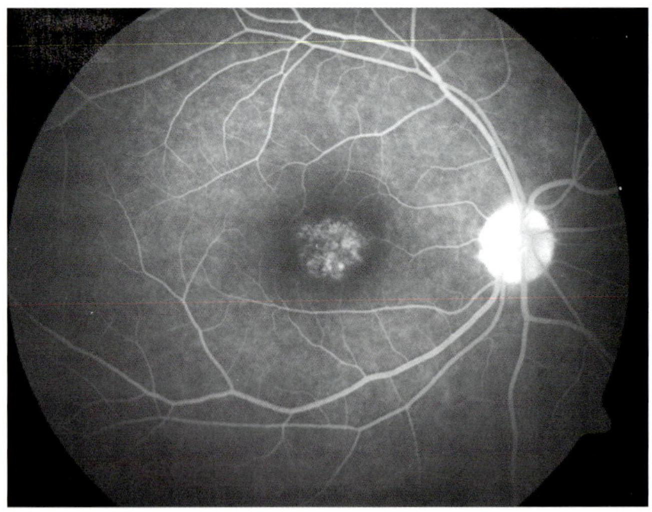

Late phase shows fading of the hyperfluorescence

CASE 2 (*Continued*)

Left Eye of the Patient

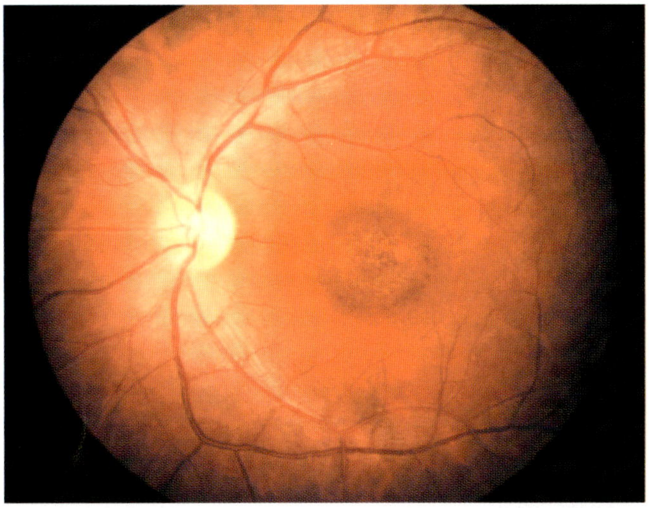

Fundus photograph of the left eye showing an atrophic lesion at the fovea

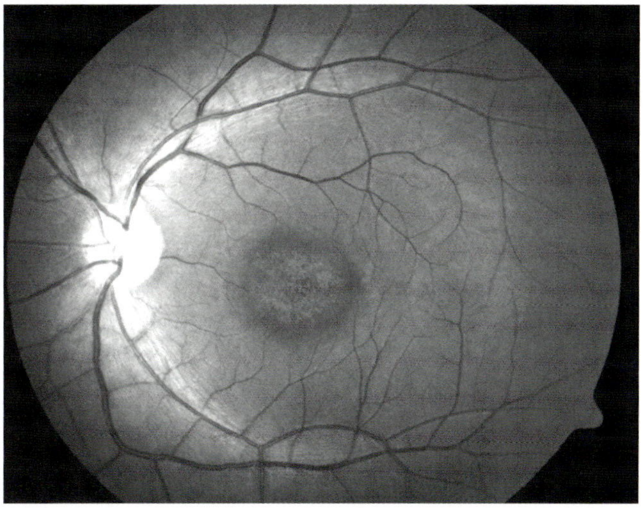

Red free photograph of the left eye

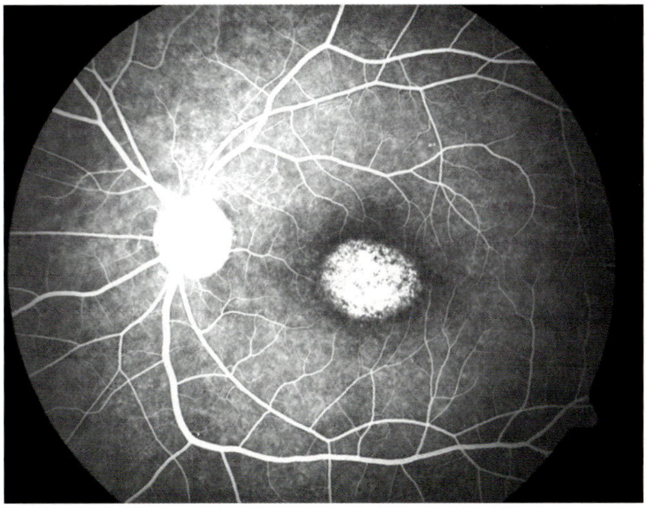

Arteriovenous phase of the angiogram showing transmitted irregular hyperfluorescence within the atrophic lesion

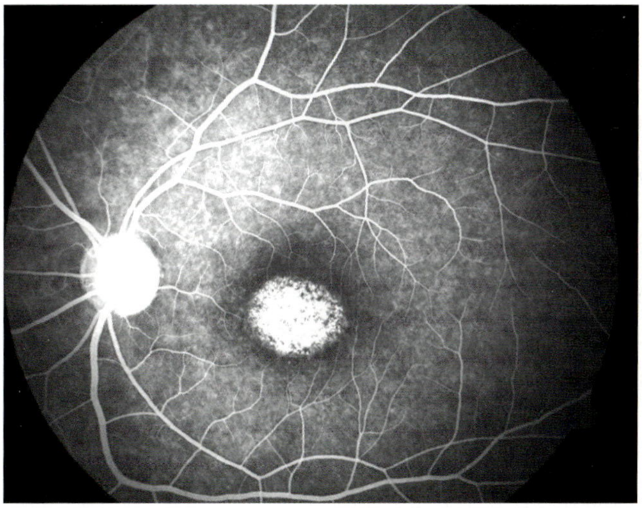

Increase in the hyperfluorescence seen as the angiogram proceeds

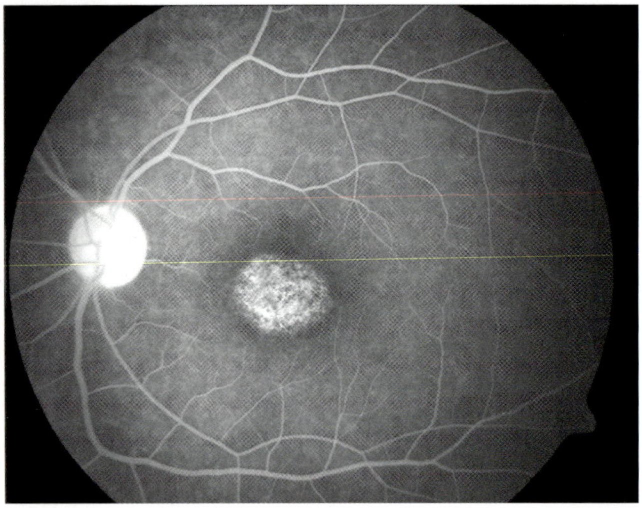

Late phase shows fading of the hyperfluorescence

COMMENT

Angiogram is showing transmission defects due to RPE alterations at the fovea.

Fluorescein angiogram picks up even very subtle RPE alterations.

CASE 3

A 21-year-old male presented with history of reduced vision in both eyes of four years duration. Visual acuity was 6/60; N6 in both eyes. The electroretinogram showed reduced cone responses.

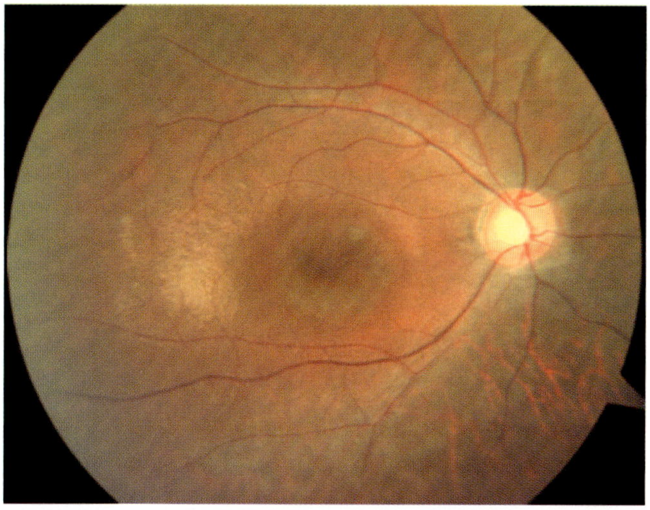

Fundus photograph showing a bull's eye like lesion at the fovea. A reflective Mizuo-like sheen is seen temporal to this lesion

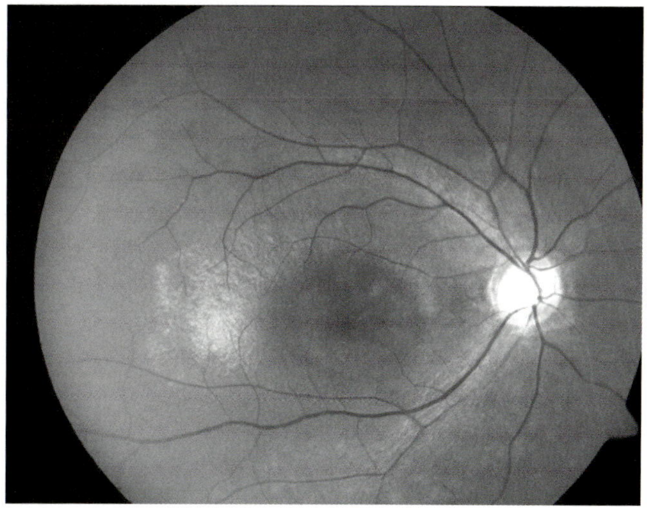

Red free photograph of the right eye

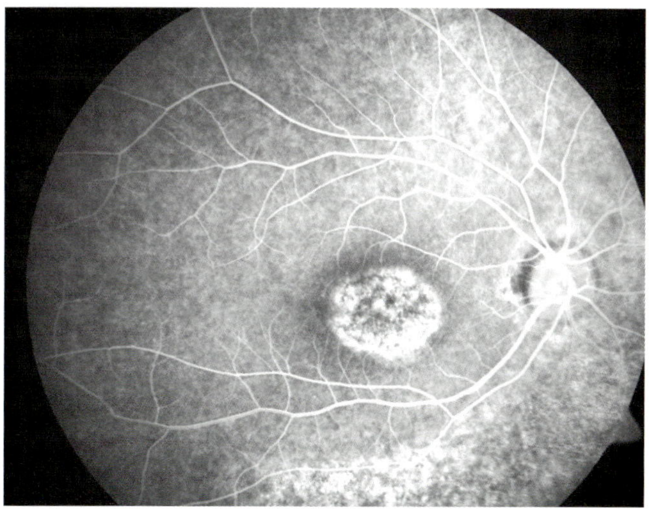

Early arteriovenous phase showing stippled hyperfluorescence within the atrophic foveal lesion

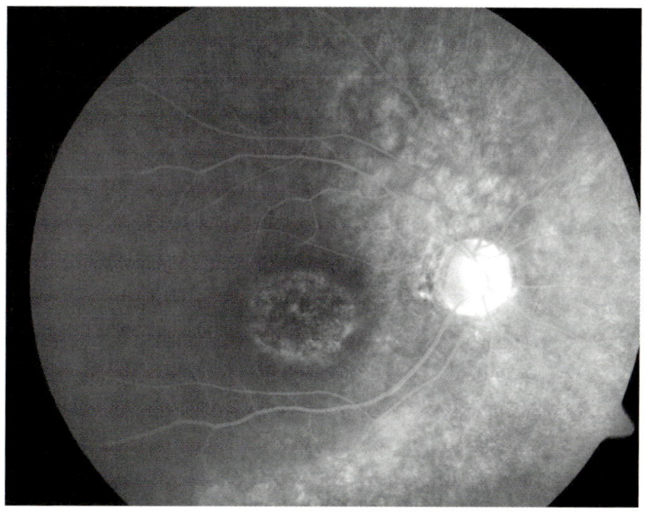

Increase in the transmitted hyperfluorescence is seen in the arteriovenous phase

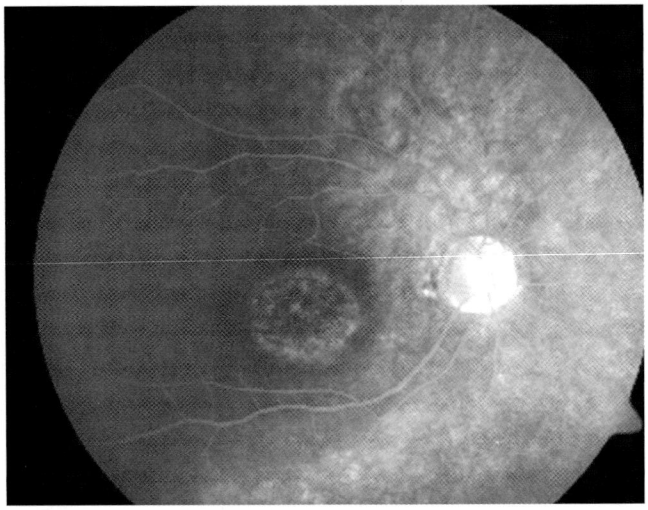

Fading of the hyperfluorescence is seen in the late phase

CASE 3 (*Continued*)

Left Eye of the Patient

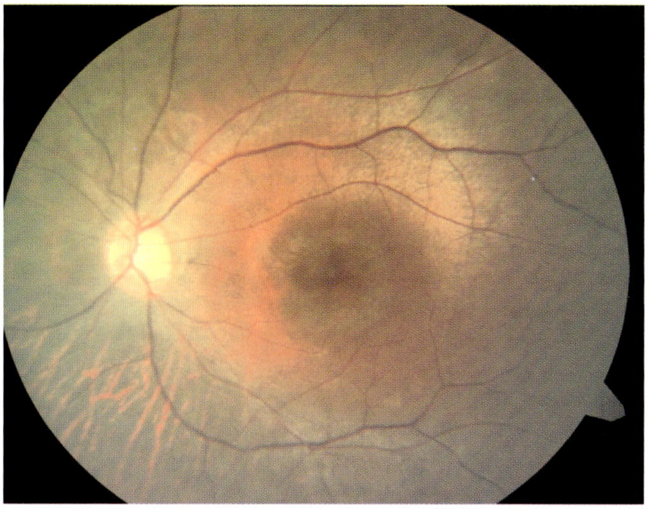

Fundus photograph of the left eye showing a bull's eye like lesion at the fovea with a Mizuo-like sheen superotemporal to it

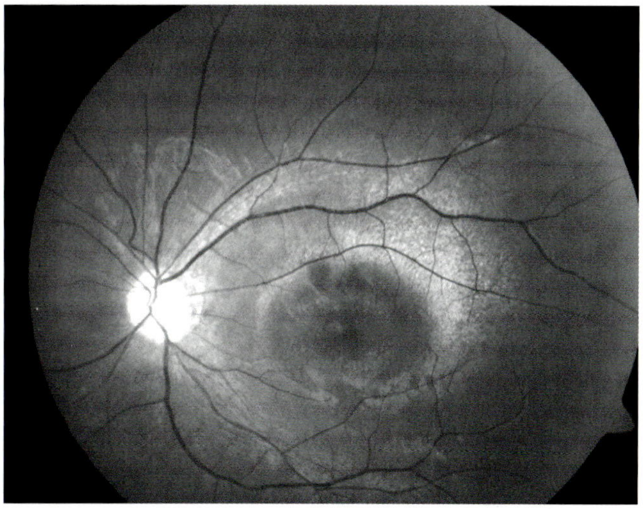

Red free photograph of the left eye

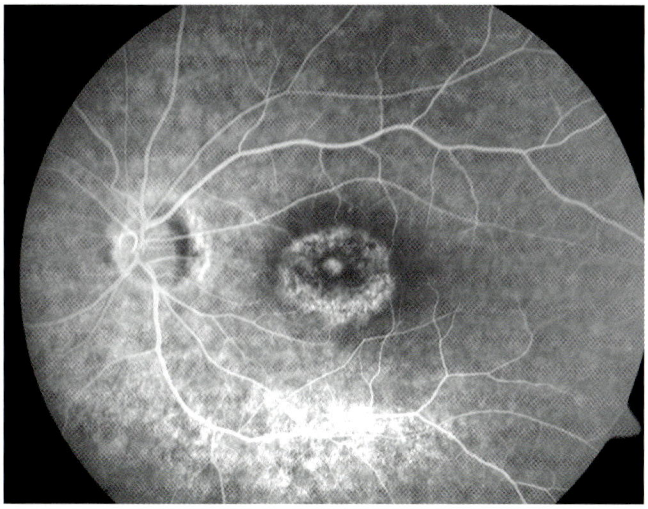

Arteriovenous phase showing an annular hyperfluorescent ring with central hypofluorescence at the fovea

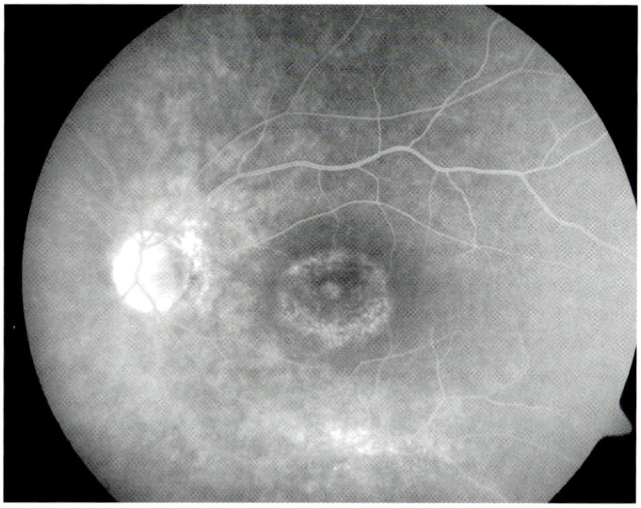

Late phase shows fading of the hyperfluorescence

COMMENT

A Mizuo-like shiny reflex is seen in a small subgroup of patients with cone dystrophy. This is more commonly seen in the temporal macula. No changes are seen in the angiogram at the site of the reflex.

57 Chapter

Other Heredomacular Dystrophies

PATTERN DYSTROPHY

CASE 1

A 26-year-old male presented with history of distortion of vision for the past one year. Visual acuity was 6/6; N6 in both eyes.

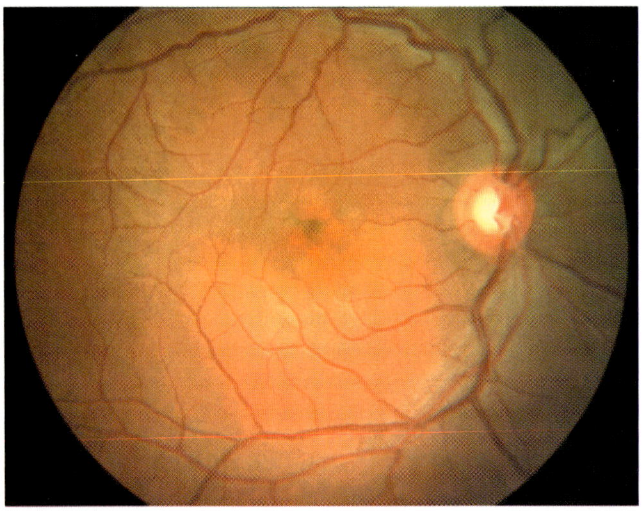

Fundus photograph of the right eye showing irregular subretinal deposits at the fovea

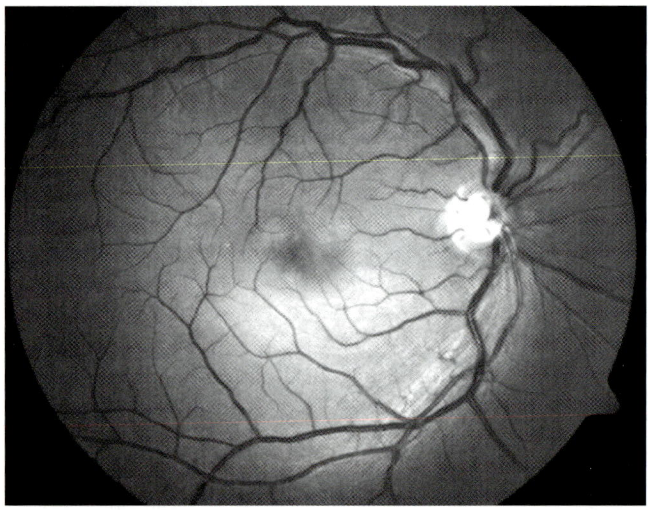

Red free photograph of the right eye

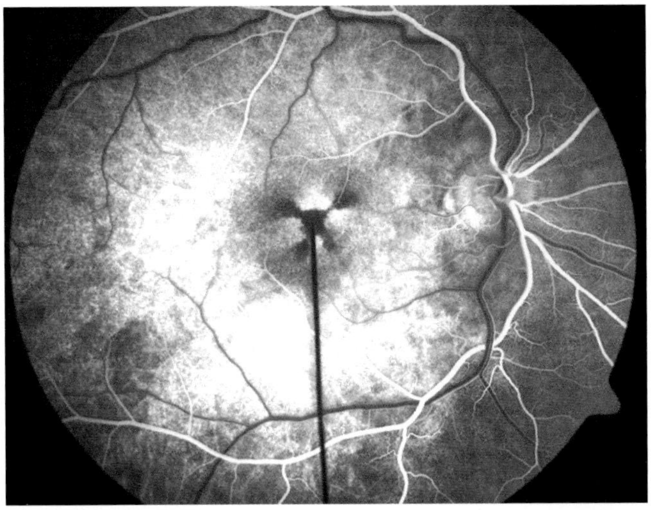

Arterial phase showing a central area of hypofluorescence with radiating spokes

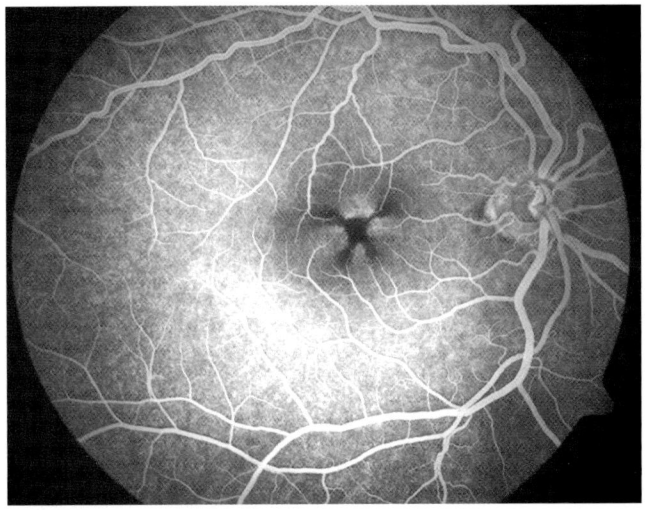

The pattern is quite well seen in the arteriovenous phase

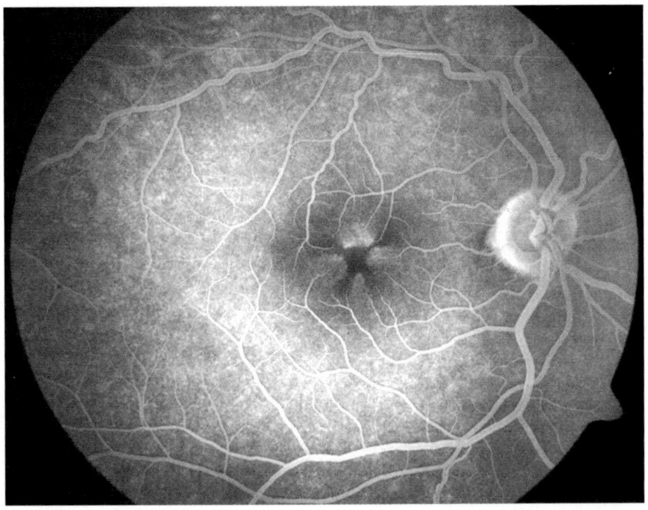

Late phase of the angiogram shows persistence of the hyperfluorescent pattern

CASE 1 (*Continued*)

Left Eye of the Patient

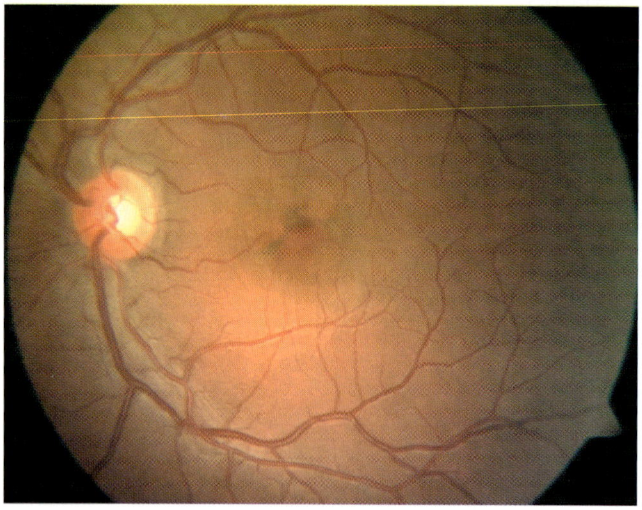

Fundus photograph of the left eye showing subretinal deposits at the fovea

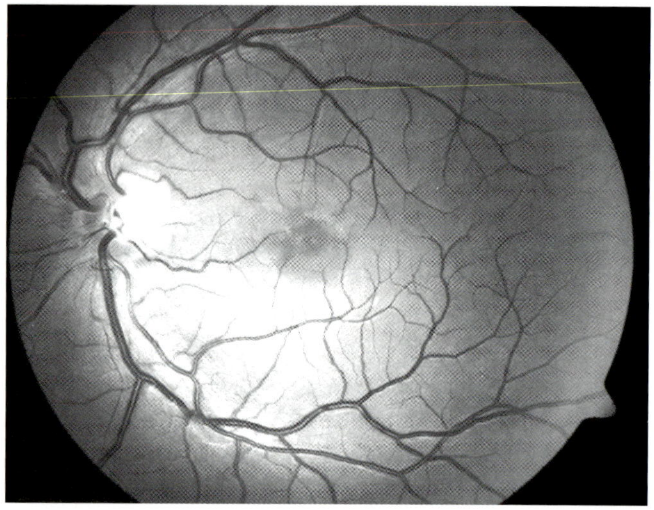

Red free photograph of the left eye

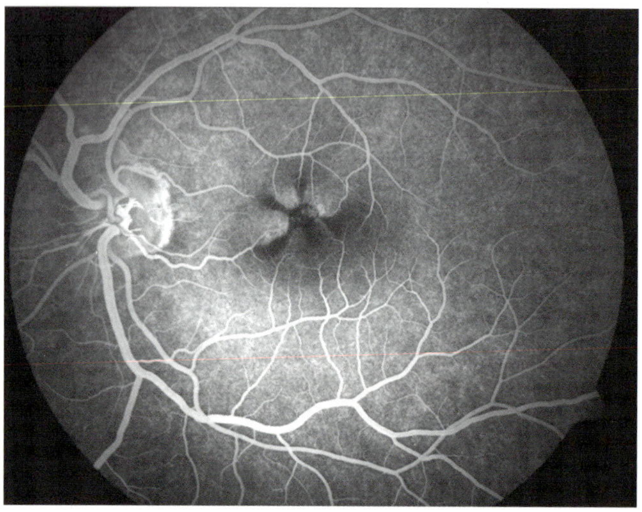

A pattern similar to that seen in the right eye is noted at the fovea in the arteriovenous phase of the angiogram

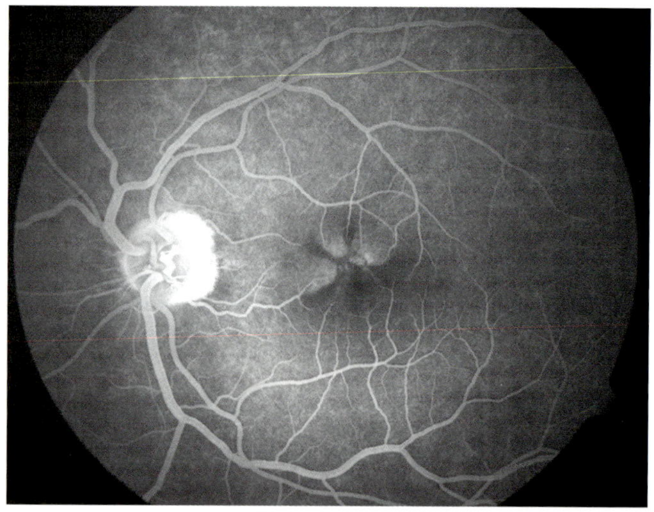

Late phase angiogram picture showing persistence of hypofluorescence at the fovea

COMMENT

There is deposition of a yellow-orange material in the subretinal space in pattern dystrophy. This blocks the background choroidal fluorescence giving rise to the pattern seen angiographically.

FOVEAL SCHISIS

CASE 2

An 18-year-old male presented with a history of reduced vision for distance in both eyes for the past one year. Visual acuity was 6/12; N8 in the right eye and 6/18; N8 in the left eye.

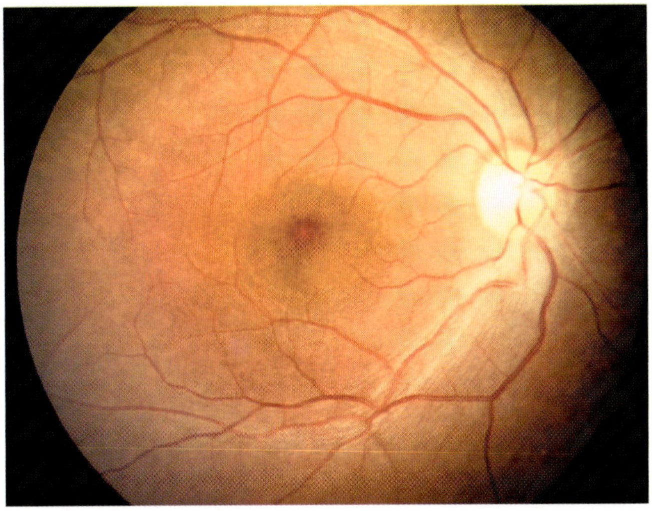

Fundus photograph of the right eye showing foveal schisis

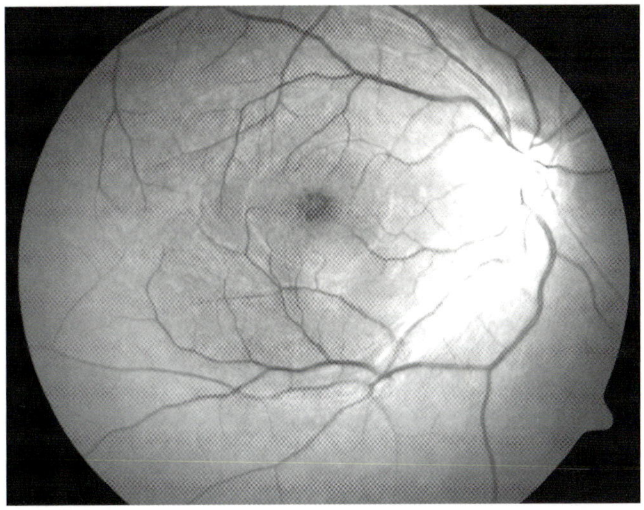

Red free photograph of the right eye showing a central large foveal cyst

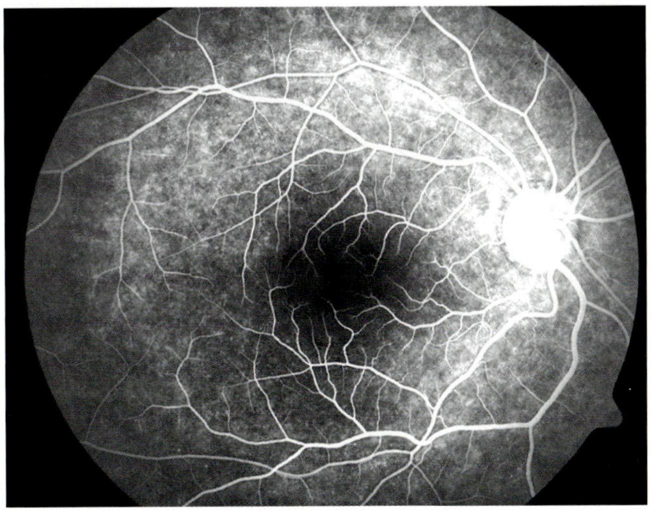

No leakage or accumulation of the dye is seen in the arteriovenous phase of the angiogram

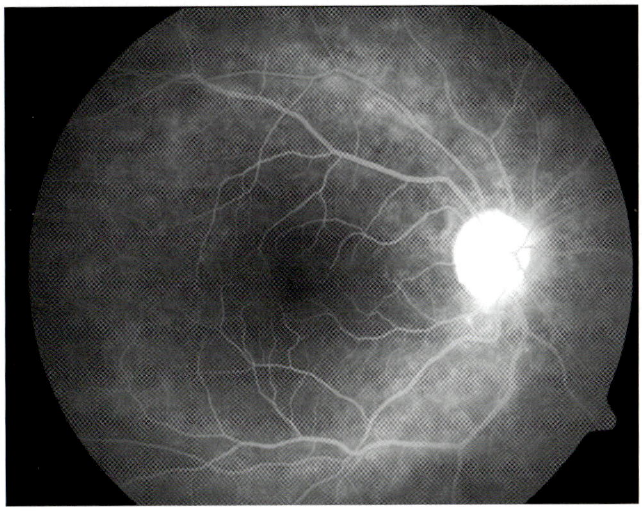

The area of foveal schisis does not show any abnormal fluorescence even in the late film

CASE 2 (*Continued*)

Left Eye of the Patient

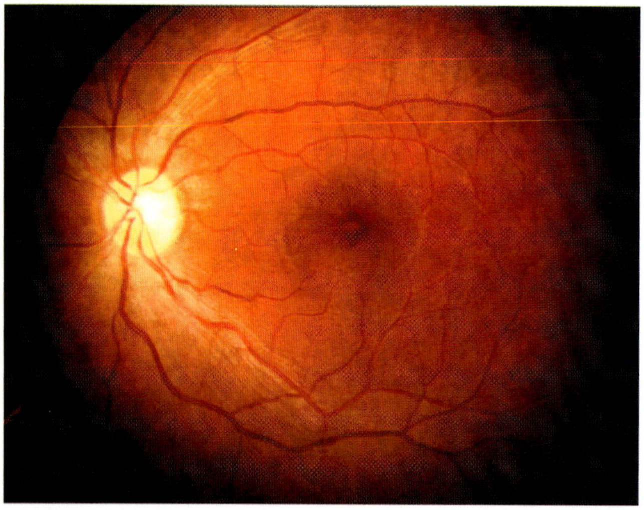

Fundus photograph of the left eye showing foveal schisis

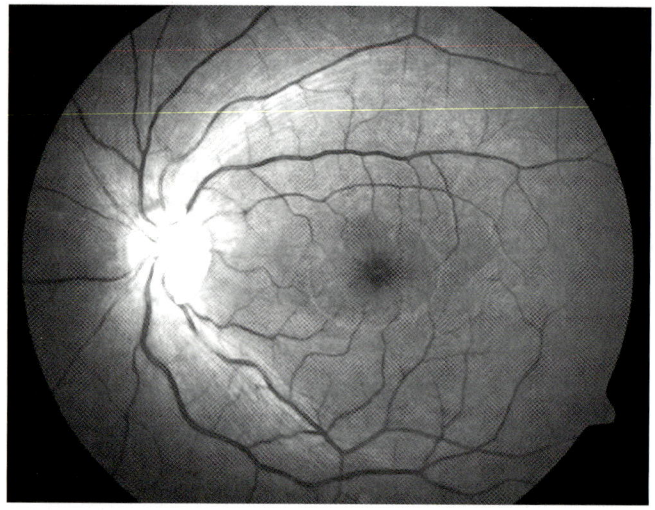

Red free photograph showing the foveal microcysts

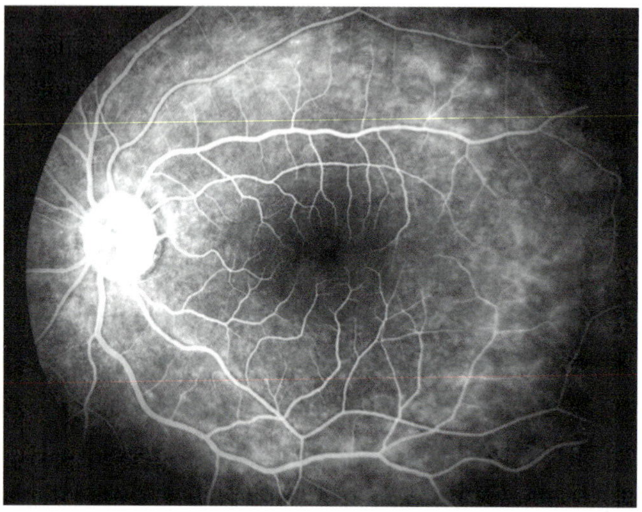

Arteriovenous phase not showing any abnormal fluorescence at the fovea

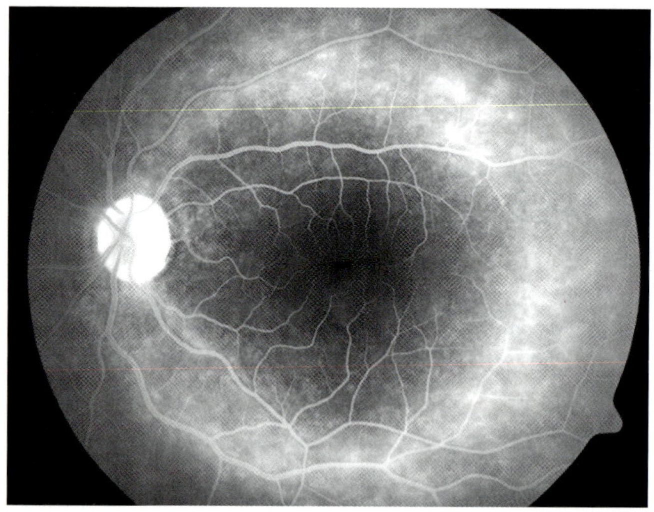

Late phase angiogram not showing any dye accumulation in the cysts

COMMENT

Unlike in cystoid macular edema, no pooling of the dye is seen in eyes with foveal schisis.

Angiogram is usually normal or may show a few transmission defects at the fovea.

FOVEAL HYPOPLASIA

CASE 3

A 17-year-old male presented with reduced vision in both eyes since early childhood. Visual acuity was 3/60 in both eyes.

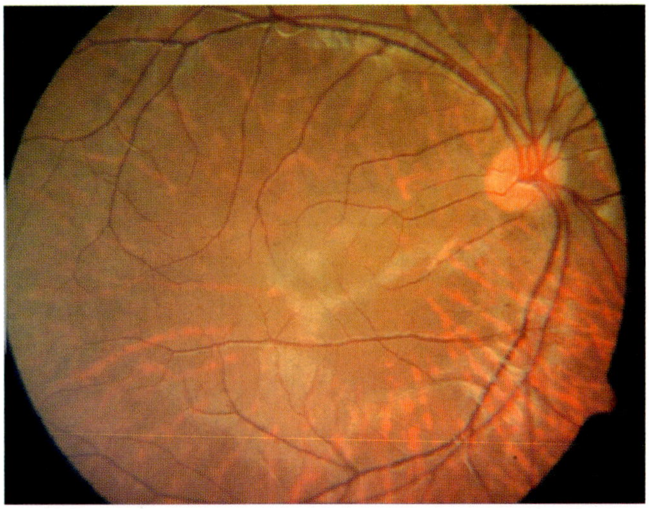

Fundus photograph of the right eye showing absence of a well-formed fovea

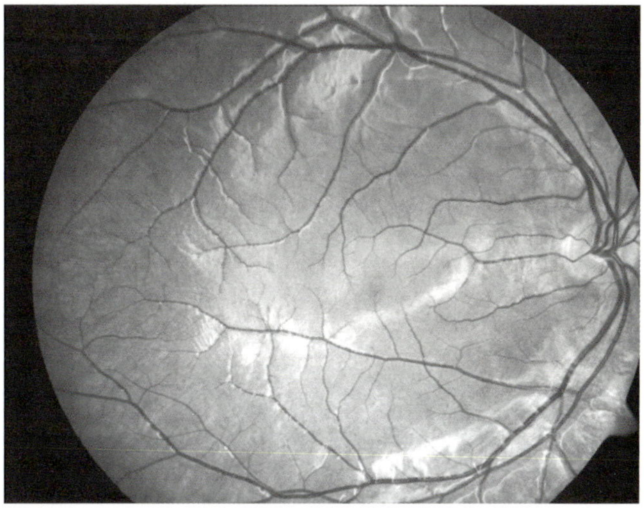

Red free photograph shows lack of a foveal avascular zone

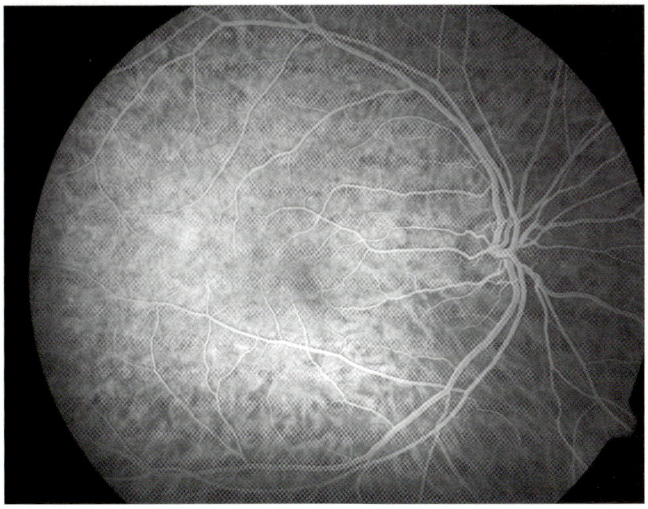

Arteriovenous phase does not show a foveal avascular zone. The normal hypofluorescence at the fovea is absent

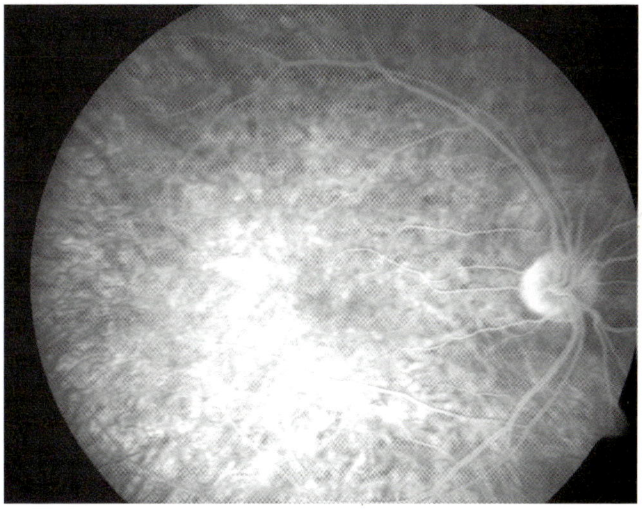

Late phase angiogram

CASE 3 (*Continued*)

Left Eye of the Patient

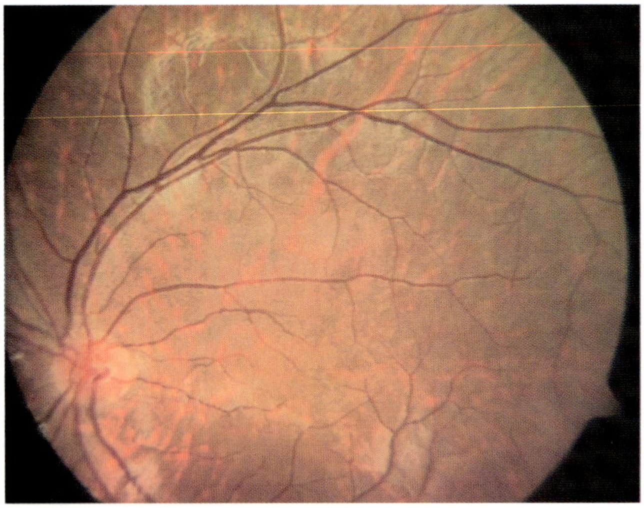

Fundus photograph of the left eye does not show a foveal reflex

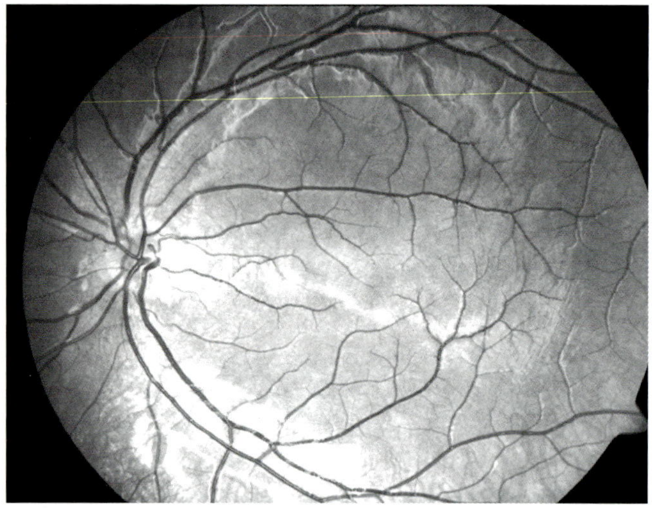

Red free photograph shows absence of a capillary free zone at the center of the macula

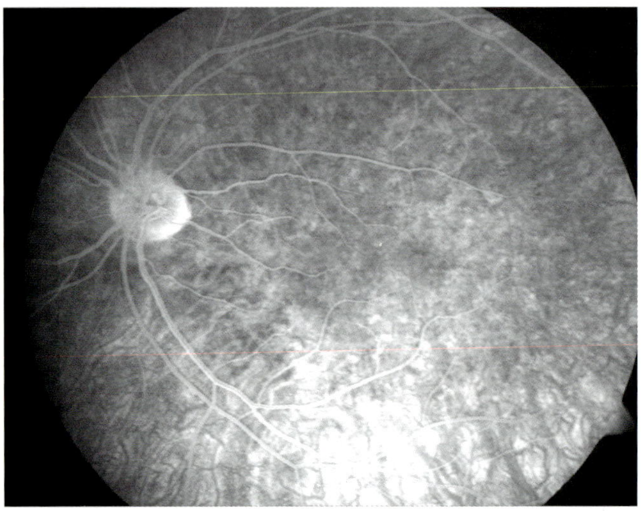

Arteriovenous phase shows lack of a foveal avascular zone or a parafoveal capillary plexus. The normal foveal hypofluorescence is absent

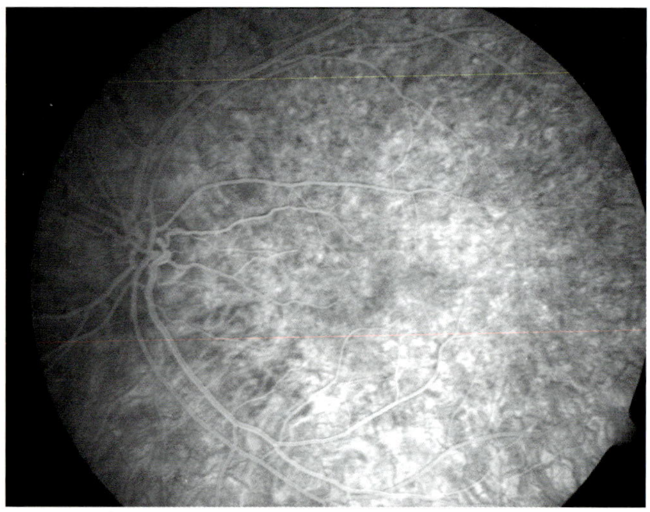

Late phase of the angiogram

COMMENT

The FAZ in foveal hypoplasia is either absent or ill-formed. Blood vessels may be seen traversing the normal site of the fovea.

CLINICAL NUGGETS

1. Heredomacular dystrophies are familial, bilaterally symmetrical disorders occurring at the posterior pole.
2. History, clinical features, color vision, visual fields, electrodiagnostic tests, and fluorescein angiography are useful investigative tools in patients with heredomacular dystrophies.

BIBLIOGRAPHY

1. Anmarkrud N. Fundus Fluorescein angiography in Fundus flavimaculatus and Stargardts disease. Acta Ophthalmol 1979;57:172-82.
2. Ayazi S, Fagan R. Pattern dystrophy of the pigment epithelium. Retina 1981;1:287-9.
3. Curry HF Jr, Moorman LT. Fluorescein photography of vitelliform macular degeneration. Arch Ophthalmol 1968;79:705-9.
4. Deutman A F, van Blommestein JDA, Henkes H E et al. Butterfly-shaped pigment dystrophy of the fovea. Arch Ophthalmol 1970;83:558-69.
5. Franceschetti A, François J. Fundus flavimaculatus. Arch Ophthalmol 1965;25:505.
6. Klien BA, Krill AE. Fundus flavimaculatus: clinical functions and histopathologic observations. Am J Ophthalmol 1967;64:3.
7. Krause U, Vainio-Mattila B, Eriksson A, Forsius. Fluorescein angiographic studies on X-chromosomal retinoschisis. Acta Ophthalmol 1970;48:794.
8. Miller SA. Fluorescence in Bests vitelliform dystrophy, lipofuschin and fundus flavimaculatus. Br J Ophthalmol 1978;62:256-60.
9. Morse PH, MacLean AL. Fluorescein fundus studies in hereditary vitelloeruptive macular degeneration. Am J Ophthalmol 1968;66:485-94.
10. Uliss AE, Moore AT, Bird AC. The dark choroid in posterior retinal dystrophies. Ophthalmology 1987; 94(11):1423-7.
11. von Ruckmann A, Fitzke FW, Bird AC. In vivo fundus autofluorescence in macular dystrophies: Arch Ophthalmol 1997;115(5):609-15.

Chapter 58

Ocular Albinism

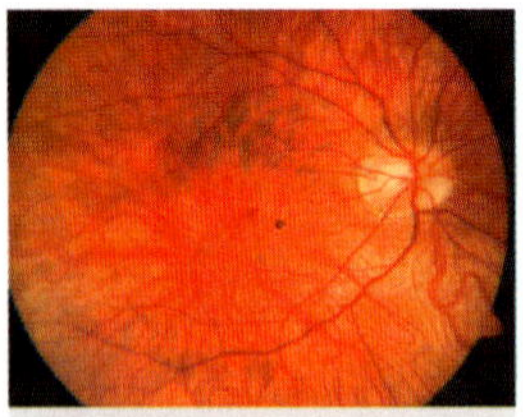

- Albinism is a group of disorders associated with an inborn error of amino acid metabolism affecting the production of melanin.
- Oculocutaneous albinism comprises of ocular involvement along with the skin and hair involvement. This can be either tyrosinase negative (complete) or tyrosinase positive (incomplete).
- Ocular albinism is characterized by changes restricted to the ocular structures.
- Oculocutaneous albinism is autosomal recessive while the ocular albinism is usually X-linked; though autosomal recessive inheritance is also known.
- Presenting features include poor vision and pendular nystagmus which reduces with increasing age. Retinal changes associated with albinism include a depigmented fundus, foveal hypoplasia and optic disc hypoplasia.

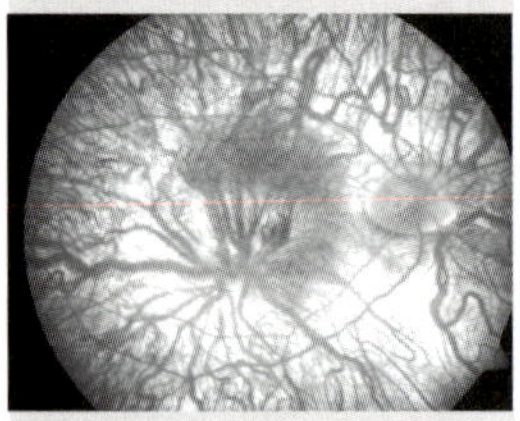

- Increased visibility of the choroidal vessels is noted due to lack of masking by the overlying pigment.
- Foveal hypoplasia may be evident by absence of a well formed foveal avascular zone.
- Late phase shows the choroidal and retinal vessels silhouetted against the background fluorescence from scleral staining.

CASE 1

A 19-year-old female with ocular albinism presented with history of strabismus since early childhood. Her brother was noted to have similar complaints. Visual acuity was 6/24; N6 in the right eye and 6/18; N6 in the left eye.

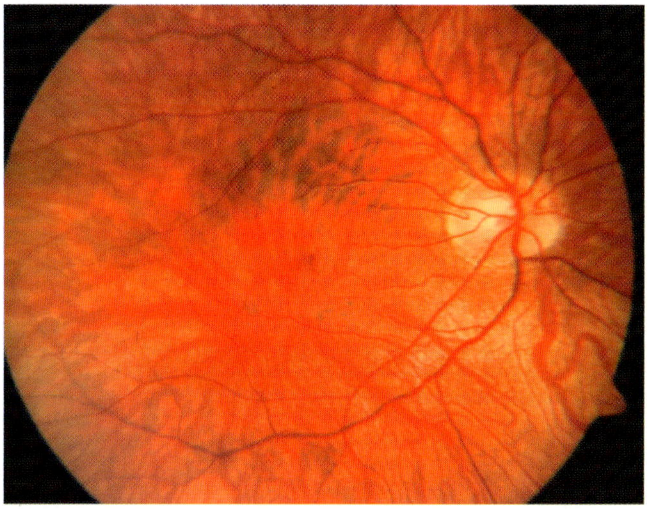

Fundus photograph of the right eye showing a markedly depigmented fundus. Few patches of pigmented RPE are seen in the macula

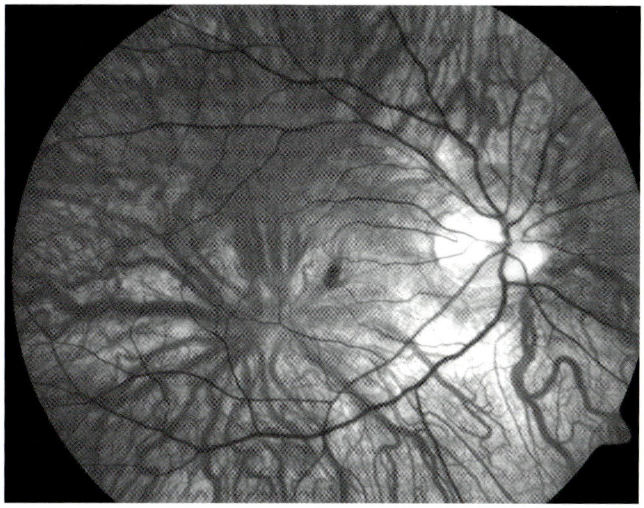

Red free photograph shows increased visibility of the larger choroidal vessels due to lack of pigment in the more anterior layers

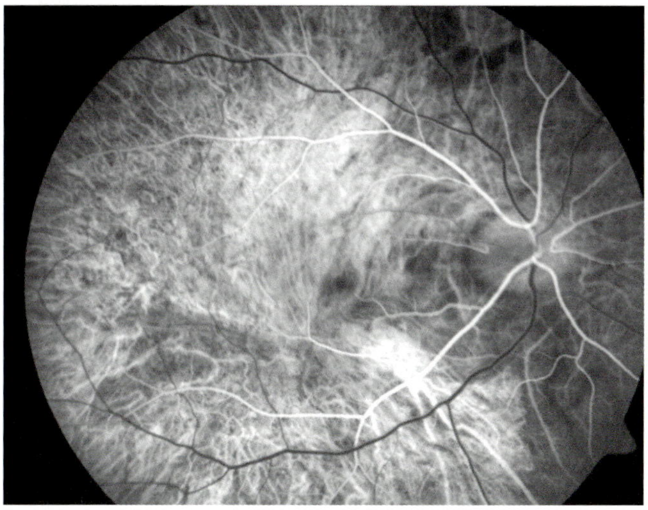

Arterial phase of the angiogram shows increased visibility of the larger choroidal vessels due to lack of blockage by the normally pigmented RPE. The choroidal details are blurred in the few areas of preserved RPE in the macula

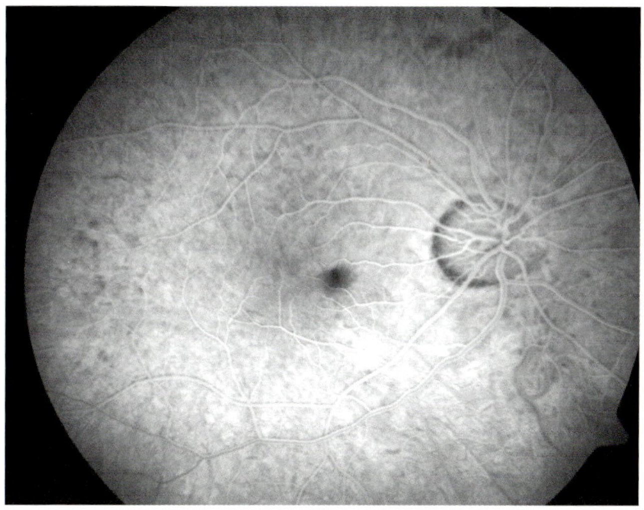

A diffuse choroidal fluorescence is seen due to leakage of dye from the choriocapillaris. Note the retinal vessels are not clearly visualized due to lack of contrast

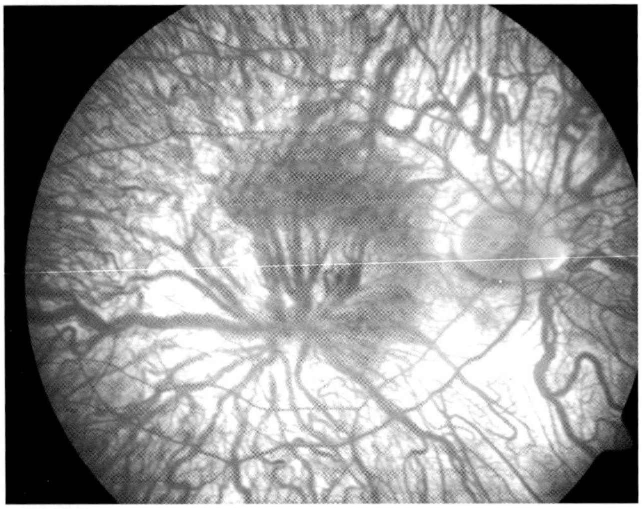

Late phase shows the relatively hypofluorescent larger choroidal vessels and the retinal vessels silhouetted against the background fluorescence due to scleral staining

COMMENT

There is increased visibility of the large choroidal vessels as the pigment in the RPE, which normally blocks the choroidal fluorescence, is deficient.

CASE 1 (*Continued*)

Left Eye of the Patient

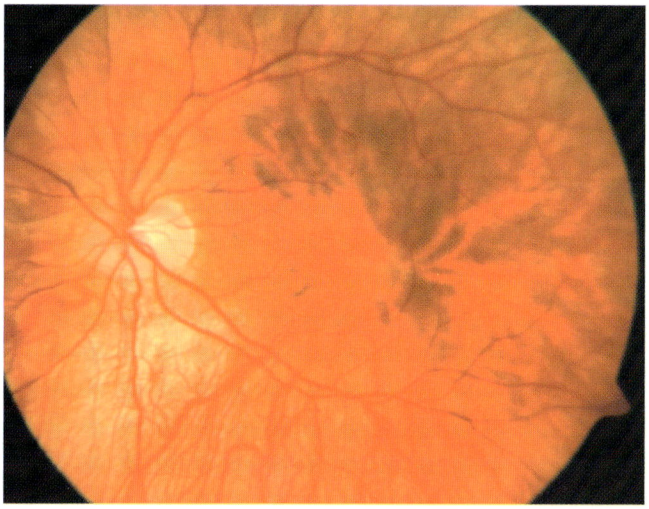

Fundus photograph of the left eye showing the depigmented fundus. Areas of normal pigmented RPE is noted in the macula

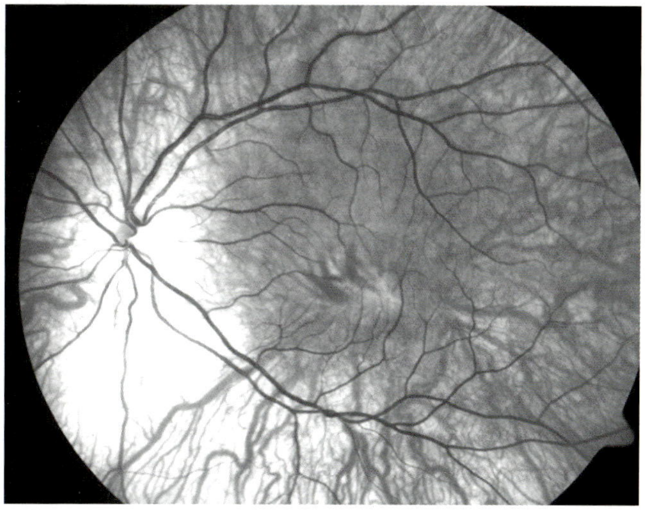

Red free photograph of the left eye

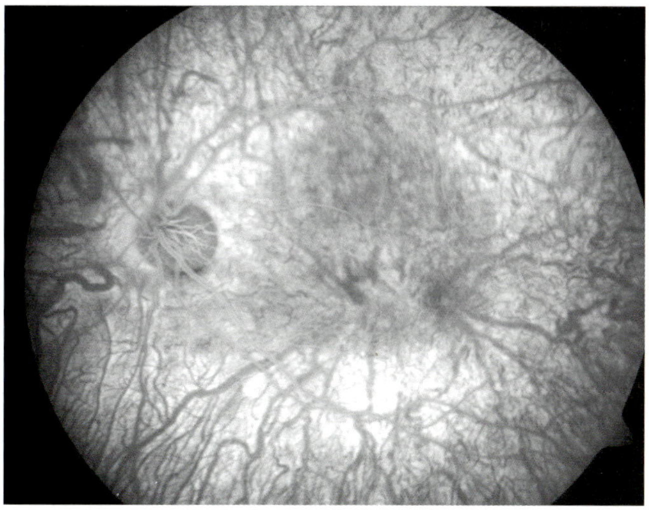

Arteriovenous phase of the angiogram showing increased visibility of the larger choroidal vessels due to lack of blockage by the pigment. It is difficult to appreciate the retinal vessels due to lack of contrast. The normal foveal hypofluorescence is absent

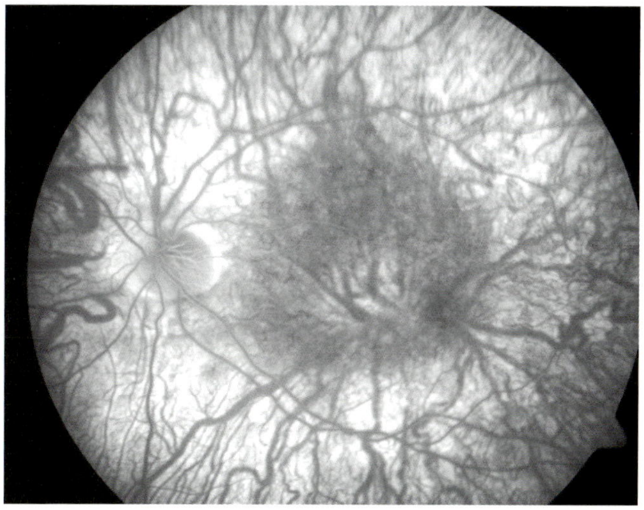

Late phase showing the choroidal and retinal vessels silhouetted against the background scleral staining. The areas of pigmented RPE in the macula is seen to block this background fluorescence

COMMENT

The normal hypofluorescence that is seen at the fovea is absent due to the reduced pigment in the RPE.

Foveal hypoplasia is commonly associated with ocular albinism and is characterized by absent or an ill formed FAZ.

CLINICAL NUGGETS

1. Albinism is a group of inherited disorders characterized by absent or deficient pigmentation.
2. Skin, hair and eyes are involved in oculocutaneous albinism; abnormal pigmentation primarily involves the eyes in ocular albinism.

BIBLIOGRAPHY

1. Gregor. The perifoveal vasculature in albinism. Br J Ophthalmol 1978;62:554-7.
2. Spedick MJ, Beauchamp GR. Retinal vascular and optic nerve abnormality in albinism. J Pediatric Ophthalmology Strabismus 1986;23:58-63.

Chapter 59

Retinitis Pigmentosa and Allied Disorders

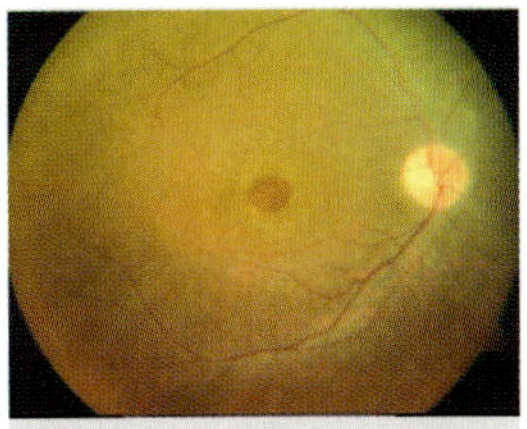

- Retinitis pigmentosa (RP) is characterized by arteriolar attenuation, disc pallor and bony spicule pigmentation in the mid-peripheral fundus.
- Mottled retinal pigment epithelial changes are seen throughout the fundus.
- In early stages of retinitis pigmentosa, fundus findings are better delineated on fluorescein angiogram.

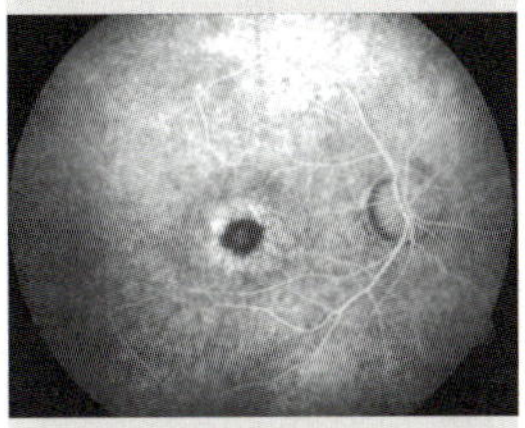

- The angiographic appearance in retinitis pigmentosa depends on the severity of the retinal changes.
- In early RP, the choroidal flush is normal, with a mottled hyperfluorescence seen more prominently in the mid-peripheral retina.
- As the disease progresses, patches of choriocapillary non-filling are noted.
- In advanced disease, due to loss of the choriocapillaris the choroidal flush may be absent.
- Leakage of dye from the retinal capillary causes increased staining of the retinal tissue in the late phase. This may be confined to the macular area or in the region of the vascular arcades, or it may be widespread. It is difficult to determine whether most of the fluorescein staining is derived from leaking retinal capillaries or choriocapillaris through the abnormal RPE.
- Cystoid macular edema is seen in a small percentage of patients of RP.
- An increased retinal circulation time is seen.

CASE 1

A 40-year-old female presented with history of decreased vision in the left eye for the past one year. Visual acuity was 6/36; N36 in the left eye. Right eye had similar fundus findings. Electroretinogram showed markedly reduced responses in both eyes.

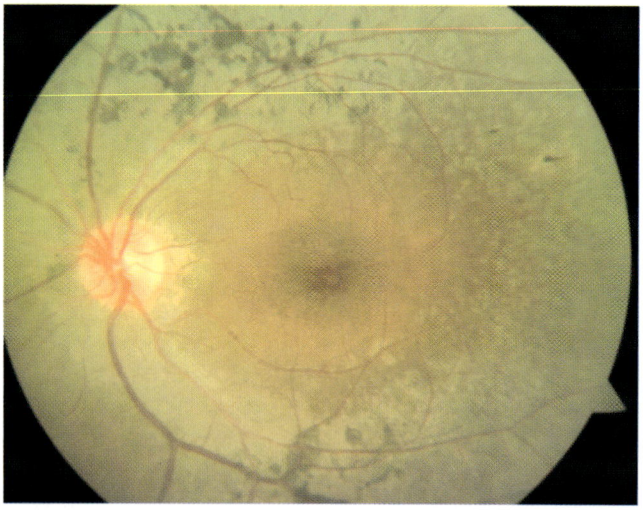

Fundus photograph of the left eye showing RPE alteration and pigment clumping along the arcades. The peripheral retina was relatively unaffected

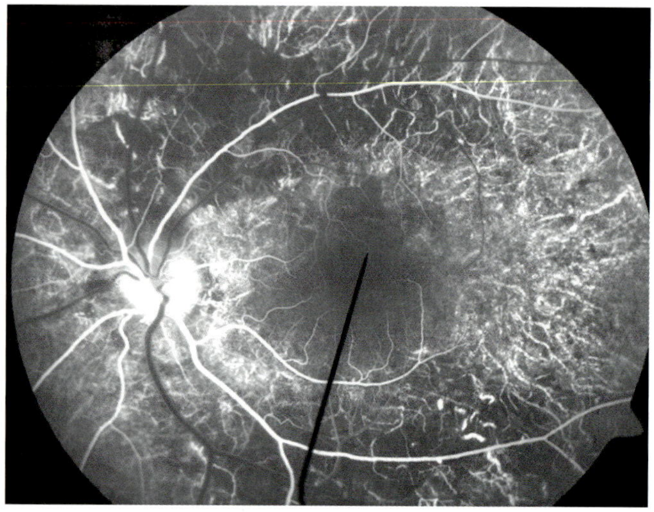

Arterial phase of the angiogram showing large choroidal vessels in areas of RPE and choriocapillaris atrophy

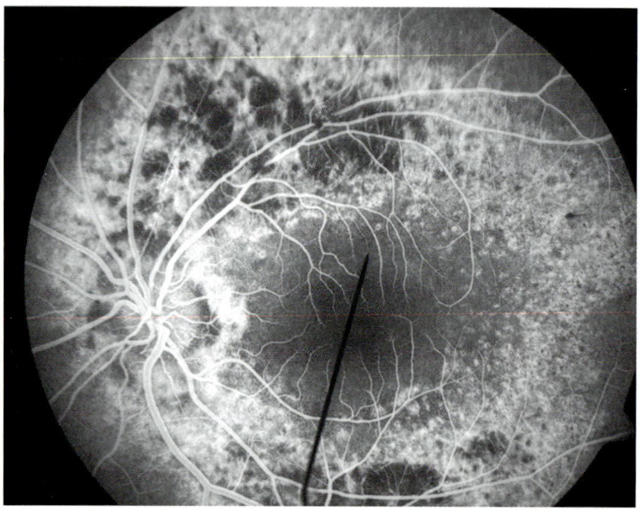

Transmitted fluorescence is seen in the affected areas

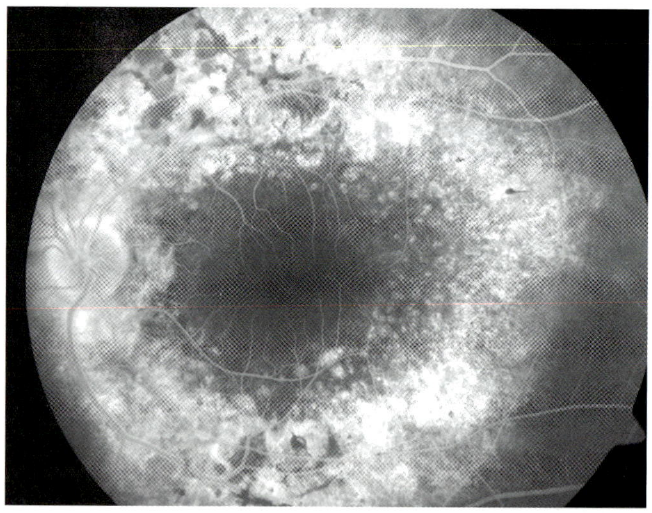

Late phase angiogram showing the background scleral staining as hyperfluorescence through the overlying atrophied layers

COMMENT

Fluorescein angiography is useful to assess the status of the choriocapillaris in RP.
Early hyperfluorescence through the window defects in the RPE suggests intact choriocapillaris.
Delayed hyperfluorescence indicates atrophy of the choriocapillaris.
Fluorescein angiography can thus be of prognostic value in patients with RP.

CASE 2

A 45-year-old female presented with a history of night blindness for the past fifteen years. She noticed floaters in front of both eyes for the last three months. Examination did not reveal any inflammatory process in the eye. Visual acuity was 6/9; N18 in both eyes.

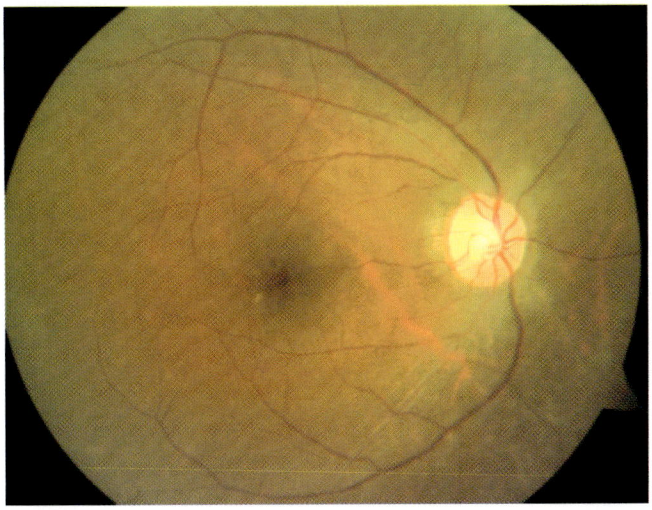

Fundus photograph of the right eye showing attenuated arterioles. Retinal thickening was noted at the fovea on biomicroscopic examination

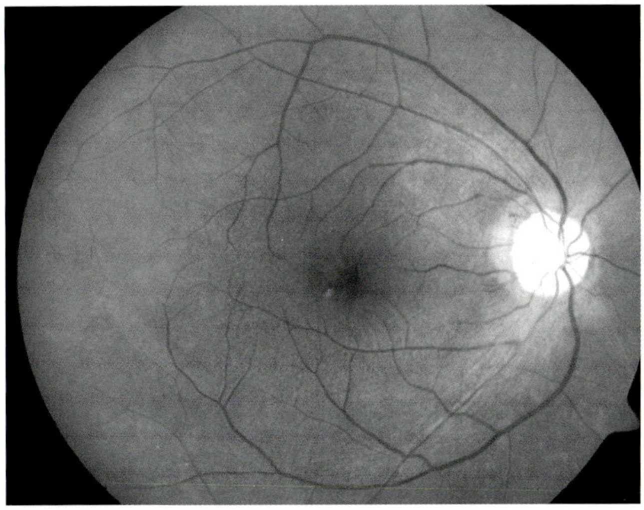

Red free photograph of the right eye

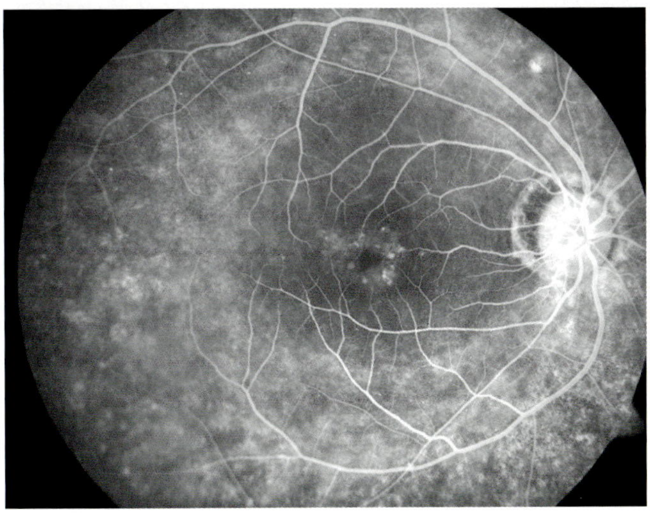

Arteriovenous phase showing dilation of the parafoveal capillaries with minimal leakage of the dye. Irregular hyperfluorescence due to transmission defect is seen elsewhere in the fundus

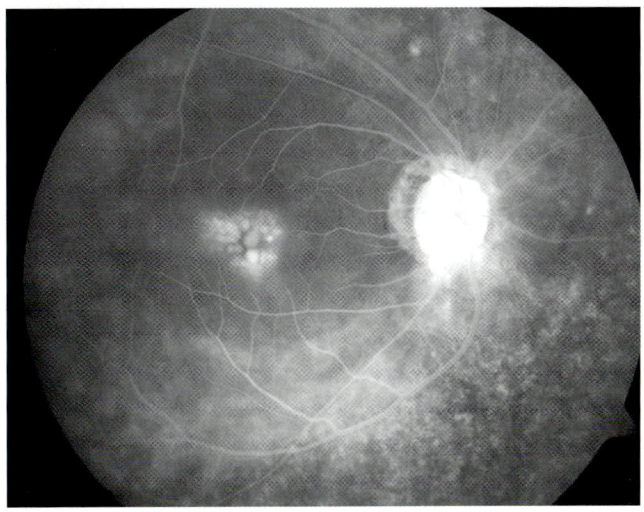

Late phase shows accumulation of the dye in cystoid spaces at the fovea. Minimal staining of the retina is also evident along the inferotemporal arcade

CASE 2 (*Continued*)

Left Eye of the Patient

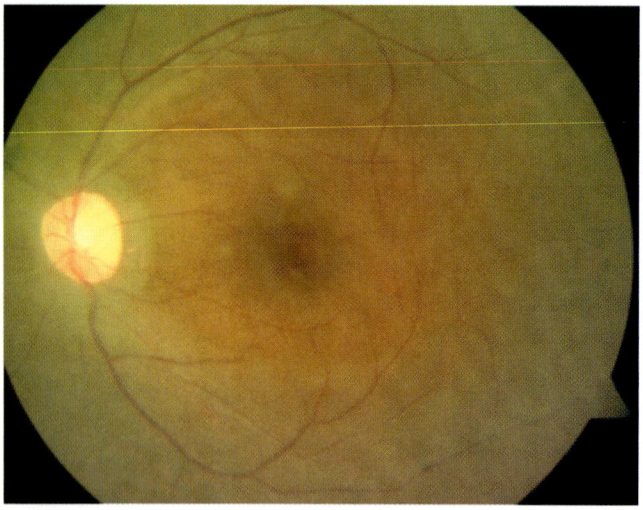

Fundus photograph of the left eye showing arteriolar attenuation and RPE alterations beyond the arcade. Cystoid changes were seen clinically at the fovea

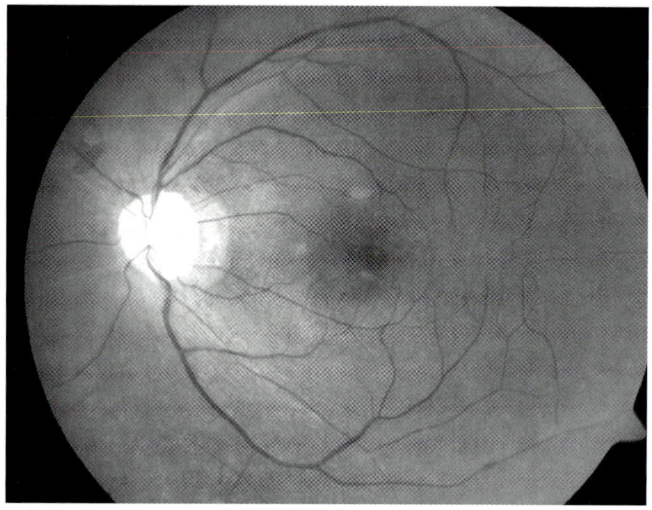

Red free photograph of the left eye

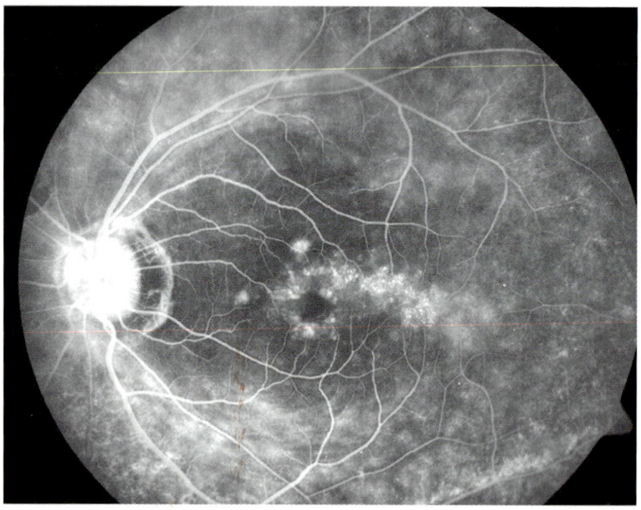

Arteriovenous phase showing leakage of the dye from the capillaries around the fovea. Widespread irregular hyperfluorescence is seen due to window defects

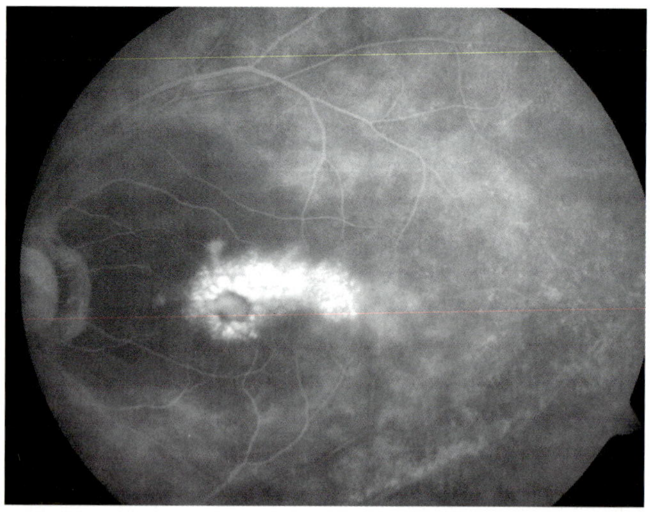

Late phase showing cystoid macular edema

COMMENT

A small percentage of patients with RP develop cystoid macular changes. The leakage is most likely from the parafoveal and perifoveal capillaries.

CASE 3

A 19-year-old male presented with progressive decrease of vision in dim illumination for the past four years. Visual acuity was 6/36; N18 in both eyes. Electroretinogram showed grossly reduced responses.

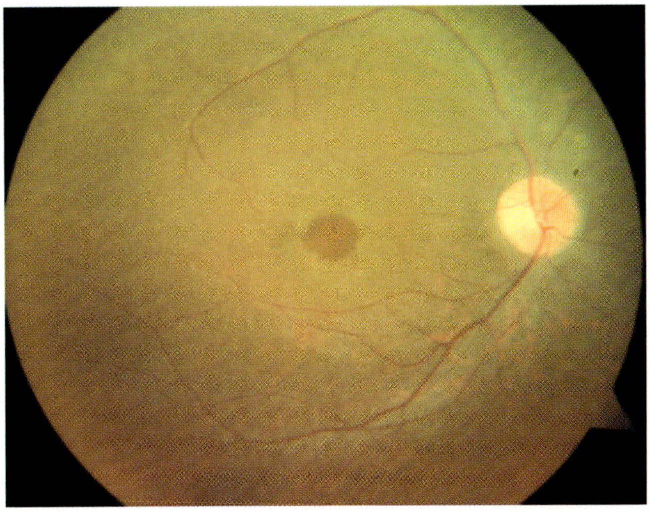

Fundus photograph of the right eye showing an annular atrophy around the fovea. Arteriolar attenuation and widespread RPE alteration are also seen

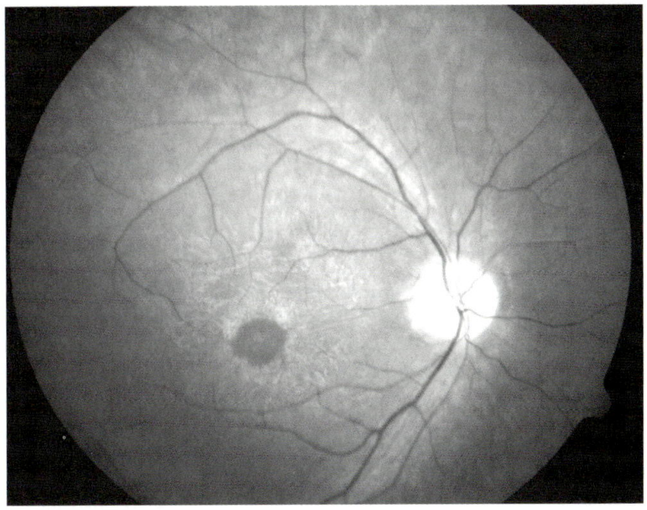

Red free photograph of the right eye

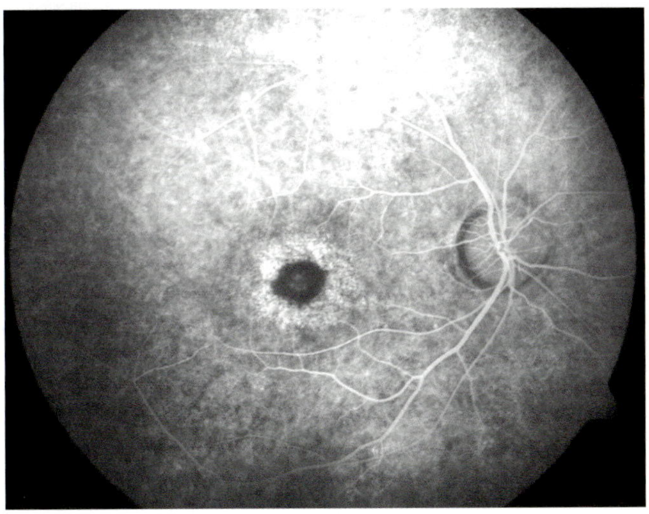

Hyperfluorescence due to transmission defect is seen at the atrophic ring around the fovea. Elsewhere in the fundus, irregular stippled hyperfluorescence due to RPE atrophy is seen. The normal hypofluorescence at the fovea is accentuated by the surrounding hyperfluorescence

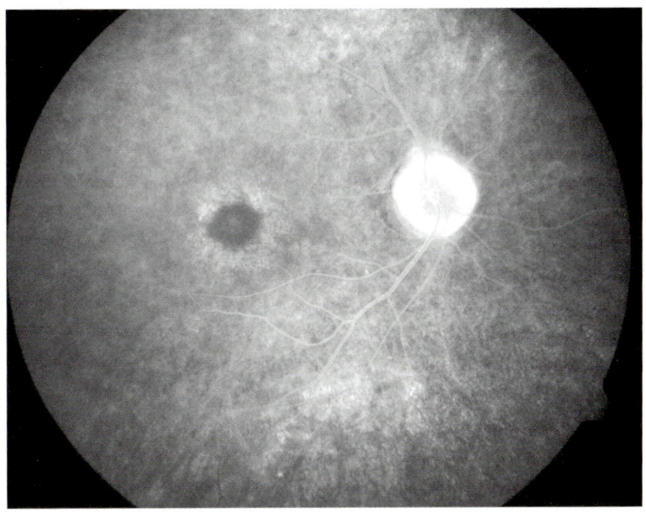

Late phase angiogram shows fading of the hyperfluorescence

CASE 3 (*Continued*)

Left Eye of the Patient

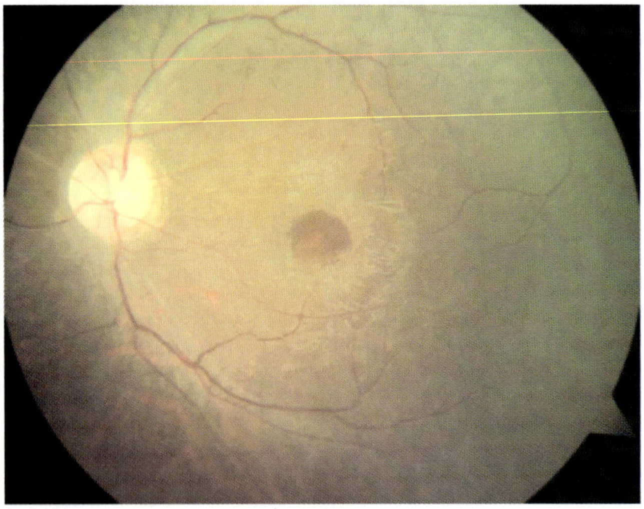

Fundus photograph of the left eye showing similar changes as that in the right eye

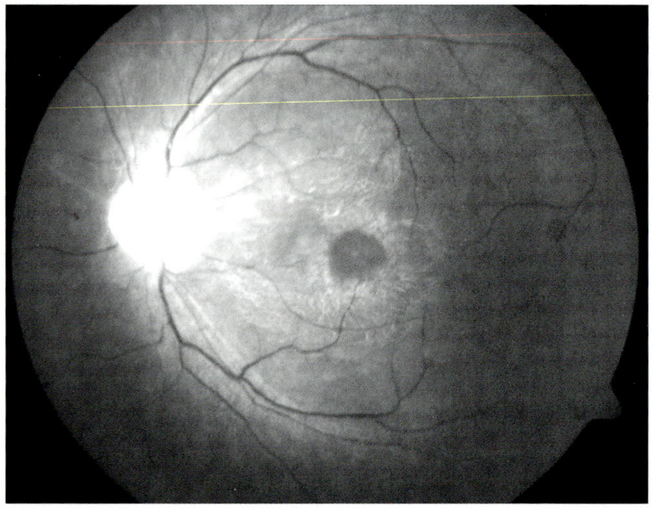

Red free photograph of the left eye

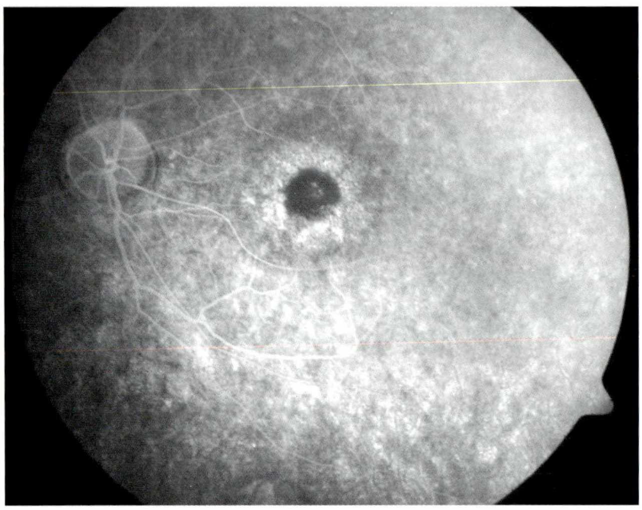

Arteriovenous phase showing hyperfluorescence due to transmission defects. The annular atrophy around the fovea is well made out

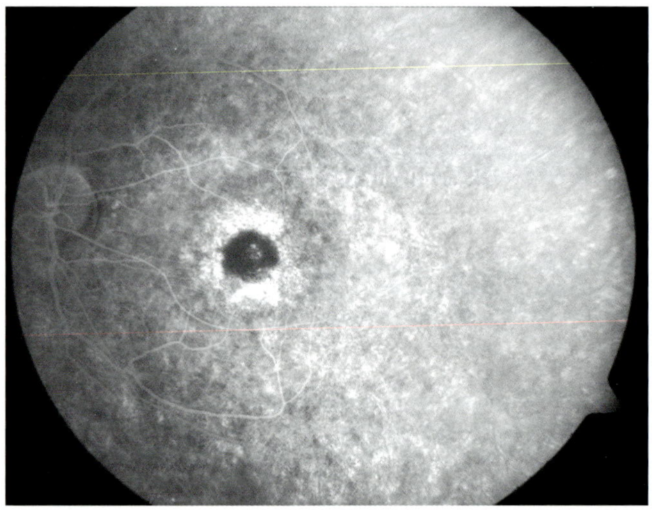

Some fading of the hyperfluorescence is seen in the late film

COMMENT

Development of atrophic changes at the macula is an important cause of reduction in the central vision in patients with RP. Bull's eye like lesion due to atrophic changes in the parafoveal region can occur.

CASE 4

A 37-year-old female presented with history of difficulty in dim illumination for the past one year. Visual acuity was 6/6; N6 in both eyes. Electroretinogram showed unrecordable responses.

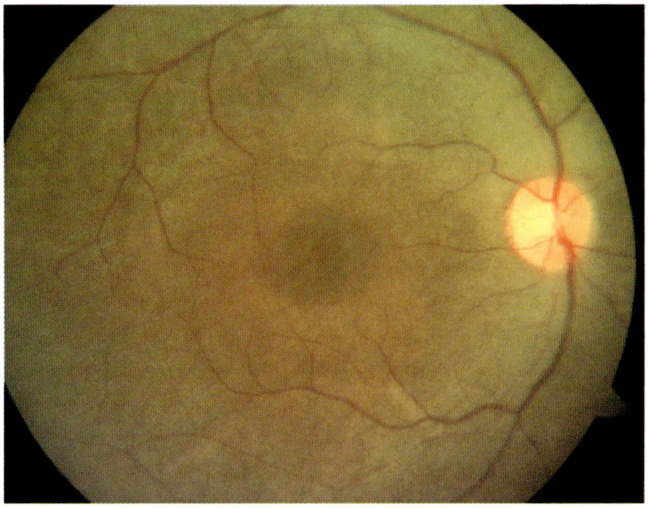

Fundus photograph of the right eye showing arteriolar attenuation and RPE alterations along the arcade

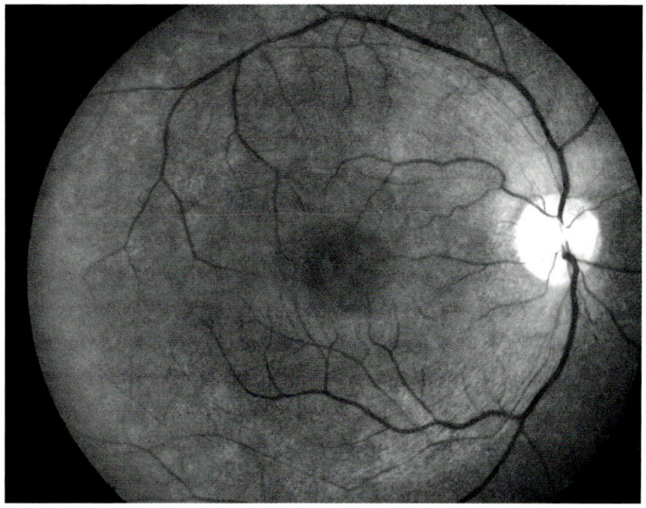

Red free photograph of the right eye

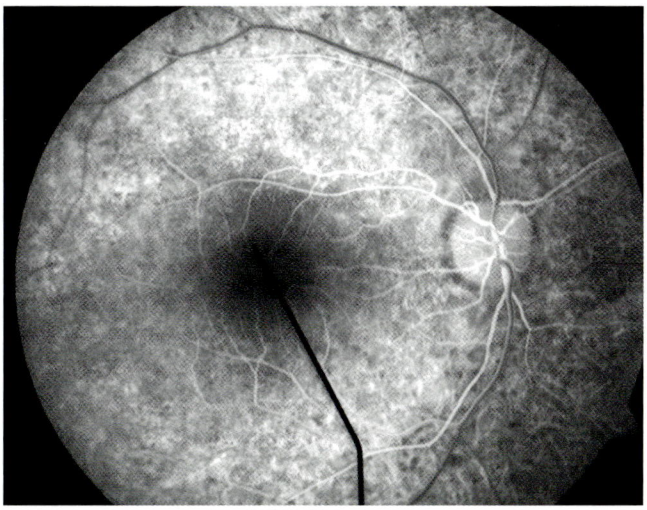

Early arteriovenous phase showing widespread irregular stippled hyperfluorescence

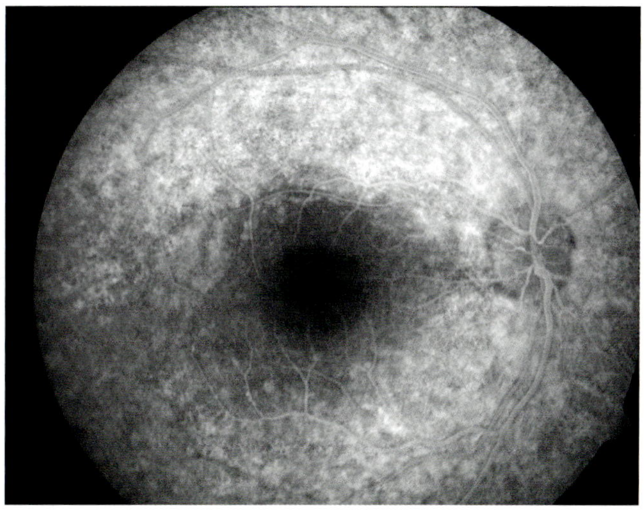

Increase in the transmitted fluorescence is seen in the arteriovenous phase

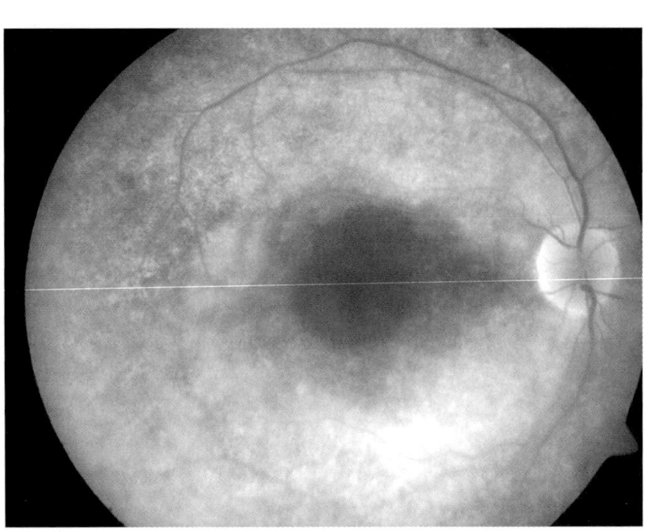

Late phase angiogram showing increased staining of the retina inferotemporal and superotemporal to the disc

CASE 4 (*Continued*)

Left Eye of the Patient

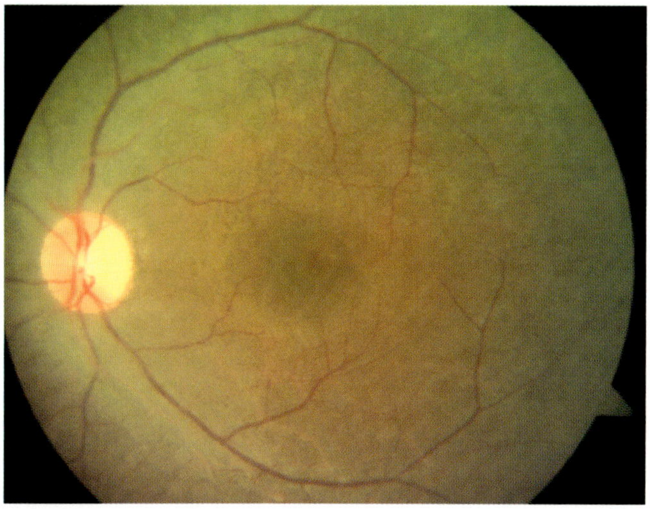

Fundus photograph of the left eye showing similar changes as in the right eye

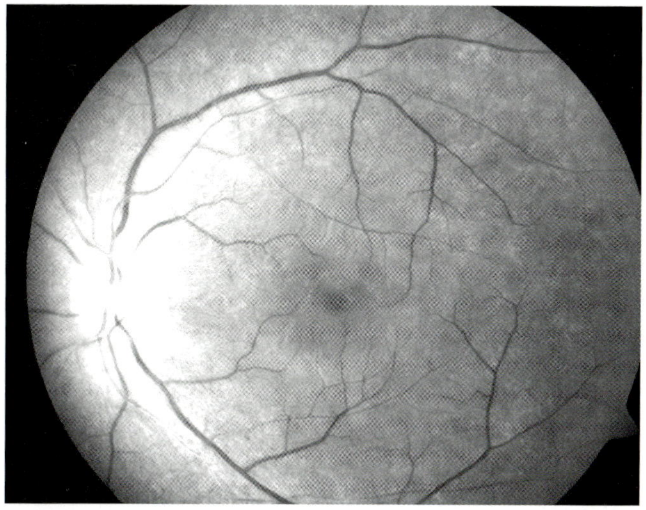

Red free photograph of the left eye

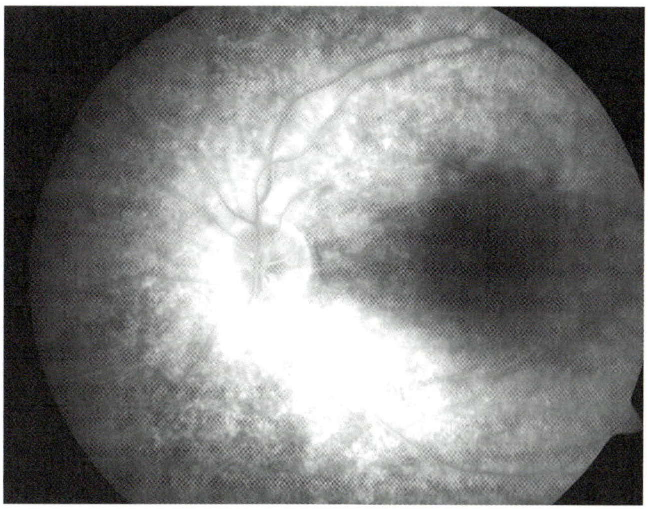

Arteriovenous phase showing transmitted fluorescence throughout the fundus. Normal hypofluorescence at the fovea is seen

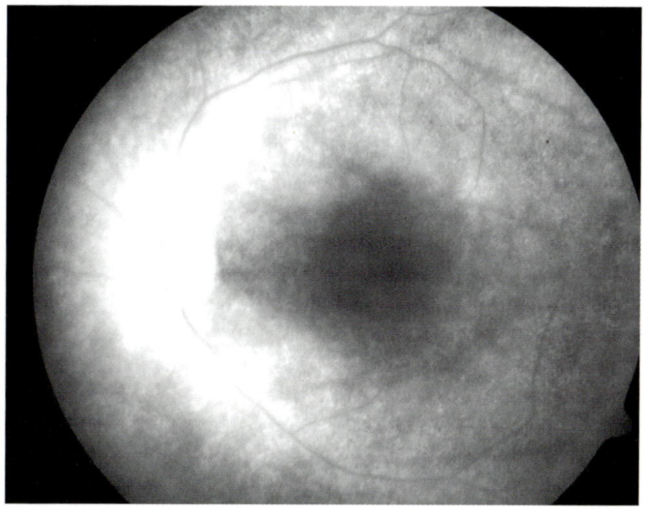

Late phase angiogram showing some staining of the retina along the arcades

COMMENT

Leakage of the dye into the retinal tissue can occur either from the retinal blood vessels or from choriocapillaris through the defects in the RPE layer. Late phase angiogram shows diffuse staining of the retina in these cases.

CASE 5

A 15-year-old child was brought for examination with a history of night blindness since early childhood. Visual acuity was 6/18; N6 in both eyes. Electroretinogram showed unrecordable responses.

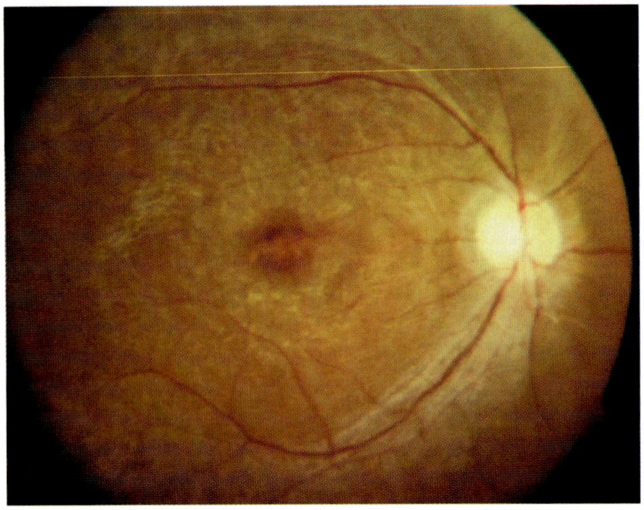

Fundus photograph of the right eye showing annular atrophy around the fovea. Arteriolar attenuation and widespread RPE alteration is also seen

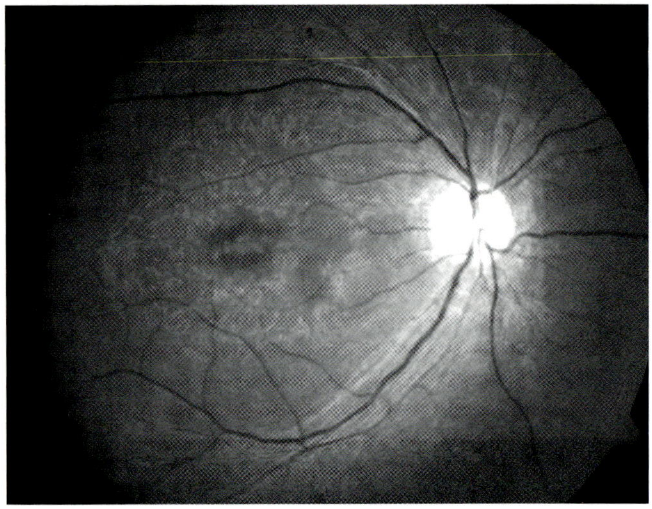

Red free photograph of the right eye

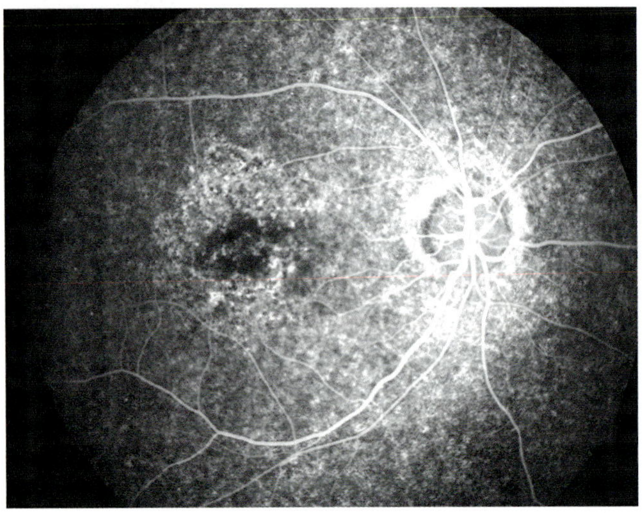

Hyperfluorescence due to transmission defect is seen at the atrophic ring around the fovea. Elsewhere in the fundus, irregular stippled hyperfluorescence is seen. Transmission defect is also evident at the foveal center

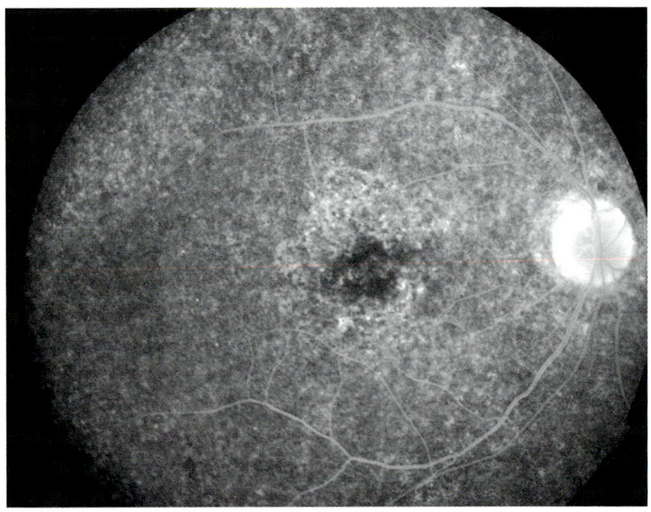

Late phase angiogram shows some fading of the hyperfluorescence

CASE 5 (*Continued*)

Left Eye of the Patient

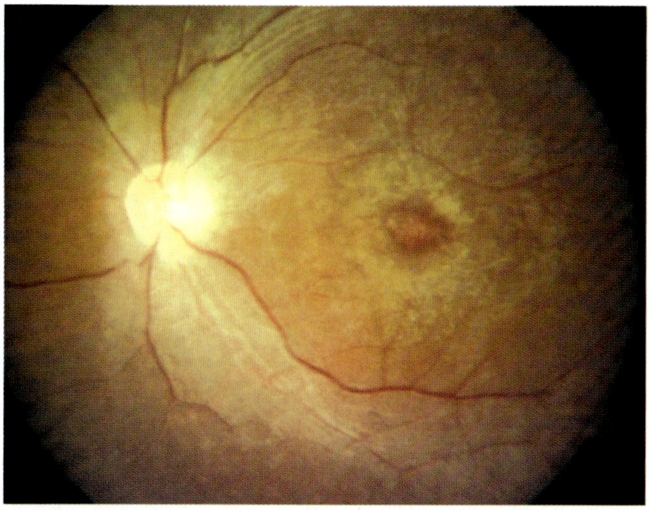

Fundus photograph of the left eye showing similar changes as that in the right eye

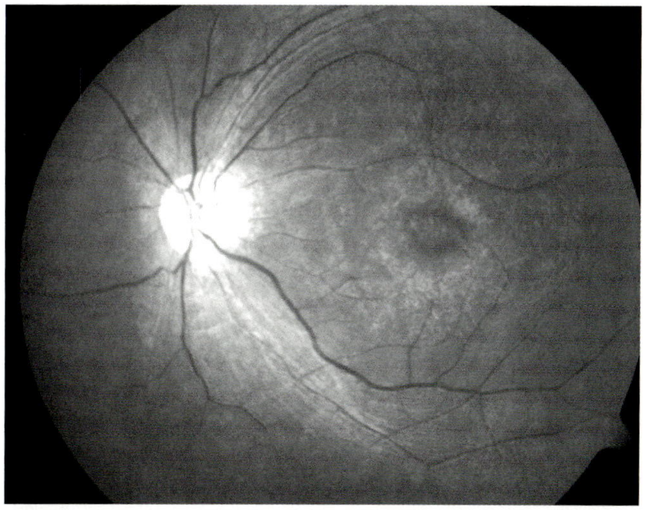

Red free photograph of the left eye

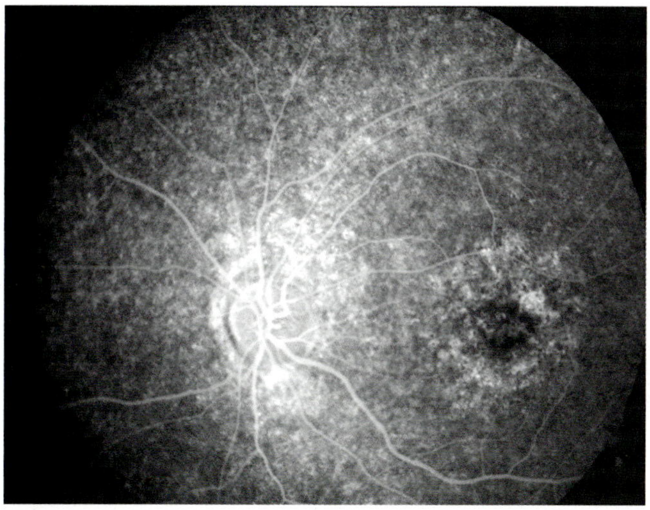

Arteriovenous phase showing hyperfluorescence due to transmission defects. Transmission defects are also seen at the foveal center

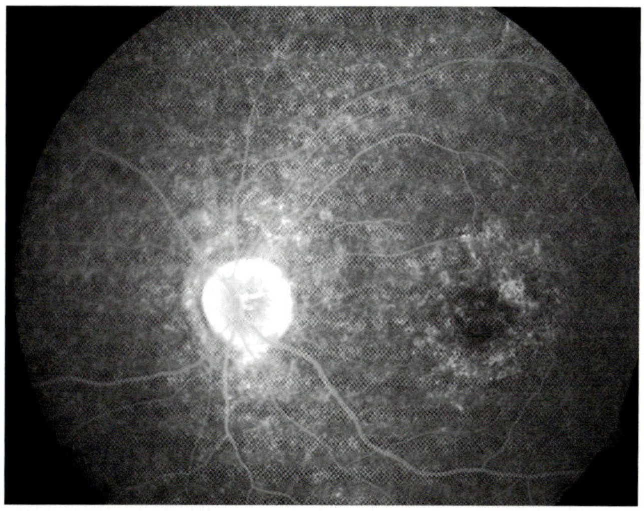

Fading of the hyperfluorescence is seen in the late film

COMMENT

The diffuse RPE alterations occurring in RP are seen on the angiogram as stippled transmitted fluorescence throughout the fundus.

CHOROIDEREMIA

CASE 6

A 31-year-old male presented with a history of night blindness since early childhood. He complained of decreased vision in the right eye for the past 15 days. Visual acuity was 6/12; N10 in the right eye and 6/9; N6 in the left eye.

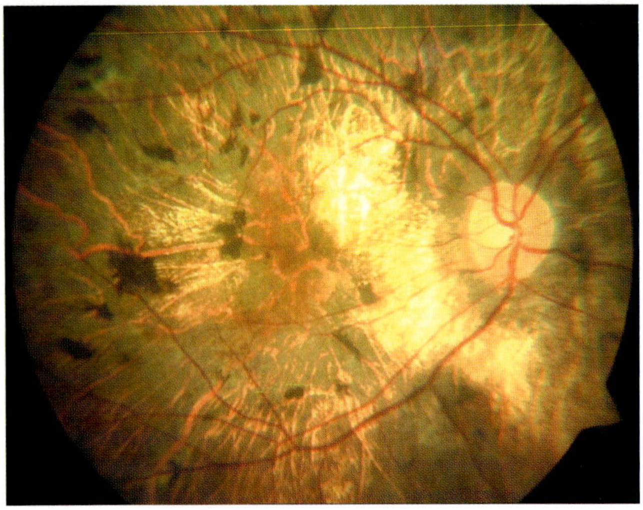

Fundus photograph of the right eye shows extensive atrophy of the RPE and choriocapillaris. A strip of RPE is preserved at the fovea; pigment clumps are seen

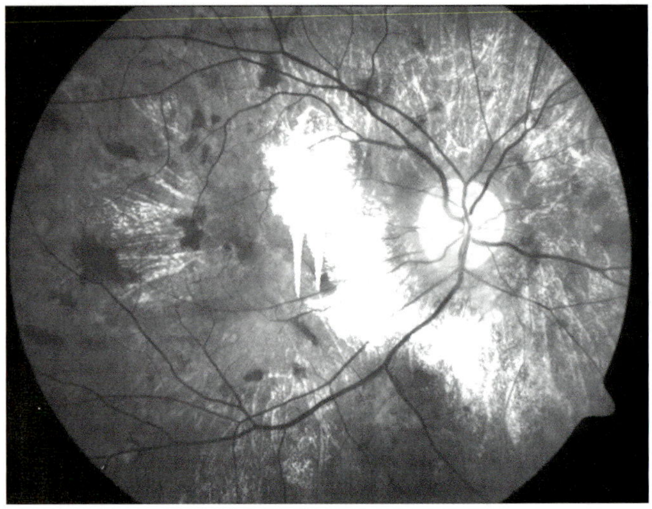

Red free photograph of the right eye

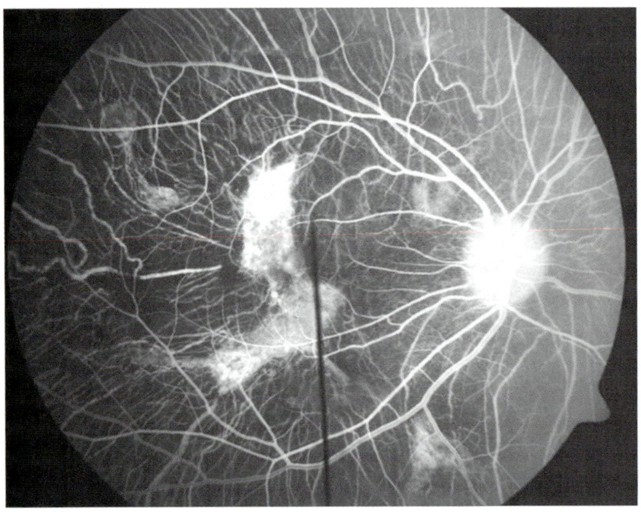

Arteriovenous phase showing the absence of the choriocapillaris except for a vertical strip at the fovea. The large choroidal vessels are seen

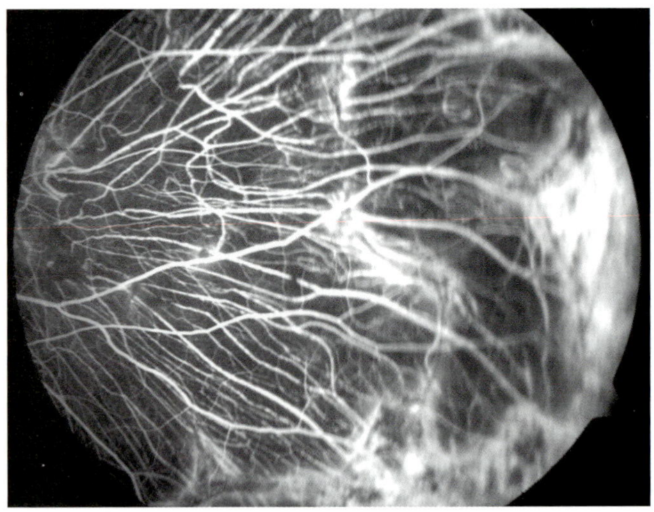

Peripheral fundus in the arteriovenous phase showing large choroidal vessels due to absence of overlying RPE and choriocapillaris

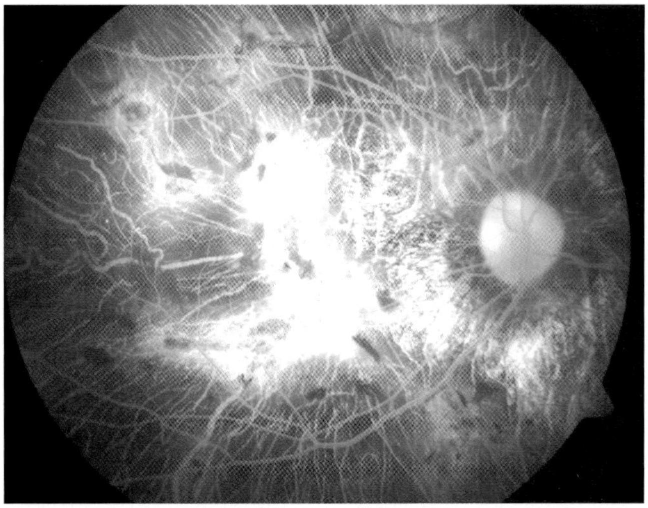

Late phase angiogram showing very minimal staining of the sclera in the areas of atrophy

CASE 6 (*Continued*)

Left Eye of the Patient

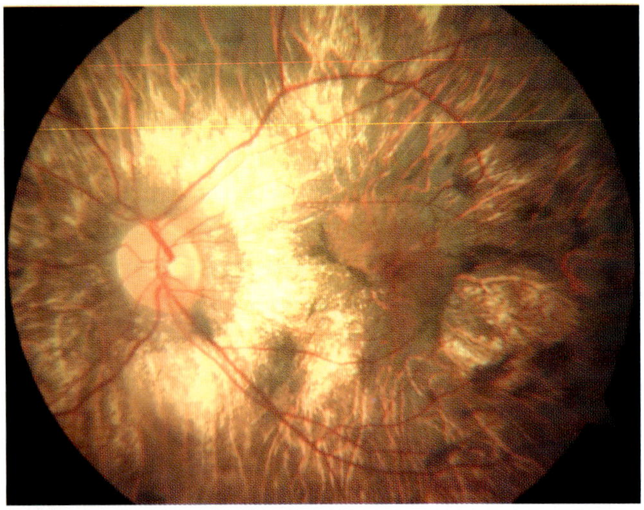

Fundus photograph of the left eye showing absence of RPE and choriocapillaris except for a small patch at the fovea

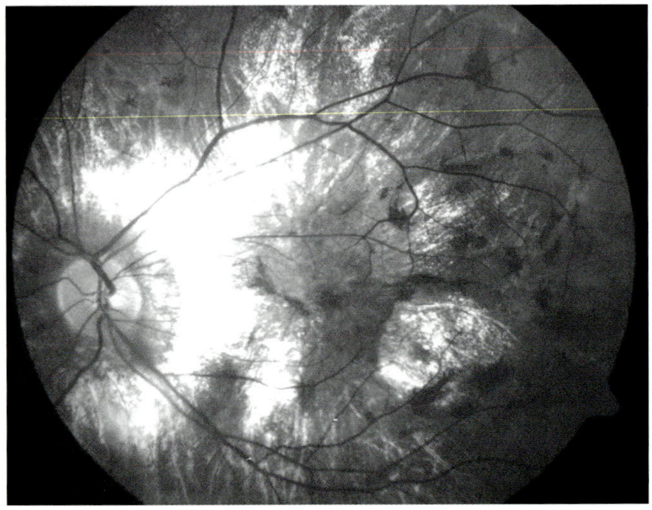

Red free photograph of the left eye

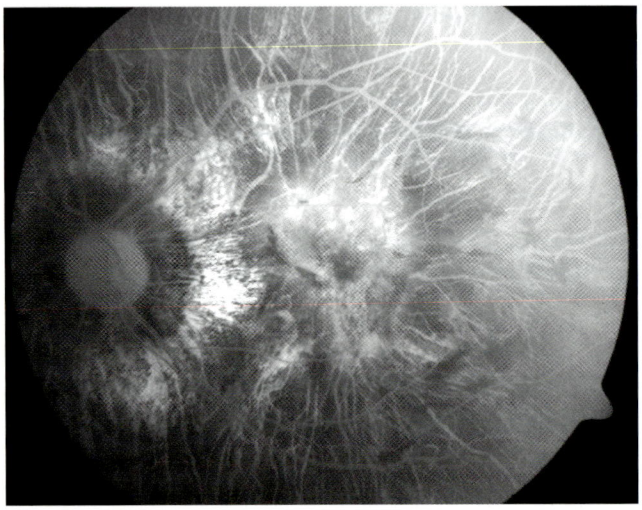

Late phase showing the central patch of preserved RPE

COMMENT

Diffuse loss of the choriocapillaris is the hallmark of choroideremia.

The normal prominent scleral staining that occurs in the late phase is not seen in this condition as the leakage of dye is minimal from the atrophic choriocapillaris.

GYRATE ATROPHY

CASE 7

A 25-year-old female presented with history of reduced night vision. Visual acuity was 6/9; N6 in both eyes. The serum ornithine levels were raised.

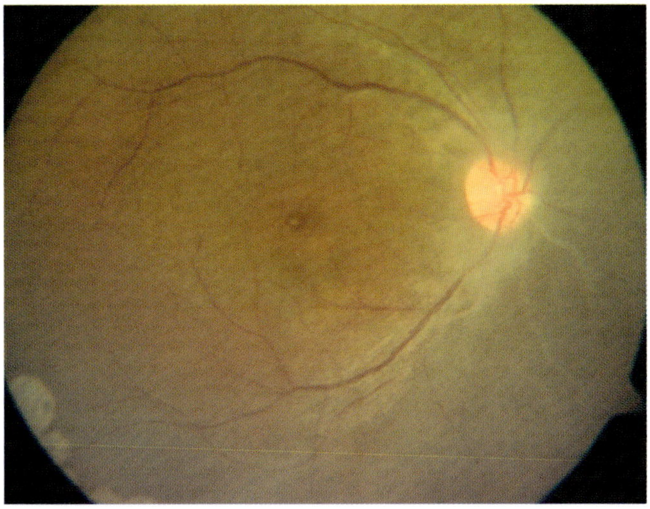

Fundus photograph of the posterior pole of the right eye of the patient. Discrete atrophic patches were seen in the midperiphery of the fundus

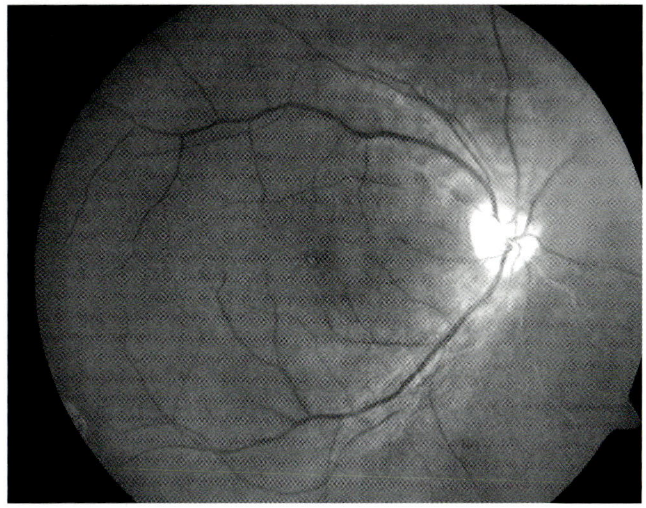

Red free photograph of the right eye

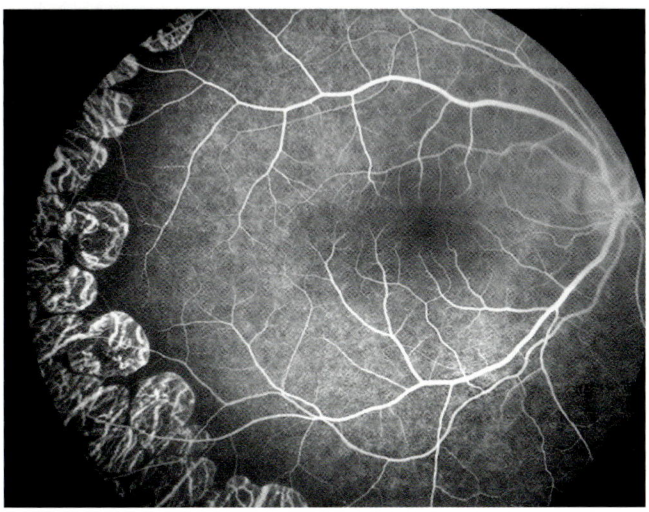

Mid arteriovenous phase showing the discrete chorioretinal atrophic patches in the midperiphery. The large choroidal vessels are seen within the lesions

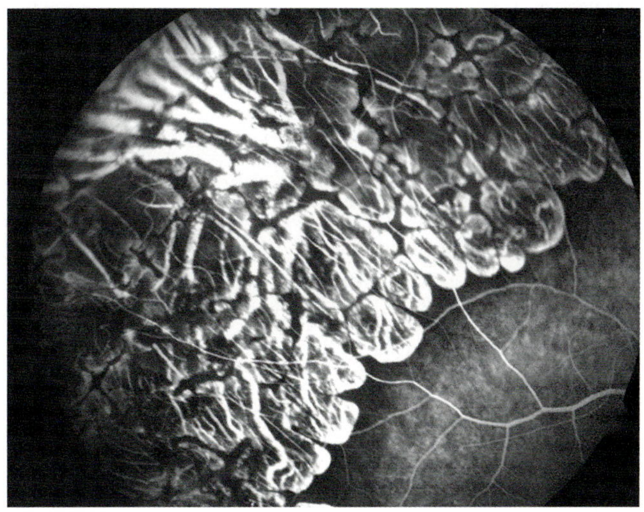

Atrophic patches seen in the superotemporal mid-periphery

COMMENT

Gyrate atrophy is characterized by the loss of discrete patches of RPE and choriocapillaris.

CASE 7 (*Continued*)

Left Eye of the Patient

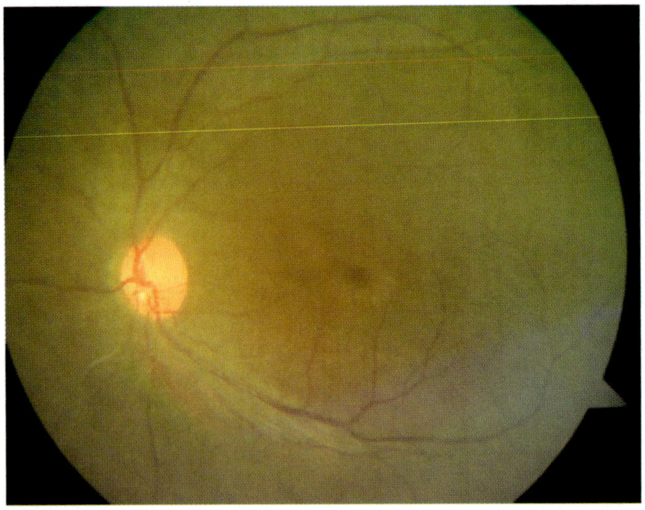

Fundus photograph of the left eye

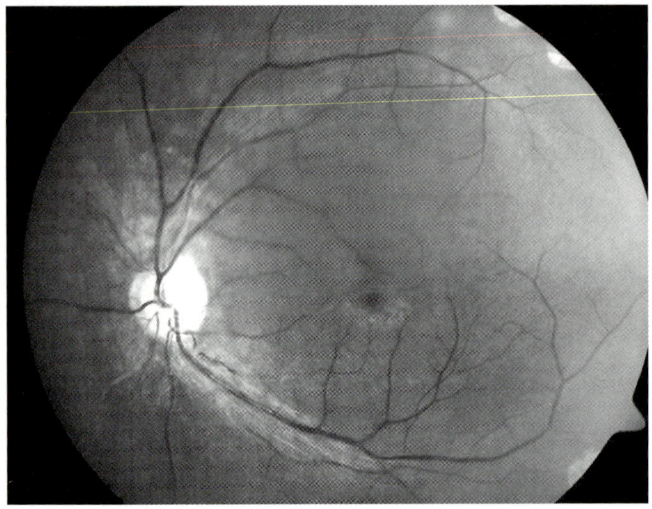

Red free photograph of the left eye

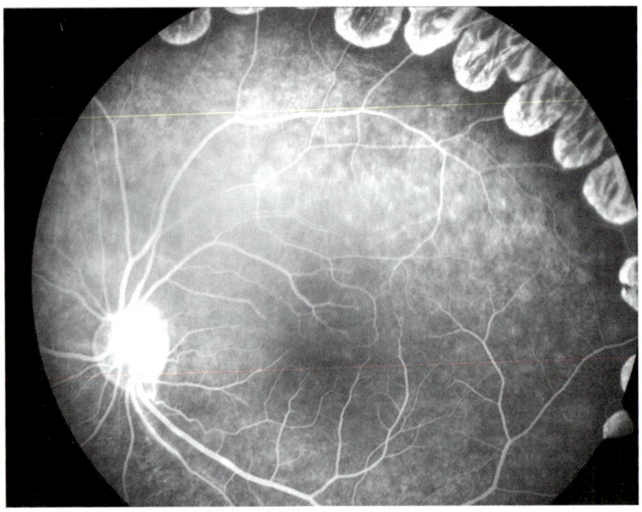

Arteriovenous phase showing the atrophic patches temporally

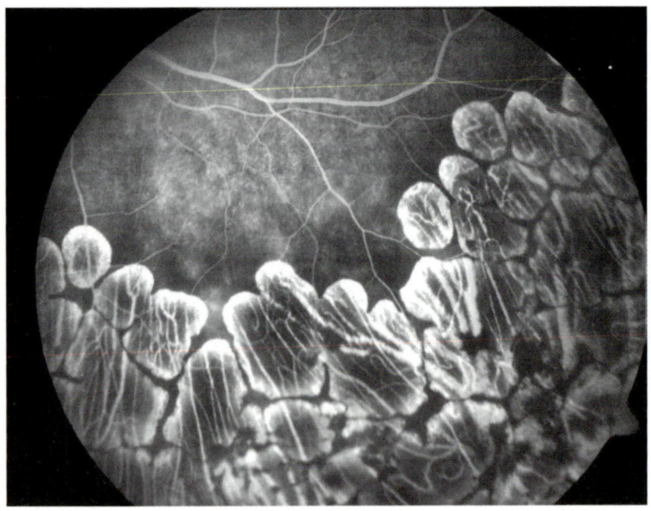

The discrete atrophic patches seen in the inferotemporal quadrant

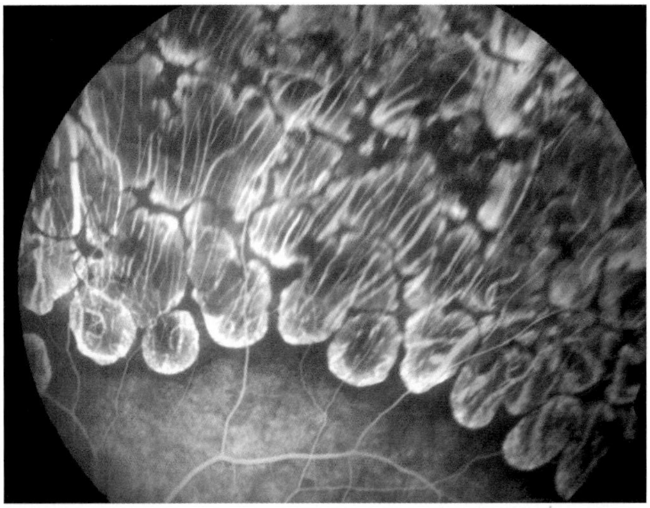

Superotemporal quadrant showing the discrete atrophic patches

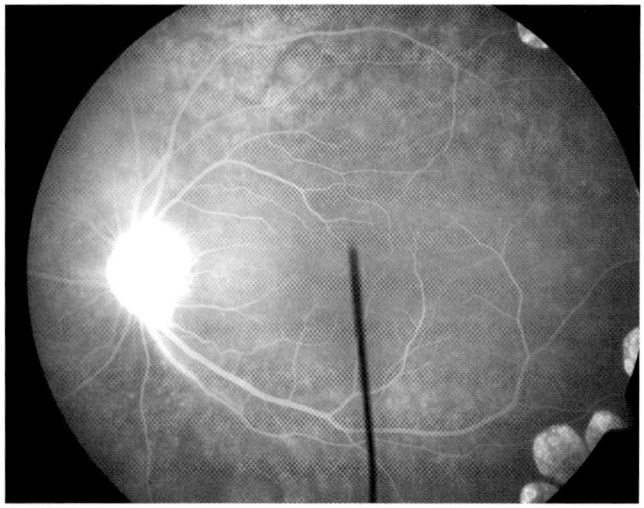

Late phase angiogram showing the normal posterior pole

PIGMENTED PARAVENOUS CHORIORETINAL ATROPHY

CASE 8

A 43-year-old male was referred with a diagnosis of retinitis pigmentosa in both eyes. Visual acuity was 6/9; N6 in both eyes. There was no history of night vision difficulty.

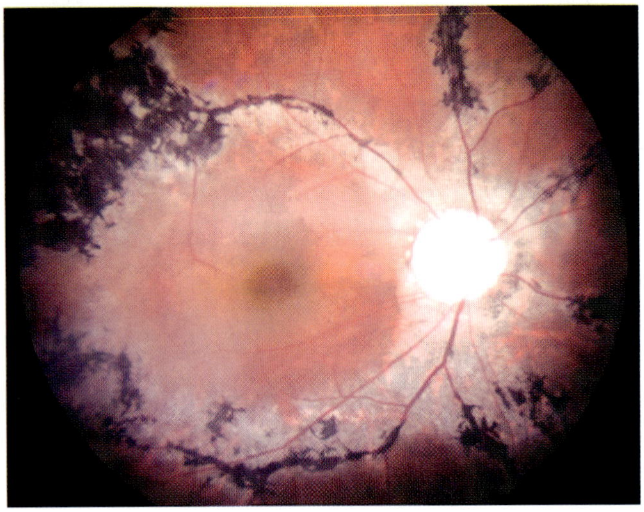

Fundus photograph of the right eye showing chorioretinal atrophy with associated pigment migration along the major retinal veins

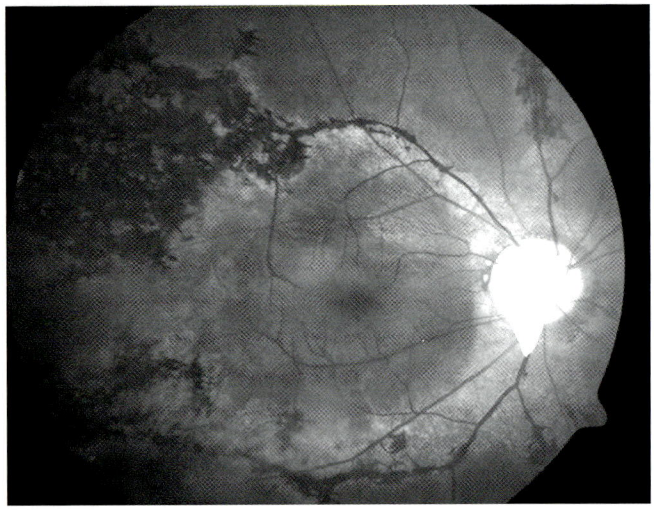

Red free photograph of the right eye

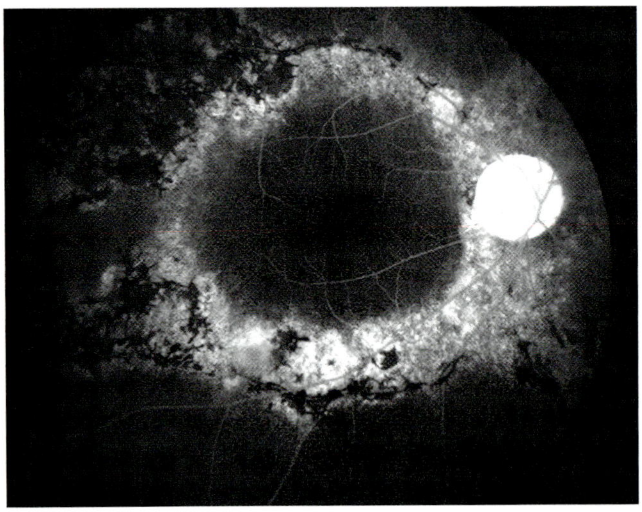

Increased hyperfluorescence due to transmission defects and areas of blocked fluorescence due to pigment are seen along the arcades

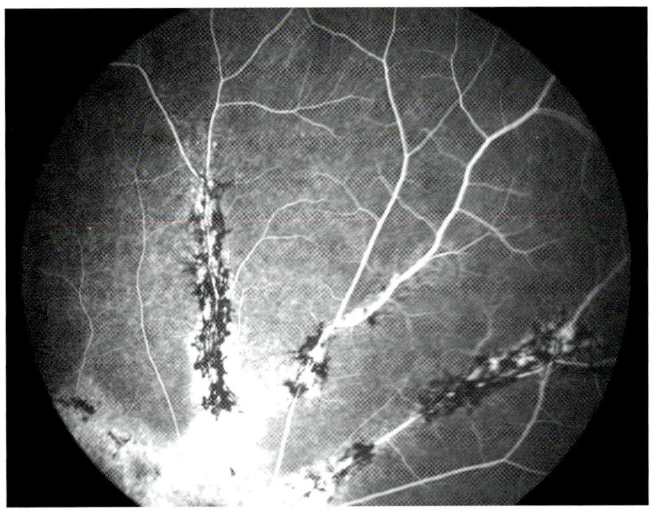

Similar areas are seen along the veins in the superonasal quadrant

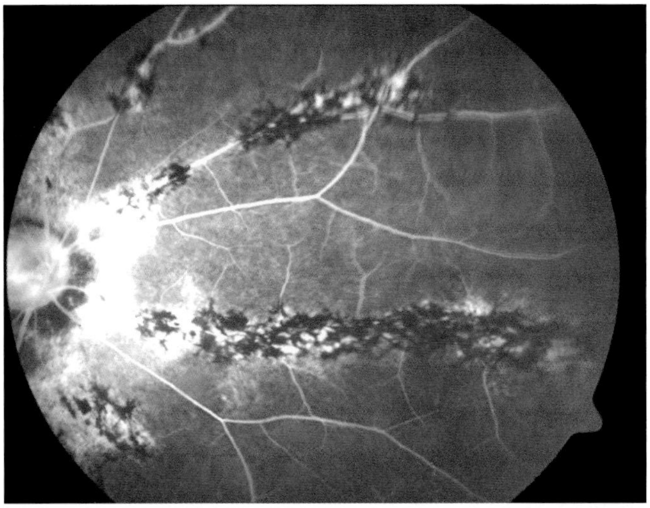

Nasal quadrant

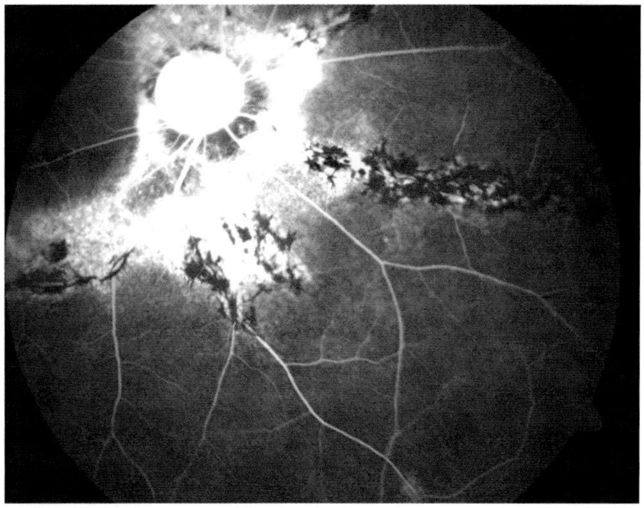

Inferonasal quadrant

CASE 8 (*Continued*)

Left Eye of the Patient

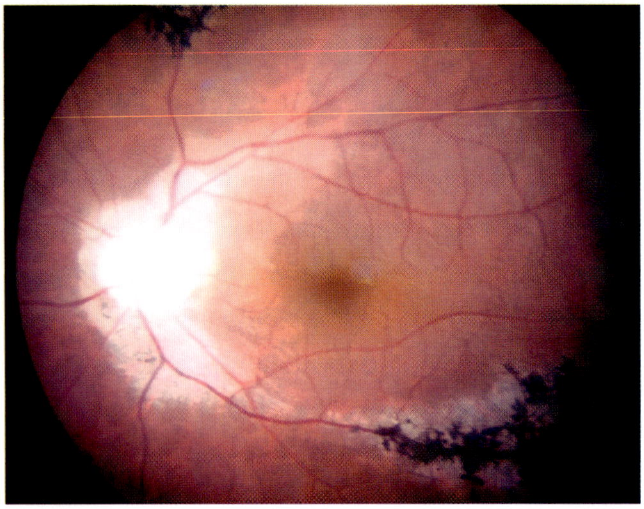

Fundus photograph of the left eye showing chorioretinal atrophy and pigmentary changes along the inferotemporal vessels

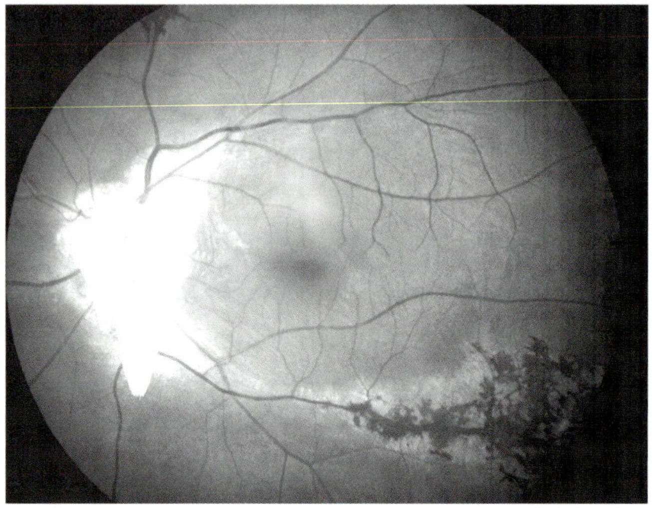

Red free photograph of the left eye

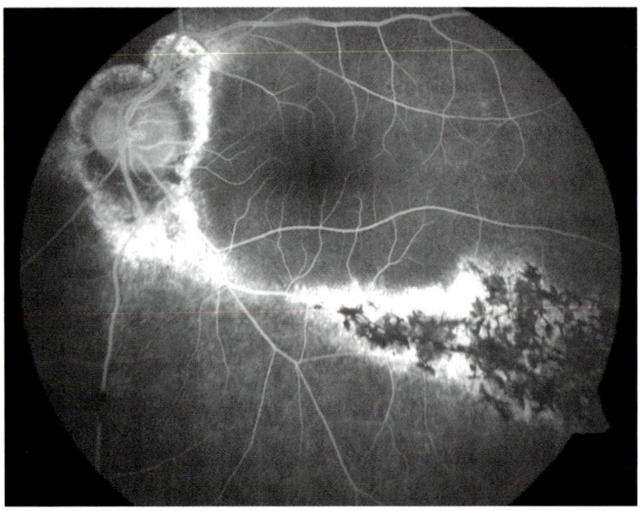

Areas of transmitted fluorescence with areas of blocked fluorescence are seen around the disc and along the inferotemporal vein

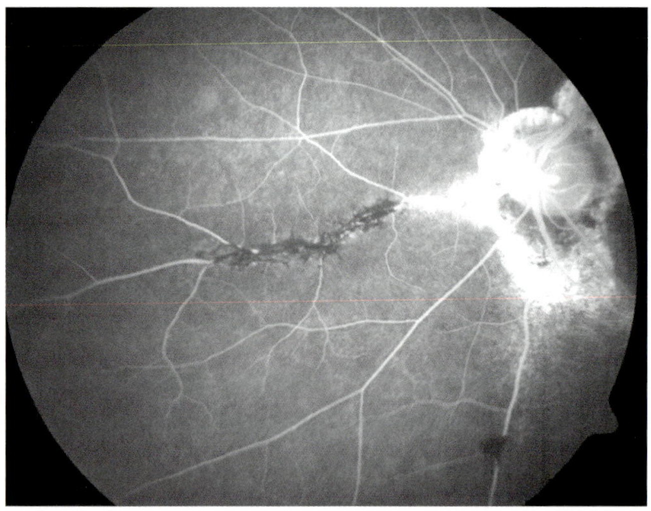

Similar changes seen extending along the vein in the nasal quadrant

FUNDUS ALBIPUNCTATUS

CASE 9

A 27-year-old male presented with history of night vision difficulty since early childhood. There was no worsening of the symptoms overs the years. Visual acuity was 6/6; N6 in both eyes. Electroretinogram showed reduced responses which improved after prolonged dark adaptation.

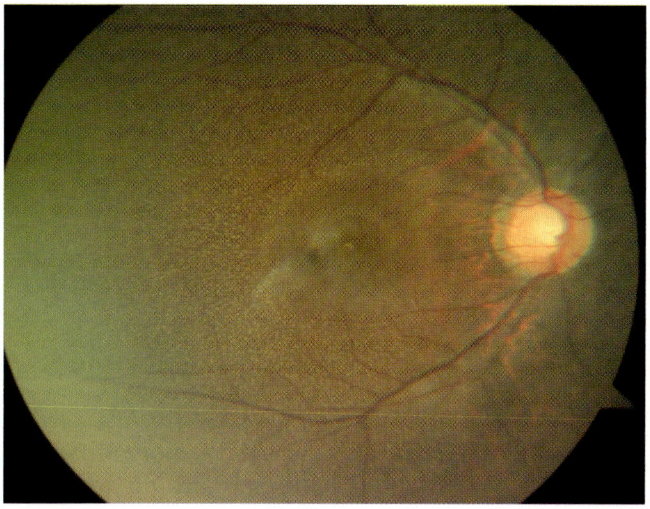

Fundus photograph of the right eye. Innumerable tiny white dots were seen scattered throughout the fundus

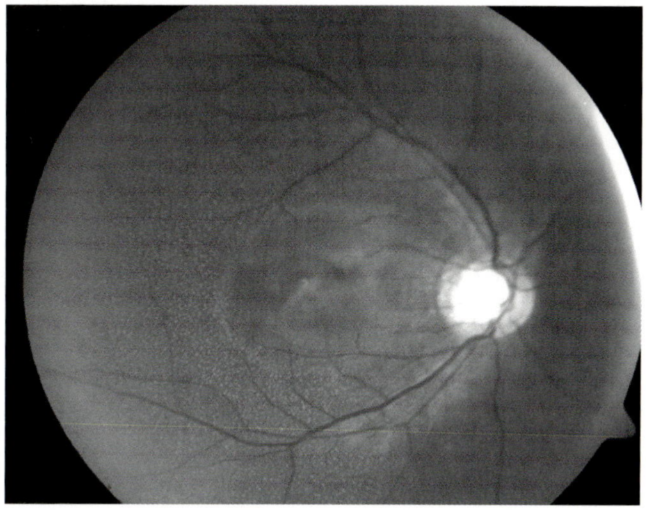

Red free photograph showing the fine dots in the temporal region

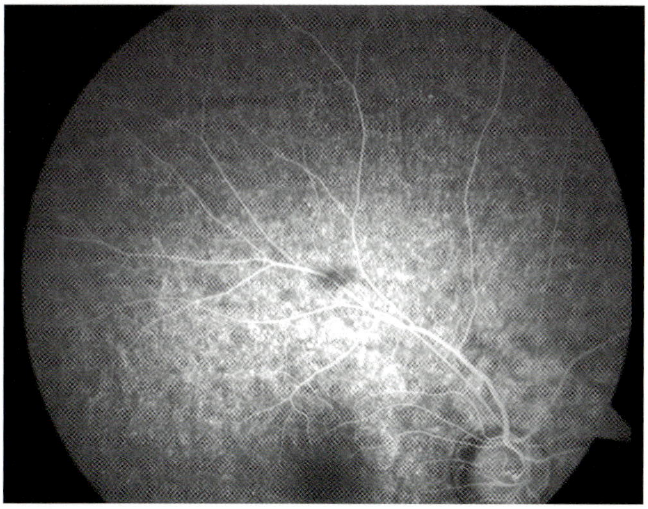

A fine stippled hyperfluorescence due to transmission defect is seen throughout the fundus in the mid arteriovenous phase

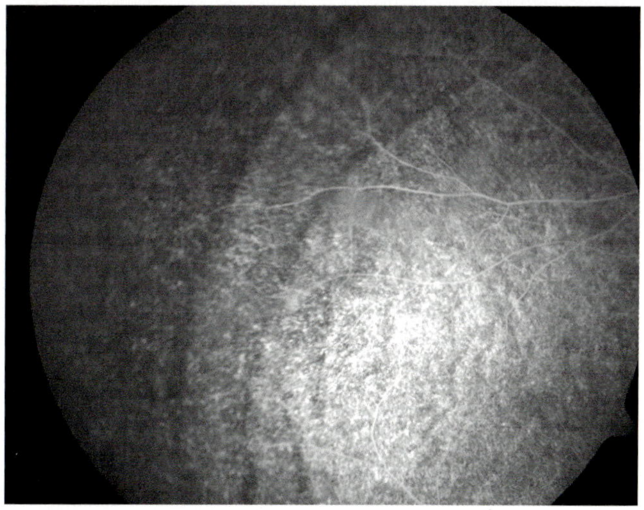

Stippled hyperfluorescence is seen in the temporal periphery in the late arteriovenous phase

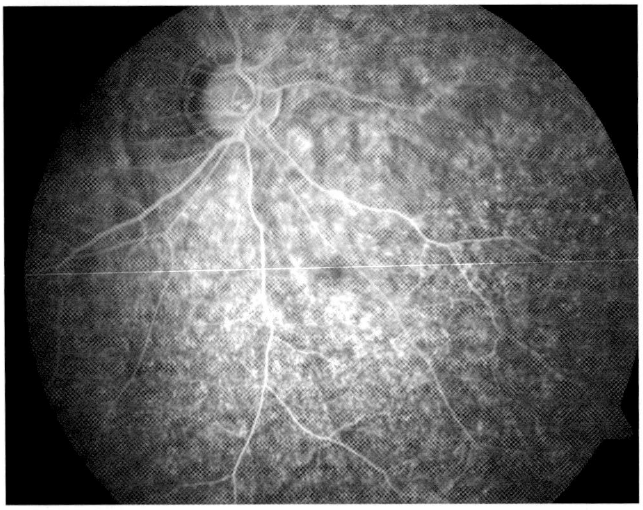

Similar stippled hyperfluorescence is seen in the inferonasal periphery

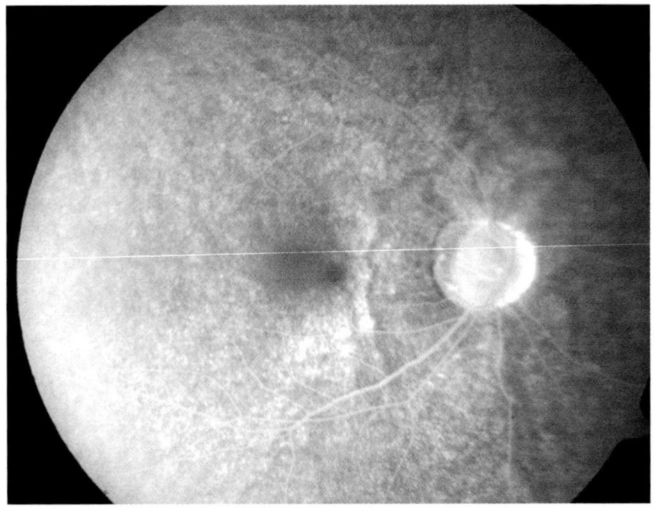

Fading of the hyperfluorescence is seen in the late phase

CASE 9 (*Continued*)

Left Eye of the Patient

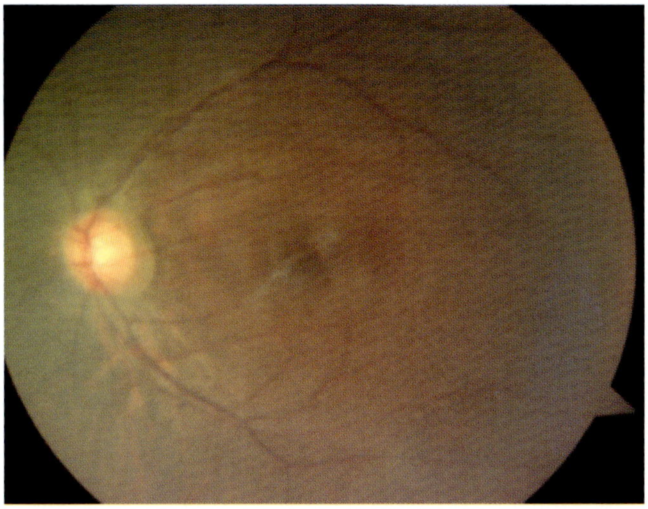

Fundus photograph of the left eye. Changes similar to those in the right eye were seen

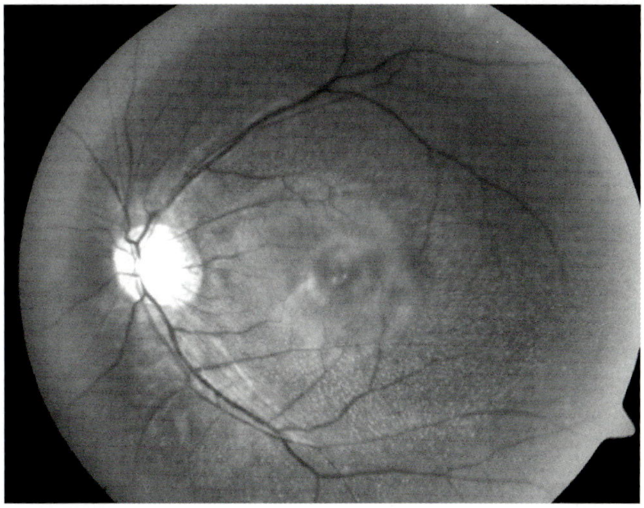

Red free photograph of the left eye

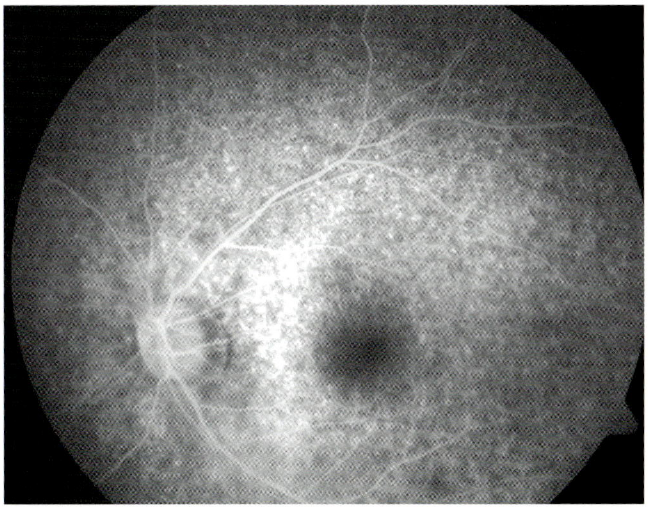

Stippled hyperfluorescence due to transmission defect is seen throughout the posterior pole

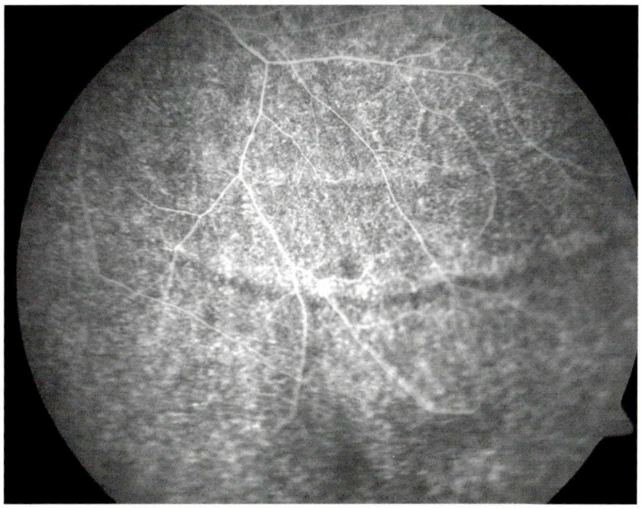

Stippled hyperfluorescence is seen in the inferior periphery

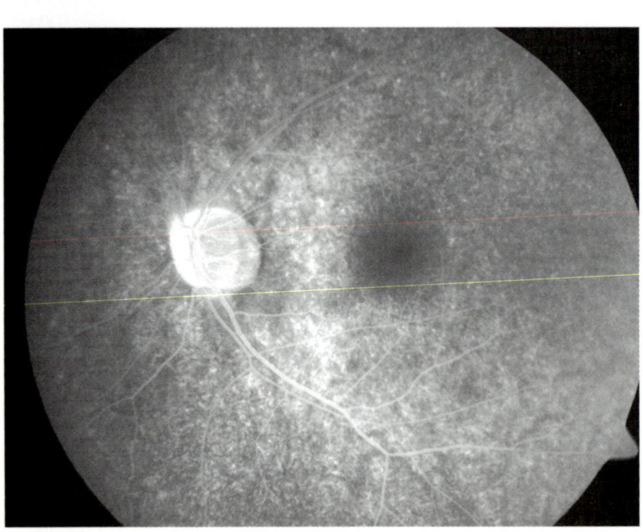

Fading of the hyperfluorescence is seen in the late film

COMMENT

Stippled hyperfluorescence seen in fundus albipunctatus does not exactly correspond to the innumerable tiny flecks seen clinically.

BENIGN FLECK RETINA

CASE 10

A 32-year-old female came for a routine eye examination. She was asymptomatic and had a visual acuity of 6/6; N6 in both eyes. Fundus examination showed innumerable flecks scattered throughout the fundus.

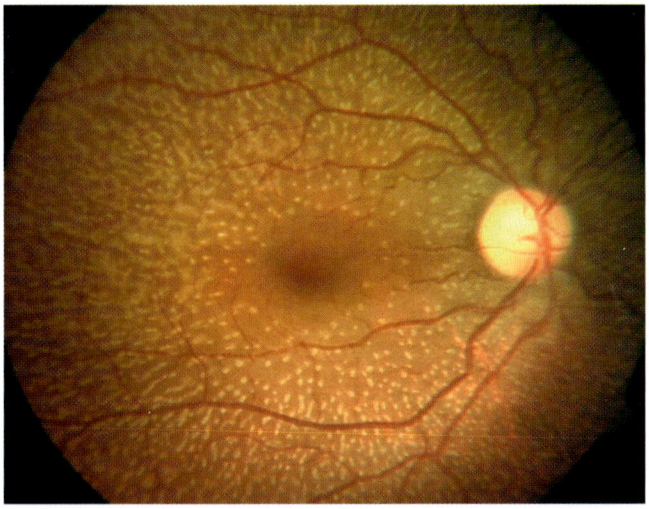

Fundus photograph of the right eye shows innumerable yellow-white flecks seen throughout the posterior pole. The fovea is spared

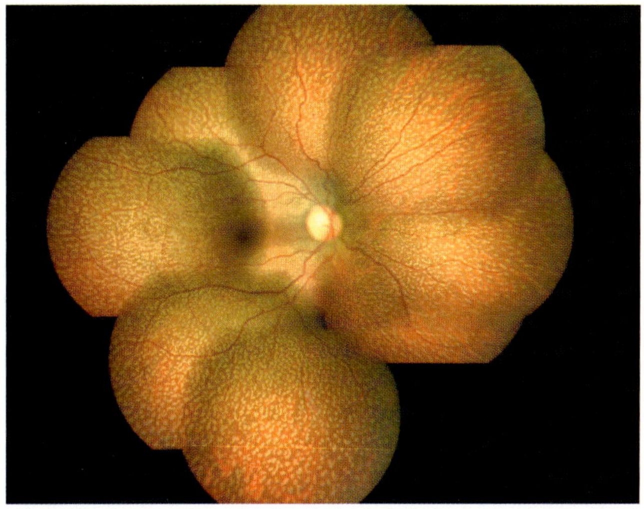

Color montage photograph of the right eye showing the flecks scattered throughout the fundus

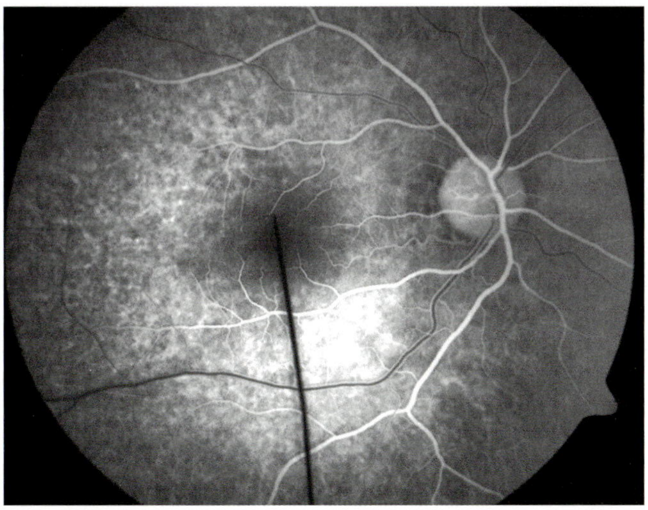

Early arteriovenous phase shows irregular hyperfluorescence, more marked temporally

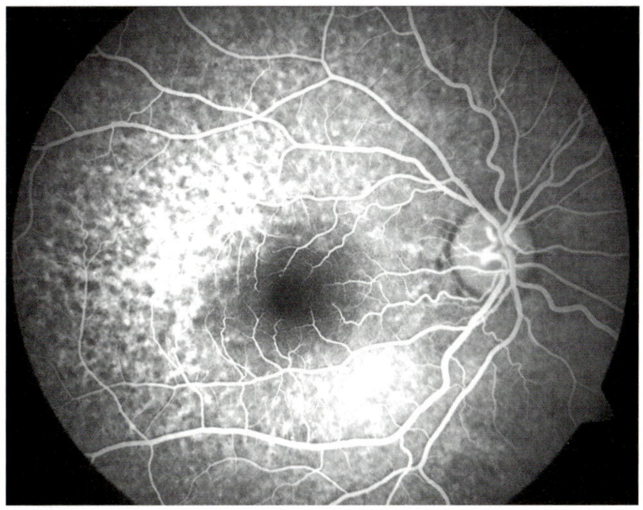

Mid arteriovenous phase shows increased irregular hyperfluorescence due to transmission defect

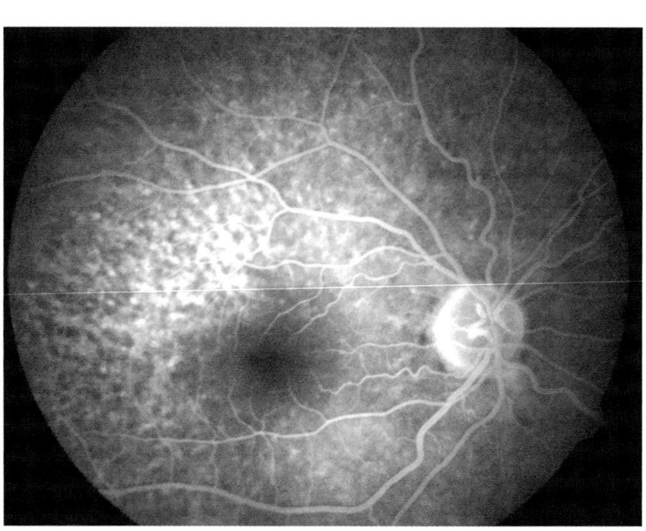

Late phase showing fading of the hyperfluorescence

CASE 10 (*Continued*)

Left Eye of the Patient

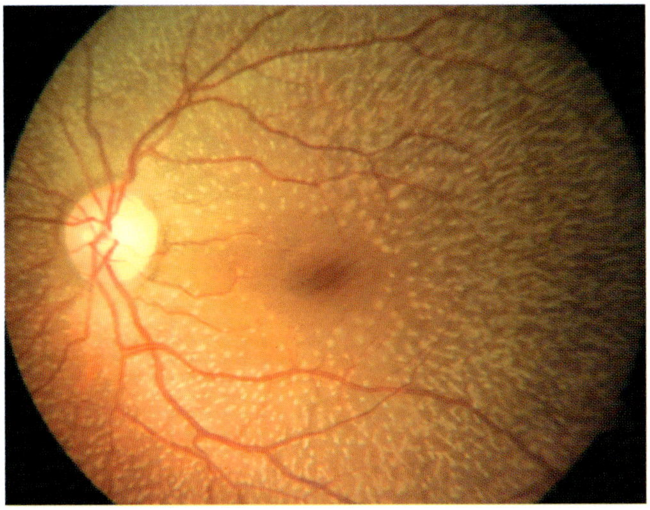

Fundus photograph of the left eye showing the flecks at the posterior pole

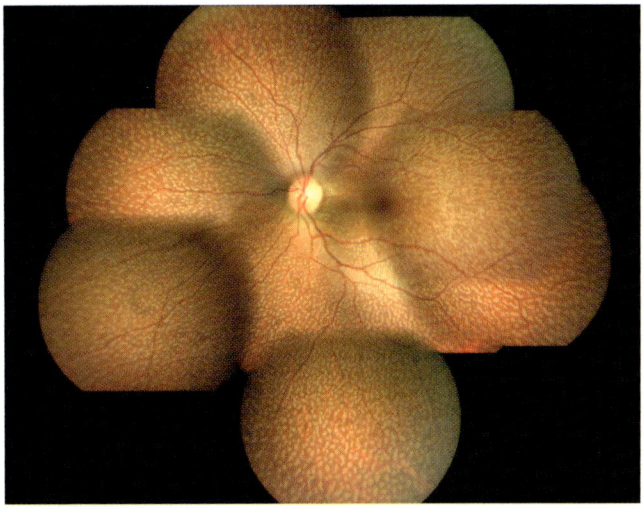

Color montage photograph of the left eye showing the flecks scattered throughout the fundus

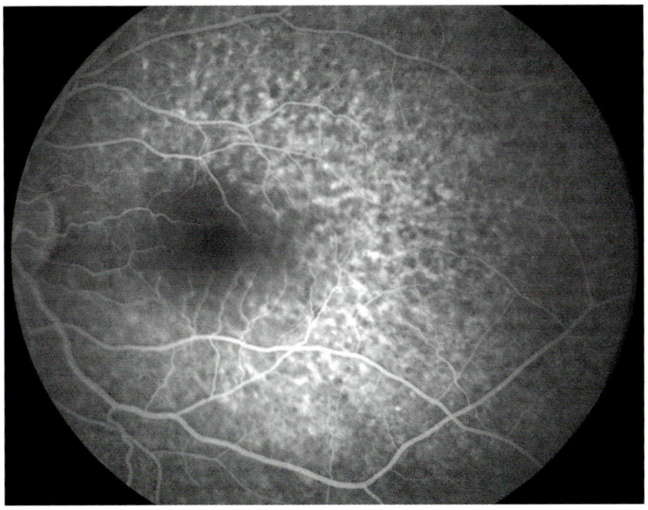

Irregular transmitted fluorescence seen in the arteriovenous phase of the angiogram

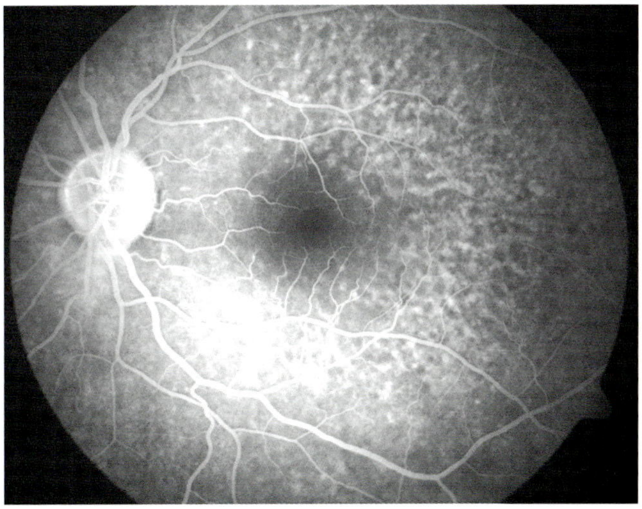

Fading of the hyperfluorescence is seen in the later phase of the angiogram

COMMENT

This entity has been called 'Benign flecked retina' and probably represents a variant of fundus albipunctatus. Affected patients are asymptomatic with normal visual acuity. Electrophysiological tests are relatively unaffected.

CLINICAL NUGGETS

1. Posterior subcapsular cataract, macular degeneration and cystoid macular edema are important causes for loss of central vision in patients with RP.
2. In RP, approximately 16-18% loss of ERG amplitudes per year is seen.
3. In RP, approximately 4.6% of the remaining visual field loss occurs per year.

BIBLIOGRAPHY

1. Khan JA, I de CH, Strickland MP. Coat's –type RP Surv Ophthalmol 1988;32:317-32.
2. Newsome DA. Retinal fluorescein leakage in retinitis pigmentosa. Am J Ophthalmol 1986;101:354-60.
3. Piermarocchi S, Segato T, Midena E. Retinal fluorescein leakage in RP. Am J Ophthalmol 1986;102:674.
4. Ronald E Carr. The generalized heredoretinal disorders in vitreoretinal diseases, the essentials. (Ist edn); (Eds: CD Regillo; GC Brown and HW Flynn) page 309.
5. Spallone A. Retinal fluorescein leakage in RP. Am J Ophthalmol 1986;102:408.

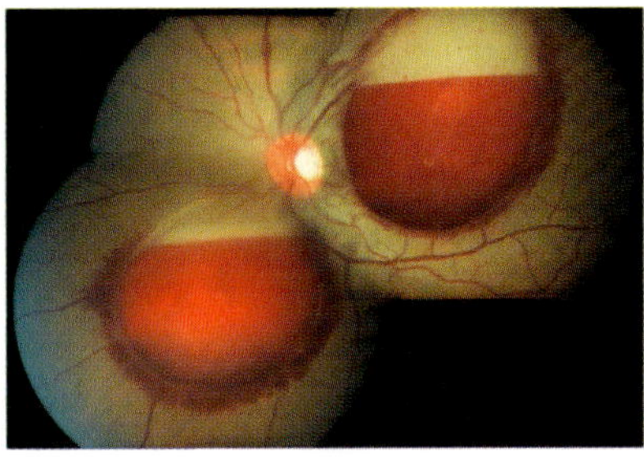

Section 6

Optic Nerve Disorders

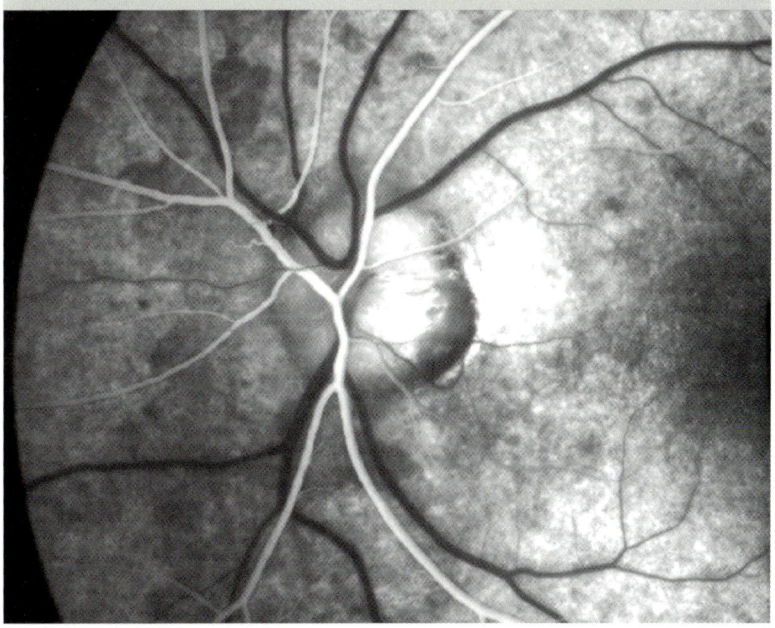

Chapter 60 Optic Nerve Disorders

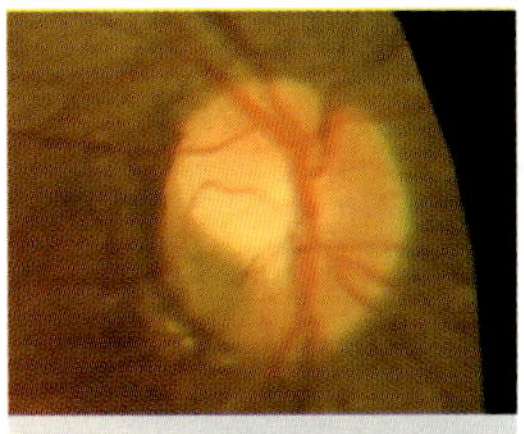

- The conditions included in this section are:
  - Optic disc pit
  - Optic nerve head drusen
  - Papilledema
  - Neuroretinitis
  - Optic neuritis
  - Leber's hereditary optic neuropathy (LHON)
  - Anterior ischemic optic neuropathy (AION).

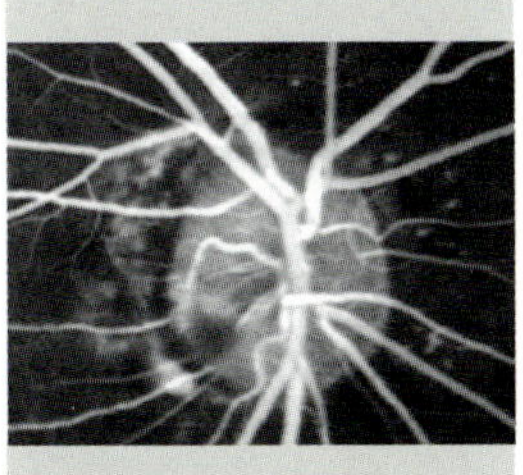

- Optic Pit
  - Early hypofluorescence is seen at the pit due to absence of vessels in the optic pit. Late staining of the tissue in the optic pit is seen.
- Optic Nerve Head Drusen
  - Autofluorescence is seen in the pre-injection photograph. Late staining of the optic nerve head drusen is seen.
- Papilledema
  - Dilatation of the disc capillaries with leakage of the dye is seen in the early phase of the angiogram. Late staining of the disc is seen.
- Neuroretinitis
  - Dilated disc capillaries with leakage of the dye is seen in the early part of the angiogram. Late staining of the disc occurs.
- Optic Neuritis
  - Dilated disc capillaries which leak dye resulting in staining of the disc is seen in the late phase.
- Leber's Hereditary Optic Neuropathy (LHON)
  - Dilated and tortuous capillaries are seen in the peripapillary region. No abnormal staining of the disc is seen in the late phase.
- Anterior Ischemic Optic Neuropathy (AION)
  - Differential filling of the disc capillaries in the upper and lower half of the optic disc is seen.

CASE 1

A 22-year-old male presented with reduced vision in the left eye for the past four months. Visual acuity was 6/18; N12.

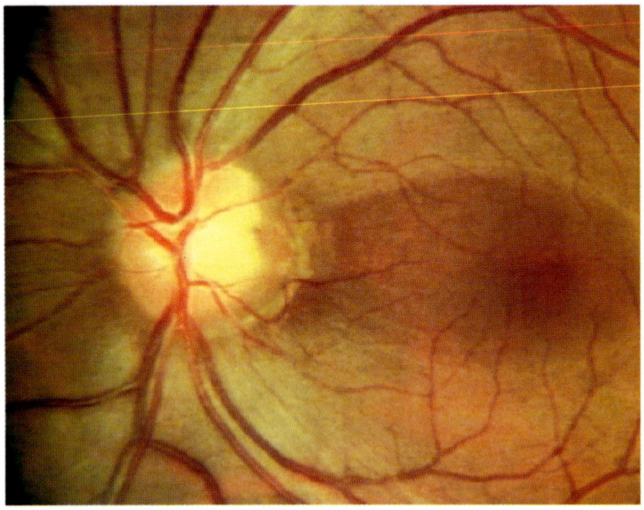

Fundus photograph of the left eye showing an optic pit in the temporal part of the disc. Note the flask shaped elevation of the retina temporal to the disc

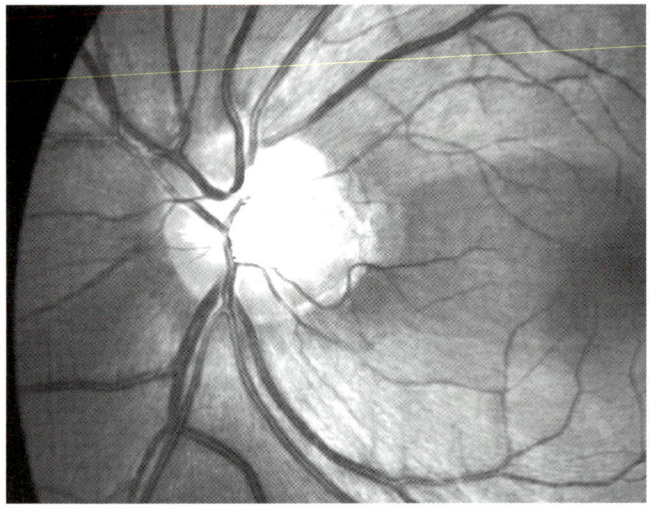

Red free photograph of the left eye

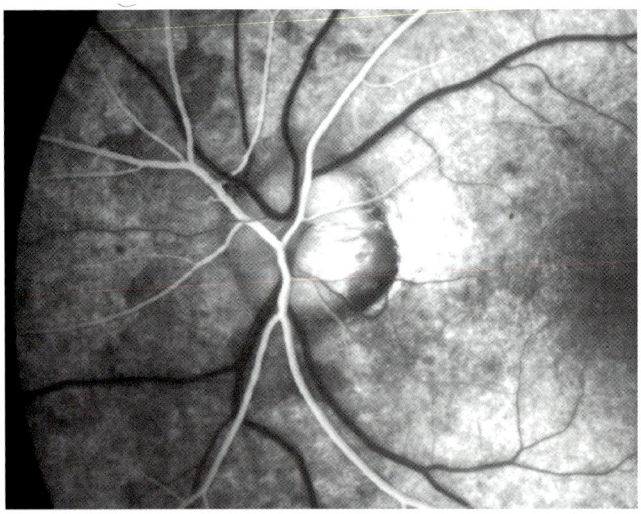

Arterial phase of the angiogram showing hypofluorescence in the region of the optic pit

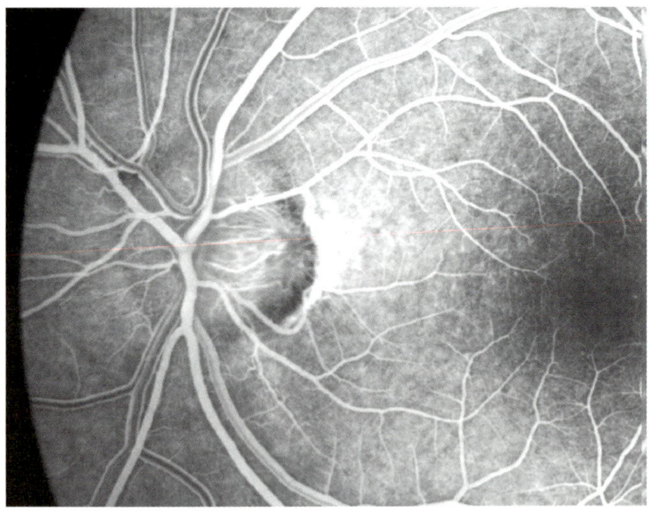

The hypofluorescence at the optic pit is persisting in the early arteriovenous phase of the angiogram

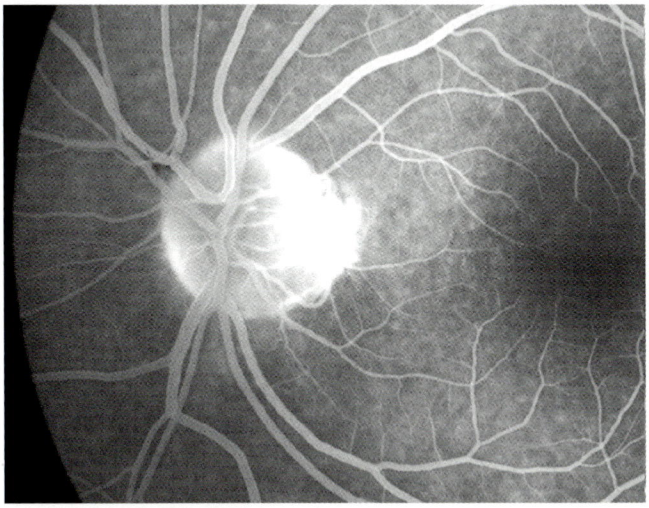

Hyperfluorescence due to staining is seen at the optic pit in the late phase. Note there is no leakage of dye into the sensory retinal elevation

COMMENT

Optic pit appears hypofluorescent in the early phase due to absence of vessels in the pit. Late hyperfluorescence is due to staining of the tissue at the pit.

No leakage of the dye is seen from the pit into the sensory retinal elevation.

CASE 2

A 45-year-old male patient had come for a routine eye check-up. Visual acuity was 6/18; N18 in the right eye. Left eye was normal.

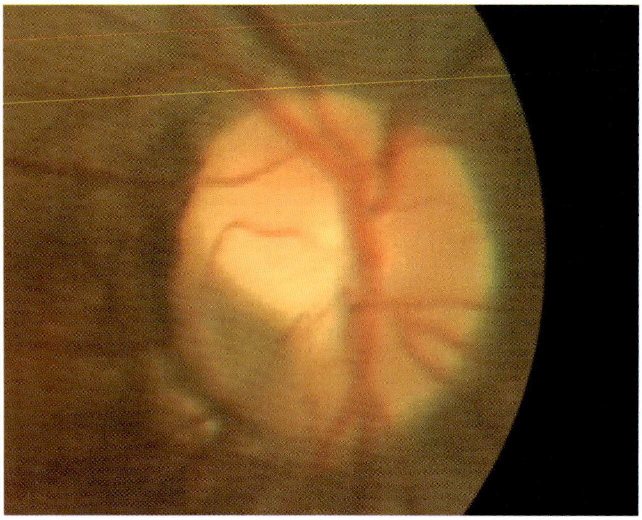

Fundus photograph of the right eye showing the optic pit in the inferotemporal part of the disc

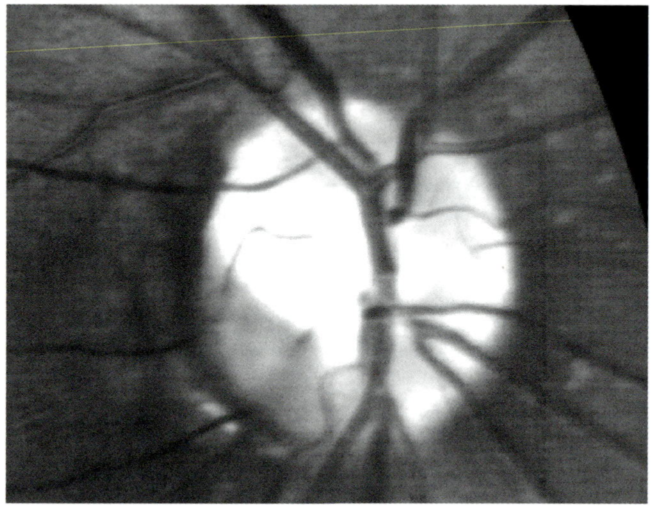

Red free photograph of the right eye

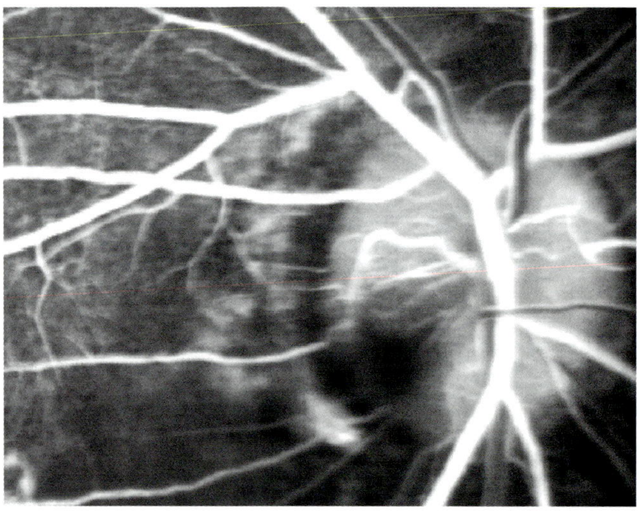

Hypofluorescence is seen at the optic pit in the early arteriovenous phase

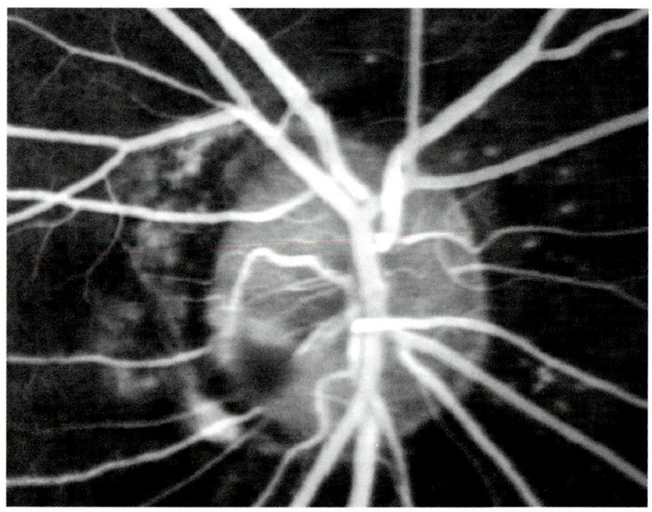

Minimal hyperfluorescence is seen at the optic pit in the mid arteriovenous phase of the angiogram

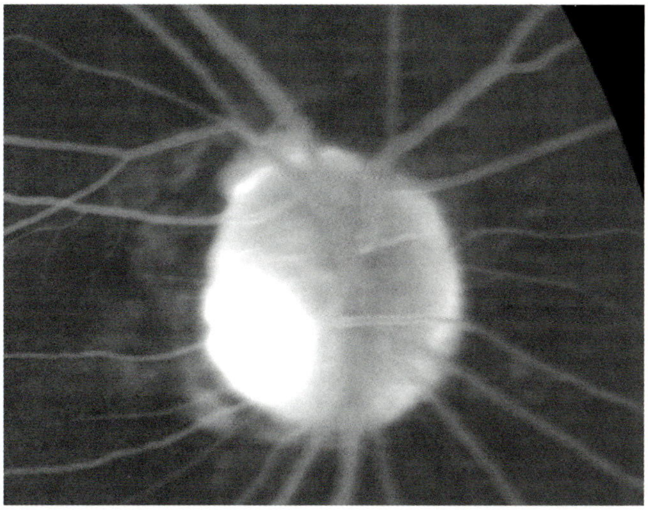

Increased staining of the tissue at the optic pit is seen in the late phase of the angiogram

COMMENT

Case shows the typical angiographic picture of the optic pit.

OPTIC NERVE HEAD DRUSEN

CASE 3

A 24-year-old female was referred with a diagnosis of papillitis in the left eye. Visual acuity was 6/6; N6 in both eyes. Nodular elevation of the disc was seen. Ultrasound examination showed a high reflective echo at the optic nerve head, suggestive of an optic nerve head drusen.

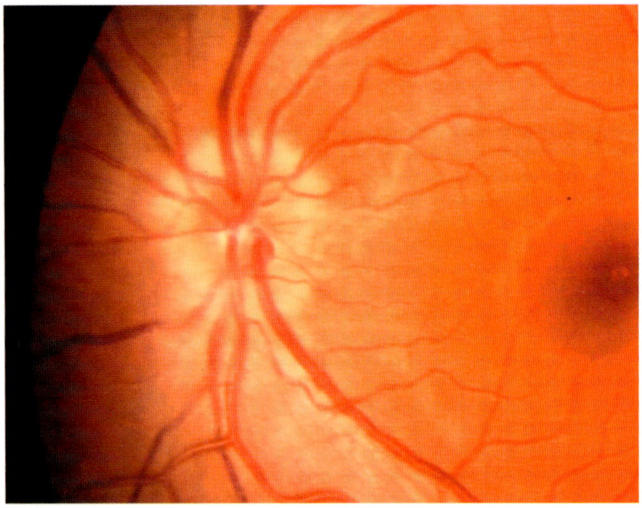

Fundus photograph of the left eye showing the nodular elevation along the disc margin

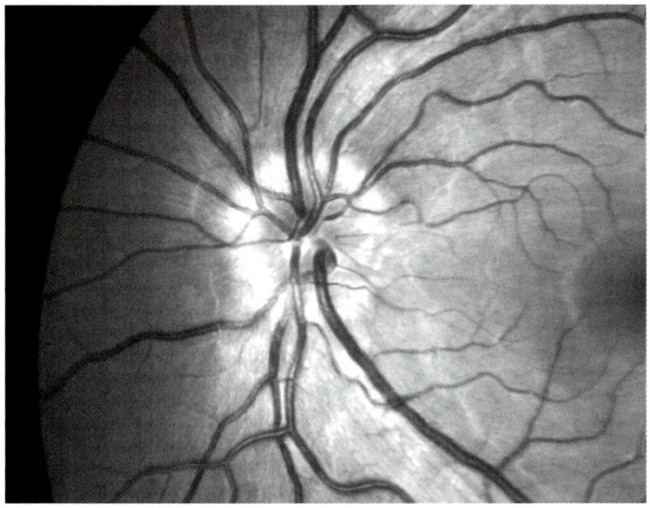

Red free photograph of the left eye. Note the crowding of the vessels at the disc

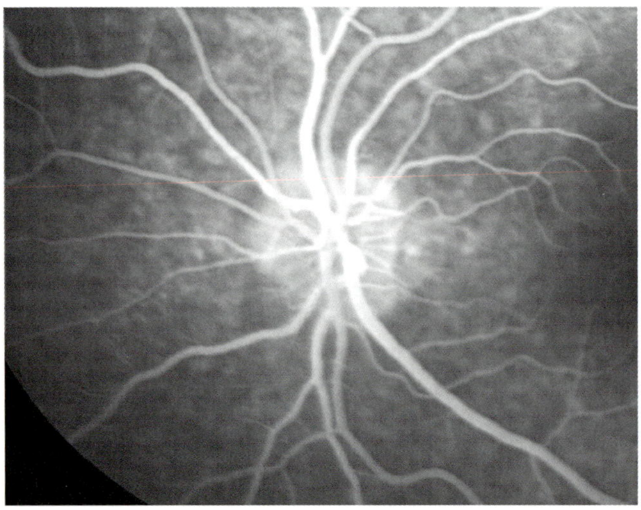

Irregularity along the disc margin is seen in the mid arteriovenous phase of the angiogram

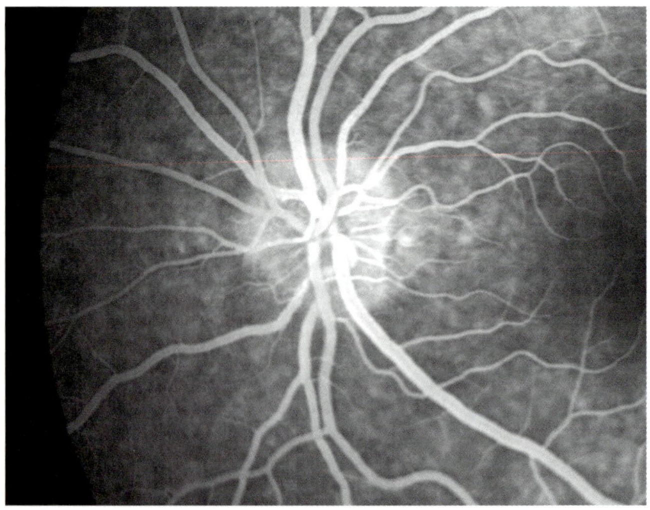

Late arteriovenous phase of the angiogram showing the irregularity along the disc margin. Note that there is no dilatation of the disc capillaries

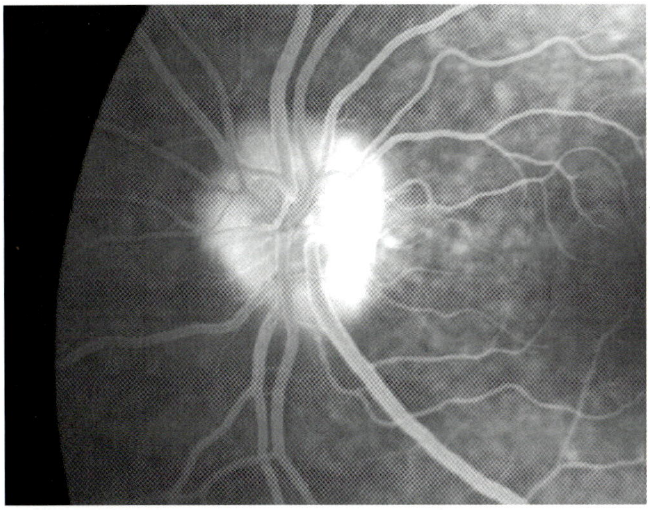

Late phase showing the increased staining of the disc drusen

COMMENT

Optic nerve head drusen shows autofluorescence in pre-injection photograph.

PAPILLEDEMA

CASE 4

A 26-year-old female, diagnosed to have idiopathic intracranial hypertension was found to have papilledema in both eyes and referred for an ophthalmic checkup. Visual acuity was 6/6; N6 in both eyes.

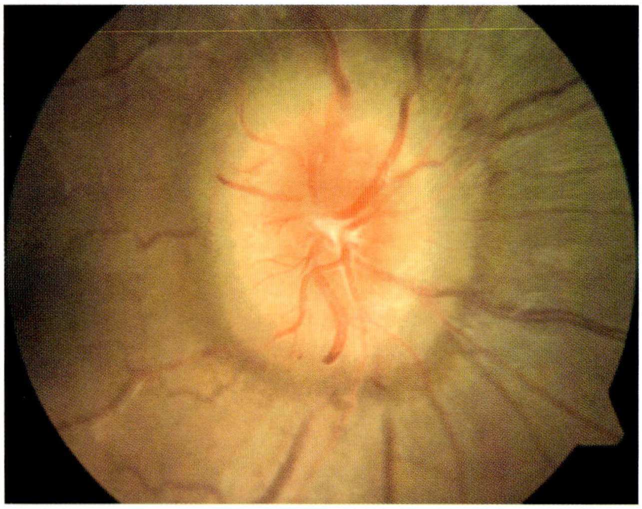

Fundus photograph of the right eye showing the swollen hyperemic disc

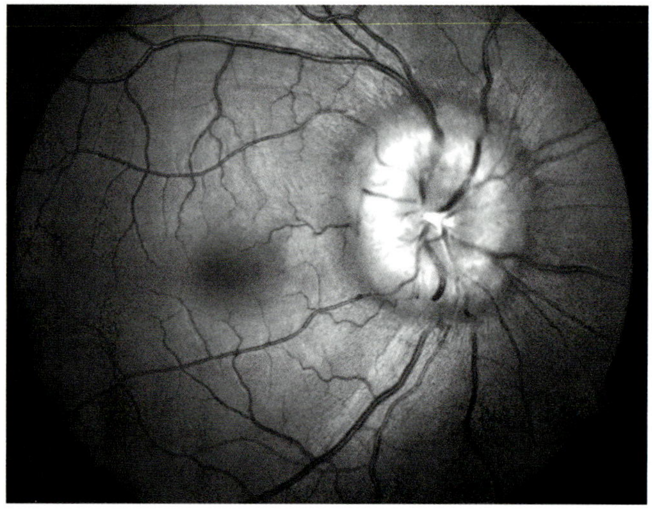

Red free photograph of the right eye

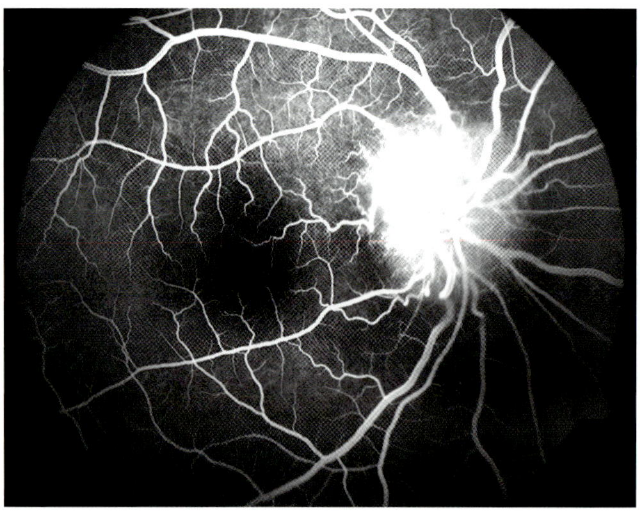

Mid arteriovenous phase of the angiogram showing dilation of the disc capillaries. The margins of the disc are blurred

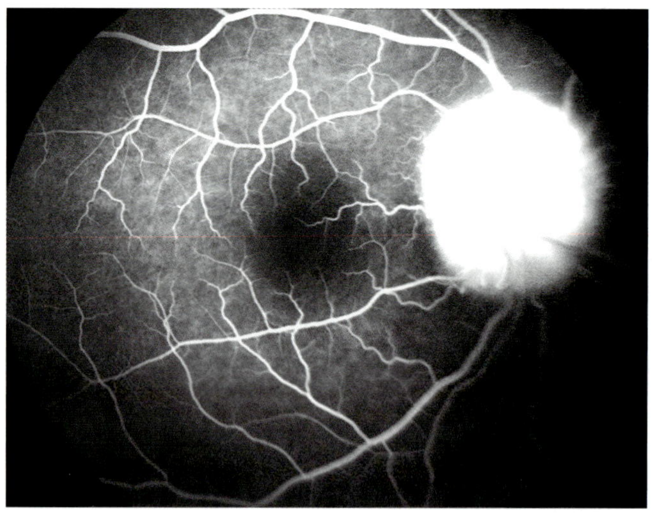

Late phase of the angiogram showing increased staining of the disc

CASE 4 (*Continued*)

Left Eye of the Patient

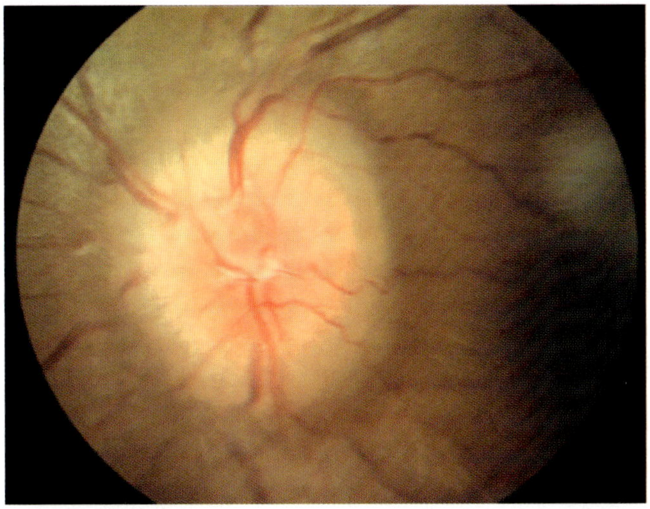

Fundus photograph of the left eye showing the swollen disc. The margins of the disc are blurred

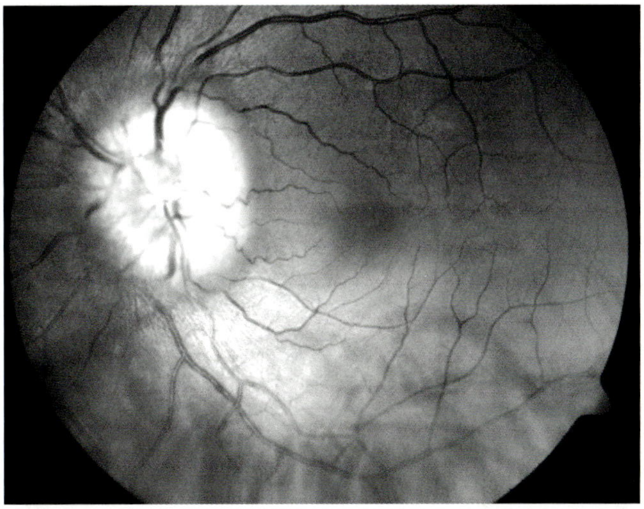

Red free photograph of the left eye

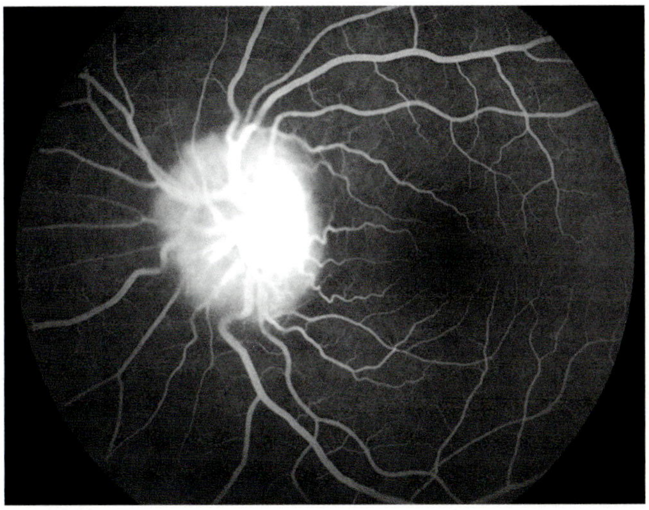

Increased fluorescence of the disc and dilated disc capillaries are seen in the arteriovenous phase of the angiogram

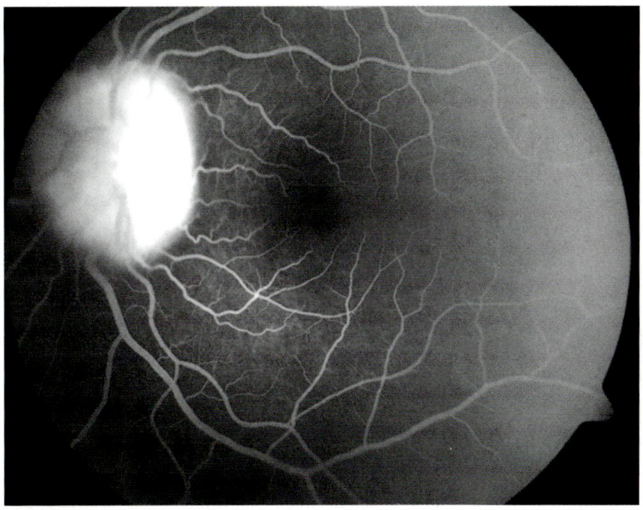

Late phase of the angiogram showing increased staining of the disc

COMMENT

Leakage of the dye from the dilated disc capillaries is seen in papilledema; late staining of the disc is also seen.

NEUROREТINITIS

CASE 5

A 19-year-old female presented with reduced vision in the right eye of three days duration. Visual acuity was 3/60 in the right eye. Vitreous cells were noted in the right eye. Left eye was normal.

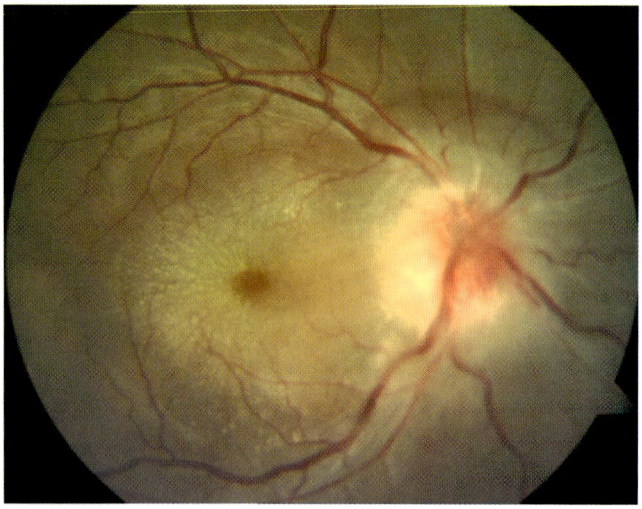

Fundus photograph of the right eye showing a swollen, hyperemic disc with marked exudation in the macula. A macular star is seen

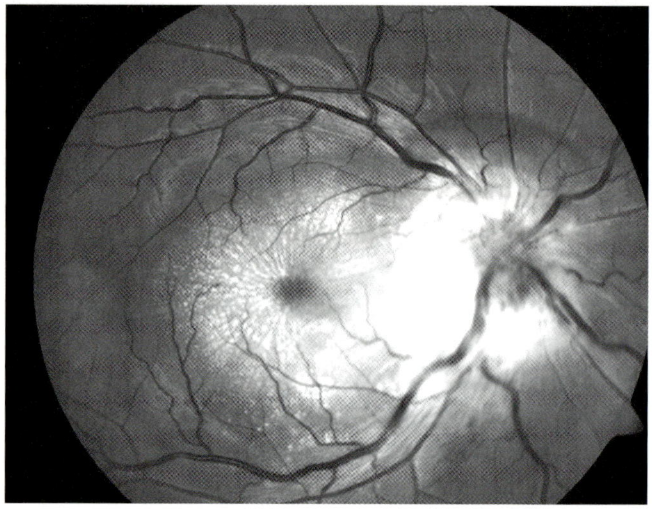

Red free photograph of the right eye showing the macular star

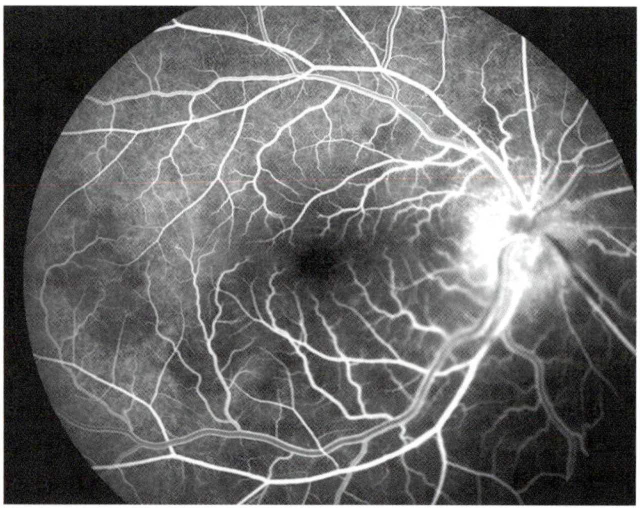

Early arteriovenous phase showing the dilated disc capillaries

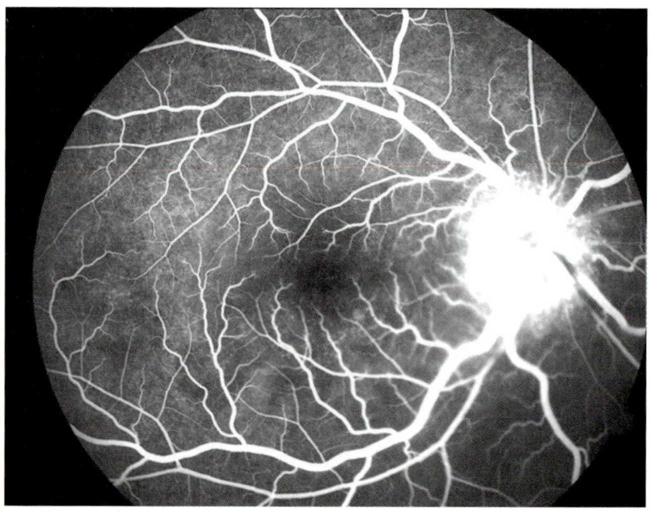

Late arteriovenous phase showing leakage of the dye from the disc capillaries. Note that no leakage is seen from the macular retinal vessels

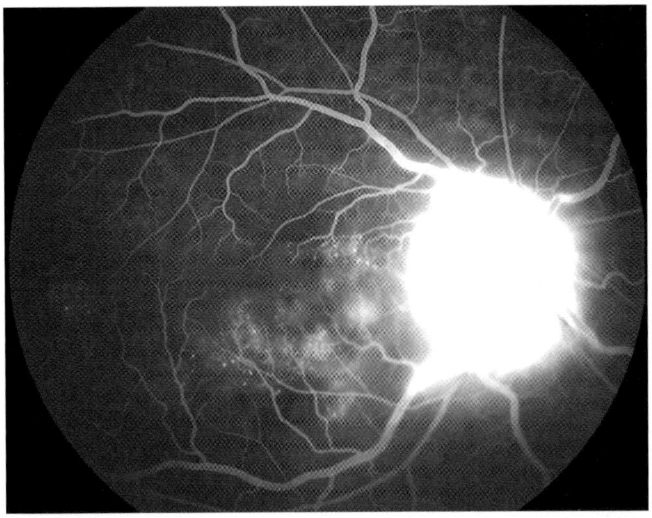

Marked staining of the optic nerve head is seen in the late phase

COMMENT

Dilatation of the disc capillaries with leakage of the dye and late staining of the disc is seen in patients with neuroretinitis.

The lipid exudation is most likely from the disc capillaries as no leakage is seen from the macular retinal vessels.

OPTIC NEURITIS

CASE 6

A 32-year-old female with multiple sclerosis, presented with sudden onset drop in vision in the right eye of one day duration. Visual acuity was 2/60 in the right eye.

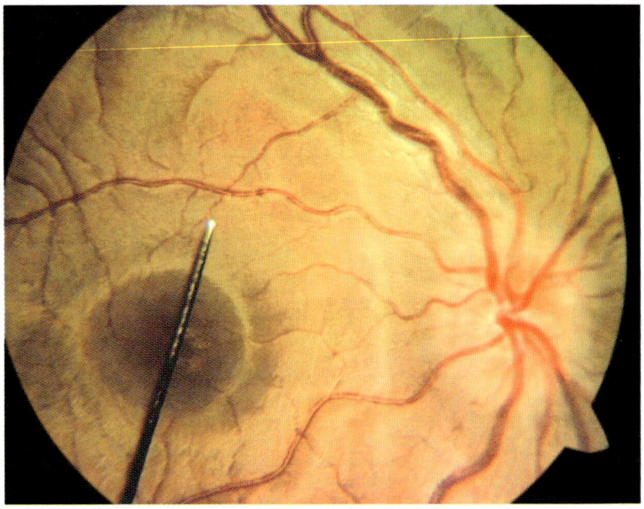

Fundus photograph of the right eye showing a swollen, hyperemic disc. The disc margins are blurred

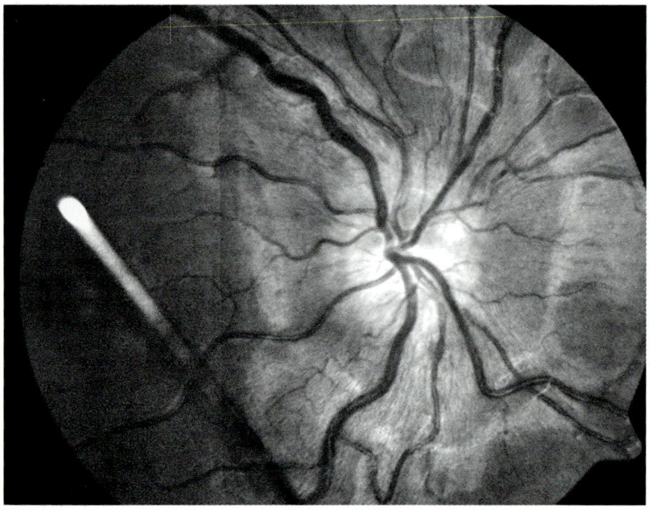

Red free photograph of the right eye

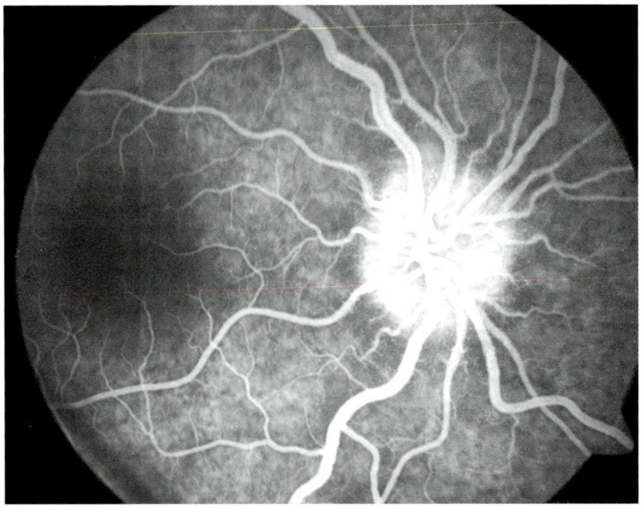

Marked dilatation of the disc capillaries is seen in the arteriovenous phase of the angiogram

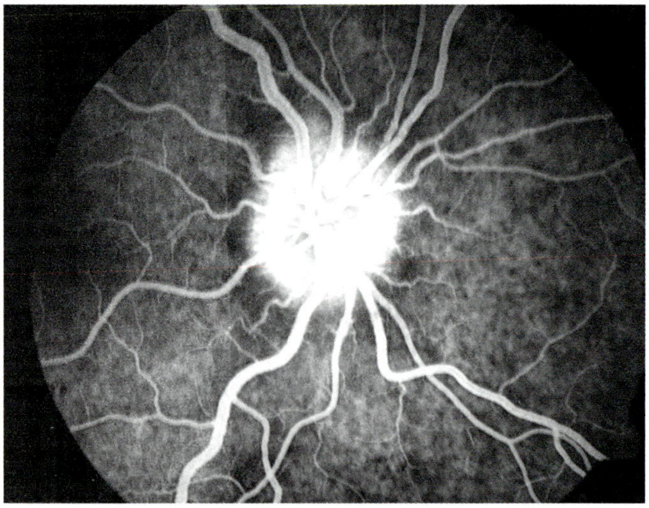

Increased staining of the disc is seen in the late phase

COMMENT

Lipid exudation is not common in patients with optic neuritis occurring in demyelinating disorders.

LEBER'S HEREDITARY OPTIC NEUROPATHY (LHON)

CASE 7

A 14-year-old male presented with reduced vision in both eyes of one month duration. Visual acuity was 3/60 in both eyes. CT scan was normal. Serum lactate, pyruvate and ammonia were found to be raised.

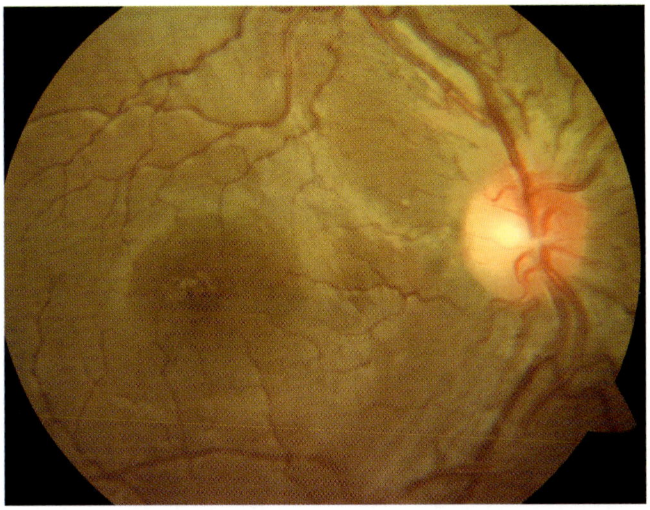

Fundus photograph of the right eye. Dilated capillaries are seen in the peripapillary region

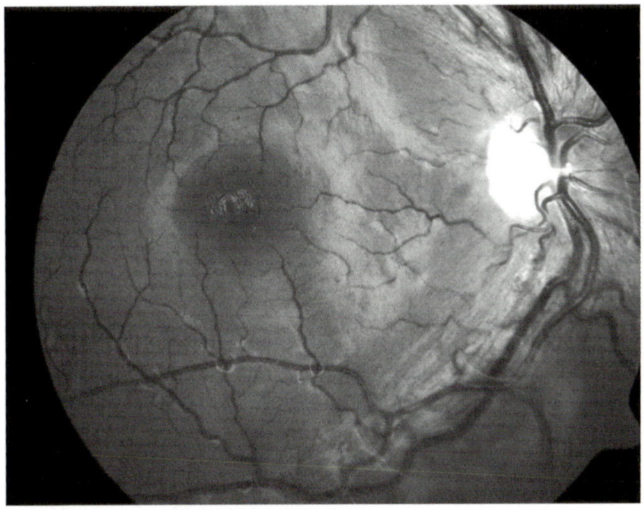

Red free photograph of the right eye

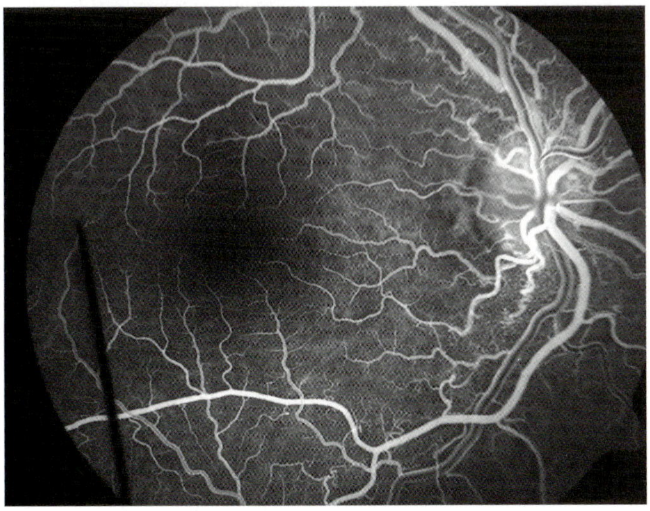

Dilated and tortuous capillaries are seen around the disc in the early arteriovenous phase

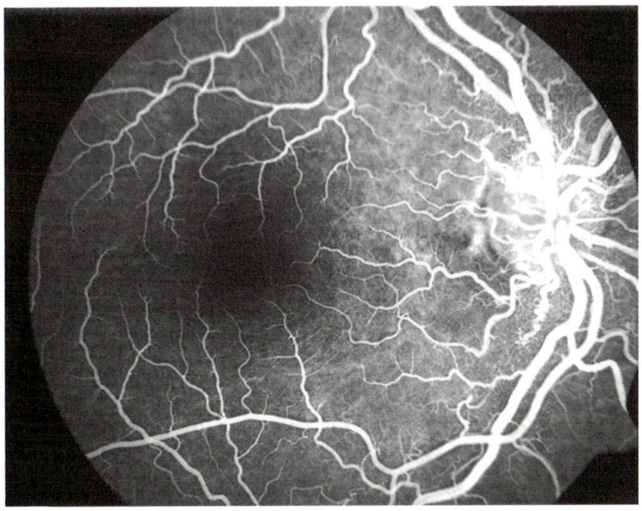

No leakage of the dye is seen from the dilated capillaries in the late arteriovenous phase

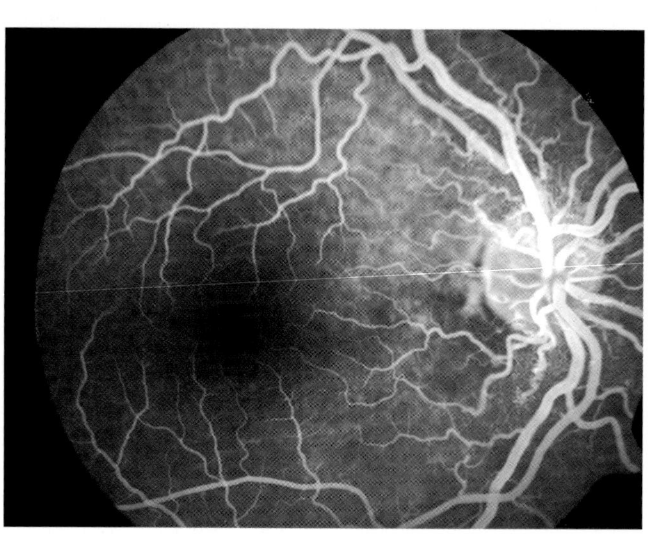

Late phase showing normal disc fluorescence. No abnormal staining of the disc is seen

CASE 7 (*Continued*)

Left Eye of the Patient

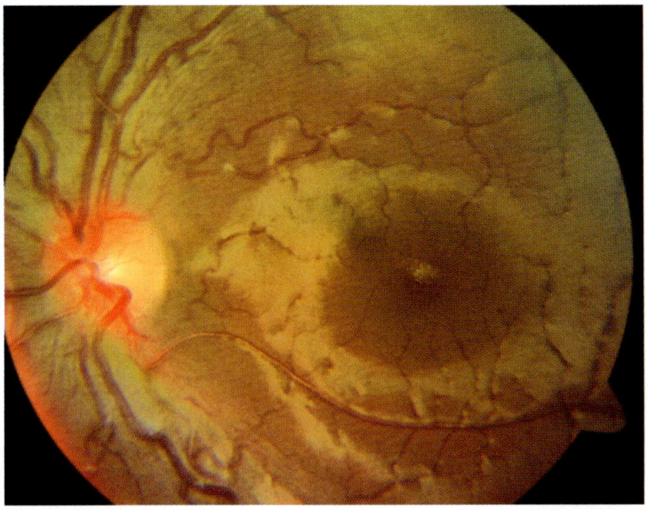

Fundus photograph of the left eye showing the dilated peripapillary capillaries

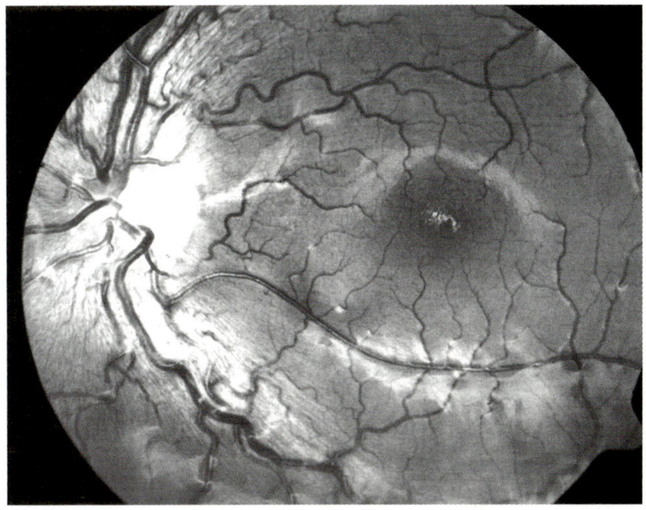

Red free photograph of the left eye

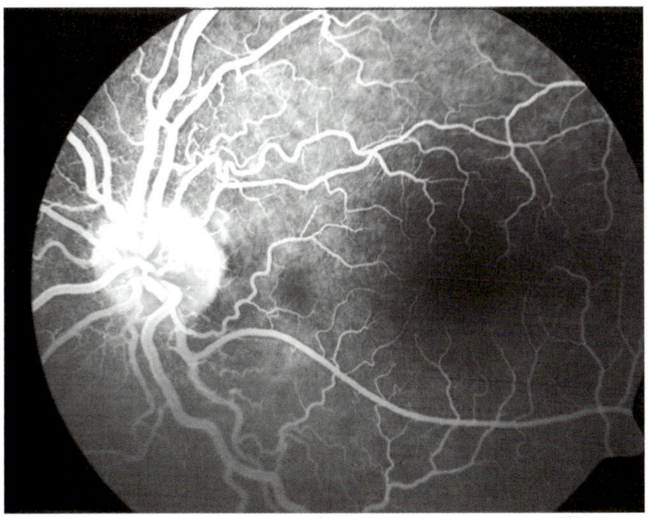

Arteriovenous phase showing the dilated and tortuous capillaries around the disc

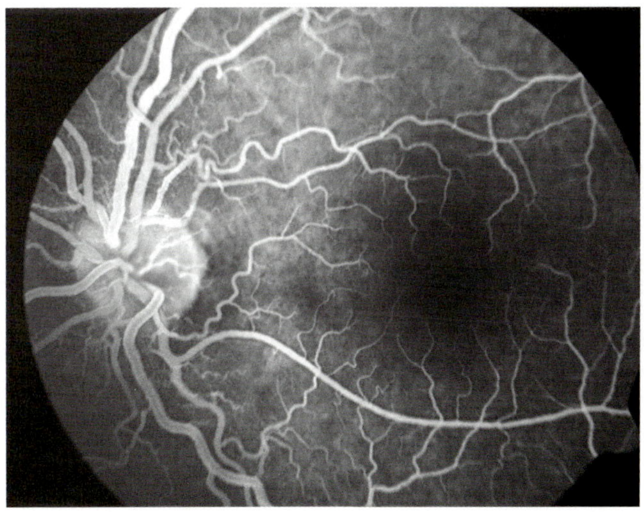

No abnormal staining of the disc is seen in the late phase

COMMENT

Leber's hereditary optic neuropathy is characterized by the presence of telangiectatic vessels in the peripapillary region. Typically, no abnormal staining of the disc is seen in the late phase.

ANTERIOR ISCHEMIC OPTIC NEUROPATHY (AION)

CASE 8

A 50-year-old diabetic male presented with an inferior altitudinal field defect in the left eye. Visual acuity was 6/18; N10.

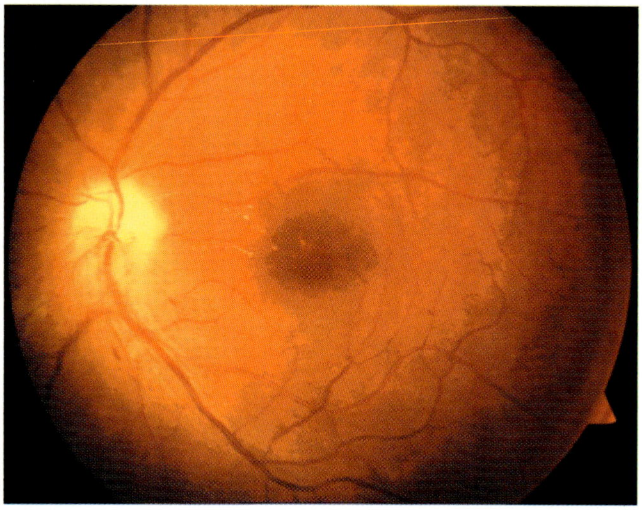

Fundus photograph of the left eye showing pallor in the upper half of the disc. Microaneurysms and hard exudates due to diabetic retinopathy are seen in the macula

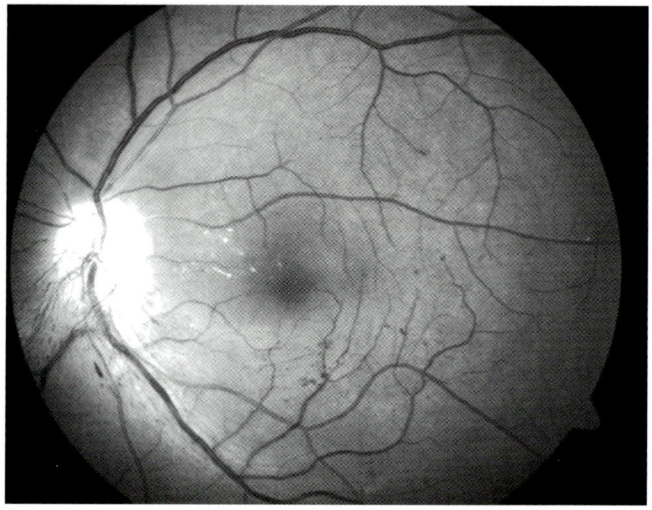

Red free photograph of the left eye

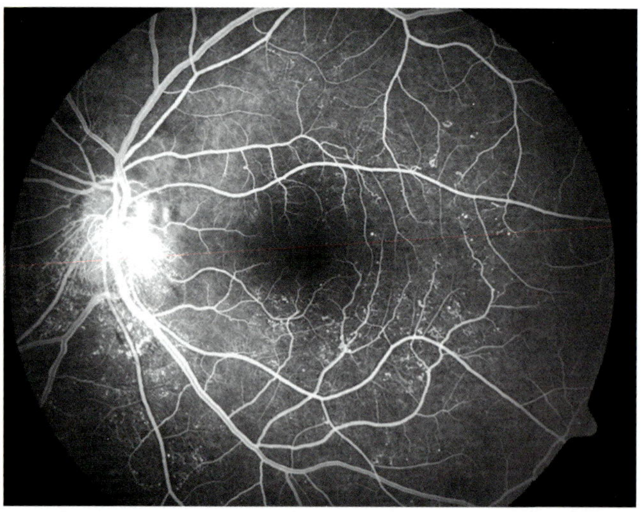

Filling of the disc capillaries is seen in the lower half. The upper half of the disc shows relative hypofluorescence. Microvascular abnormalities are seen in the macula

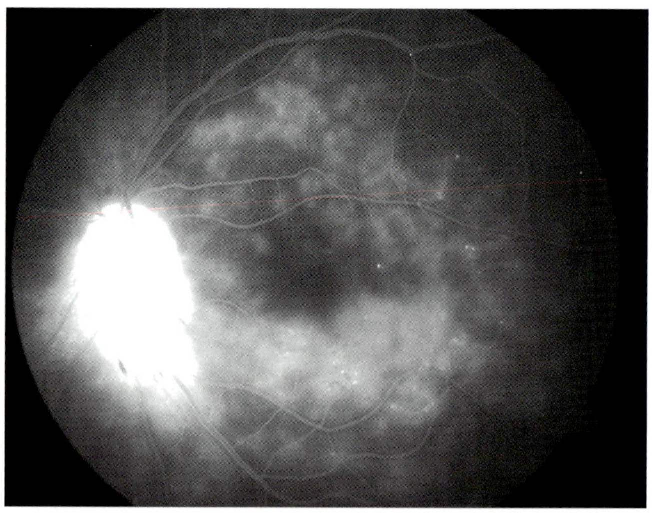

Increased staining of the disc is seen. Retention of dye is seen in the macula, indicative of macular edema

COMMENT

Differential filling of the disc capillaries is seen in AION.

CLINICAL NUGGET

Visual acuity, pupillary reaction, color vision, visual fields and visual evoked potential are useful for assessement of the optic nerve function.

BIBLIOGRAPHY

1. Arnold AC, Helper RS. Fluorescein angiography in acute nonarteritic anterior ischemic optic neuropathy. Am J Ophthalmol 1994;117:222-30.
2. Boghen DR, Glaser JS. Ischemic optic neuropathy: The clinical profile and natural history. Brain 1975;98:689-708.
3. Bonnet M. Serous macular detachment associated with optic nerve pits. Graefe's Arch Clin Exp Ophthalmol 1991;229:526-32.
4. Brown GC, Shields JA, Goldberg RE. Congenital pits of the optic nerve head. II. Clinical Studies in humans. Ophthalmology 1980;87:51-65.
5. Kelley JS. Autofluorescence of the optic nerve head. Arch Ophthalmol 1974;92:263-64.
6. Mustonen E. Pseudopapilledema with and without verified optic disc drusen: A clinical analysis II. Acta Ophthalmol 1983;61:1057-66.
7. Mustonen E. Pseudopapilledema with and without verified optic disc drusen clinical analysis I. Acta Ophthalmol 1983;61:1037-56.
8. Oosterhuis JA, Boen-Tan TN. Fluorescein angiography in papilledema and pseudopapilledema. Ophthalmologica 1969;159:96-110.
9. Papilledema. In Walsh and Hoyt's Clinical Neuro-ophthalmology, 5th edn. The Essentials. Editors: Miller NR, Newman NJ, Baltimore, Williams and Wilkins, chapter 1999;6,166-195.
10. Sanders MD. A classification of papilledema based on a fluorescein angiographic study. Trans Ophthalmol Soc UK 1969;89:177-92.
11. Yen MY, Wei YH, Liu JH. Peripapillary fluorescein leakage in 11778 Leber's optic neuropathy. J Neuro-ophthalmol 1996;16(3):178-81.

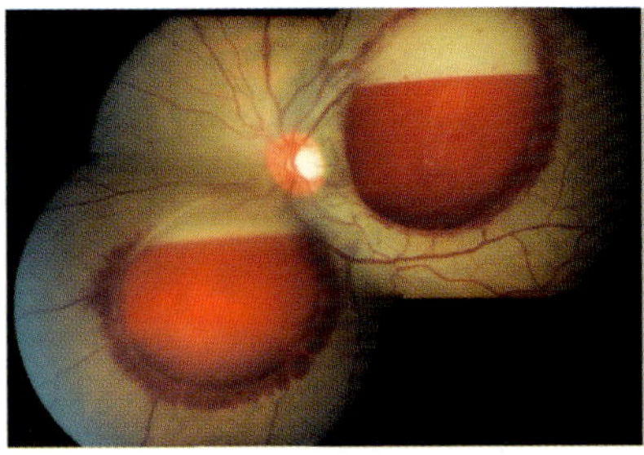

7 Section

Tumors

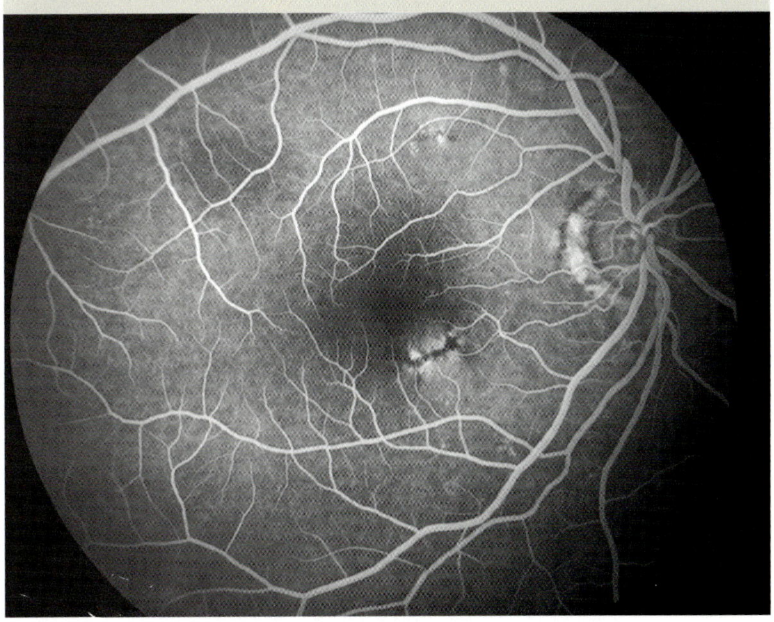

61 Chapter

Choroidal Nevus

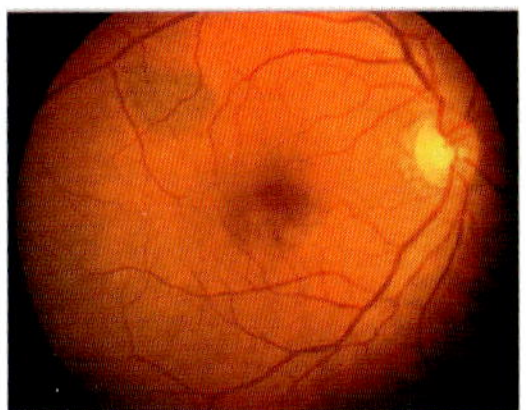

- Choroidal nevus appears as a flat, brown to slate gray lesion occurring more commonly in the postequatorial region.
- The degree of pigmentation can vary with some being amelanotic.
- Histopathologically, these are variably pigmented placoid lesions located in the outer choroid.
- The choriocapillaris are generally spared.
  Drusen and RPE alterations are features of chronicity.

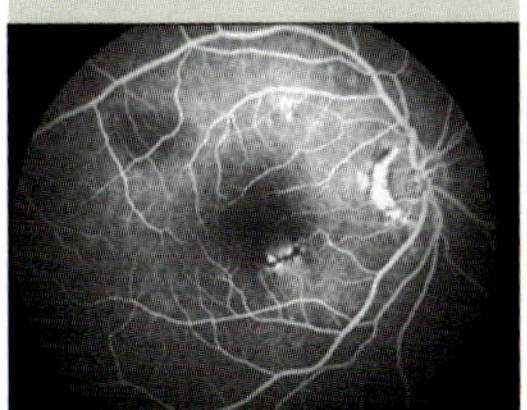

- Angiographic appearance depends on the degree of pigmentation of the nevus, its exact location in the choroid and changes in the overlying retinal pigment epithelium.
- If the nevus is confined to the outer choroid, sparing the choriocapillaris, the fluorescein angiogram may be relatively normal.
- If the choriocapillaris is partially involved, it may show up as a relatively hypofluorescent lesion.
- If changes in the overlying retinal pigment epithelium are present, it may show up as hyperfluorescent transmission defects within the hypofluorescent lesion.

CASE 1

A 48-year-old male underwent a fluorescein angiogram for RPE alterations close to the fovea. Visual acuity was 6/6; N6 in both eyes.

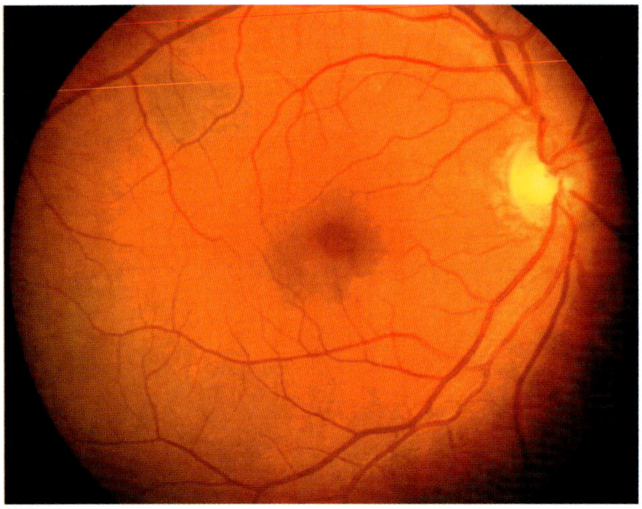

Fundus photograph of the right eye showing a choroidal nevus superotemporal to the fovea. Few RPE alterations are seen just inferonasal to the foveal center

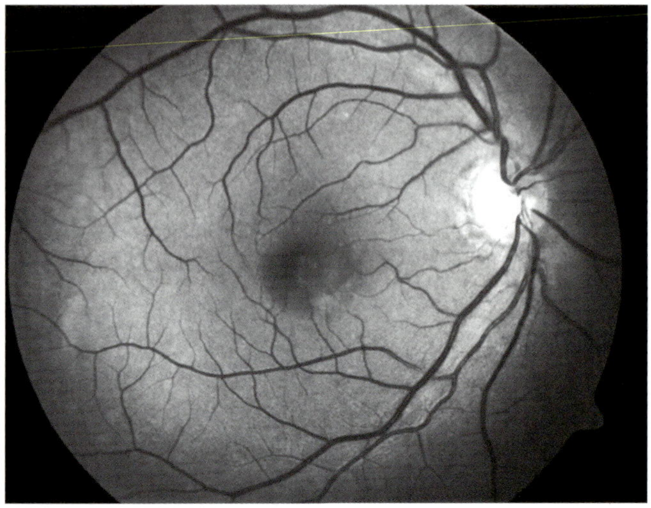

The right eye showing the RPE alterations inferonasal to the fovea in the red free photograph

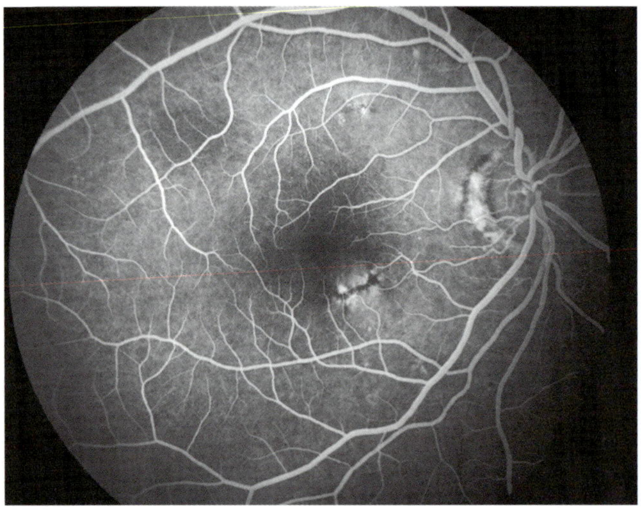

Hyperfluorescence due to transmission defects is noted inferonasal to the fovea

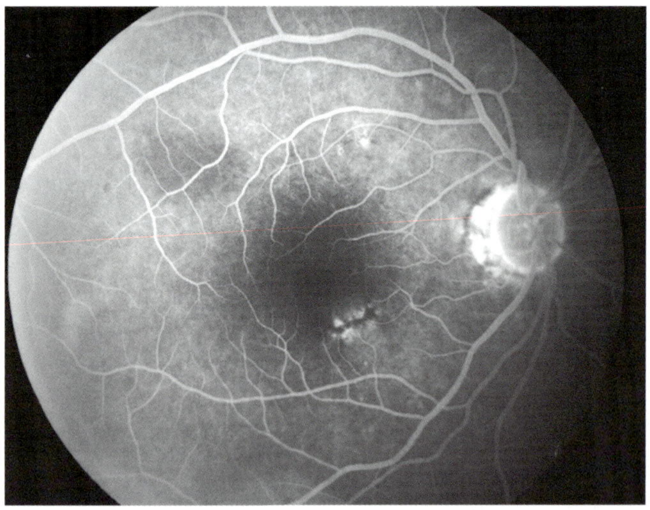

The faint hypofluorescence of the nevus persists in the late phase. The transmission defect has faded

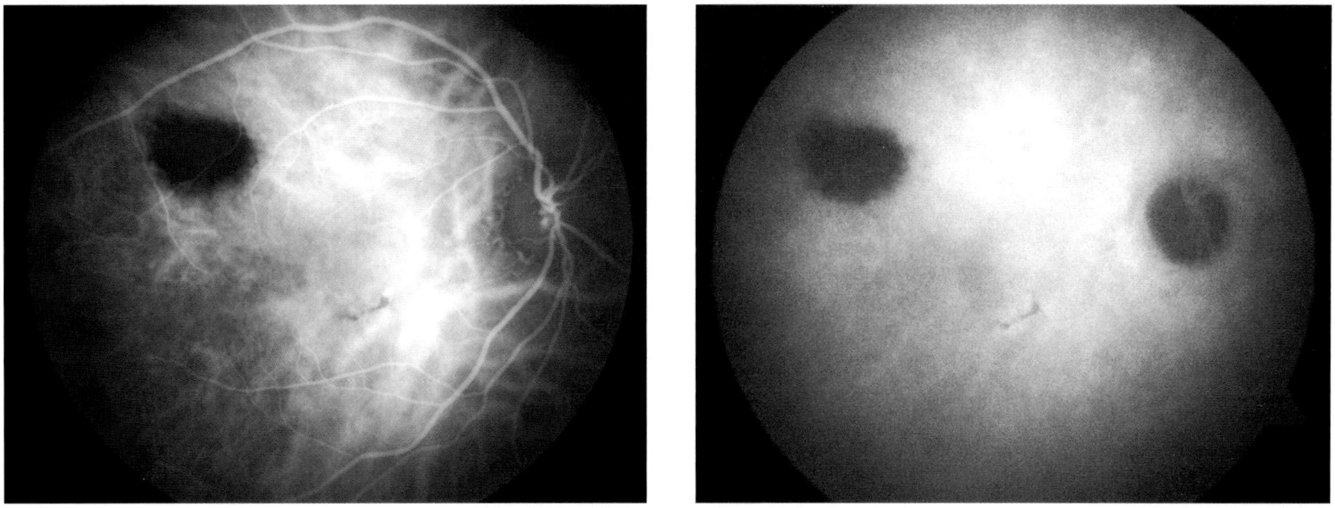

Indocyanine green angiogram delineates the nevus better in both the early and the late phase

COMMENT

Choroidal nevus shows blocked choroidal fluorescence through all phases of the angiogram. It is better delineated in the ICG angiogram.

62 Chapter

Melanocytoma

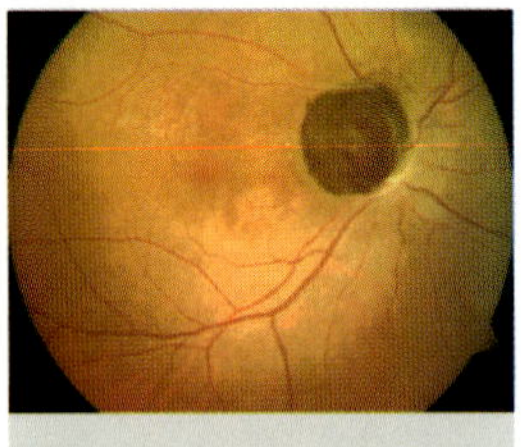

- It is a benign tumor arising from the optic nerve head.
- It is said to be derived from the uveal dendritic melanocytes.
- It appears as dark pigmented mass lesion on the optic nerve head.
- Malignant transformation of the melanocytoma is rare.
  Melanocytoma may be associated with neuroretinitis, retinal vascular occlusion, secondary (melanomalytic) glaucoma and compressive optic neuropathy.

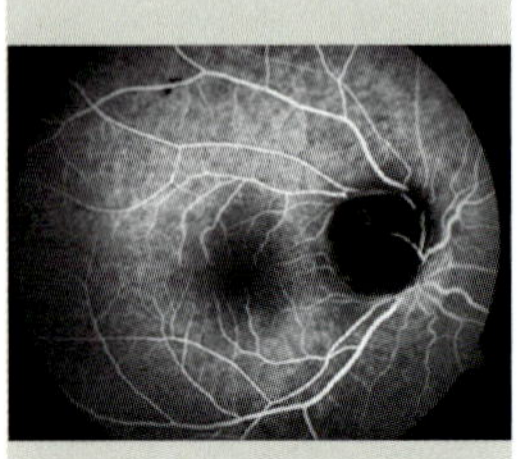

- Blocked disc fluorescence is seen through all phases of the angiogram.

CASE 1

A 33-year-old female presented with history of reduced vision in the right eye. Visual acuity was 6/12; N6.

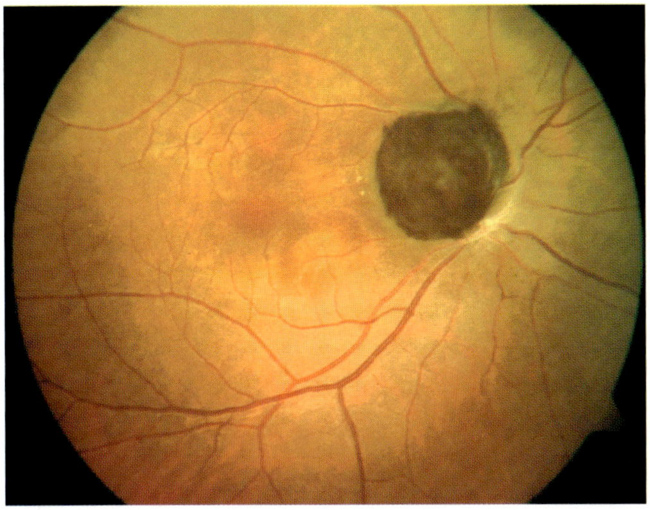

Fundus photograph of the right eye showing a typical melanocytoma at the optic nerve head

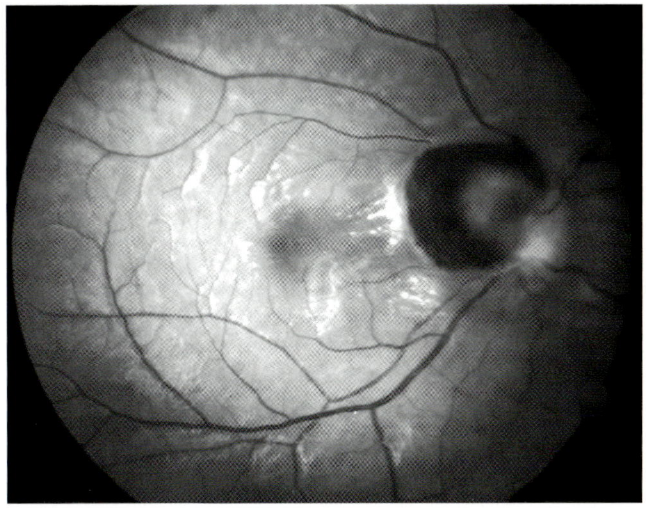

Red free photograph of the right eye

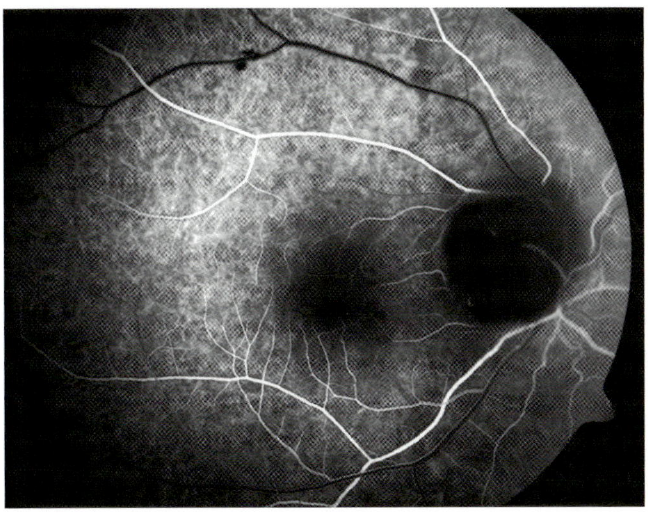

A blocked fluorescence due to the melanocytoma is seen in the early arteriovenous phase. An arteriole is seen coursing over the tumor

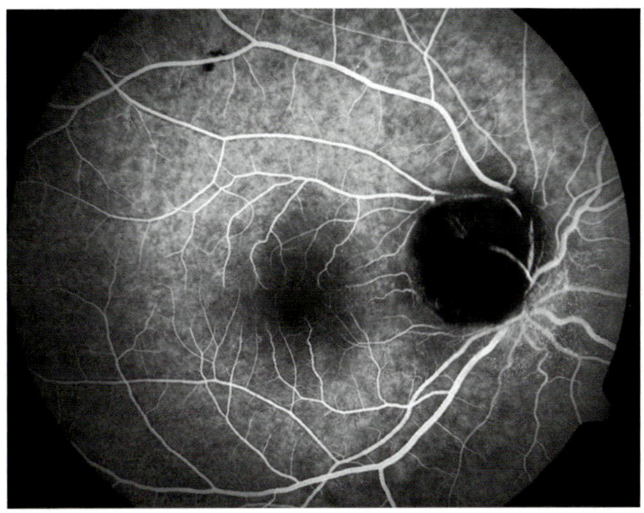

Arteriovenous phase showing the blocked fluorescence at the disc

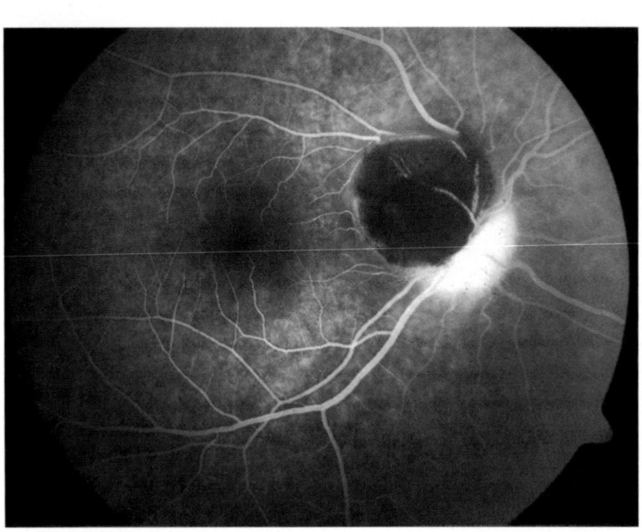

Hypofluorescence is seen to persist in the late phase of the angiogram

COMMENT

The pigment in the tumor blocks the underlying disc fluorescence through all phases of the angiogram.

BIBLIOGRAPHY

Rishi P, Ramesh V. Central retinal artery occlusion secondary to optic disc melanocytoma. Retinal cases and brief reports. Published ahead of print 30 Sep 2011.

63 Chapter

Malignant Melanoma

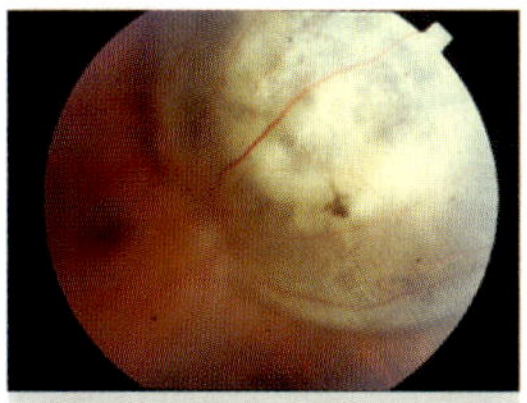

- Malignant melanoma is the most common primary intraocular tumor.
- It presents as a dark pigmented elevated ovoid mass lesion.
- The degree of pigmentation can vary.
- Some of the tumors may be amelanotic.
- It may assume a mushroom shape if it breaks through the Bruch's membrane.
- Overlying orange pigmentation may be seen.

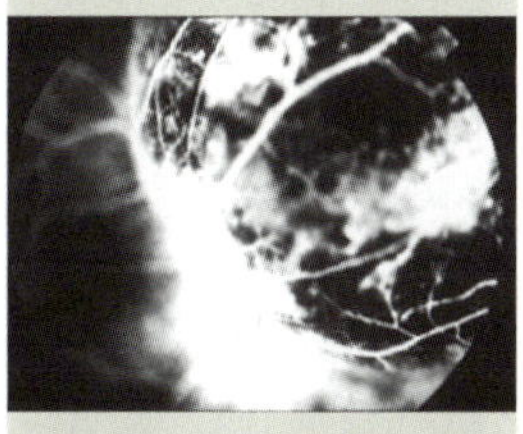

- The fluorescein angiographic picture of a malignant melanoma can vary depending on the size of the tumor and the degree of pigmentation.
- A small melanoma shows mottled hyperfluorescence in the arteriovenous phase. Increased staining of the mass lesion is seen in the late phase of the angiogram.
- Larger melanomas may show filling up of the large tumor vessels (double circulation–simultaneous filling up of the normal retinal vessels and the tumor vessels).
- Late diffuse staining of the mass lesion is seen.

CASE 1

A 32-year-old male was detected to have a mass lesion in the right eye and referred for further management. Visual acuity was 6/18; N8.

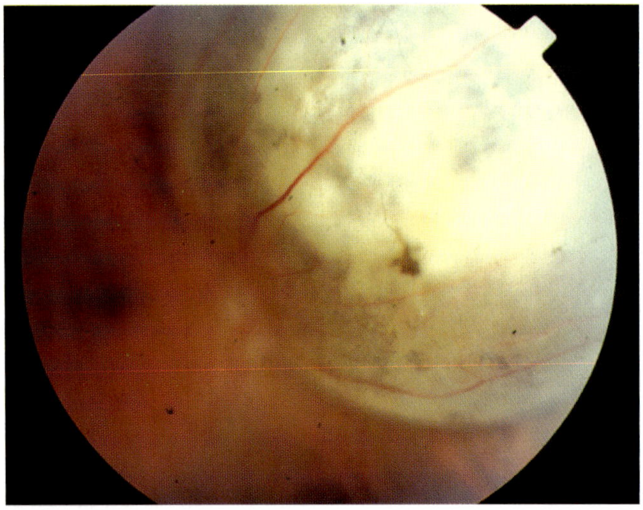

Fundus photograph of the right eye showing a dome shaped, pigmented, subretinal mass lesion in the peripapillary region

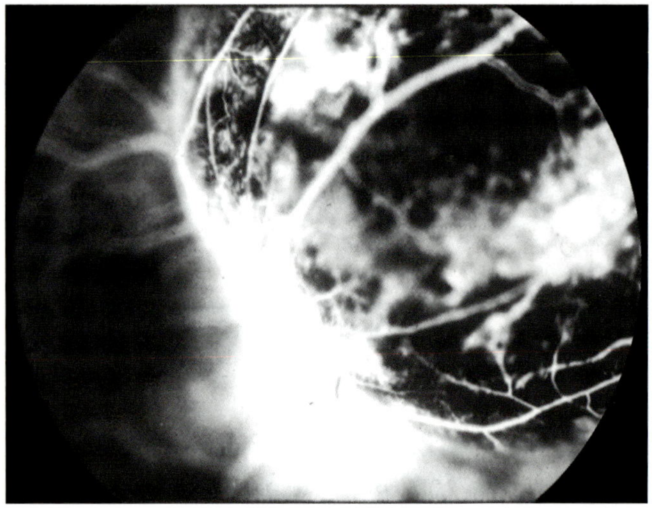

Arteriovenous phase of the angiogram showing patchy speckled hyperfluorescence over the mass lesion. The tumor vessels are made out within the mass lesion

COMMENT

Mottled hyperfluorescence in the mass lesion is seen in the early phase of the angiogram. Leakage of the dye from the tumor vessels occurs as the angiogram progresses leading to diffuse staining in the late phase.

In less pigmented tumors, both the retinal and tumor vessels are readily evident—this is called double circulation.

COMS Classification of Tumor Size

	Small	Medium	Large
Apical height	1.5–2.4 mm	2.5–10 mm	>10
Basal diameter	5–16 mm	≤16 mm	>16 mm

64 Chapter Choroidal Hemangioma

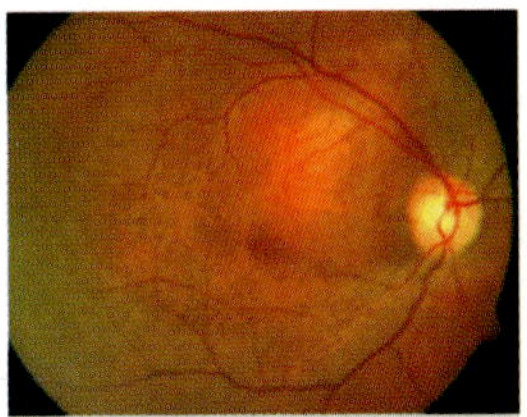

- Choroidal hemangioma is a vascular hamartoma and can either be circumscribed or diffuse.
- Circumscribed choroidal hemangioma is seen as a well defined red-orange, slightly elevated dome shaped lesion usually located at the posterior pole.
- It may be associated with a serous retinal detachment and CNVM.
- Histopathologically it may show a cavernous, capillary or a mixed type of a hemangioma. Large, thin walled, blood filled vascular channels are seen. Cystic changes are commonly seen in the outer retinal layers overlying the tumor.

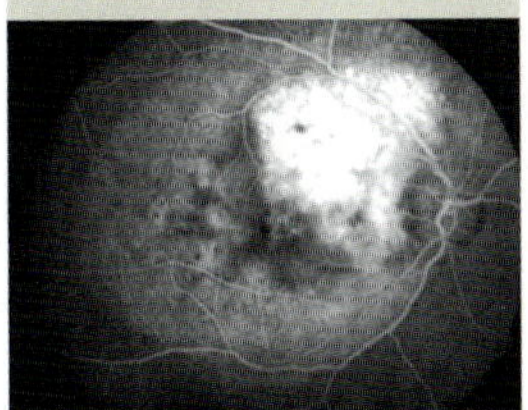

- Arterial and early arteriovenous phase may show the reticular vascular pattern due to the large choroidal vessels within the tumor.
- The arteriovenous phase shows stippled hyperfluorescence.
- Increased staining and leakage is seen in the late phase of the angiogram.

CASE 1

A 34-year-old male was referred for a mass lesion detected in the left eye. Visual acuity was 6/6; N6.

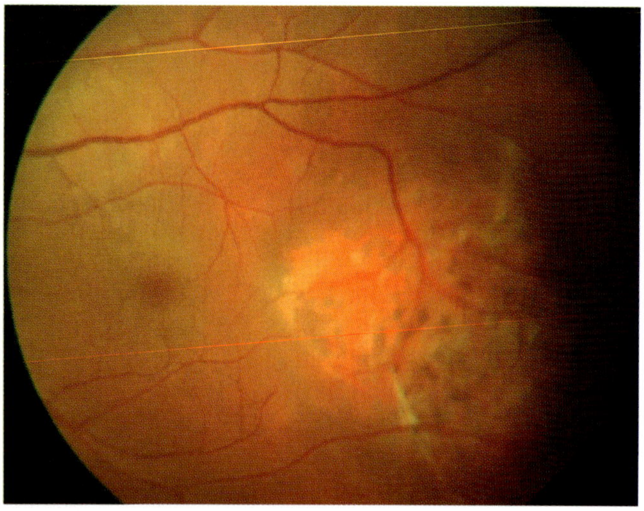

Fundus photograph of the left eye showing a red orange, minimally elevated mass lesion temporal to the macula. Note extensive pigment overlying the mass lesion and a subretinal gliotic band

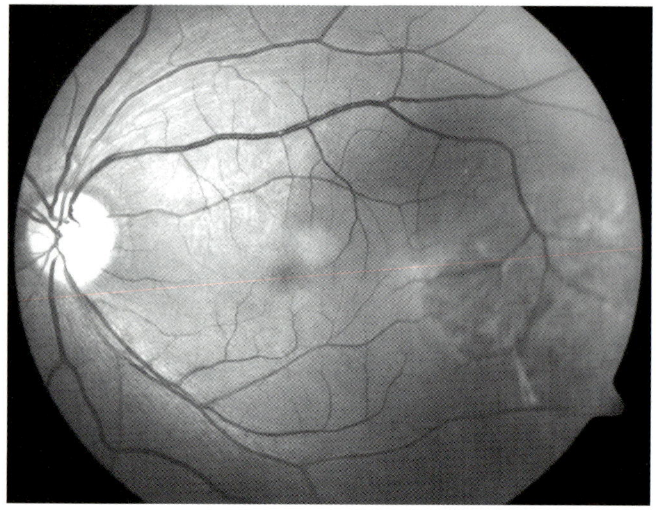

Red free photograph of the left eye

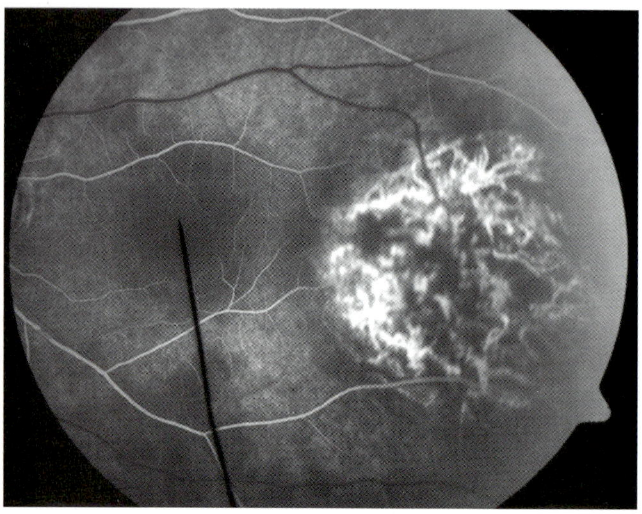

Arterial phase showing intense hyperfluorescence of the tumor indicating its choroidal origin and vascularity

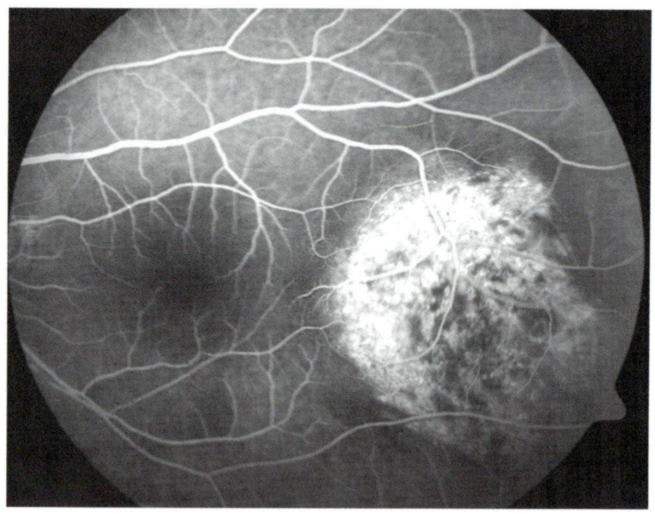

Mid arteriovenous phase showing increase in hyperfluorescence indicating leakage of the dye. Note patches of blocked fluorescence due to pigment

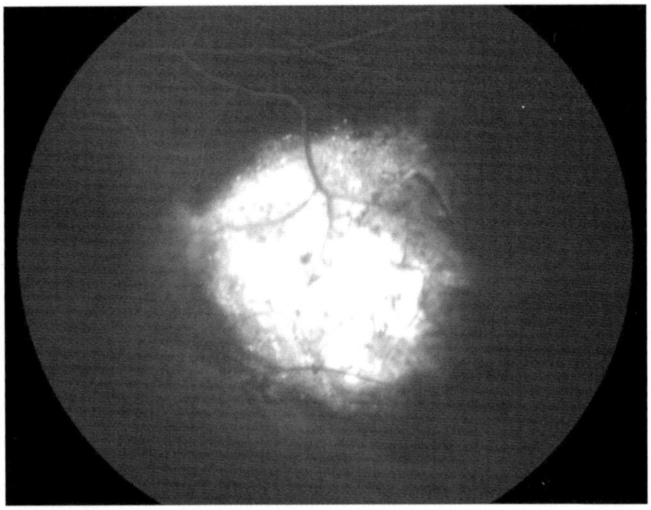

Late phase angiogram showing leakage of the dye from the tumor vessels

COMMENT

Choroidal hemangioma shows early hyperfluorescence with late leakage of the dye and staining of the tumor.

BIBLIOGRAPHY

1. Sharma T, Krishnan T, Gopal L, Nagpal A, Khetan V, Rishi P. Transpupillary thermotherapy for circumscribed choroidal hemangioma. Ophthalmic Surg Lasers Imaging 2011;42(5):360-8.
2. Boixadera A, Garcia-Arumi J, Martinez–Castillo V, et al. Prospective clinical trial evaluating the efficacy of photodynamic therapy for symptomatic circumscribed choroidal hemagioma. Ophthalmology 2009;116(1):100-5.

65
Chapter

Choroidal Osteoma

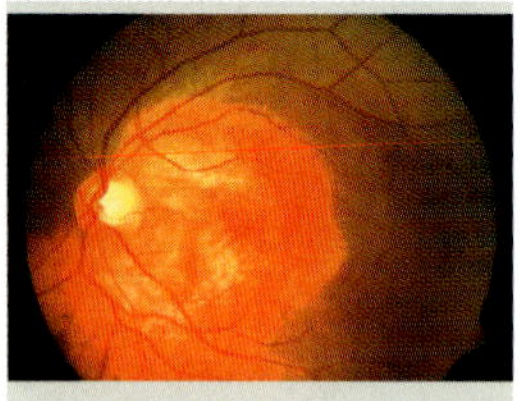

- Choroidal osteoma is a rare benign tumor of choroid, mostly unilateral and commonly seen in females in second to third decade of life.
- It is a choriostoma of choroid composed of mature bone which can be present subretinal, preretinal or at both locations. Most common location is juxta or parapapillary but can be seen in the macular area.
- Most patients are asymptomatic but can have symptoms if a choroidal neovascular membrane develops in the subfoveal location or due to the development of spontaneous subretinal hemorrhage, subretinal fluid and decalcification with RPE degeneration.
- Its appearance varies from yellow-white to orange-red flat lesion (<2 mm) depending on the overlying thinning and depigmentation of retinal pigment epithelium and thickness of calcium plaque with variable pigment deposits.
- It has well defined scalloped margins with pseudopod like projections. It can be associated with overlying subretinal fluid or hemorrhage suggestive of choroidal neovascular membrane.

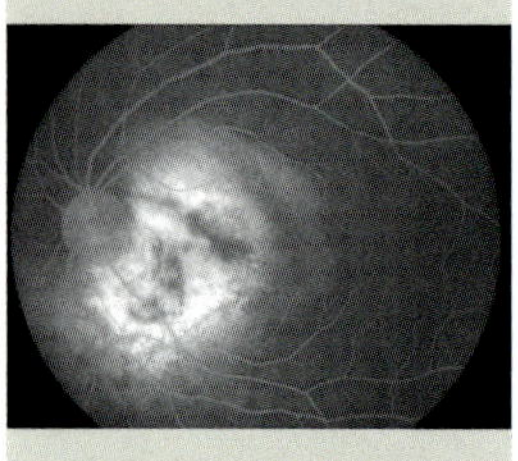

- Fluorescein angiogram shows mild patchy early hyperfluorescence with diffuse late staining in the area of the osteoma.
- Presence of early lacy pattern of hyperfluoresence with leakage of fluorescein in late phases is suggestive of choroidal neovascular membrane.
- Blocked fluorescence is seen in presence of hemorrhage and pigment clumping.
- Multiple pinpoint leakage sites may be seen suggestive of RPE defects.

CASE 1

An 18-year-old female presented with history of gradual loss of vision in the left eye of 6 months duration. BCVA in left eye was 6/36; N18. She was diagnosed of 'resolved chorioretinitis', elsewhere.

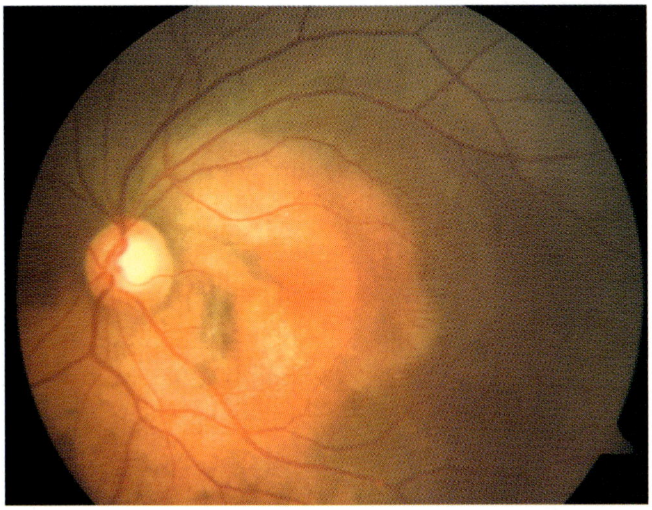

Fundus photograph shows the orange-red subretinal lesion in the macular and peripapillary area with areas of pigment hyperplasia temporal to disc and a subretinal, fibrotic lesion suggestive of scarred subretinal neovascular membrane

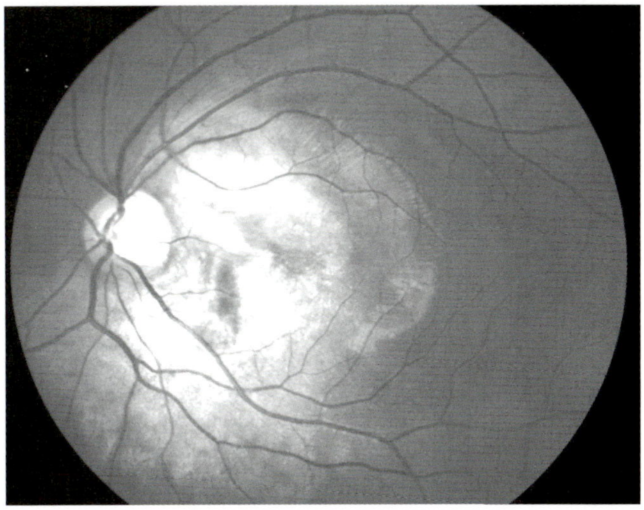

Red free photograph highlights the subretinal fibrotic lesion

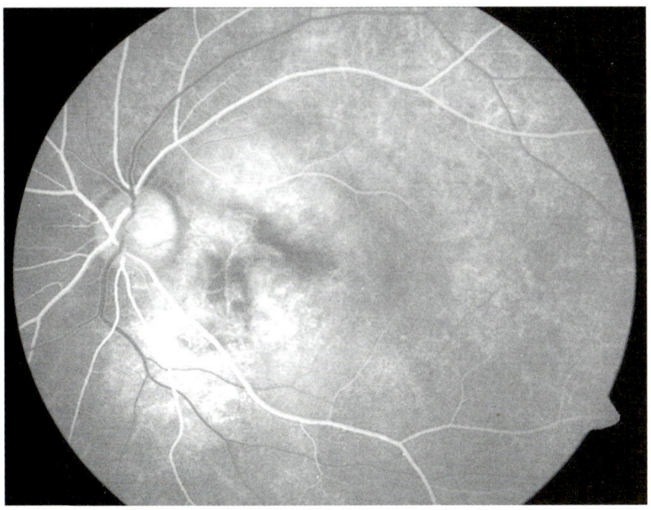

Early A-V phase angiogram shows a lacy pattern of hyperfluorescence in the temporal peripapillary area suggestive of a subretinal neovascular membrane. Hypofluorescent areas temporal to it signify blocked fluorescence due to pigment hyperplasia. There a few pinpoint areas of hyperfluorescence over a generalized granular hyperfluorescence signifying RPE window defects over the choroidal osteoma

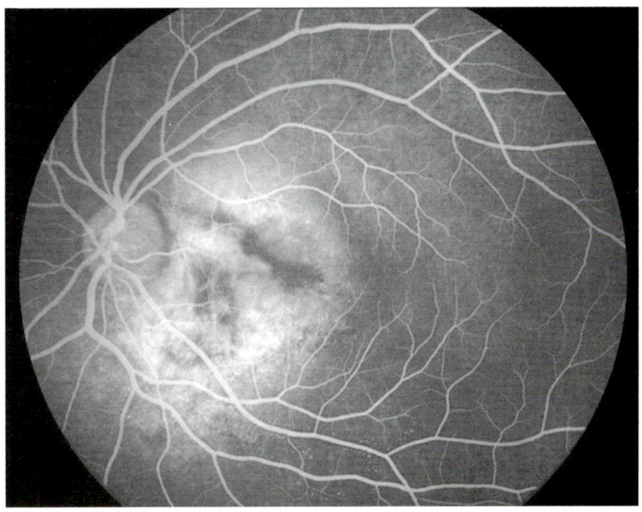

Mid A-V phase shows staining of the subretinal neovascularization in the parapapillary area and increase in the hyperfluorescence in the area of choroidal osteoma

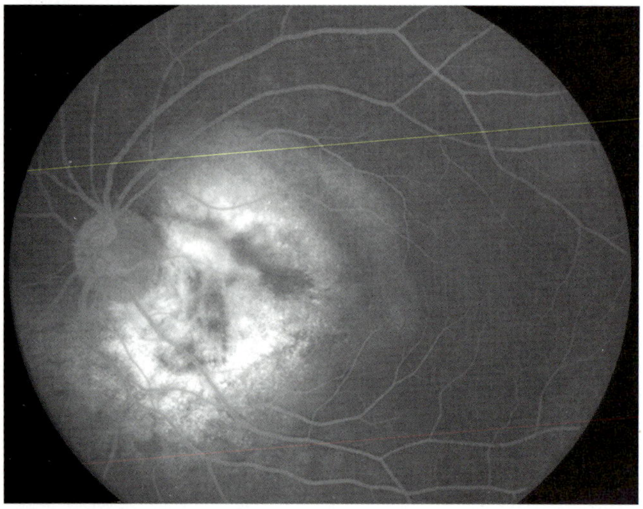

Late phase- faint staining of the choroidal osteoma is seen. Note the black silhouette in the inferior margin of the lesion representing the vasculature of the osteoma

COMMENT

FFA helps in identifying, localizing and monitoring the treatment of CNVM secondary to osteoma.

Indocyanine green angiography can help in identifying the vascular remodeling of the Haversian system of choroidal osteoma over a period of time.

Choroidal osteoma should be borne as a differential in diagnosis in a young female patient with spontaneous choroidal hemorrhage.

Ultrasound and CT scan can be used to confirm a choroidal osteoma and to differentiate from a malignant choroidal tumor like choroidal melanoma.

CLINICAL NUGGETS

1. Optical coherence tomography is useful for monitoring response to treatment of CNVM in osteoma.
2. OCT also helps in prognosticating the visual prognosis by demonstrating the photoreceptor atrophy and retinal thinning that occur over the decalcifying osteoma.
3. Anti- VEGF therapy is successful in the resolution of CNVM secondary to osteoma.
4. Laser treatment for CNVM can stimulate decalcification and vascular remodeling of the choroidal osteoma.

BIBLIOGRAPHY

1. Barkeh Hanim Jumaat. Bone in the eye. Am J Ophthalmol 2003;135:254-56.
2. David J. Choroidal osteoma, observations from a community setting. browning. Ophthalmol 2003; 110:1327-34.
3. Shields CL. Optical coherence tomography of choroidal osteoma in 22 cases. Ophthalmol 2007;114: e54-e58.

66

Chapter

Retinoblastoma

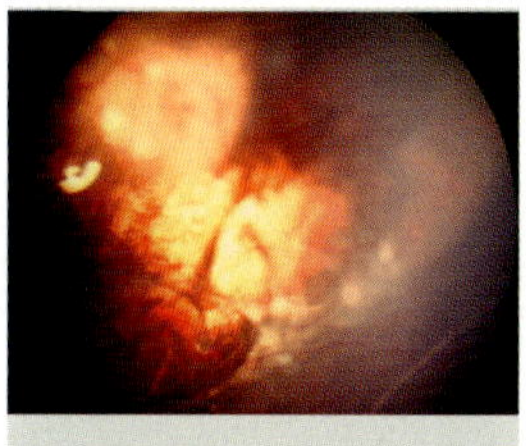

- It is the most common intraocular malignancy of childhood.
- It can be unilateral or bilateral.
- It starts as a small transparent lesion in the retina. Later on it becomes more opaque with development of tumor vessels.
- The growth of the tumor can be towards the subretinal space (exophytic) or towards the vitreous (endophytic). Rarely it may be diffuse.

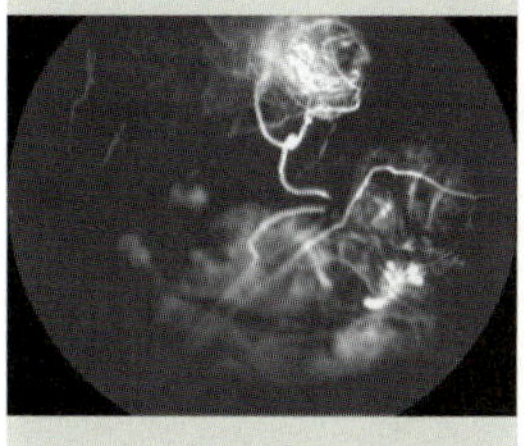

- Early phase shows filling of the tumor vessels with leakage of the dye seen in the later phases.
- Late hyperfluorescence of the tumor is seen.

CASE 1

An 8-year-old child with retinoblastoma was referred for reactivation of the tumor in the right eye. Left eye had been enucleated six year back and he had undergone cryotherapy, radiation and chemotherapy for the tumor in the right eye. Visual acuity was 6/12; N6.

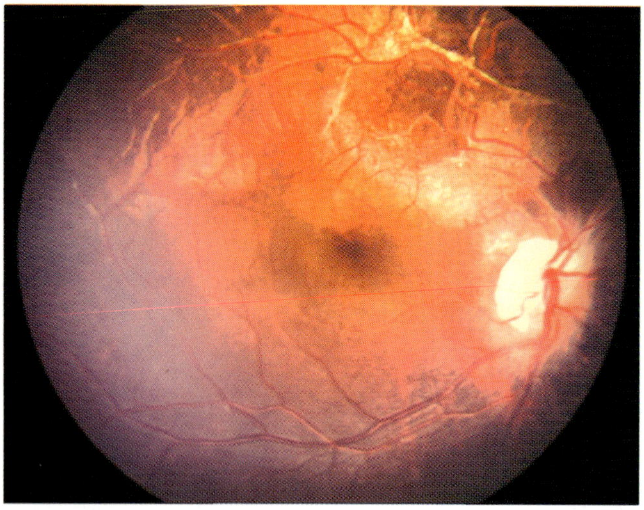

Fundus photograph of the right eye showing chorioretinal atrophy along the superotemporal arcade

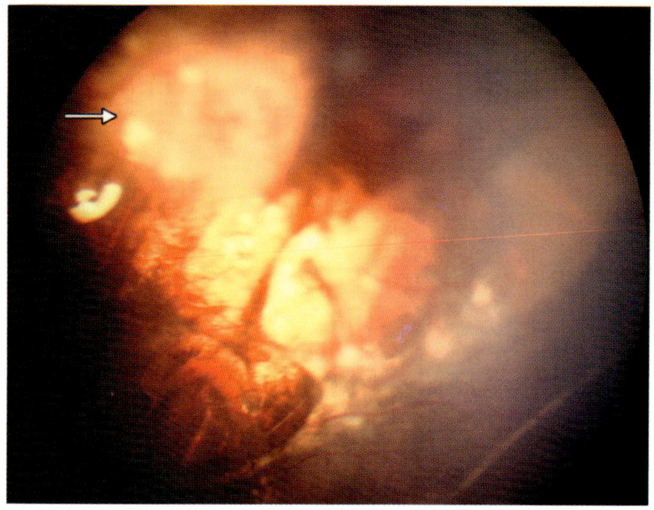

Fundus photograph of the superotemporal periphery showing an elevated pearly white vascularized mass lesion (arrow) in the area of extensive chorioretinal atrophy

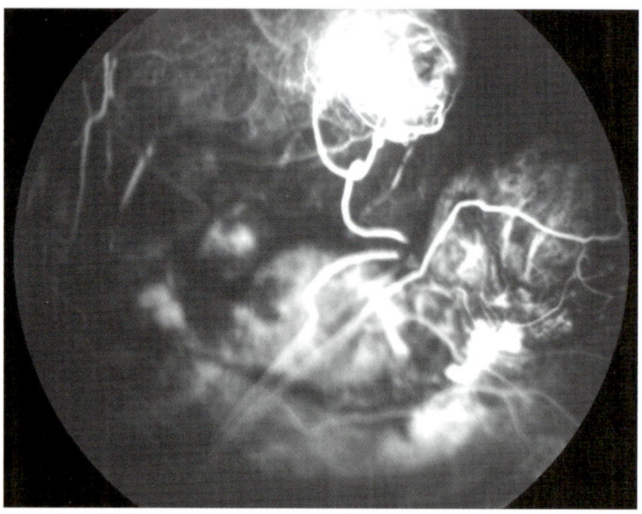

Early arteriovenous phase showing the intrinsic vasculature of the tumor vessels and its connection to the retinal circulation

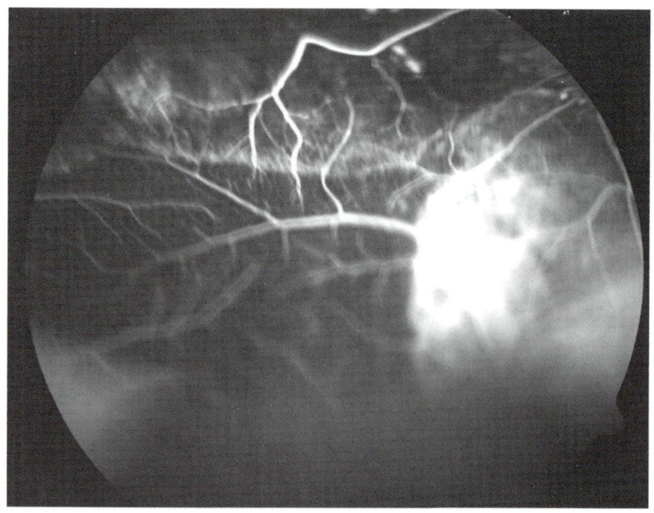

Mid arteriovenous phase showing increase in hyperfluorescence due to leakage of the dye

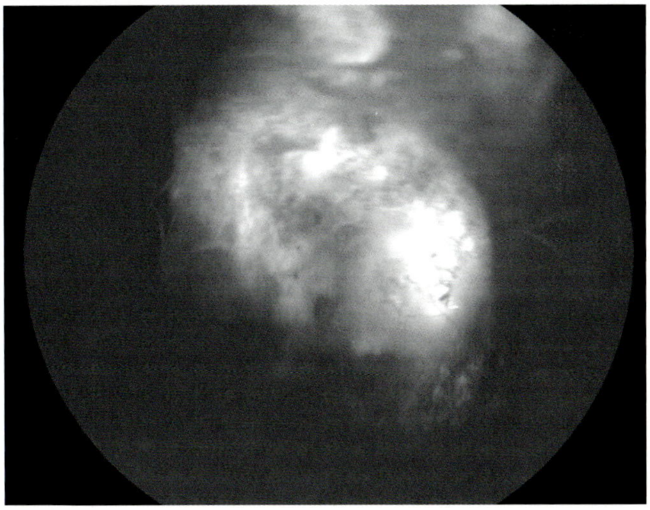

Late phase shows leakage of the dye from the tumor

COMMENT

Early filling of the tumor vasculature with subsequent leakage of the dye is seen in retinoblastoma.

International Intraocular Retinoblastoma Classification (IIRC)

Group A—very low risk

Eyes with small discrete tumors away from critical structures

All tumors are 3 mm or smaller, confined to the retina, and located at least 3 mm from the foveola and 1.5 mm from the optic nerve.

No vitreous or subretinal seeding is allowed.

Group B—low risk

Eyes with no vitreous or subretinal seeding and discrete retinal tumor of any size or location.

Retinal tumors may be of any size or location not in Group A.

No vitreous or subretinal seeding allowed.

A small cuff of subretinal fluid extending no more than 5 mm from the base of the tumor is allowed.

Group C—moderate risk

Eyes with only focal vitreous or subretinal seeding and discrete retinal tumors of any size and location.

Any seeding must be local, fine and limited so as to be theoretically treatable with a radioactive plaque.

Retinal tumors are discrete and of any size and location.

Up to one quadrant of subretinal fluid may be present.

Group D—high risk

Eyes with diffuse vitreous or subretinal seeding and/or massive, nondiscrete endophytic or exophytic disease Eyes with more extensive seeding than Group C.

Massive and/or diffuse intraocular disseminated disease may consist of fine or "greasy" vitreous seeding or avascular masses.

Subretinal seeding may be plaque-like. Includes exophytic disease and more than one quadrant of retinal detachment.

Group E—very high risk

Eyes that have been destroyed anatomically or functionally by the tumor.

Eyes with anyone or more of the following:

- Irreversible neovascular glaucoma
- Massive intraocular hemorrhage
- Aseptic orbital cellulitis
- Tumor anterior to anterior vitreous face
- Tumor touching the lens
- Diffuse infiltrating retinoblastoma
- Phthisis or pre-phthisis.

67

Chapter

Retinal Angiomatosis

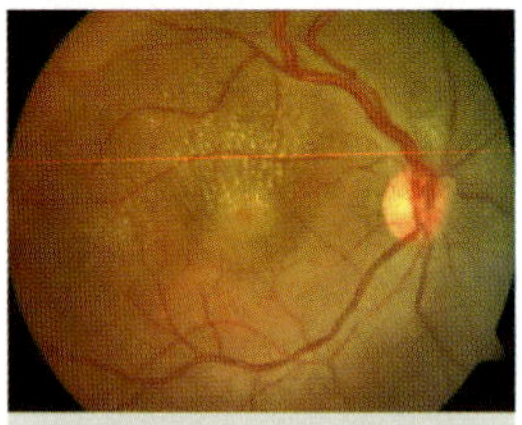

- It is usually diagnosed in children or young adults.
- It can occur as a solitary tumor without any systemic associations or as a part of the von Hippel-Lindau (VHL) syndrome.
- It appears as a reddish-pink tumor in the retina or on the optic disc.
- Associated feeder vessels are seen.
- It may be associated with extensive subretinal fluid, lipid exudation, fibrosis and combined retinal detachment. Fluorescein angiography is mandatory to pick up peripheral lesions.

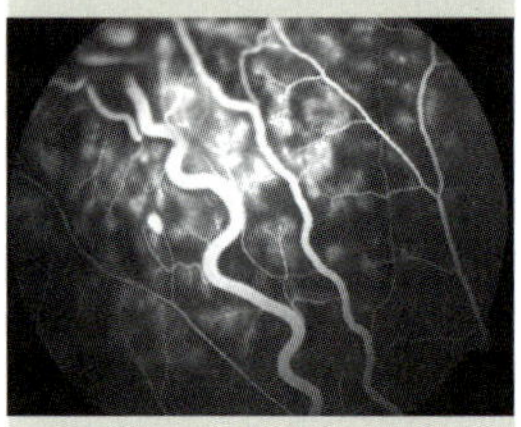

- Capillary hemangioma shows rapid filling of the tumor mass in the early phase of the angiogram.
- Leakage of the dye with intense hyperfluorescence is seen in the late phase.

CASE 1

A 15-year-old male patient presented with history of loss of vision in the left eye for the past three years. He had been diagnosed to have a retinal angioma with exudative retinal detachment in the left eye and had undergone cryotherapy in the past. Visual acuity was 6/5; N6 in the right eye and no perception of light in the left eye. He was found to have retinal angiomas in the right eye.

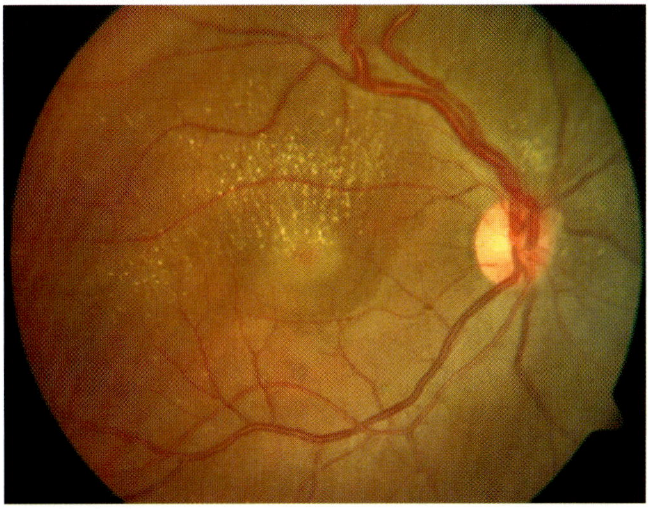

Fundus photograph of the right eye showing dilated twin feeder vessels with exudates at the macula

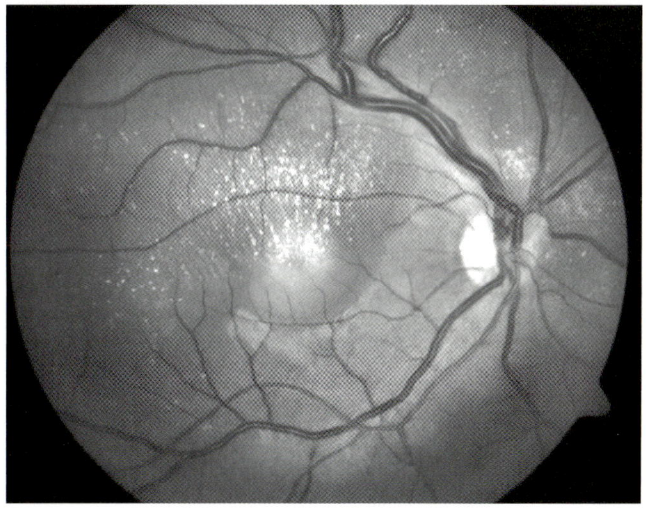

Red free photograph of the right eye

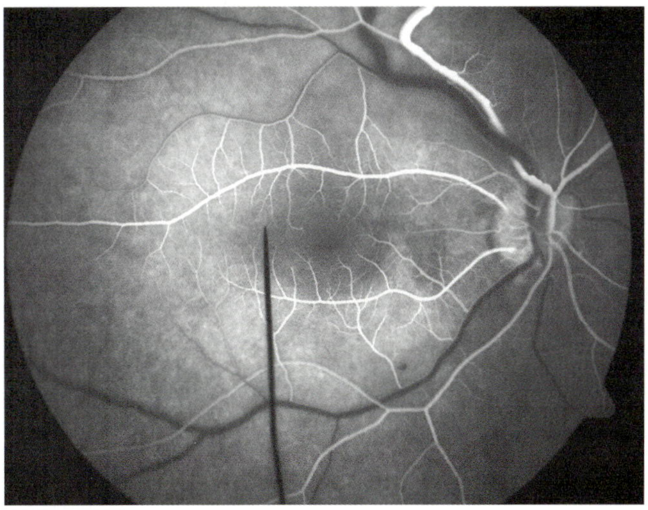

Arterial phase helps to differentiate the feeder arteriole from the venule

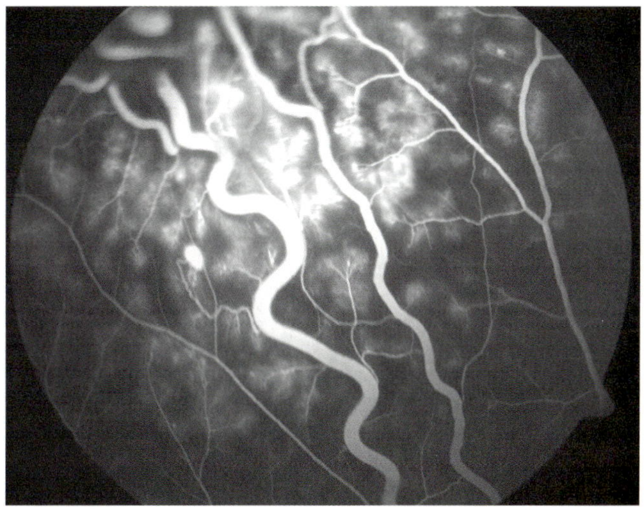

Rapid flow through the angioma is reflected in early filling of the draining venule in the arteriovenous phase of the angiogram

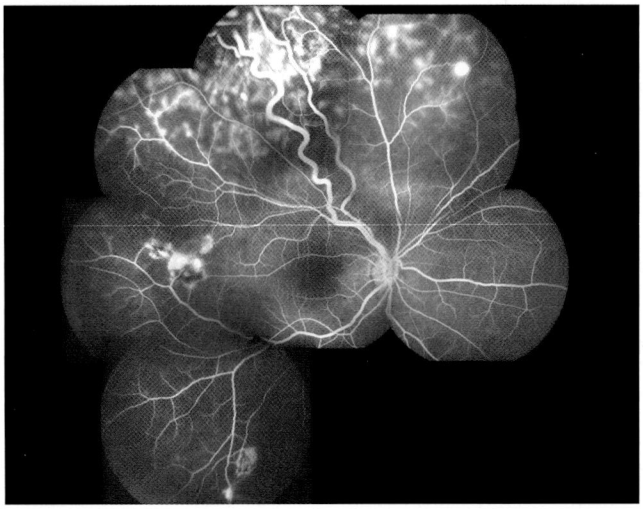

The multiple capillary hemangiomas are evident in this montage

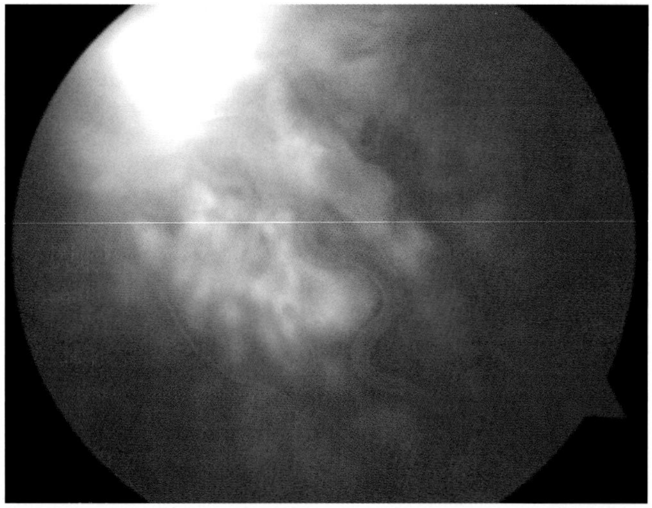

Profuse leakage of the dye from the tumor vessels is seen in the late phase of the angiogram

Astrocytic Hamartoma

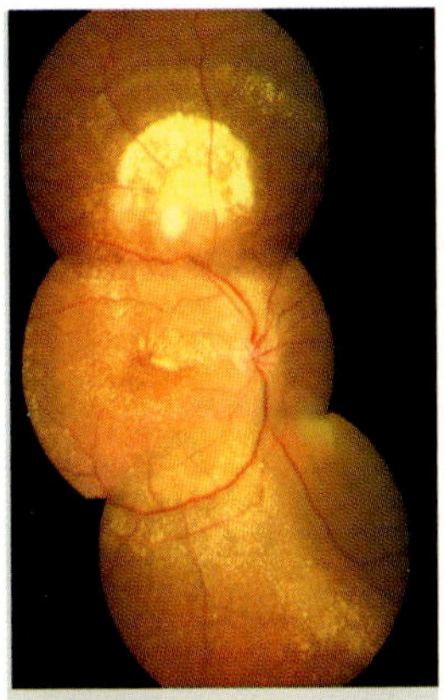

- It is a benign proliferation of astrocytes which is either seen in young and associated with phacomatoses or may affect older individuals and is then acquired.
- Usually these are solitary, peripapillary, lobulated, whitish lesions resembling a mulberry with variable amounts of calcification.
- These tumors can appear as subtle thickening of nerve fibre layer to a huge mass.
- They can rarely cause exudation or bleeding through tiny vessels within the tumor.

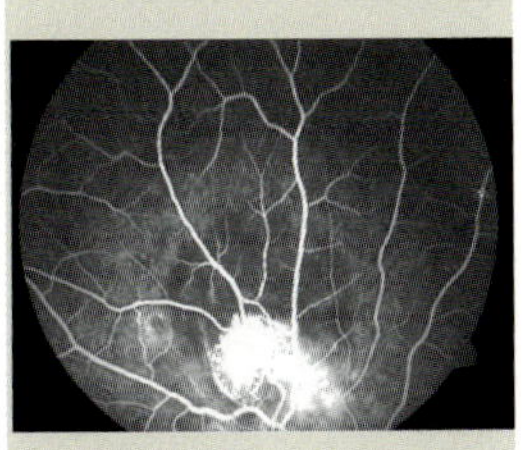

- Astrocytic hamartomas have been classified into three types based on angiography.
- Arterial phase of the angiogram shows hypofluorescence due to blockage of underlying choroidal vessels by the mass itself.
- The abnormal tumor vessels fill up all the along the mass lesion.
- Fine, tortuous vessels fill up along with the retinal vessels as well.

CASE 1

A 30 year-old lady presented to us with sudden, painless loss of vision in the right eye for the past one month. Her BCVA was 6/18; N10 in right eye. Left eye was normal and fundus was unremarkable.

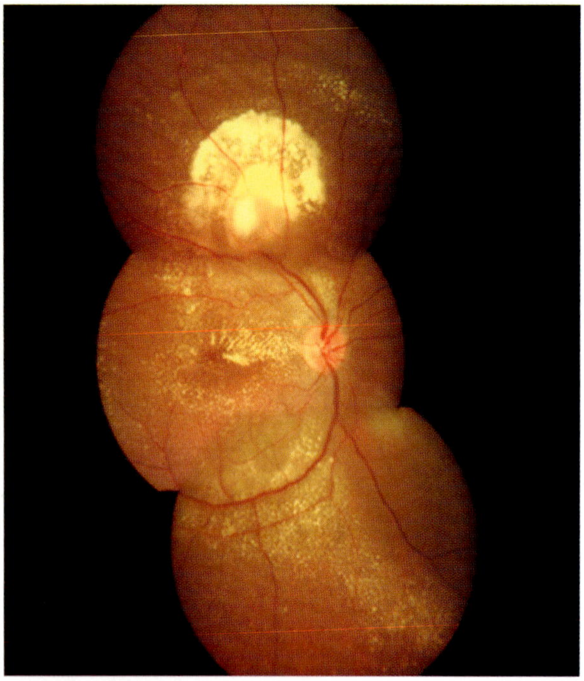

Fundus photo shows presence of peripapillary yellowish mass lesion superiorly with multiple hard exudates all around the mass and presence of macular star

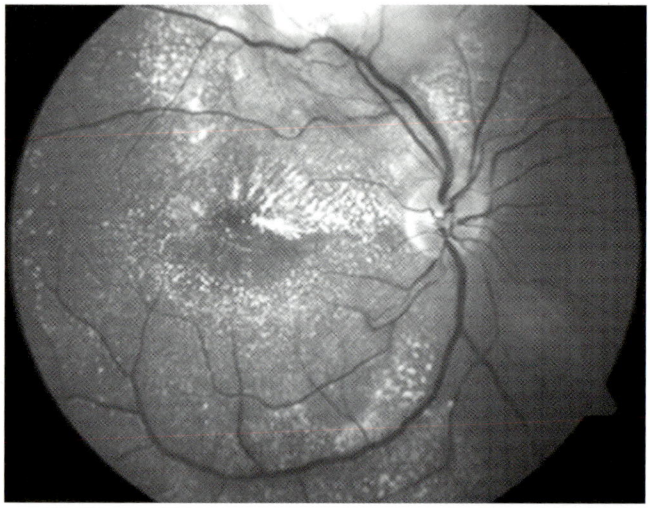

Red free photograph of the same eye shows the dense exudation over the posterior pole. Inferior edge of the mass is just visible along the superotemporal arcade

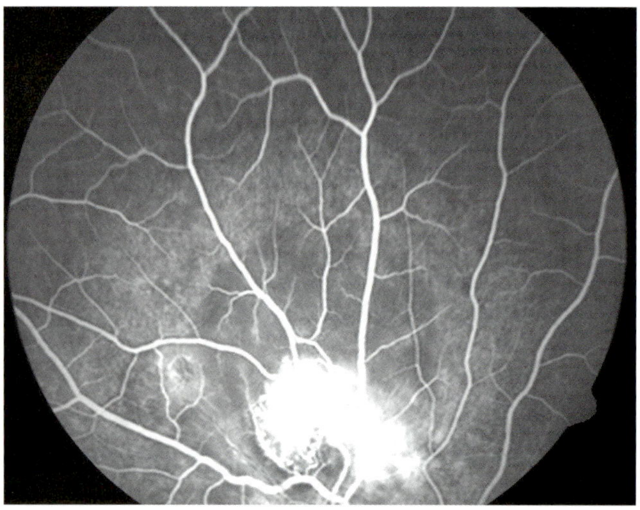

Arterial phase of the angiogram showing hypofluorescence due to blockage of underlying choroidal vessels all along the mass lesion. The abnormal tumor vessels are filling up as well by the mass itself. Fine, tortous vessels fill up along with the retinal vessels

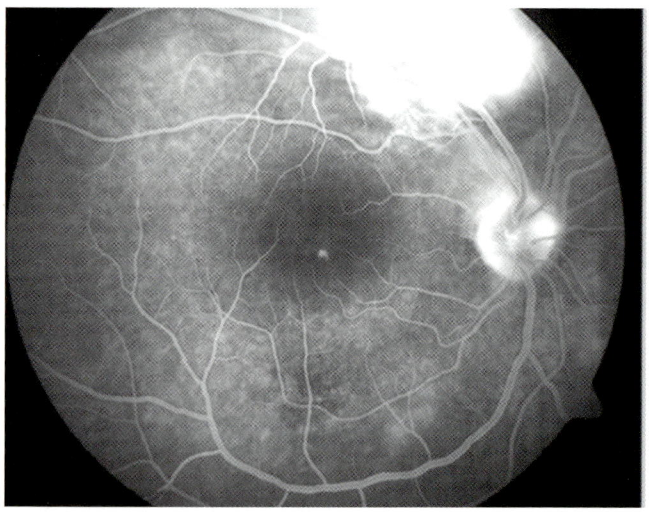

Mid phase of the angiogram showing a prominent network of vessels over superficial part of the tumor with profuse leakage

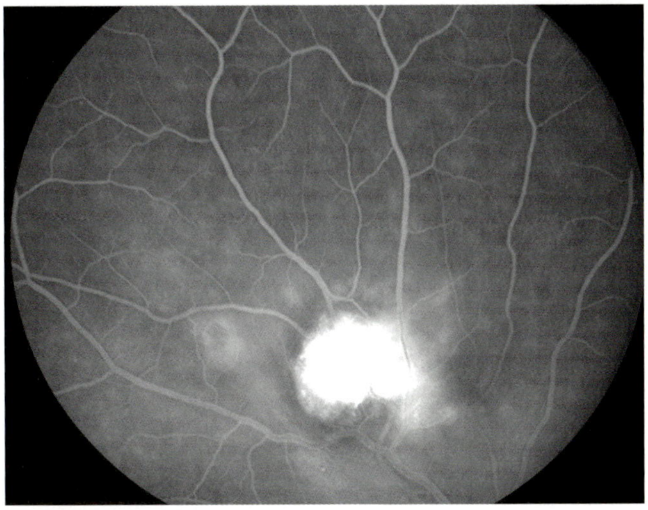

Late phase of the angiogram showing intense and diffuse homogeneous staining of the mass

CLINICAL NUGGETS

1. Astrocytomas have been classified into three types based on angiography. Type 1 being the subtle ones which are difficult to pick upon examination but clearly show blocked fluorescence on FFA and ICG both.
2. It may be the presenting feature in cases of phacomatoses, hence needs a high index of suspicion.
3. It can be differentiated from angioma by absence of feeder vessel and more superficial location.
4. Cavernous hemangioma mostly seen in a similar peripapillary location can be differentiated by its typical capping sign, tendency to fill more slowly and minimal leakage unlike a hamartoma.

BIBLIOGRAPHY

1. Brodsky MC, Safar AN. Optic Disc Tuber. Arch Ophthalmol. 2007;125(5):710-3.
2. Giles J, Singh AD, Rundle PA, Noe KP, Rennie IG. Retinal astrocytic hamartoma with exudation. Eye 2005;19: 724-25.
3. Grenga PL, Sagoo MS, Malagola R. Recurrent vitreous haemorrhage from sporadic retinal astrocytic hamartoma. Eye 2007;21:682-4.
4. Mennel S, Meyer CH, Eggarter F, Peter S. Autofluorescence and angiographic findings of retinal astrocytic hamartomas in tuberous sclerosis. Ophthalmologica. 2005;219(6):350-6.
5. Sachdeva, et al. Astrocytic hamartoma of the optic disc and multiple café-au-lait macules in a child with neurofibromatosis type 2. Ophthalmic Genetics, Ophthalmic Genetics 2010;31(4):209-14.

69 Chapter

Other Tumors

OPTIC NERVE HEMANGIOMA

CASE 1

A 49-year-old male presented with reduced vision in the right eye for the past five years. Visual acuity was 6/60; N36 in the right eye.

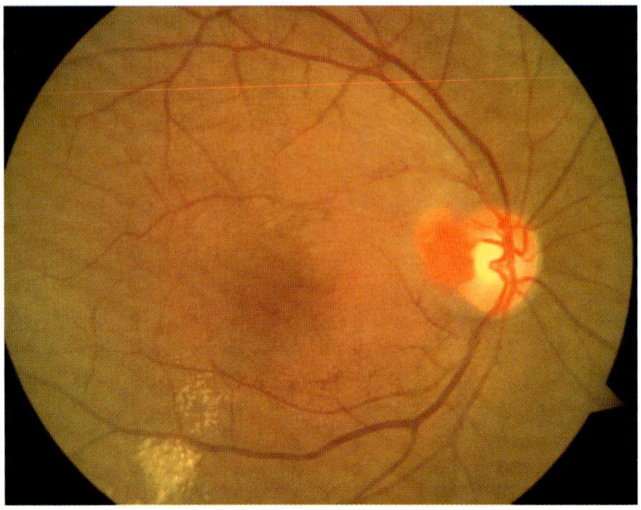

Fundus photograph of the right eye showing a orange-red well defined lesion at the disc margin. Hard exudates are seen along the inferotemporal arcade indicating exudation from the tumor

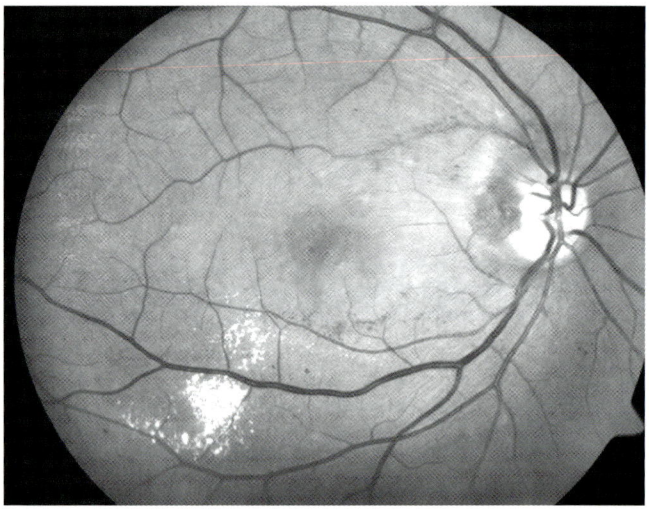

Red free photograph of the right eye

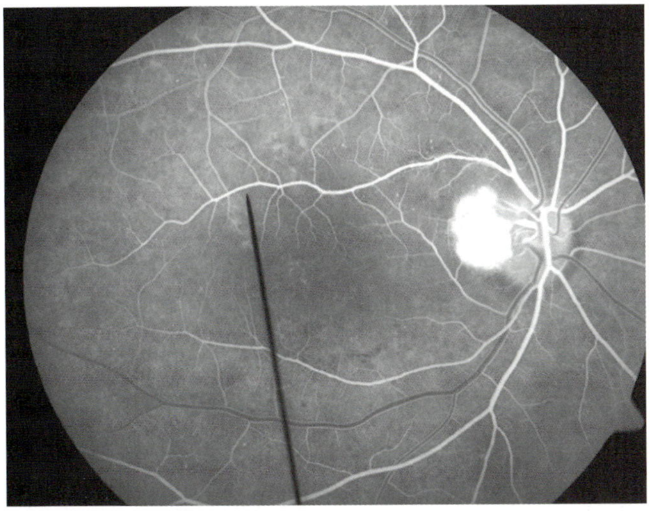

Lesion shows intense hyperfluorescence in the early arteriovenous phase indicating the vascular nature of the lesion

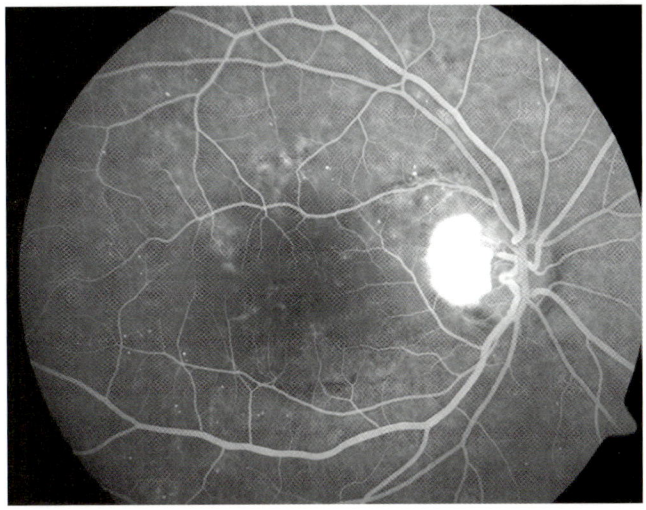

Late arteriovenous phase showing increased area of hyperfluorescence due to leakage of the dye. Note intraretinal dye leakage, presumed to be due to vascular 'steal' by the tumor

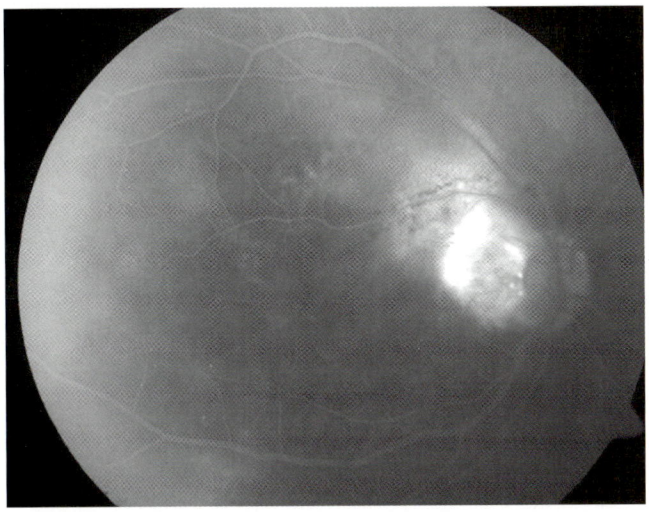

Late phase angiogram shows dye leakage from the tumor and increased intraretinal dye leakage

COMMENT

The vascular nature of the lesion gives rise to the intense hyperfluorescence seen on the angiogram.

RETINAL CAVERNOUS HEMANGIOMA

CASE 2

A 31-year-old female presented with complaints of occasional headache for the past three months. Visual acuity was 6/6; N6 in both eyes.

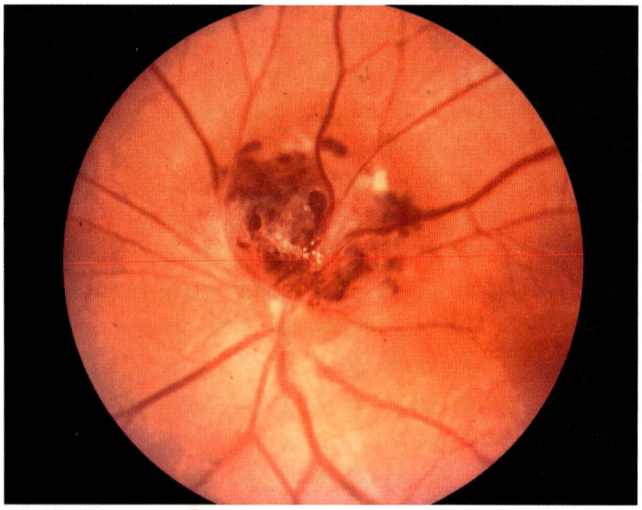

Fundus photograph of the left eye showing a cluster of grapes like appearing cavernous hemangioma of the optic nerve head

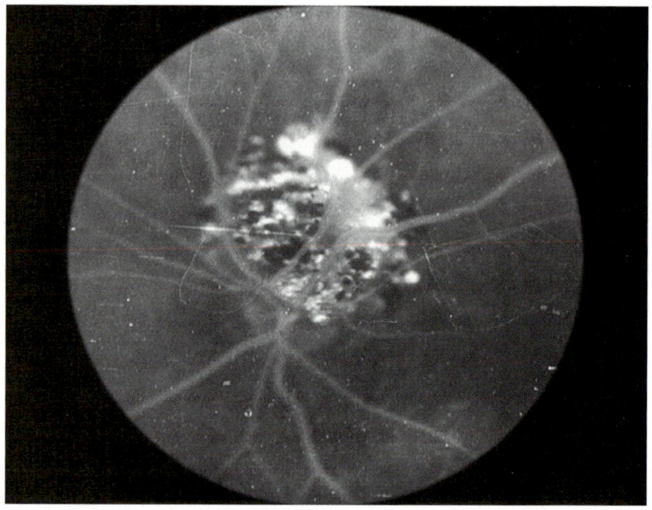

Late phase showing the classical picture of cavernous hemangioma. The dye has filled the upper half of the saccular aneurysms while the lower half remains hypofluorescent

COMMENT

The dark red color of the hemorrhage within the tumor indicates a sluggish circulation. Sedimentation of cellular elements and supernatant serum is seen as a fluid level in each globular lesion. The fluorescein dye enters only the upper supernatant plasma; the sedimented cellular elements in the lower half do not allow fluorescein to percolate, causing it to remain hypofluorescent.

COMBINED HAMARTOMA

CASE 3

A 43-year-old male patient was referred with a diagnosis of choroiditis in the right eye. He complained of reduced vision noted for the last 3 months. Visual acuity was 6/9; N8 in the right eye and 6/6; N6 in the left eye. Left eye was normal.

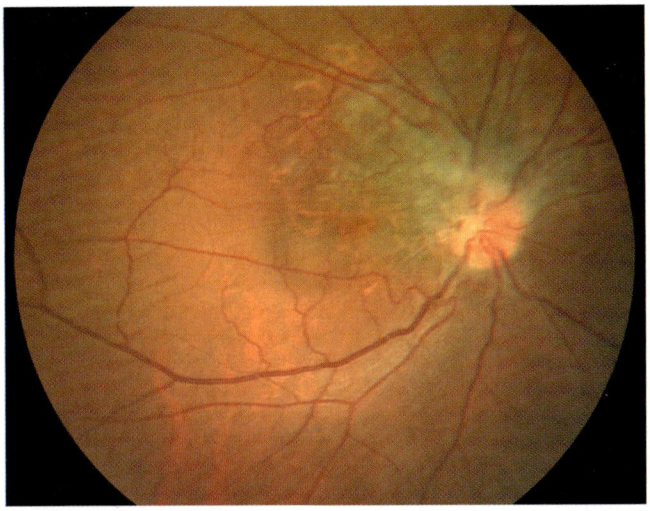

Fundus photograph of the right eye showing a hyperpigmentation at the level of the RPE. Glial proliferation involving the retina is seen, causing tortuosity of retinal vasculature and blurring of disc margin

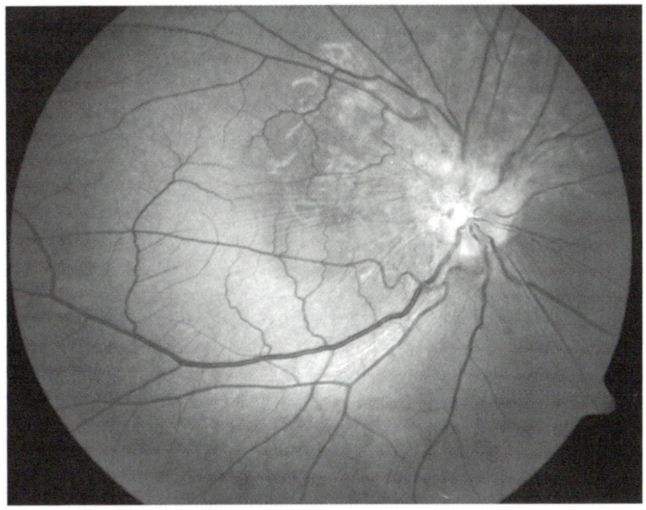

Red free photograph of the right eye

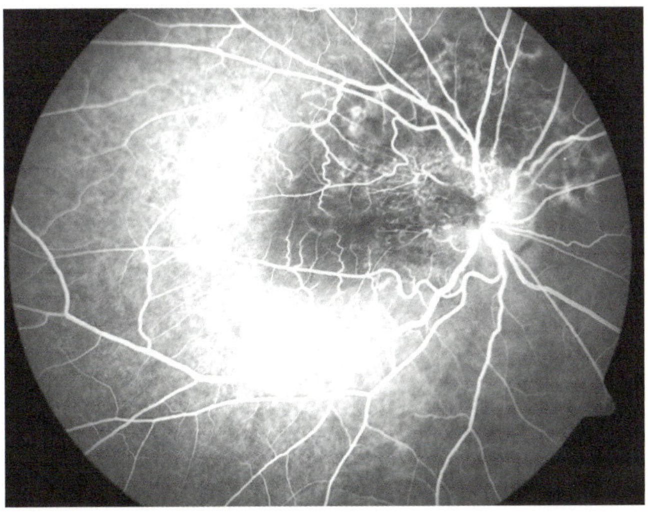

Mid arteriovenous phase shows a well defined patch of blocked choroidal fluorescence. Distortion of the retinal vasculature is well made out

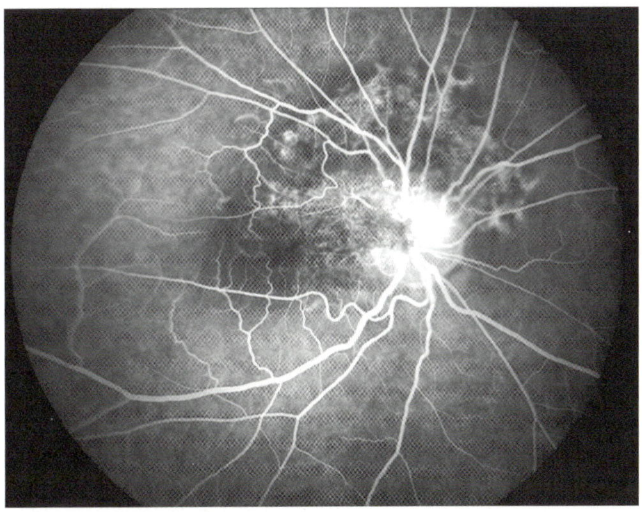

Late arteriovenous phase showing increased hyperfluorescence due to leaking abnormal vessels in the tumor

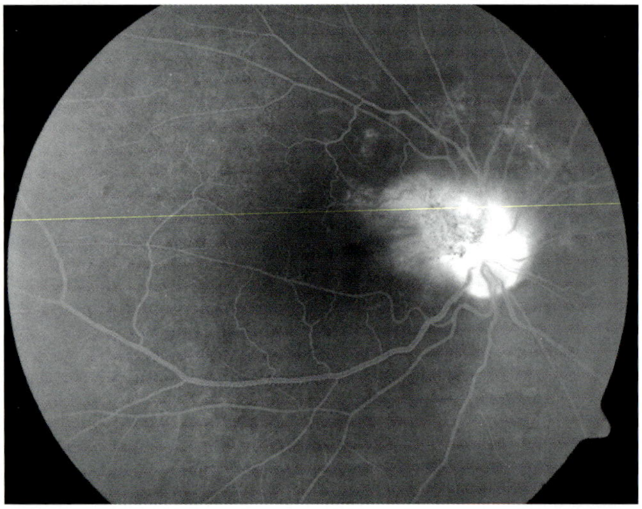

Late phase shows increased staining of the tumor tissue

COMMENT

The blocked choroidal fluorescence occurs due to the increased pigmentation of the RPE. The distortion of the vessels is better made out in the angiogram than in the fundus photograph.

CLINICAL NUGGETS

1. Ultrasonography, CT scan and MRI are useful investigative tools in the management of ocular tumors.
2. Combined hamartoma is an uncommon benign tumor causing papillary and retinal distortion characterized by proliferation of vascular, RPE and glial tissue.
3. Cause of reduced vision are direct involvement of fovea, papillomacular bundle or optic nerve, intra/ subretinal exudation from vascular components of lesion, ERM, CNVM and vitreous hemorrhage.

BIBLIOGRAPHY

1. Alegret A, Cebulla C, Dubovy S, et al. Photodynamic therapy and vitrectomy for a large optic nerve hemangioma with neovascularization and retinal detachment: a clinicopathologic correlation. RETINAL cases and Brief Reports: Winter 2009-Volume 3-Issue 1-pp 93-95.
2. Edwards WC, Layden WE, MC Donald R. Fundus fluorescein angiography of malignant melanoma of the choroid. Am Journal of Ophthalmol. 1969;68:797-808.
3. Flindall RJ, Gass JDM. A histopathologic and fluorescein angiographic correlative study of malignant melanomas of the choroid. Can J Ophthalmol. 1971;6:258-67.
4. Gass JDM. Fundus fluorescein angiography: An aid in the differential diagnosis of intraocular tumors. Inter Ophthalmol Clin 1972;12:85-120.
5. Hayreh SS. Choroidal melanomata. Fundus fluorescein angiography and histopathologic study. Br J Ophthalmol 1970;54:145-60.
6. Horst H, Hugo N. Presumed Combined Hamartoma of the Retina and Retinal Pigment Epithelium with Preretinal Neovascularization. Am J Ophthalmol 2003; 136:1157-59.
7. Joffe L, Shields JA, Osher R, et al. Clinical and follow-up studies of melanocytomas of the optic disc. Ophthalmol 1979;86:1067-78.
8. Norton EWD, Gutman F. Fundus fluorescein angiography of choroidal hemangioma. Arch Ophthalmol 1967; 78:121-5.
9. Nortan EWD, Smith JL, Curtin VJ. Fundus fluorescein angiography; An aid in differential diagnosis of posterior ocular lesion. Trans American Acad Ophthalmol and Otolaryngol 1964;68:755-65.
10. Shields CL, Archana T, Kimberly H, Paola V, Cesare P, Shields JA. Combined Hamartoma of the Retina and Retinal Pigment Epithelium in 77 consecutive patients. Visual outcome based on macular versus extramacular tumor location. Ophthalmology 2008;115:2246-52
11. Sheilds JA. Current approaches to the diagnosis and management of choroidal melanoma. Surv. Ophthalmol 1977;21:443-63.
12. Smith JL, David NJ, Hart LM, et al. Choroidal hemangioma fundus fluorescein photography and photocoagulation. Arch Ophthalmol 1963;9:51-4.

Self Test

1. Which of the following statements is correct?
   a. Macula lutea means red spot and is present at the center of the posterior retina
   b. The macula lutea derives its color from the presence of lipofuscin in the RPE
   c. Presence of lutein, zeaxanthin and xanthophylls in the macula lutea contributes to hypofluorescence in fluorescein angiography
   d. Macula is that area with a single layer of ganglion cells centered in between the temporal arcades and is 5-6 mm in diameter

Ans: (c)

2. The usual dose of fluorescein used in fundus fluorescein angiography is:
   a. 500 mg
   b. 25 mg
   c. 100 mg
   d. 1000 mg

Ans: (a)

3. The following are different stages in a FFA:
   a. Retinal capillaries fill up
   b. Staining of the disc
   c. Laminar retinal venous flow
   d. Arterial phase with filling of retinal arteries
   e. Filling of cilioretinal artery

   Find correct sequence of events:
   1. e, d, a, c, b
   2. a, d, c, e, b
   3. e, d, c, a, b
   4. d, e, a, b, c

Ans: (1)

4. Which of the following statements is true:
   a. Autofluorescence is caused by melanin in the RPE
   b. Pseudofluorescence is caused by non-fluorescent light passing through the exciter and barrier filters
   c. Blocked fluorescence cannot be caused by media opacities.
   d. Hyperfluorescence due to window defects does not fade in the late phase of angiogram

Ans: (b)

5. Which of the following statements is the most correct:
   a. If the patient develops vomiting after fluorescein injection, the FFA cannot be done and will have to be deferred
   b. History of vomiting with sodium fluorescein is an absolute contraindication for future FFA testing
   c. If the patient develops vomiting during testing, it most often occurs around 30 seconds when most of the angiography details are already obtained for clinical interpretation
   d. Nausea and vomiting are most seen with larger volumes of fluorescein injection and are not dependent on speed of injection of the dye

Ans: (c)

6. Indications for indocyanine green angiography include all *except*:
   a. Retinal angiomatosis proliferans
   b. Polypidal choroidal vasaculopathy
   c. Retinal capillary angiomas
   d. Choroidal neovascular membranes.

Ans: (c)

7. Which of the following statements regarding human retinal blood supply is true?
   a. The central retinal artery enters the ventromedial aspect of the optic nerve 12 cm posterior to the globe

b. Retinal blood vessels supply the retinal layers from the internal limiting membrane to the outer nuclear layer
c. Retinal blood vessels permeate the retinal layers from the internal limiting membrane to the inner nuclear layer
d. The human retina is fully vascularized by 32 weeks of gestation

Ans: (c)

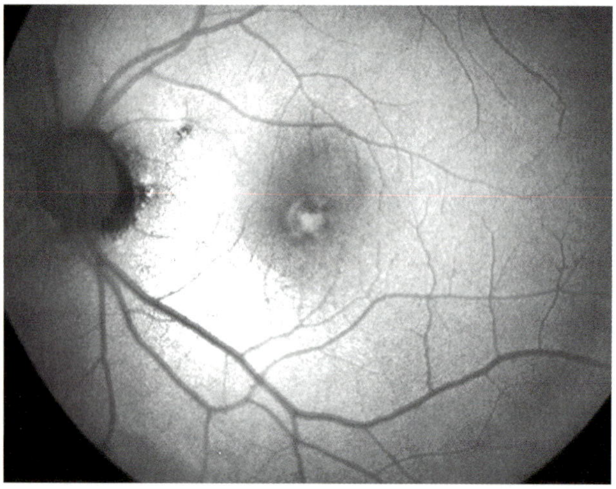

8. The picture above:
   a. Is a red free photograph of the left eye
   b. Is the late phase of fundus fluorescein angiography showing late choroidal filling
   c. Is the early phase of a ICG angiography
   d. Is an autofluorescence image of the left eye
   e. Is the recirculation phase of ICG –A

Ans: (d)

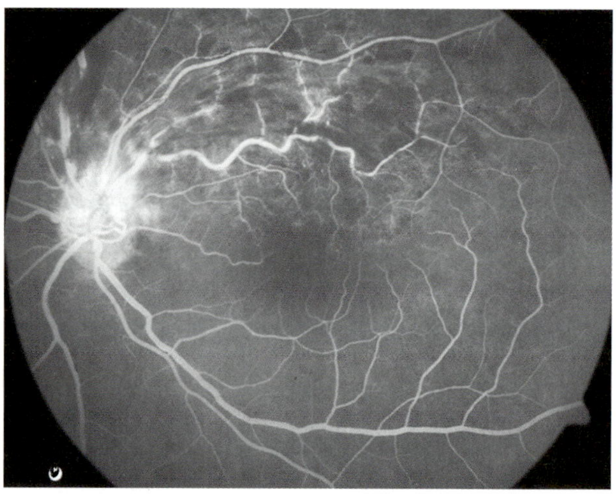

9. All the following statements regarding the FFA shown above are true *except*:
   a. Picture taken is that of the late venous phase of angiography
   b. Shows extensive neovascularization of the disc which is leaking and is best adviced to receive sector photocoagulation
   c. Signs of cystoid macular edema are best appreciated in the late phase of angiography
   d. Shows tortuosity and dilation of the superotemporal branch retinal vein

Ans: (b)

10.

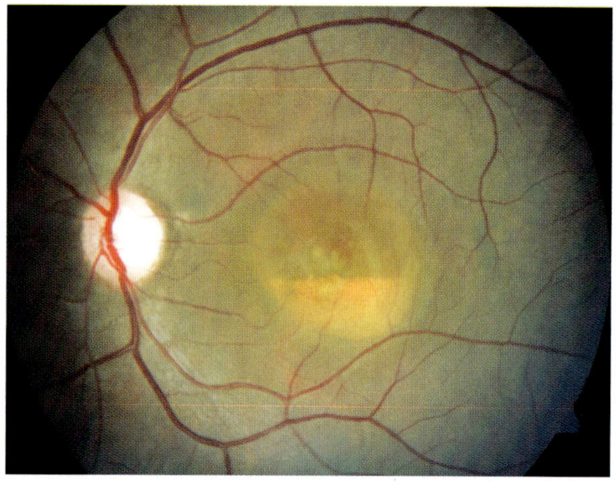

The most relevant investigative modality which will help us diagnose this condition is:
a. Electro-oculogram
b. Electroretinogram
c. Fundus fluorescein angiography
d. Indocyanine green angiography

Ans: (a)

11.

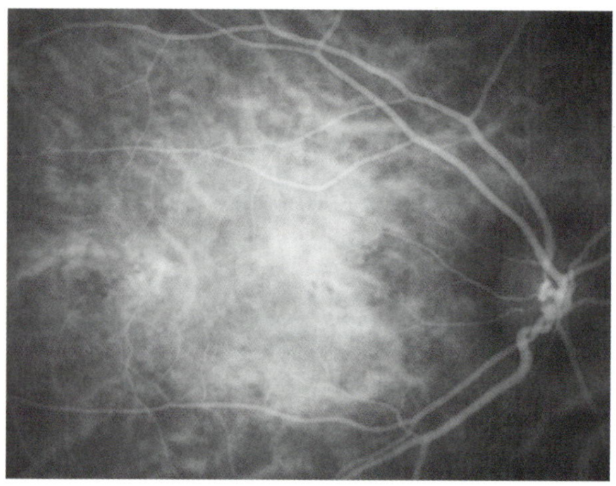

All the statements regarding the above are false *except*:

a. History of allergy to iodine must be elicited prior to procedure
b. This test can be done only with special ultraviolet video cameras
c. This fluorescence is usually emitted in the 435 nm range
d. The picture above is most probably a case of albinism

Ans: (a)

12. The binding of fluorescein to serum protein is:
 a. 50%
 b. 60-70%
 c. 70-80%
 d. 90%

Ans: (c)

13. The fluorescein seen in the angiogram is constituted by:
 a. Free fluorescein
 b. Bound fluorescein
 c. Both free and bound fluorescein
 d. Only 1% of the injected amount

Ans: (a)

14. The dark appearance of FAZ is not because of:
 a. Avascularity
 b. Melanin in RPE
 c. Increased xanthophyll
 d. Increased lipofuscin

Ans: (d)

15. 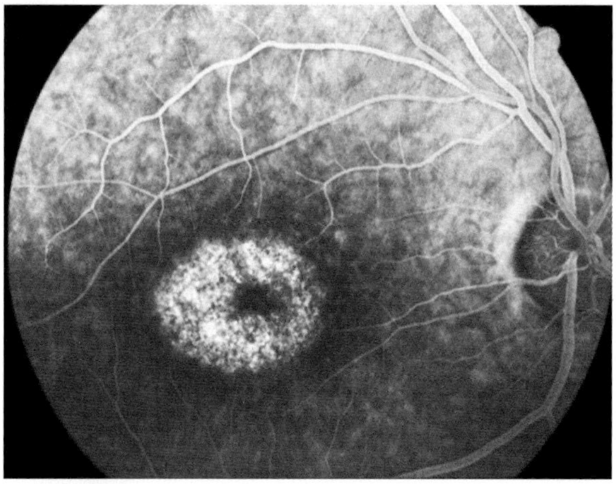

The above angiogram depicts:
 a. Leakage with cystoids macular edema
 b. Leakage with classic CNVM
 c. Window defects due to RPE atrophy
 d. Staining of scarred CNVM

Ans: (c)

16. 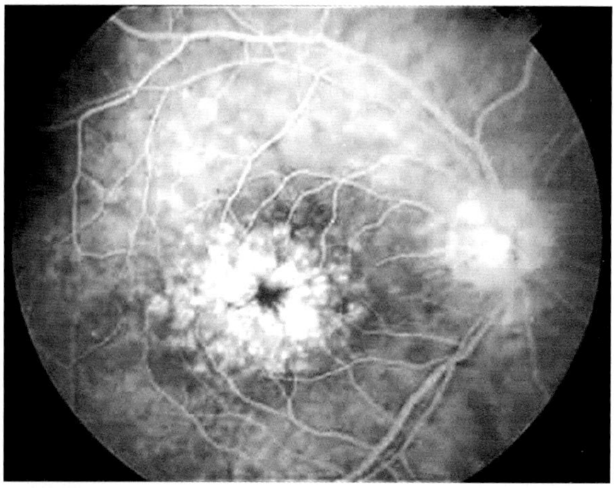

What is not true about the above angiogram?
 a. The condition can be associated with traction on macula
 b. Seen best in late stages of FFA
 c. Disc staining can be associated
 d. Staining is the underlying mechanism

Ans: (d)

17. Which of these is the cause of inadequate details of choroidal circulation during FFA:
 a. Melanin in RPE
 b. High molecular weight of fluorescein
 c. Inadequate binding of fluorescein to plasma proteins
 d. All of the above

Ans: (a)

18. 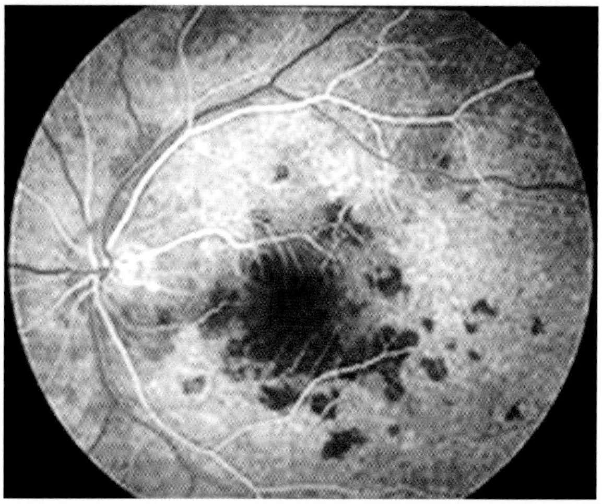

The angiogram depicts

a. Areas of capillary dropout
b. Areas of blocked fluorescence
c. Both of above
d. Cannot be commented on basis of this single picture

Ans: (b)

19. Which statement is not correct:

a. Early choroidal fluorescence is faint, patchy and irregular
b. Choroidal flush is seen before patchy choroidal filling
c. Choroidal filling starts 12-15 seconds after injection in older patients.
d. Filling of cilioretinal artery occurs simultaneously with appearance of choroidal flush

Ans: (d)

20. Autofluorescence is not exhibited by:

a. Crystalline lens
b. Myelinated nerve fibres
c. Lipofuscin
d. Xanthophyll

Ans: (d)

21. Which of above is incorrect regarding sodium fluorescein dye:

a. It is an inorganic dye
b. It has molecular weight of 376 Daltons
c. It is metabolized by the liver and excreted by the kidneys

Ans: (a)

22.

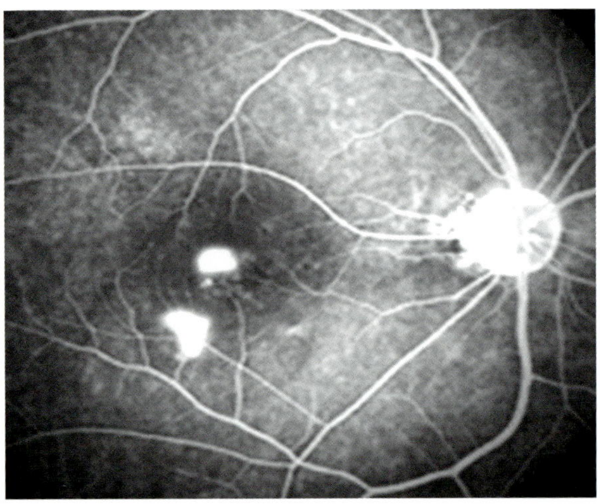

The mechanism of hyperfluorescence in above angiogram is:

a. Leakage
b. Staining
c. More pictures of different phases are needed to comment

Ans: (b)

23.

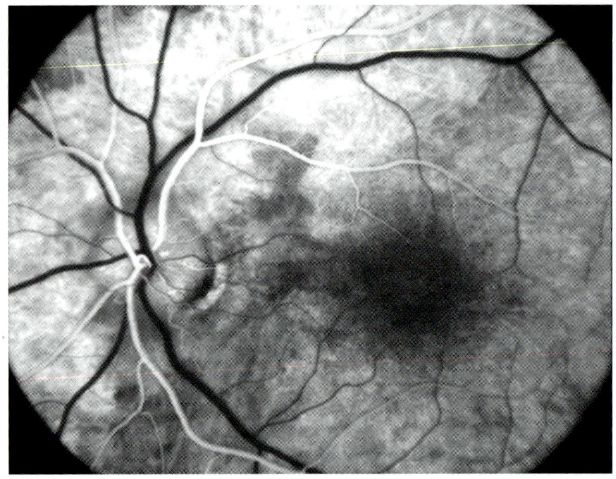

Which phase is depicted in the above angiogram

a. Red free photo
b. Retinal arterial phase
c. Autofluorescence photograph
d. Late recirculation phase

Ans: (b)

24.

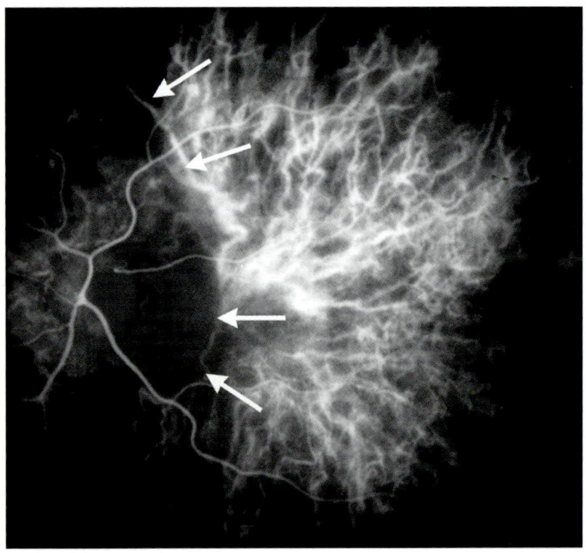

The above ICG represents

a. Choroidal rupture
b. Choroidal watershed
c. Dilated feeder vessels
d. Blocked cyanescence

Ans: (b)

25. Arterial phase of FFA lasts for approx:

a. 2-3 seconds
b. 10-12 seconds

   c. 20-30 seconds
   d. 6-7 seconds

Ans: (b)

26. Which of these is not correct regarding late phase of FFA:
   a. There is gradual elimination of dye from the choroidal and the retinal circulation.
   b. Staining of the disc is the normal finding.
   c. Any areas of late hyperfluorescence suggest an abnormality

Ans: (c)

27. The fluorescein present in serum and urine after FFA can give false positive results in following laboratory tests:
   a. Benedict's test for glucose determination in urine
   b. Catecholamines determination
   c. Serum bilirubin determination
   d. All of the above

Ans: (d)

28. Fluorescein can easily pass through which layer(s):
   a. Endothelium of choriocapillaries
   b. Retinal pigment epithelium
   c. Endothelium of retinal capillaries
   d. Bruch's membrane

Ans: (a), (d)

29. Which of the following is a correct statement:
   a. Some leakage at the edges of the optic disc from choroidal capillaries in late phases is a normal finding
   b. Disc staining alone and not disc leakage is a normal finding on FFA
   c. Late leakage can be seen from optic nerve head in disc drusen
   d. Scleral staining will be masked and less seen in conditions like choroideremia and gyrate atrophy

Ans: (a)

30. Which statement is true regarding ICG angiography:
   a. Vertical water-shed zone is more clearly seen in the old age
   b. Vertical watershed is better defined on ICGA than horizontal watershed zone
   c. After administration, ICG dye is metabolized only by the liver and then excreted into bile
   d. Indocyanine green (ICG) is a water-soluble tricarbocyanine dye

Ans: (d)

Glossary

Arterial phase: Appearance of fluorescein dye in the retinal arterioles to its first appearance in the retinal veins.

Arteriovenous phase: The stage of fluorescein angiogram when fluorescein dye is present in the retinal arteries and veins; this stage begins with retinal venous laminar filling.

Autofluorescence: Preinjection fluorescence produced by lesions that naturally fluoresce when exposed to excitatory blue light.

Background fluorescence: A complete sheet of fluorescence beneath the retinal vessels that has a ground-glass pattern; it varies according to the filling pattern of the choroid and density of the retinal pigment epithelium.

Barrier filter: A filter used to transmit fluorescein light and prevent transmission of reflected light from the fundus.

Blocked fluorescence: A form of hypofluorescence that occurs when tissue or fluid obscures retinal or choroidal vascular fluorescence.

Capillary dropout: Non-perfusion of retinal capillaries.

Choroidal phase: The stage of fluorescein angiogram when dye first enters the choroidal vasculature. It precedes retinal arterial phase.

Collateral vessels: An anastomotic vascular communication that develops in response to vascular obstruction. It joins obstructed vessels to open vessels or bypasses a blocked area in a single vessel.

Cystoid edema: Accumulation of dye in discrete spaces in the outer plexiform layer.

Exciter filter: An absorption filter that selectively transmits light of the wavelengths needed to cause the fluorescence. It is placed between the light source and the fundus.

Feeder vessel: Inflow channels to an abnormal frond of vessel in the retina or to a tumor.

Hot spot: A focal area of intense hyperfluorescence beneath a pigment epithelium detachment indicative of choroidal neovascularization.

Hyperfluorescence: An abnormal increase in fluorescence produced by vascular leakage, vascular changes or window defects.

Laminar flow: The fluorescent flow seen along the walls of veins, caused by the slower, nonturbulent movement of blood along the vessel wall.

Light bulb fluorescence: A discrete area of hyperfluorescence seen in the late stages of a fluorescein angiogram at the site of a retinal macroaneurysm.

Pooling: Late hyperfluorescence produced by leakage into an anatomical space.

Pseudofluorescence: Preinjection fluorescence that emanates from highly reflective surfaces in the fundus, and that is produced by poorly matched filters.

Red free photo: A photograph using a green filter that eliminates the normal red reflex of the fundus and increases fundus contrast.

Staining: Late hyperfluorescence produced by leakage of fluorescein into tissues.

Telangiectasia: A retinal vascular disorder consisting of variable degrees of capillary dilatation and aneurysm formation.

Transmitted fluorescence: Early hyperfluorescence produced by accentuation of normal choroidal fluorescence through defects in the retinal pigment epithelium (Window defects).

Vascular filling defects: Hypofluorescence produced by delay or absence in perfusion of the retinal or choroidal vasculature.

Index

Page numbers followed by *f* refer to figure